Mental Health Services

WITHDRAWN

Mental Health Services

A Public Health Perspective
Third Edition

Edited by

BRUCE LUBOTSKY LEVIN, DrPH, MPH
Associate Professor & Head
Graduate Studies in Behavioral Health Program
Editor-in-Chief
Journal of Behavioral Health Services & Research
Louis de la Parte Florida Mental Health Institute & College of Public Health
University of South Florida

KEVIN D. HENNESSY, PhD
Senior Advisor
Office of Applied Studies
Substance Abuse and Mental Health Services Administration

JOHN PETRILA, JD, LLM
Professor
Department of Mental Health Law & Policy
Louis de la Parte Florida Mental Health Institute
University of South Florida

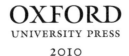

OXFORD
UNIVERSITY PRESS
2010

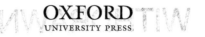

OXFORD
UNIVERSITY PRESS

Oxford University Press, Inc., publishes works that further
Oxford University's objective of excellence
in research, scholarship, and education.

Oxford   New York
Auckland   Cape Town   Dar es Salaam   Hong Kong   Karachi
Kuala Lumpur   Madrid   Melbourne   Mexico City   Nairobi
New Delhi   Shanghai   Taipei   Toronto

With offices in
Argentina   Austria   Brazil   Chile   Czech Republic   France   Greece
Guatemala   Hungary   Italy   Japan   Poland   Portugal   Singapore
South Korea   Switzerland   Thailand   Turkey   Ukraine   Vietnam

Published by Oxford University Press, Inc.
198 Madison Avenue, New York, New York 10016

www.oup.com

Oxford is a registered trademark of Oxford University Press

Library of Congress Cataloging-in-Publication Data

Mental health services: a public health perspective /
edited by Bruce Lubotsky Levin, Kevin D. Hennessy, John Petrila. —3rd ed.
p. ; cm.
Includes bibliographical references and index.
ISBN 978-0-19-538857-2 (alk. paper)
1. Mental health services—United States.   2. Mental health policy—United States.
I. Levin, Bruce Lubotsky. II. Hennessy, Kevin D. III. Petrila, John.
[DNLM: 1. Mental Health Services—organization & administration—United States.
2. Health Policy—United States.   3. Mental Disorders—United States.
4. Mental Health Services—economics—United States.
WM 30 M5531625 2010]
RA790.6.M445 2010
362.20973–dc22
2009041119
35798642

Printed in the United States of America
on acid-free paper

CONTENTS

ABBREVIATIONS

AAGP	American Association for Geriatric Psychiatry
ACT	Assertive Community Treatment
ADA	Americans with Disabilities Act
ADHD	attention-deficit/hyperactivity disorder
AHCPR	Agency for Health Care Policy and Research
AHRQ	Agency for Healthcare Research and Quality
AoA	Administration on Aging
CASSP	Child and Adolescent Service System Program
CATIE	Clinical Antipsychotic Trials of Intervention Effectiveness
Child STEPs	MacArthur Foundation Child System and Treatment Enhancement Projects
CIDI	Composite International Diagnostic Interview
CIT	Crisis Intervention Teams
CJ-DATS	Criminal Justice Drug Abuse Treatment Studies
CMHBG	Community Mental Health Block Grant
CMHCs	community mental health centers
CMHI	Children's Mental Health Initiative
CMHS	Center for Mental Health Services
CMS	Centers for Medicare and Medicaid Services
CPES	Collaborative Psychiatric Epidemiology Surveys
CSAT	Center for Substance Abuse Treatment
CUtLASS	Cost Utility of the Latest Antipsychotic Drugs in Schizophrenia Study
DATOS	Drug Abuse Treatment Outcomes Studies
DHHS	U.S. Department of Health and Human Services

EBM	evidence-based medicine
EBT	evidence-based treatment
ECA	Epidemiologic Catchment Area
EMRs	electronic medical records
ERISA	Employment Retirement and Security Act
ESMH	expanded school mental health
EST	empirically supported treatment
FDA	Food and Drug Administration
FERPA	Family Educational Right to Privacy Act
FQHCs	Federally Qualified Health Centers
HCFA	Health Care Financing Administration
Health IT	health information technology
HEDIS	Health Plan Employer Data and Information Set
HIPAA	Health Insurance Portability and Accountability Act
HMO	Health Maintenance Organization
HRSA	Health Resources Services Administration
HSRR	Health Services and Sciences Research Resources
HUD	U.S. Department of Housing and Urban Development
IDEA	Individuals with Disabilities Education Act
IMD	Institutions for Mental Disease
IOM	Institute of Medicine
MBHOs	managed behavioral health care organizations
MCO	managed care organization
MedPAC	Medicare Payment Advisory Commission
MHCs	mental health courts
MHSIP	Mental Health Statistical Improvement Program
MHT-SIG	Mental Health Transformation-State Incentive Grants
MMA	Medicare Prescription Drug, Improvement, and Modernization Act
NAMBHA	National Alliance of Multi-Ethnic Behavioral Health Associations
NAMHC	National Advisory Mental Health Council
NAMI	National Alliance on Mental Illness
NASMHPD	National Association of State Mental Health Program Directors
NCCBH	National Council for Community Behavioral Healthcare
NCS	National Comorbidity Survey
NCS-R	National Comorbidity Survey Replication
NESARC	National Epidemiologic Survey on Alcohol and Related Conditions
NIAAA	National Institute on Alcohol Abuse and Alcoholism
NIATx	Network for the Improvement of Addiction Treatment
NIDA	National Institute on Drug Abuse
NIH	National Institutes of Health
NLAAS	National Latino and Asian American Survey
NNED	National Network to Eliminate Disparities in Behavioral Health

NREPP	National Registry of Evidence-Based Programs and Practices
NSAL	National Survey of American Life
NSDUH	National Survey on Drug Use and Health
N-SSATS	National Survey of Substance Abuse Treatment Services
OAA	Older Americans Act
OBRA	Omnibus Budget Reconciliation Acts
PACE	Program for All-Inclusive Care for the Elderly
PASRR	Preadmission Screening and Resident Review
PBM	Pharmacy Benefit Manager
PDP	Prescription Drug Plan
POS	Point of Service
PPO	Preferred Provider Organization
RTI	Response to Intervention
SAMHSA	Substance Abuse and Mental Health Services Administration
SAP	Student Assistance Program
SBHC	school-based health center
SCAP	socio-cultural assessment protocols
SCHIP	State Children's Health Insurance Program
SED	severe emotional disturbance
SIM	Sequential Intercept Model
SMH	school mental health
SMHA	state mental health agency
SMI	severely mentally ill, severe mental illness
SPMI	Severe, persistent mental illness
SSDI	Social Security Disability Income
SSI	Supplemental Security Income
SSRI	Selective Serotonin Reuptake Inhibitor
TOPS	Treatment Outcome Prospective Study
TSIGs	Transformation Systems Improvement Grants
URS	Uniform Reporting System
VA	Department of Veterans Affairs
WHCoA	White House Conference on Aging
WHO	World Health Organization
WHO-DAS	WHO Disability Assessment Schedule
WMH	World Mental Health

CONTRIBUTORS

Sergio Aguilar-Gaxiola, M.D., Ph.D., is Professor of Internal Medicine, School of Medicine, University of California (UC), Davis. He is the Founding Director of the Center for Reducing Health Disparities at UC Davis Health System and is Co-Chair of the National Institutes of Health's Community Engagement Key Function Committee for the Clinical and Translational Science Awards. Dr. Aguilar-Gaxiola is the Coordinator for Latin America and the Caribbean of the World Health Organization's World Mental Health Surveys Consortium, and his research includes cross-national epidemiologic studies on patterns and correlates of mental disorders and understanding and reducing health disparities in underserved populations.

Jordi Alonso, M.D., Ph.D., is the head of the Health Services Research Unit of the Institut Municipal d'Investigació Mèdica (IMIM-Hospital del Mar). He is a Professor at the Pompeu Fabra University (UPF), Barcelona, where he is the Director of the Master's Program in Public Health and also an Associate Professor at Johns Hopkins Bloomberg School of Public Health. Dr. Alonso has published over 400 scientific articles in the area of health outcomes research.

William A. Anthony, Ph.D., is Director of Boston University's Center for Psychiatric Rehabilitation and a Professor in the College of Health and Rehabilitation Sciences at Boston University. In 1992, Dr. Anthony received the Distinguished Service Award from the President of the United States for his efforts "in promoting the dignity, equality, independence and employment of people with disabilities." He has written extensively on the topic of psychiatric rehabilitation, and has authored or co-authored over 100 articles in professional journals, 16 textbooks, and several dozen book chapters.

Lori Ashcraft, Ph.D., is the Executive Director for the Recovery Innovations Recovery Opportunity Center. She has developed several curricula to help individuals with psychiatric experiences move beyond recovery by finding their purpose, making their own unique contribution, and using their experiences to help others grow and recover, skills based on her own personal experiences of having struggled with severe depression most of her life. Previously, Dr. Ashcraft served as the Deputy Director for Community Programs in the California Department of Mental Health, Director for Adult Services for the Arizona Regional Behavioral Health Authority, and Executive Director of the Recovery Education Center.

Stephen J. Bartels, M.D., M.S., is Professor of Psychiatry and Professor of Community & Family Medicine at Dartmouth Medical School. He is the Director of Dartmouth's Centers for Health and Aging and oversees the Center for Aging Research, the Northern New England Geriatric Education Center, and the Dartmouth-Hitchcock Center for Senior Health, as well as serving as the Medical Director for New Hampshire's Bureau of Elder Services. Dr. Bartels has authored or co-authored over 130 peer-reviewed articles, monographs, and book chapters, and has served in a variety of national leadership roles in the field of geriatrics.

Crystal R. Blyler, Ph.D., is a Social Science Analyst with the Substance Abuse and Mental Health Services Administration. An experimental psychologist by training, Dr. Blyler has served for the past 10 years as a project officer for evaluations of the federal Center for Mental Health Services' discretionary grant portfolio, including: transformation of state mental health systems, supported employment, consumer-operated services, disability work incentives, and comprehensive services for transition-aged youth with serious mental illnesses and emotional disturbances.

Robert W. Burke, Ph.D., is an Associate Professor in the Department of Teacher Education at Miami University in Oxford, Ohio, where he teaches courses in the Early Childhood Education Preparation Program. In his previous work with children and families, he served as an elementary school teacher in grades K-5 for twelve years as well as an additional seven years as a caseworker in both mental health and juvenile justice agencies. His teaching, research, and service agendas examine the intersection of individual, group, and political dynamics of teaching and learning at kindergarten to sixth-grade levels, with a particular focus on the "Psychosocial Curriculum" that encompasses the mental health dimensions inherent in teachers' and students' shared lives in classrooms.

Tina Crenshaw, Ph.D., M.S.Ed., M.L.S., is a psychologist affiliated with the National Center for Posttraumatic Stress Disorder within the U.S. Department of Veterans Affairs. She has worked previously as a psychologist, librarian, research writer, and electronic information resource manager. Dr. Crenshaw holds advanced degrees in clinical psychology, educational psychology, and library science.

Karen J. Cusack, Ph.D., is an Assistant Professor in the Department of Psychiatry and a Research Fellow at the Cecil G. Sheps Center for Health Services Research at the University of North Carolina at Chapel Hill. Previously, Dr. Cusack completed a National Research Service Award postdoctoral fellowship jointly sponsored by the University of North Carolina at Chapel Hill and Duke University. His research focuses on post-traumatic stress disorder and substance abuse, cognitive-behavioral interventions, and the intersection of mental health and criminal justice, areas in which she has published extensively.

Faith B. Dickerson, Ph.D., M.P.H., is Director of Psychology at the Sheppard Pratt Health System. She also heads the Sheppard Pratt Stanley Research Program and chairs the Sheppard Pratt Institutional Review Board. Dr. Dickerson holds adjunct appointments in the Department of Psychiatry at the University of Maryland and at the Johns Hopkins School of Medicine, and her research interests focus on health services for persons with serious mental illness and the role of infectious agents and other environmental factors in schizophrenia and bipolar disorder.

Marisa Elena Domino, Ph.D., is an Associate Professor of Health Economics in the Department of Health Policy and Administration at the University of North Carolina at Chapel Hill. Dr. Domino's research interests include the economics of mental health, agency relationships among physicians, patients, and insurers, the diffusion of new technologies, and the public provision of health care and health insurance to low income populations. She has published scholarly work on the impact of managed care on treatment selection for depression in both public and private settings, the impact of managed care on the field of psychiatry, behavioral health carve-outs, and the effect that Medicare Part D has on individuals with severe mental illness.

Thomas W. Doub, Ph.D., is the Chief Operating Officer for Centerstone Research Institute in Nashville, Tennessee. He works with academic researchers and clinicians across the United States toward the goal of providing access to the most innovative mental health and addiction treatments. Dr. Doub oversees Centerstone's community mental health research portfolio, and directs efforts to implement these findings into clinical practice.

Joel F. Farley, R.Ph., Ph.D., is an Assistant Professor in the Division of Pharmaceutical Outcomes and Policy in the Eshelman School of Pharmacy at the University of North Carolina at Chapel Hill. Dr. Farley's research focuses on the impact of Medicaid prescription managed care policies on economic and clinical outcomes in vulnerable patient populations. Currently, he is examining Medicaid data to assess the effect of prescription benefit changes on patterns of care for individuals with schizophrenia.

Paul Flaspohler, Ph.D., is an Assistant Professor of Clinical Psychology and the Director of Program Development and Evaluation for the Center for School-Based Mental Health Programs at Miami (Ohio) University. In addition to applied work in community development and program evaluation, he assists schools and communities identifying needs and developing solutions for community problems. Dr. Flaspohler's current projects include the Evidence-Based Practices for School-Wide Prevention Programs (funded by the Health Foundation of Great Cincinnati) and the development of a network of University-Community partnerships support-ing expanded School Mental Health (EPIC).

Howard H. Goldman, M.D., Ph.D., is Professor of Psychiatry at the University of Maryland School of Medicine, where he directs the Mental Health Systems Improvement Collaborative. Dr. Goldman was the Senior Scientific Editor of *Mental Health: A Report of the Surgeon General*, and he is the Editor of *Psychiatric Services*.

Junius J. Gonzales, M.D., M.B.A., is founding Dean of the College of Behavioral & Community Sciences and Executive Director of the Louis de la Parte Florida Mental Health Institute at the University of South Florida. Dr. Gonzales is a psy-chiatrist and health services researcher who previously served as Principal and Scientist at Abt Associates, as well as Chief of the Services Research & Clinical Epidemiology Branch and Acting Director for the Division of Services & Intervention Research at the National Institute of Mental Health.

Jan Goodson, B.S., is Director of Grant Writing for the Centerstone Research Institute. She oversees the development and submission of all grant proposals to government and private sector funders in order to sustain, enhance, and expand the prevention, treatment, and research of mental health and substance abuse disorders in Tennessee and Indiana. Ms. Goodson is Grant Professional Certified by the American Association of Grant Professionals.

Julie Goldstein Grumet, Ph.D., is a clinical psychologist currently with the Washington, D.C., Department of Mental Health. Dr. Grumet is the Prinicipal Investigator on a federally funded grant from the Substance Abuse and Mental Health Services Administration on the prevention of youth suicide. She has exten-sive experience in providing school-based mental health prevention, intervention, early intervention, and treatment to minority youth.

Sharon Green-Hennessy, Ph.D., is an Associate Professor of Psychology at Loyola University Maryland, where she teaches graduate seminars on child and adolescent psychopathology and its treatment. Prior to joining Loyola, Dr. Green-Hennessy held a joint Instructor appointment in the Departments of Psychiatry at Johns Hopkins School of Medicine and Kennedy Krieger Institute. Dr. Green-Hennessy is a licensed psychologist in Maryland, with research interests in access and barriers to mental health care among children and adolescents, child maltreat-ment, attachment theory, and the psychological assessment of children.

Ardis Hanson, M.L.S., is Director of the Research Library at the Louis de la Parte Florida Mental Health Institute at the University of South Florida (USF). Her interest in the use of technology to enhance research led Ms. Hanson to develop the Web site for the Library and the Institute in 1993 and, as Institute Webmaster, she has created a number of specialized research resources for Institute and Internet users. Ms. Hanson is an editor and author of texts in library and information sci-ences and is currently pursuing her doctoral degree in health and organizational communication at USF.

Kevin D. Hennessy, Ph.D., is a Senior Advisor within the Substance Abuse and Mental Health Services Administration (SAMHSA), where he provides leadership and guidance on issues of health care financing, workforce development, and translating research to practice for mental health and substance use services. Dr. Hennessy is a practicing clinical psychologist who previously served in the Office of the Assistant Secretary for Planning and Evaluation of the U.S. Department of Health and Human Services, and as a Senior Policy Advisor to the President's New Freedom Commission on Mental Health. He is currently an Associate Editor of the *Journal of Behavioral Health Services and Research*.

Jill G. Hensley, M.A., currently serves as the Program Manager for the Substance Abuse and Mental Health Administration's (SAMHSA) Fetal Alcohol Spectrum Disorders (FASD) Coordinating Center, which oversees efforts to implement evidence-based practices to prevent, diagnose, and address FASD across state, local, and juvenile court settings. Previously she served as Project Director for SAMHSA's Co-Occurring Center for Excellence (COCE), a technical assistance and training center addressing co-occurring mental health and substance abuse disorders. Ms. Hensley has over 20 years of research, policy, and program experience in the areas of mental health and substance abuse treatment, HIV/AIDS, and criminal justice.

Michael Hogan, Ph.D., is Commissioner of Mental Health in New York. Dr. Hogan chaired the President's New Freedom Commission on Mental Health in 2002–2003 and was appointed as the first behavioral health representative on the Board of the Joint Commission in 2007. He previously served as Director of the Ohio Department of Mental Health and Commissioner of the Connecticut Department of Mental Health, as well as President of the National Association of State Mental Health Program Directors (NASMHPD) and NASMHPD's Research Institute.

Ronald C. Kessler, Ph.D., is a Professor of Health Care Policy at Harvard Medical School, where he leads a program in psychiatric epidemiology. Dr. Kessler is the Principal Investigator of the U.S. National Comorbidity Surveys and a Co-Director of the WHO World Mental Health Survey Initiative. He is a member of the Institute of Medicine and the National Academy of Sciences, and the ISI Web of Knowledge has rated Dr. Kessler the most highly cited researcher in the world in the field of psychiatry for each of the past nine years.

Sing Lee, M.B., B.S., FRCPsych, is a Professor at the Department of Psychiatry and the Director of the Hong Kong Mood Disorders Center, Faculty of Medicine, the Chinese University of Hong Kong. He is also lecturer at the Department of Social Medicine, Harvard Medical School, and the Asia-Pacific Coordinator of the World Mental Health Initiative. Dr. Lee's principal research interest is mental health and social change in Chinese society.

H. Stephen Leff., Ph.D., is a Senior Vice President at the Human Services Research Institute (HSRI) and Associate Professor in the Harvard Medical School Department of Psychiatry at the Cambridge Health Alliance. He directs The Evaluation Center at HSRI, a program to provide technical assistance nationally for the evaluation of adult mental health systems change, and has developed Web-based needs assessment and resource allocations tools for mental health planning. Dr. Leff's research interests and work focus on mental health systems evaluation and planning, evidence-based practices, the measurement of cultural competency, fidelity measurement, and the linking of mental health evaluation and planning activities.

Bruce Lubotsky Levin, Dr.P.H., M.P.H., is Associate Professor and Head of the Graduate Studies in Behavioral Health Program at the Louis de la Parte Florida Mental Health Institute & the College of Public Health, both at the University of South Florida (USF). Dr. Levin is also Editor-in-Chief of the *Journal of Behavioral Health Services & Research* and Director of the USF Graduate Certificate in Mental Health Planning, Evaluation, & Accountability Program. He is Senior Editor of texts in women's mental health, mental health, and public health for pharmacists, with research interests in managed behavioral health care, mental health policy, graduate behavioral health education, and mental health informatics.

Anne Lezak, M.P.A., is Principal of ADL Consulting, as well as a Senior Writer for Advocates for Human Potential, Inc., with an expertise in mental health policy and planning, homelessness, children's mental health, and systems of care. Over the past 20 years, she has authored major reports, monographs, technical assistance materials, and grant submissions for a host of federal, state and national organizations.

Theodore C. Lutterman, B.A., is Director of Research Analysis at the National Association of State Mental Health Program Directors' Research Institute (NRI). Mr. Lutterman has over 25 years experience working with state mental health agencies in the design, development, and implementation of national data compilation and research projects. Mr. Lutterman also directs the federally funded State Data Infrastructure Coordinating Center, which produces the State Mental Health Authority Revenue/Expenditure Study, the State Profiling System, and the Client Level Data Pilot Study.

Ronald W. Manderscheid, Ph.D., is Director of Mental Health and Substance Use Programs at the Global Health Sector of SRA International, and an Adjunct Professor at the Department of Mental Health, Bloomberg School of Public Health, Johns Hopkins University. At SRA, Dr. Manderscheid develops new demonstration and research projects around mental health and substance use services, programs, and systems, using a public health framework. Previously, Dr. Manderscheid served as Branch Chief, Survey and Analysis Branch, for the federal Center for Mental Health Services in the Substance Abuse and Mental Health Services Administration, where he served as Principal Editor for eight editions of *Mental Health, United States.*

Noel A. Mazade, Ph.D., is the founding Executive Director of the National Association of State Mental Health Program Directors' Research Institute, Inc. Previously, he held managerial positions with the National Institute of Mental

Health, North Carolina Mental Health Legislative Study Commission, and the Oakland County (Michigan) Mental Health Services Board. He has held faculty appointments in psychiatry, public health, and social work at Harvard University, the University of North Carolina at Chapel Hill, and the University of Maryland.

Dennis McCarty, Ph.D., is a Professor in the Department of Public Health & Preventive Medicine at Oregon Health & Science University. He collaborates with policymakers in state and federal government and with community-based programs to examine the organization, financing, and delivery of publicly funded treatment services for alcohol and drug use disorders, and currently leads the national evaluation for the Network for Improvement of Addiction Treatment (NIATx), and directs the Oregon/Hawaii Node of the National Drug Abuse Treatment Clinical Trials Network (CTN). Previously, Dr. McCarty directed the Massachusetts Bureau of Substance Abuse Services for the Massachusetts Department of Public Health.

Kathleen Ries Merikangas, Ph.D., is Senior Investigator and Chief of the Genetic Epidemiology Branch in the Intramural Research Program at the National Institute of Mental Health (NIMH). Prior to joining the NIMH in 2002, Dr. Merikangas was Professor of Epidemiology and Public Health, Psychiatry, and Psychology and the Director of the Genetic Epidemiology Research Unit in the Department of Epidemiology and Public Health at the Yale University School of Medicine. Dr. Merikangas has authored or co-authored more than 300 scientific publications and has presented lectures throughout the United States and in more than 20 countries.

Rebecca Morris, M.P.A., is President of Gallais Communications, which specializes in health issues. Previously, while serving as Director of Communications for Advocates for Human Potential, Inc., she had lead writing/editing responsibilities on a contract supporting the Substance Abuse and Mental Health Services Administration's (SAMHSA's) Behavioral Health Workforce Development Initiative. Ms. Morris has written and edited a wide variety of health-related monographs, working papers, briefings, conference documentation, and other reports for agencies and organizations such as the U.S. Department of Health and Human Services, U.S. Department of Justice, the U.S. Office of National Drug Control Policy, the Annie E. Casey Foundation, and The Medical Foundation.

Dennis P. Morrison, Ph.D., is Chief Executive Officer (CEO) of Centerstone Research Institute, where he oversees all research and information technology activities for Centerstone, the largest community mental health care organization in the United States. Previously, he served as the CEO of the Center for Behavioral Health (CBH) in Bloomington, Indiana. Under his leadership, CBH received the Ernest A. Codman Award in 2003, the Nicholas E. Davies Award in 2006, and the Negley Award in 2007.

Noosha Niv, Ph.D., is currently the Associate Director of the Education and Dissemination Unit of the Desert Pacific Mental Illness Research, Education and Clinical Center. She conducts clinical and health services research examining the treatment needs, utilization, and outcomes among individuals with severe mental illness, substance abuse disorders, and co-occurring disorders, as well as the influence of environmental and cultural factors on psychopathology and treatment outcomes. Dr. Niv received her doctoral degree in clinical psychology and completed a postdoctoral fellowship, both from the University of California, Los Angeles.

Fred C. Osher, M.D., is the Director of Health Systems and Health Services Policy at the Council of State Governments Justice Center and serves as a senior medical consultant to the Substance Abuse and Mental Health Services Administration's Co-Occurring Center of Excellence. Dr Osher is a community psychiatrist with clinical, research, and policy interests in effective services for persons with serious mental illnesses and co-occurring substance use disorders, and he has published extensively in the areas of homelessness, community psychiatry, co-occurring disorders, and effective approaches to justice involving persons with behavioral health disorders. Dr. Osher has a history of public-sector service at local, state, and federal levels, including the federal Center for Mental Health Services and the National Institute of Mental Health.

Airia Sasser Papadopoulos, M.P.H., is an Assistant in Research in the Department of Mental Health Law and Policy at the Louis de la Parte Florida Mental Health Institute, University of South Florida. Ms. Papadopoulos currently coordinates a state-funded study of Medicaid-funded behavioral health services. She is studying for a Ph.D. in Applied Anthropology with research interests that include racial disparities in mental health, particularly in the diagnosis and treatment of depression among African Americans, and the connection between depression and obesity among adolescents.

Carl E. Paternite, Ph.D., is Professor and Chair of the Department of Psychology at Miami University in Oxford, Ohio, where he has been on the faculty for 30 years. He is the founding and current director of the Center for School-Based Mental Health Programs in the Department of Psychology and also directs the Ohio Mental Health Network for School Success, a joint venture of the Ohio Department of Mental Health and the Ohio Department of Education. Dr. Paternite has particular expertise in approaches to involve educators more fully within school mental health efforts; public policy advocacy and moving policy to action; school mental health workforce development issues; and formative evaluation of school mental health programs; and he has published extensively in edited books and peer-reviewed journals.

John Petrila, J.D., L.L.M., is a Professor in the Department of Mental Health Law & Policy at the University of South Florida. He is a member of the MacArthur Foundation Research Network on Mandated Community Treatment and Past President of the International Association of Forensic Mental Health Services. He is also co-editor of *Behavioral Sciences and Law*, and publishes frequently on mental health law and policy issues.

Bernadette E. Phelan, Ph.D., is a Senior Research Advisor at the National Association of State Mental Health Program Directors' Research Institute and concurrent President of Phelan Research Solutions, Inc. She has experience in the field of behavioral health as an evaluator, researcher, and grant Principal Investigator. Previously, Dr. Phelan was the Chief of Research and Special Projects for the Division of Behavioral Health within the Arizona Department of Health Services, as well as Assistant Director of the Arizona Medical Board.

Allison D. Redlich, Ph.D., is an Assistant Professor in the School of Criminal Justice at the State University of New York at Albany. She conducts research on Mental Health Courts and other forms of criminal justice diversion and is a nationally recognized expert with extensive publications on police interrogations and false confessions, particularly with vulnerable populations such as persons with mental illness and juveniles. Dr. Redlich serves on the executive committee of the American Psychology-Law Society (Division 41 of the American Psychological Association), as well as on the editorial boards of three journals.

Traci Rieckmann, Ph.D., is a Research Assistant Professor in the Center for Substance Abuse Research and Policy in the Department of Public Health and Preventive Medicine at Oregon Health & Science University. Dr. Rieckmann's research focuses on the organization and delivery of drug abuse treatment services, primarily in the translation of research to practice and the implementation of evidence-based practices, as well as assessing disparities in access and retention in care and adapting practices for American Indian/Alaskan native communities. Her clinical work has focused primarily on adolescents and adults with substance abuse and co-occurring disorders.

Steven S. Sharfstein, M.D., M.P.A., is President and Chief Executive Officer of the Sheppard Pratt Health System, where he has worked for 22 years. He is also Clinical Professor and Vice Chair of Psychiatry at the University of Maryland, and previously served in various positions at the National Institute of Mental Health. A practicing clinician for more than 30 years, he is best known for his extensive research and writing on the economics of practice, and public mental health policy.

Tevfik Bedirhan Üstün, M.D., is the Coordinator of Classifications, Terminologies, and Standards in the World Health Organization (WHO). Dr. Üstün is also the Co-Director of the WHO World Mental Health Survey Initiative and is currently responsible for the WHO's Family of International Classifications (ICD, ICF and other health classifications), standardized health terminologies, and health information standards. He has authored or co-authored more than 200 articles and several books on psychiatry, primary care, classifications, and health assessment.

Aricca D. Van Citters, M.S., has over ten years of experience in the evaluation of mental health services and interventions for older adults. She has specialized in health care quality improvement, health promotion, and the implementation and dissemination of evidence-based practices. Ms. Van Citters has an extensive background in conducting outcomes evaluations and has provided technical assistance in implementing geriatric mental health services, developed curriculum for educating early career investigators in community-based geriatric mental health research, and developed educational materials for implementing effective late-life depression programs.

Philip S. Wang, M.D., Dr.P.H., is the Deputy Director of the National Institute of Mental Health (NIMH). Prior to joining NIMH, he served on the faculty at Harvard Medical School, where his research focused on effectiveness trials, pharmacoepidemiology, pharmacoeconomics, and health services research.

Mark D. Weist, Ph.D., is a Professor at the University of Maryland, School of Medicine, and serves as the Director of the Center for School Mental Health, one of two federally funded national centers providing leadership in the advancement of school mental health policies and programs in the United States. Dr. Weist is an internationally known children's mental health expert who has published extensively, advised national research and policy committees, testified before Congress, and presented to the President's New Freedom Commission on Mental Health on issues of school mental health, trauma, violence and youth, and evidence-based practice. He and other colleagues have founded the journal *Advances in School Mental Health Promotion.*

Alexander S. Young, M.D., M.S.H.S., is Director of the Health Services Unit of the Department of Veterans Affairs Desert Pacific Mental Illness Research, Education and Clinical Center, and Professor at the UCLA Department of Psychiatry. He is a national expert and has published extensively regarding the evaluation and improvement of mental health care quality, and the use of health informatics. Dr. Young has received numerous honors, including the American Psychiatric Association 2000 Early Career Health Services Research Award, and the National Alliance for the Mentally Ill 2002 Exemplary Psychiatrist Award.

Samuel H. Zuvekas, Ph.D., is Senior Economist and Deputy Director, Division of Social and Economic Research in the Center for Financing, Access and Cost Trends at the Agency for Healthcare Research and Quality (AHRQ). His research interests include the economics of mental health and substance abuse, health care finance and expenditures, and access to care. Dr. Zuvekas currently serves as chair of the World Psychiatric Association's Section on Mental Health Economics and is a member of the editorial boards of the *Journal of Mental Health Policy and Economics* and the *Journal of Behavioral Health Services & Research.*

FOREWORD

CONTEXT IS everything—particularly where mental health services are concerned. *Mental Health Services, third edition*, picks up the context where the excellent second edition left off—reflecting its subtitle, *A Public Health Perspective*. Written by an array of authorities, this new compilation of chapters is so compelling because of the importance of the public health perspective and the way the book reflects the policy context of changing times. The second edition of 2004 was a product of a field moving on after the failures of health care reform, followed by the landmark Surgeon General's reports on mental health, the Institute of Medicine's *Quality Chasm* report, and the tragedy of September 11, 2001. The third edition of 2010 is the product of its time, embodied in the work of the President's New Freedom Commission on Mental Health and its emphasis on parity, transformation, and recovery.

Parity in Medicare and private insurance became law after bills passed through the U.S. Congress were signed by President George W. Bush in his final year in office. It will be up to the new administration of President Barack Obama and its new effort at health care reform to sustain the emphasis on parity, transformation, and recovery in mental health services.

Parity implies integration. Equal coverage is predicated on the view that mental health services should be valued just like the rest of health services, and sometimes the best approach is to integrate the two. This issue is discussed in various places in the book, beginning with the explicit discussion of financing and parity and continuing in chapters on delivering services to various populations and in various settings, including in primary care. The focus is no longer on the specialty mental health services sector but on the broad array of human services sectors, where people who experience a mental disorder find themselves as they pursue their lives in their communities.

Transformation also implies integration—but at a different level. It means recognizing the role of mental health in mainstream public policy. This issue is discussed in separate chapters devoted to mental health services and the law, criminal justice, and education. Public policies related to housing and employment are featured in chapters on mental health services for children and adults in a range of treatment settings. Mental health concerns are integrated into the concerns of many areas of mainstream public policy.

Recovery is now woven into the fabric of the book, as it has been woven into the field. The second edition introduced the concept with a chapter on the recovery movement. The third edition also has a chapter devoted to this topic, but now the issue of recovery pervades the discussion of most of the chapters on treatments and mental health services policy.

The relevance of these themes and others are explored in a section of each chapter on "Implications for Mental Health." This is a welcomed feature of each contribution to the third edition. Although the implications pertain mostly to the mental health services in the United States, there are parts of the book that have a global focus and are relevant to the context in other countries.

Mental Health Services, third edition employs several organizing frameworks. Following a set of introductory chapters in Part I on "Services Delivery Issues," the text takes a public health perspective in Part II, on "Selected Populations and Treatment Settings." Part II is further subdivided into a developmental and life cycle presentation of chapters on specific selected populations (such as children and older adults) and a systems framework for looking at various treatment settings (such as various specialty mental health settings and primary care, as well as schools and the criminal justice system). Part III is a potpourri of interesting "Special Issues," such as disparities and recovery. Overall, this organizing framework advances the goal of presenting a public health perspective.

The book is well edited and balanced, as well as accessible to a wide range of readers. The references are current and cover the entire field of mental health services. The narrative encourages the reader to explore these references to learn the deep background of many of the book's assertions and discussions. The Table of Contents only hints at the topics covered within the book's 23 chapters: Evidence-based practices and empirically supported treatments are the focus of many of these chapters. The authors explore the scientific basis for such a determination and review what is known about their implementation. The role of coercion and leverage is presented, as is a discussion of client-centered care and shared decision-making within the context of a recovery orientation for mental health services. Chapters present the history of mental health services delivery and financing along with discussions of practical knowledge about clinical matters throughout the life cycle. To accomplish this mix of themes and data takes a multidisciplinary group of authors and a skilled team of editors to match them. This book succeeds in every way in combining these various aspects of the public health perspective on mental health services.

The material in *Mental Health Services, third edition* is up-to-date and authoritative. The authors are among the world's experts in their respective fields. The presentation is scientific and, where appropriate, it is clinically relevant and informed by practice. There is no better text on this topic for graduate students in public health, social work, community psychology, psychiatric nursing, and other trainees in community mental health, including psychiatric residents. It is also useful as a handbook and reference for researchers and other academics, practitioners, administrators, and policymakers, anyone with a professional affiliation with mental health and substance abuse services delivery.

We can hope that this book will have many such readers, and that they will learn from its ideas and conclusions about how to improve mental health services for all of us.

Howard H. Goldman, M.D., Ph.D.
Professor of Psychiatry
University of Maryland School of Medicine
Baltimore, MD 21227

PREFACE

THIS NEW *Third Edition* of *Mental Health Services: A Public Health Perspective* is being completed in the midst of public debate over President Obama's health care reform proposals. Debate over health care is hardly new. The *First Edition* of this text was published in 1996, shortly after the rejection of President Clinton's health care reform proposal. The *Second Edition* of this text was published in 2004, shortly after President Bush's New Freedom Commission on Mental Health had issued its final report decrying the state of public mental health in the United States.

This brief timeline illustrates three points central to the reasons we have developed this text as well as this new *Third Edition*. First, health care is an issue of the highest importance in the United States. Second, there is broad dissatisfaction with virtually every aspect of the health care systems in the United States, including access, cost, and outcomes. And third, mental health delivery systems, in particular, have changed fundamentally in the last two decades in ways that make it essential to consider mental health care not as an isolated specialty sector but as an important part of public health.

This new *Third Edition*, like its predecessors, examines the critical issues in the organization, financing, delivery, and evaluation of mental health services in the United States. It covers issues that lie at the heart of all public health sectors, such as epidemiology, treatment, and policy, examining those issues in the context of people with mental disorders. It also includes topics of special concern to mental health administrators, policymakers, planners, evaluators, and treatment professionals, such as criminal justice, co-occurring disorders, and the economics of psychopharmacology. In addition, this new *Third Edition* has been reorganized to add new chapters on specific treatment sectors that provide mental health services, including state mental health agencies, community mental health providers, and specialty hospitals and psychiatric units within general hospitals. There are also new chapters on workforce development and the global burden of mental disorders.

Like the previous two editions, the development and organization of the *Third Edition* has been influenced by the experiences of the editors. One editor of this volume (BLL) has developed and teaches in the Graduate Studies in Behavioral Health Program, a collaborative teaching initiative between the Florida Mental Health Institute (now an academic component of the USF College of Behavioral and Community Sciences) and the College of Public Health, both at the University of South Florida. This program is one of only several of the 41 accredited schools of public health in the United States and Puerto Rico offering a concentration in behavioral health (i.e., alcohol, drug abuse, and mental health services). Another editor of this volume (JP) has taught graduate courses in health care law and disability law and also provides legal consultation to public mental health systems across the United States. The editors of this text have also served as administrators in public mental health systems (JP) and in the federal government (KDH), and provide mental health services directly in a variety of clinical settings (KDH). All of the editors have worked with mental health professionals and mental health services researchers throughout the United States.

These varied experiences have convinced us that it is impossible to understand issues in mental health services unless those issues are considered within the context of a public health framework. This means that an interdisplinary approach to the topic is essential. The result is that the *Third Edition*, like the previous two, draws from nationally prominent academicians, researchers, and other experts from a variety of backgrounds and disciplines. Each expert understands his or her mental health/substance abuse specialty, but also appreciates the broader public health context in which that specialty exists. These experts have made it possible to provide an integrated text that can be used by graduate students in public health, social work, psychiatric nursing, psychology, applied anthropology, and public administration. We also have designed the book as a reference and handbook for administrators, researchers, practitioners, and policymakers who work with mental health issues at the local, state, or national levels. In brief, it can also be used by any individual or organization involved in some aspect of mental health systems delivery in the United States in the twenty-first century.

Organization of the Third Edition

The *Third Edition* is divided into three major parts: Part I—Services Delivery Issues; Part II—Selected Populations and Treatment Settings; and Part III—Special Issues.

Part I, Services Delivery Issues, includes five chapters that provide information regarding the defining characteristics of mental health systems. In Chapter 1, we provide an overview of the changes in public mental health systems over the last two decades, and place those changes in a broader public health framework. Chapter 2, written by Samuel H. Zuvekas, discusses financing of mental health and substance abuse services and the impact of managed care. In Chapter 3, Petrila and Levin describe the impact of the legal system on mental health services, organizations, and client rights. Chapter 4, by Kevin Hennessy, discusses quality assurance. Finally, Rebecca Morris and Anne Lezak discuss the role of workforce development, a new topic for this book.

Part II of this new edition is divided into two sections. Section A deals with the special populations that have emerged as key areas of focus in service delivery. Chapter 6, by Philip S. Wang and colleagues, addresses the global impact of mental disorders, reminding the reader that the issues discussed in this text are not confined to the United States. In Chapter 7, Ron Kessler and colleagues provide the latest data available on the epidemiology of mental disorders. After the overviews provided in Chapters 6 and 7, the next five chapters focus on specific populations. Sharon Green-Hennessy writes about children and adolescents in Chapter 8, while Alex Young and Noosha Niv focus on adults in Chapter 9. In Chapter 10, Steven Bartels and Aricca D. Van Citters discuss issues involving older adults. Dennis McCarty and Traci Rieckmann explore treatment systems for alcohol and drug use disorders in Chapter 11, while Fred Osher and colleagues focus in Chapter 12 on the public health implications of co-occurring addictive and mental disorders.

Section B of Part II provides an overview of the specific treatment settings in which mental disorders are most commonly assessed and treated. Chapter 13, by Ted Lutterman and colleagues, discusses the current status of state mental health agencies in America. Tom Doub and colleagues focus on community mental health centers in Chapter 14, and, in Chapter 15, Faith Dickerson and Steve Sharfstein discuss specialty pychiatric hospitals and psychiatric units within hospitals. In Chapter 16, Ron Manderscheid examines the essential but sometimes overlooked topic of the integration of primary care and specialty mental health services. Mark Weist and colleagues explore school mental health issues in Chapter 17, while, in Chapter 18, Alison Redlich and Karen Cusack conclude Part II with an overview of efforts to address the increased numbers of people with mental disorders entering the criminal justice system.

The final Part of this *Third Edition* text is devoted to Special Issues in mental health. Junius Gonzales and Airia Sasser Papadopoulos begin with an examination, in Chapter 19, of disparities in access and treatment. In Chapter 20, Bill Anthony and Lori Ashcraft provide an updated overview of the recovery movement, while in Chapter 21, Marissa Domino and Joel Farley look at the economic issues in the use of psychotropic medications. Ardis Hanson and Bruce Lubotsky Levin discuss the increasingly important topic of informatics in Chapter 22. In Chapter 23, Stephen Leff and Crystal Blyler conclude this new *Third Edition* of the text with a practical approach to evaluating mental health systems and system change.

It is, of course, impossible to include every possible topic in a book devoted to mental health services in a single volume. However, in our view, this *Third Edition* underscores the importance of continuing to rely on a multidisciplinary approach to study and understand mental health issues within a public health framework.

Throughout the development and preparation of this *Third Edition* text, there have been a number of individuals who have provided sage counsel, continuing support, and/or significant encouragement. At USF, we are grateful to Ms. Ardis Hanson for numerous valuable suggestions and for the preparation of the subject index for this *Third Edition* text. In addition, we would like to acknowledge the efforts of Ms. Annie DeMuth, a graduate student in the USF College of Public Health, for her significant efforts in copyediting every chapter in this text. We also would like to extend our deep appreciation to Ms. Molly Hildebrand and Mr. Craig Allen Panner at Oxford University Press for their many helpful suggestions during the copyediting and production of this new *Third Edition* text. Finally, we are ultimately grateful to our families for their continuing love and immeasurable support during the lengthy preparation of this *Third Edition* text.

Bruce Lubotsky Levin
Kevin D. Hennessy
John Petrila

Mental Health Services

Part I

SERVICES DELIVERY ISSUES

Chapter 1

A PUBLIC HEALTH APPROACH TO MENTAL HEALTH SERVICES

Bruce Lubotsky Levin, DrPH, MPH; Ardis Hanson, MLS;
Kevin D. Hennessy, PhD; and John Petrila, JD, LLM

Introduction

While the roots of epidemiology can be traced to John Snow and the 1854 cholera outbreak in England (Snow, 1855), C.-E.A. Winslow provided one of the earliest and most fundamental definitions of public health in America:

> Public health is the science and art of preventing disease, prolonging life, and promoting physical health and efficiency through organized community efforts . . . which will ensure to every individual a standard of living adequate for the maintenance of health . . . to enable every citizen to realize his [and her] birthright of health and longevity. (Winslow, 1920, pp. 6–7)

In 1988, the Institute of Medicine's (IOM) Committee for the Study of the Future of Public Health published the book *The Future of Public Health*, which examined public health programs and the coordination of services across U.S. government agencies and within state and local health departments. The Committee defined the *substance* of public health as "organized community efforts aimed at the prevention of disease and promotion of health" (IOM, 1988, p. 41) and defined the *mission* of public health as "the fulfillment of society's interest in assuring conditions in which people can be healthy" (IOM, 1988, p. 40).

The IOM Committee also identified three core functions of public health: 1) assessment; 2) policy development; and 3) assurance (of providing necessary public health services in the community). Subsequently, the U.S Public Health Service convened the Public Health Functions Steering Committee, a national work group chaired by the Surgeon General, which developed 10 essential public health services needed to carry out the basic public health core functions in a community:

1. Monitor health status to identify community health problems;
2. Diagnose and investigate identified health problems and health hazards in the community;
3. Inform, educate, and empower people about health issues;
4. Mobilize community partnerships to identify and solve health problems;
5. Develop policies and plans that support individual and community health efforts;
6. Enforce laws and regulations that protect health and ensure safety;
7. Link people to needed personal health services and assure the provision of health care;
8. Assure a competent public health and personal health care workforce;
9. Assess effectiveness, accessibility, and quality of personal and population-based health; and
10. Research for new insights and innovative solutions to health problems (Public Health Functions Steering Committee, 1994, p. 1).

Thus, while there are a variety of definitions and functions of public health, common elements include a population-based approach that emphasizes health promotion and disease prevention. Furthermore, a public health approach involves formal activities undertaken within government, combined with efforts by private and voluntary organizations and individuals working together to focus on maintaining the health of populations. This public health framework of problem-solving includes the following elements: 1) problem identification (utilizing epidemiologic surveillance); 2) identifying risks and protective factors; 3) development, implementation, and evaluation of interventions; and 4) monitoring implementation in relation to the impact on policy and cost-effectiveness (World Health Organization [WHO], 2009).

The chapters in this text present the latest knowledge on a variety of key issues related to the organization, financing, and delivery of mental health services (see Chapters 1–5 in this volume). Specifically, this text examines the delivery of mental health services in selected at-risk populations (see Chapters 6–12 in this volume) and in selected treatment settings (see Chapters 13–18 in this volume), and also examines a number of special issues in mental health, including disparity (see Chapter 19 in this volume), recovery (see Chapter 20 in this volume), economic issues in the use of psychotropic medication (see Chapter 21 in this volume), the complexity of data (see Chapter 22 in this volume), and evaluating systems and systems change (see Chapter 23 in this volume). This first chapter highlights the burden of mental disorders on individuals and the general public, examines the complexities of existing mental health delivery systems, and emphasizes the importance of re-focusing mental health on systems integration strategies that incorporate technology and facilitate recovery.

Burden of Mental Disorders

In addition to the definition, substance, mission, and functions of public health noted above, public health may also be viewed within the larger context of health.

The World Health Organization defines health as "a state of complete physical, mental, and social well-being and not merely the absence of disease or infirmity" (WHO, 2006). Accordingly, mental health may be conceptualized as an integral part of the overall health of individuals and populations, though different cultures and ethnicities may vary in their definitions of what constitutes "mental health" and "mental illness" (see Chapter 19 in this volume on mental health disparities).

Mental disorders are common worldwide and include some of the most complex problems in public health. An estimated 450 million people throughout the world suffer from mental disorders, including alcohol and drug use disorders. Fourteen percent of the global burden of disease is attributed to mental disorders (Prince et al., 2007; Das-Munshi et al., 2008). Over 154 million people globally suffer from depression, 25 million people suffer from schizophrenia, 91 million people are affected by alcohol use disorders, and 15 million people have drug use disorders (WHO, 2003). About one half of mental disorders begin before individuals reach the age of 14 years old (WHO, 2005). Individuals with mental disorders are more at risk for medical illnesses, for communicable and non-communicable diseases, and for injury (WHO, 2001).

The World Health Organization (2001) has emphasized the magnitude of mental disorders from a global public health perspective:

> One person in every four will be affected by a mental disorder at some stage of life . . . The social and economic burden of mental illness is enormous. (p. x)

Mental disorders in the United States are also widespread, where approximately one in five adults have a diagnosable mental disorder during any 12-month period (Kessler et al., 2005). Furthermore, mental health problems in the workplace have serious consequences for worker performance, absenteeism, accidents, and overall workplace productivity (Harnois & Gabriel, 2000) (see Chapters 5, 6, 7, and 12 in this volume for a more detailed discussion on the epidemiology of mental disorders, co-occurring disorders, and workforce mental health).

In addition, the significance of the substantial burden of mental disorders on individuals and society is underscored by expenditures for mental health and substance abuse services. In 1986, expenditures for mental health and substance abuse treatment in the United States were $42 billion. By 2003, expenditures had increased to $121 billion, and expenditures for mental health and substance abuse treatment are projected to reach $239 billion by 2014 (Levit et al., 2008). While private financing of services has increased, public financing is still considered the major funding source for mental health and substance abuse services (see Chapter 2 in this volume for a more detailed discussion on insurance, financing, and managed mental health care).

Complexity Issues and Mental Health Systems

Through the 1950s, state-run mental hospitals were the primary venue for providing care to people with serious mental disorders in the United States. As de-institutionalization occurred (see Chapters 13–15 in this volume), the publicly

financed mental health system evolved from state-run hospital settings to a variety
of specialty (sector) services within a number of different organizational settings,
largely independent from public health systems. The IOM Committee for the
Study of the Future of Public Health emphasized this fragmented (or de facto)
mental health delivery system (Regier, Goldberg, & Taube, 1978), as well as the
lack of integration between public health and mental health services. Ultimately,
the IOM Committee called for the integration of future public health initiatives
with mental health initiatives, particularly in the areas of disease prevention and
health promotion (IOM, 1988).

The de facto mental health system in the United States is not an organized
system of care. Rather, it is comprised of numerous health and mental health delivery systems, as well as other systems (for example, the social welfare, justice, and
educational systems) in which individuals with mental disorders commonly find
themselves. It includes both public and private sector services, with each sector having its own agencies, funding streams, services, and operations. It provides acute
and long-term mental health care in homes, communities, and institutional settings
across the specialty mental health sector, the general medical/primary care sector,
and the voluntary care sector. Professional licensing and accreditation organizations, managed care provider entities, insurance companies, advocacy and regulatory agencies, and health care policymaking groups potentially influence how
mental health care is accessed, organized, delivered, and financed (see Chapters
13–18 in this volume for a detailed discussion of mental health services in various
treatment settings and organizations). At the same time, assessment and treatment
of mental disorders often occur in other systems whose primary missions have
little to do with the identification of mental disorders.

One such example of the complex interrelatedness of the de facto mental health
system is the provision of mental health and substance abuse services in both jails
and prisons. While the criminal justice system offers opportunities to reach vulnerable populations at-risk for mental and substance use disorders, the provision, utilization, and costs of these services are not uniformly accepted across all
communities in the United States (see Chapter 18 in this volume for a more detailed
discussion of mental health treatment in criminal justice settings).

In addition, legislation at the state and federal levels influences (and often establishes) mental health policy and, in turn, the provision of mental health services.
Adoption of these laws through legislative proviso language and through administrative and financial appropriation language also influences mental health policy
and services delivery.

Obviously, there are many factors that potentially impact the way mental health
delivery systems are organized, financed, and delivered within a given community,
region, state, or throughout America. Some of these factors may contribute to the
integration of mental health and policy within a public health framework, while
others may have the opposite effect. The continuing issue is how best to effect
change within a complex and fragmented system so as to improve the quality of life
of persons with mental and substance use disorders, and thereby improve society as
a whole. A recent example of addressing this ongoing challenge is reflected in the
charge to the President's New Freedom Commission on Mental Health (2003) to
identify policies that would transform the de facto mental health delivery system

into one system emphasizing, among other things, the prevention of mental illnesses and the promotion of a recovery orientation among both those providing and receiving services.

Technology, Recovery, and Prevention

The New Freedom Commission on Mental Health (2003) made a number of recommendations to fundamentally transform the delivery of mental health services in the United States. Of the five goals the Commission identified, three that are most pertinent to this discussion include technology, recovery, and prevention.

The use of technology has two major aims. The first addresses advancing research in the development of evidence-based practices to treat individuals with mental and substance use disorders, with the ultimate goal of preventing mental disorders and promoting recovery among individuals with mental illnesses. The second aim is the effective use of technology to maximize diffusion, early adoption, and implementation of effective practices and to improve service provision and service utilization. Technology is also relevant to workforce development issues in assuring that current and future practitioners have access to and utilize evidence-based services. In addition, technology is a critical component in developing the knowledge base in mental and substance use disorders, particularly in the areas of disparities, trauma, acute care, and long-term consequences of medications. Finally, integrated information technology (e.g., electronic health records) and communications infrastructure (e.g., telehealth systems) require substantial investments, but are critical to the effective delivery of mental health services (see Chapter 22 in this volume for a detailed discussion of the complexity of mental health data).

Mental health systems that are consumer- and family-driven are one focus of the New Freedom Commission report. The report emphasizes the need for individualized plans of care, stakeholder voices, protection and advocacy for persons with mental disorders, and improved access and accountability for mental health services. Emphasis on applied mental health research to promote recovery and resiliency is a cornerstone of transforming mental health services. The basic message of recovery from serious mental disorder for each individual is hope for the restoration of a meaningful life. This message of hope offers the possibility of an identity that is simultaneously *within* and *beyond* the limits of disability. According to Anthony (1993), recovery requires "the development of new meaning and purpose in one's life as one grows beyond the catastrophic effects of mental illness" (p. 11). What is critical about recovery as a process and as an outcome, however, is the personal meaning that each individual attaches to the concept (see Chapter 20 in this volume for a detailed discussion on the recovery movement).

Prevention is included in the Commission's recommendation for early mental health screening, assessment, and referral to services, with the emphasis on developing integrated mental health systems. With the dissemination, adoption, and implementation of evidence-based practices together with an improved workforce, a fundamental transformation of America's varied approaches to mental health care may be achieved.

Implications for Mental Health

A public health approach to mental health focuses on health promotion and disease prevention to improve the health and mental health of populations. This text uses a population approach to specific mental health services delivery issues. The chapters address prevention, promotion, and service integration within their respective topics, from mental health services for children and adolescents to financing of mental health care to developing and accessing effective information systems on mental and substance use disorders.

A public health perspective allows one to examine and address the continued fragmentation and gaps in care for children, adults, and the elderly; recovery issues surrounding unemployment, stigma, and disability for people with serious mental disorders; and the lack of a national priority for mental health and suicide prevention.

The President's New Freedom Commission on Mental Health (2003) envisioned "a future when everyone with a mental illness at any stage of life has access to effective treatment and supports—essentials for living, working, learning, and participating fully in the community" (p. 1). In meeting this very ambitious goal, it is essential that a public health approach to mental health services be adopted. Often, mental disorders are conceptualized and approached from a "problem-saturated perspective," which "services the disorders" and not the person, often disrupting the processes that emphasize abilities and "the help one needs for getting on with life" (Sullivan, 1994). On the other hand, a public health perspective integrates mental health within a broader public health framework, recognizes the enormous impact of untreated mental disorders on the population as well as the individual, and assumes recovery is possible. Finally, it focuses, as does this text, upon achieving a better life for individuals and at-risk populations with serious mental disorders and their families and obtaining appropriate assistance from the many systems of health and mental health care available to persons with mental disorders.

References

Anthony, W. A. (1993). Recovery from mental illness: The guiding vision of the mental health service system in the 1990s. *Psychosocial Rehabilitation Journal, 16*(4), 11–23.

Das-Munshi, J., Goldberg, D., Bebbington, P. E., Bhugra, D. K., Brugha, T. S., Dewey, M. E., et al. (2008). Public health significance of mixed anxiety and depression: Beyond current classification. *British Journal of Psychiatry, 192*(3), 171–177.

Harnois, G., & Gabriel, P. (2000). *Mental Health and Work: Impact, Issues, and Good Practices.* Geneva: World Health Organization.

Institute of Medicine, Committee for the Study of the Future of Public Health, Division of Health Care Services. (1988). *The Future of Public Health.* Washington, DC, National Academy Press.

Kessler, R. C., Demler, O., Frank, R. G., Olfson, M., Pincus, H. A., Walters, E. E., et al. (2005). Prevalence and treatment of mental disorders, 1990 to 2003. *New England Journal of Medicine, 352,* 2515–2523.

Levit, K. R., Kassed, C. A., Coffey, R. M., Mark, T. L., McKusick, D. R., King, E., et al. (2008). *Projections of National Expenditures for Mental Health Services and Substance Abuse Treatment, 2004–2014.* SAMHSA Publication No. SMA 08-4326. Rockville, MD: Substance Abuse and Mental Health Services Administration.

New Freedom Commission on Mental Health. (2003). *Achieving the Promise: Transforming Mental Health Care in America. Final Report.* DHHS Pub. No. SMA-03-3832. Rockville, MD: U.S. Department of Health and Human Services.

Prince, M., Patel, V., Saxena, S., Maj, M., Maselko, J., Phillips, M. R., et al. (2007). No health without mental health. *The Lancet, 370*(9590), 859–877.

Public Health Functions Steering Committee. (1994). *Public Health in America.* Washington, DC: U.S. Public Health Services. Available online at http://www.health.gov/phfunctions/public. htm. Accessed February 23, 2010.

Regier, D., Goldberg, I., & Taube, C. (1978). The de facto U.S. mental health services system: A public health perspective. *Archives of General Psychiatry, 35,* 685–693.

Snow, J. (1855). *On the Mode of Communication of Cholera.* London: John Churchill.

Sullivan, W. P. (1994). A long and winding road: The process of recovery from mental illness. *Innovations and Research, 3*(3), 19–27.

Winslow, C.-E. A. (1920). The untilled fields of public health. *Modern Medicine, 2,* 1–9.

World Health Organization. (2001). *The World Health Report, 2001: Mental Health; New Understanding, New Hope.* Geneva, Switzerland: World Health Organization.

World Health Organization (2003). *Investing in Mental Health.* Geneva, Switzerland: World Health Organization.

World Health Organization. (2005). *Preventing Chronic Diseases: A Vital Investment; WHO Global Report.* Geneva, Switzerland: World Health Organization.

World Health Organization. (2006). *Constitution of the World Health Organization.* Available online at http://www.who.int/governance/eb/who_constitution_en.pdf. Accessed November 12, 2009.

World Health Organization. (2009). *Global Campaign for Violence Prevention.* Available online at http://www.who.int/violenceprevention/approach/public_health/en/index.html. Accessed November 12, 2009.

Chapter 2

THE FINANCING OF MENTAL HEALTH AND SUBSTANCE ABUSE SERVICES: INSURANCE, MANAGED CARE, AND REIMBURSEMENT

Samuel H. Zuvekas, PhD*

Overview

Mental health services continue to move toward largely insurance-based and-financed systems of care, with even the public sector widely adopting private-sector models of insurance-based financing. Up until the 1950s, most mental health services were provided in state and local long-term psychiatric hospitals and financed primarily through state and local general revenues. The Community Mental Health Centers Act of 1963 added federal funding for more community-based services through grants to the states. But it was the passage of the Medicare and Medicaid health insurance programs in the 1960s, Medicaid in particular, that fundamentally altered the way mental health/substance abuse (MH/SA) services were financed in this country. Medicaid is jointly financed by federal and state governments, with states receiving roughly a dollar-to-dollar match. However, when the program was instituted Medicaid reimbursement was expressly prohibited in state psychiatric facilities under the Medicaid Institutions for Mental Disease (IMD) rule. Under the IMD rule, hospitals, nursing homes, and residential facilities with more than 16 beds that specialize in mental health treatment cannot receive reimbursement for residents aged 22–64 even if they are otherwise eligible for Medicaid. Thus, states had powerful incentives to provide services outside of state psychiatric facilities because only half the costs were paid by the states under

* The views expressed in this chapter are those of the author, and no official endorsement by the Agency for Healthcare Research and Quality or the Department of Health and Human Services is intended or should be inferred.

Medicaid. The Federal Social Security Disability Income (SSDI), passed in 1956, and later the Supplemental Security Income (SSI) programs in the 1970s, provided further impetus for community-based services by giving income support to those individuals disabled by mental disorders.

Private health insurance systems have also become central to the financing of MH/SA services. Most Americans under the age of 65 obtain health insurance coverage through employers and unions rather than through public insurance programs, although a significant percentage of individuals remain uninsured. The introduction of Selective Serotonin Reuptake Inhibitors (SSRIs) and other newer antidepressants, beginning in 1988, led millions more Americans into treatment over the last two decades, the majority with private health insurance coverage (Kessler et al., 2005). Prescription medications now account for one in five MH/SA services dollars, and thus, their financing is of primary importance to public and private insurance programs alike.

The movement to insurance-based MH/SA service systems has meant much tighter integration with the larger and constantly evolving health and social insurance systems. Thus, changes in the Medicaid and Medicare public insurance programs and private health plans increasingly drive how MH/SA services are organized, delivered, and financed. The principal goals of this chapter are to 1) understand how these private-sector models of insurance (including Medicare and Medicaid) operate in theory and in practice, and 2) understand the implications of the increasing strains on employer-based private health insurance and public insurance systems for the future of MH/SA services.

How Are Mental Health Services Financed Today?

Funding for MH/SA services today comes from a complex array of public and private sources, some insurance-based and some not. Table 2.1 presents the latest statistics from an ongoing project by the Substance Abuse and Mental Health Services Administration (SAMHSA) to track spending on MH/SA services (Mark et al., 2007).

Public and private health insurance plans together paid just over half of the estimated $121 billion spent on MH/SA services in 2003. Medicaid (25%) was the single most important insurance-based source, followed closely by private health insurance plans (22%) and more distantly, Medicare (7%). The other half of MH/SA services were financed from other state and local sources (24%); federal sources including Veterans Administration programs, the Indian Health Service, and the $1.6 billion in SAMHSA block grants to state and local agencies (5%); other private sources (5%); and patients and their families' own pockets (13%).

Medicaid (and to a lesser extent, private insurance) continues to grow in importance relative to traditional state and local mental health authorities. Medicaid spending surpassed other state and local sources for the first time around the turn of this millennium. Most analysts predict that the Medicaid share of MH/SA spending will continue to grow for the foreseeable future, while other state and local sources shares decline. Other state and local spending has not actually declined in absolute terms; rather, it has been growing much more slowly than Medicaid expenditures.

This trend has been described as the "Medicaidization" of MH/SA services, where increasingly, decisions about MH/SA are made within the Medicaid program rather than by state and local mental health authorities (Cunningham, 2003). However, other state and local authorities (including funding that comes through federal block grants) remain an important source of financing of MH/SA services. This is especially true of substance abuse services, where the majority of funding comes from public sources other than Medicare and Medicaid.

While the long-standing trend to largely insurance-financed MH/SA treatment systems continues, it still has not reached the levels of somatic (or physical health) care. Three-quarters of funding for non-MH/SA services comes from health insurance sources (Table 2.1). Medicaid is also a more important source of financing

Table 2.1 Distribution of Spending by Payment Source, 1993 and 2003

	1993 MHSA		*2003 MHSA*		*1993 Total*		*2003 Total*	
	Millions ($)	*Percent*	*Millions ($)*	*Percent*	*Millions ($)*	*Percent*	*Millions ($)*	*Percent*
Private—Total	26,103	37.2	46,702	38.6	484,049	56.5	892,564	55.3
Out-of-Pocket	9,090	13.0	15,977	13.2	146,948	17.2	230,483	14.3
Private Insurance	13,239	18.9	26,400	21.8	298,078	34.8	600,594	37.2
Other Private	3,774	5.4	4,325	3.6	39,023	4.6	61,487	3.8
Public—Total	44,085	62.8	74,360	61.4	372,225	43.5	721,658	44.7
Medicare	5,397	7.7	8,270	6.8	148,336	17.3	283,104	17.5
Medicaid[1]	14,143	20.1	30,101	24.9	121,612	14.2	268,629	16.6
Other Federal[2]	5,318	7.6	6,591	5.4	36,247	4.2	65,672	4.1
Other State and Local[3]	19,228	27.4	29,398	24.3	66,030	7.7	104,253	6.5
All Federal[3]	19,641	28.0	32,598	26.9	261,345	30.5	507,480	31.4
All State[4]	24,444	34.8	41,762	34.5	110,880	12.9	214,178	13.3
Total	70,189	100.0	121,062	100.0	856,274	100.0	1,614,222	100.0

Source: Table A.2 and Table A.7, Mark, Levit, McKusick, Harwood, Bouchery et al. (2007).

Notes:
1. The State Children's Health Insurance Program (SCHIP) total NHA spending was $6.6 billion in 2003. MHSA SCHIP spending was estimated at $1.1 billion or about 1 percent of total MHSA. In this table, SCHIP is distributed across Medicaid, Other Federal, and Other State and Local categories, depending on whether the SCHIP was run through Medicaid or as a separate state SCHIP program.
2. SAMHSA block grants to "State and Local" agencies are part of "Other Federal" government spending. In 2003, block grants amounted to $385 million for MH and $1,227 for SA.
3. Includes Federal share of Medicaid.
4. Includes State and Local share of Medicaid.

for MH/SA services compared to other health care services, while Medicare and private insurance plans are relatively more important in financing somatic services.

Where Do Services Dollars Go?

Treatment continues to shift from hospital- to community-based services. Only one in four MH/SA services dollars were spent in specialty psychiatric and general hospitals in 2003 (Table 2.2), and that figure is probably even less today. Because these aggregate figures also include outpatient and partial-day treatment, the amount spent on inpatient care is still less. Spending in psychiatric specialty hospitals actually declined between 1993 and 2003, after growing rapidly in the previous decade, and now accounts for only 1 in 10 of every MH/SA dollar. Much of this drop is due to the rapid growth of specialty managed behavioral health care organizations (MBHOs) over this period, which achieved cost savings primarily by restricting inpatient care (see below). Overhead costs of insurance have increased as a by-product of increased management of behavioral health services. That is, proportionately fewer dollars are going to direct patient care.

Spending on psychiatrists and other MH/SA professionals continues to grow in absolute terms, but the specialists' share of spending in percentage terms remains fairly stable (Table 2.2). Likewise, the non-psychiatric-physician share of total spending continues to grow only slightly. Estimates of aggregate spending on specialty MH/SA providers still outstrip spending on non-specialists by four to one. There are good reasons, however, to believe that these aggregate estimates understate the amount spent on primary care physicians, because MH/SA services and diagnoses are often not coded as such in the claims data that form the basis for these estimates. In fact, the majority of people receiving MH/SA services get their care from non-specialist providers, although they tend to have many fewer visits on average than people who receive services from specialists (also see Chapter 7 in this volume for more on this).

About half of the recent growth in MH/SA spending comes from prescription medications. In 1993, psychotropic medications accounted for only 6% of MH/SA spending. Now they account for about one in five services dollars. Spending on psychotropic medications now outstrips the combined spending on psychiatrists, psychologists, social workers, and other mental health professionals (Table 2.2). From 1993 to 2003, expenditures on psychotropic medications grew at an average annual rate of 19%. More recent estimates find that psychotropic medications continue to experience double-digit annual spending increases (Table 2.3).

The Growing Importance of Prescription Medications

Psychotropic medications have been around for many decades. Thorazine, first introduced in 1954, and the other typical antipsychotics that followed were a key factor behind successive waves of deinstitutionalization, as treatment shifted from psychiatric institutions to the community. However, the sustained and explosive growth in spending on psychotropic drugs over the last few decades is something

Table 2.2 Mental Health and Substance Abuse Services Spending by Type of Service, 1993 and 2003

	1993 MHSA		2003 MHSA	
	Millions ($)	*Percent*	*Millions ($)*	*Percent*
Specialty Sector	**50,156**	**71.5**	**65,986**	**54.5**
General Hospitals, Specialty Units[1]	10,226	14.6	9,458	7.8
Specialty Hospitals	13,181	18.8	12,348	10.2
Psychiatrists	5,592	8.0	10,342	8.5
Other Professionals[2]	6,703	9.5	11,006	9.1
Multi-Services Mental Health Organizations[3]	9,284	13.2	14,390	11.9
Specialty Substance Abuse Centers[4]	5,169	7.4	8,441	7.0
General Sector Providers	**11,968**	**17.1**	**23,267**	**19.2**
General Hospitals, Non-specialty Units[5]	3,240	4.6	10,828	8.9
Non-Psychiatric physicians	2,677	3.8	5,077	4.2
Free-Standing Nursing Homes	5,667	8.1	6,535	5.4
Free-Standing Home Health	384	0.5	827	0.7
Retail Prescription Medications	**4,191**	**6.0**	**23,357**	**19.3**
Insurance Admin.	**3,874**	**5.5**	**8,452**	**7.0**
Total	**70,189**	**100.0**	**121,062**	**100.0**

Source: Table A.3 and Table A.8, Mark, Levit, McKusick, Harwood, Bouchery et al. (2007).

Notes:
1. Includes specialty units of general hospitals and all MH and SA expenditures at VA hospitals
2. Includes psychologists and counselors/social workers.
3. Includes Residential Treatment Centers for Children.
4. Includes other facilities for treating substance abuse.
5. Includes general hospital non-specialty units but excludes non-specialty units of VA hospitals

new altogether. The new classes of antidepressants first introduced in the late 1990s and the atypical antipsychotic medications introduced in the 1990s were widely perceived to have fewer side effects and greater efficacy than older medications (Berndt, Bhattacharjya, Mishol, Arcelus, & Lasky, 2002). Not only did these newer, more expensive medications quickly supplant the older, cheaper (generic) medications, by itself greatly increasing spending, they also drew millions more Americans into MH/SA services systems (see Chapter 21 in this volume for more on this). Clinicians viewed the new antidepressants as easier to administer and monitor. Primary care physicians in particular were much more willing to prescribe the newer medications, and as a result, they now treat the majority of Americans with

Table 2.3 Trends in Prescription Medication Use and Expenditures in the Civilian Non-institutionalized Population, 1977–2005

Year	% of Population with Fills	Mean Expenditure Per User 2005 $	Distribution of Payments		
			Out-of-Pocket	Private Insurance	Other Sources
Psychotropic Medications					
1977[a]	9.1	$ 71	68%	15%	16%
1987[b]	7.6	$ 146	56%	27%	17%
1997[c]	10.5	$ 367	39%	37%	24%
2002[c]	13.2	$ 534	35%	39%	27%
2005[c]	14.0	$ 682	34%	35%	32%
All Medications					
1977[d]	58.2	$ 122	74%	12%	14%
1987[e]	57.3	$ 250	57%	28%	15%
1997[c]	62.1	$ 508	47%	36%	16%
2002[c]	64.4	$ 881	42%	37%	21%
2005[c]	63.1	$ 1,140	39%	39%	22%

[a]*Source:* Cafferta and Kasper (1983), based on the 1977 National Medical Care Expenditure Survey.
[b]*Source:* Zuvekas (2001), based on the 1987 National Medical Expenditure Survey.
[c]*Source:* Author's own calculations from the Medical Expenditure Panel Survey, Center for Financing Access and Cost Trends, Agency for Healthcare Research and Quality.
[d]*Source:* Kasper (1982), based on the 1977 National Medical Care Expenditure Survey.
[e]*Source:* Hahn and Lefkowitz (1992), based on the 1987 National Medical Expenditure Survey.

mental disorders. Pharmaceutical companies also invested heavily in promoting these medications both to clinicians and directly to consumers after the Food and Drug Administration (FDA) relaxed its rules on advertising in 1997. There is strong evidence that physician detailing and direct-to-consumer advertising increased use of these medications (Berndt et al., 2002; Donohue, Berndt, Rosenthal, Epstein, & Frank, 2004; Wosinska, 2005; and Meyerhoefer & Zuvekas, 2008). The introduction of these new medications likely also contributed to shifts in attitudes toward mental disorders and mental health services among Americans. Reduced stigma likely also increased sales, but these effects are much more difficult to quantify.

Financial factors played a key role as well. On the consumer side, coverage for prescription drug expenditures has improved markedly over the last few decades. Prescription drugs were not included in the original Medicare program enacted in 1965. As late as the 1970s, many private plans did not cover drug costs either. As a result, consumers paid 68% of the costs of psychotropic medications out of their own pockets in 1977 (Table 2.3). By 1987, consumers paid 56% of their psychotropic medications out of pocket, falling to 39% in 1997 and 34% in 2005. This closely mirrors trends toward improved coverage for all types of medications, not just psychotropic drugs (Table 2.3). As medications became central to the treatment of health conditions and became much more expensive, consumers demanded better coverage. In turn, the reduced out-of-pocket costs that came with better coverage likely stimulated increased medication use (Manning, Newhouse, Duan, Keeler, & Leibowitz, 1987). On the provider side, there is evidence that managed behavioral health organizations (MBHOs) helped accelerate the diffusion of these new psychotropic medications (Ling, Berndt, & Frank, 2008; see Chapter 21 in this volume for more on this).

Recent Trends in Health Insurance Coverage

As we have seen, the financing of MH/SA services increasingly depends on the health insurance coverage Americans hold. It is well established that health insurance coverage is strongly associated with access to and use of MH/SA services (Zuvekas, 1999; Frank & McGuire, 1986). Loss of health insurance coverage reduces use of MH/SA services; extending health insurance coverage improves access. Thus, changes in the health insurance system have immediate consequences for MH/SA services.

The mixed public and private nature of U.S. health care systems extends to health insurance coverage. Only those aged 65 and above have near universal coverage through the federally funded Medicare health insurance program. Working-age Americans and their children depend primarily on private insurance obtained through employers or unions to pay for their health care. About 90% of all private insurance in the non-elderly population is obtained through employers.[1] However, not all Americans have access to employment-related insurance. Some employers do not offer health insurance coverage or offer coverage only to certain types of employees. Some employees decline their employer's offer of insurance either because they are covered by other insurance or cannot or do not wish to pay the employee out-of-pocket share of the insurance premium.

The percentage of Americans who are uninsured has remained relatively stable over the last decade. Approximately 15% of the U.S. population is uninsured or 19% of the non-elderly population (Figure 2.1). This stability masks enormous changes in health insurance systems. In 1996, 69% of the non-elderly population was covered by private health insurance. By 2006, this had declined to 65% and is expected to continue to decline. Rising insurance premiums are likely a major factor in the decline. The average total cost of an employer-provided plan for a single person more than doubled from $1,992 in 1996 to $4,188 in 2006. Similarly, the average total cost of a family plan rose dramatically from $4,954 to $11,381 between 1996 and 2006. Economists generally believe that employees absorb most of these increased insurance costs in the form of lower wage increases. For example, unions have been willing to make wage concessions in return for continuing guarantees of health insurance coverage in collective bargaining agreements. However, as total premiums continue to rise, so too do the amounts employees are required to pay out of pocket for their coverage by employers. The average out-of-pocket share for a single plan was $788, and $2,890 for a family plan in 2006 (Agency for Healthcare Research and Quality [AHRQ], 2006a). This is a likely reason why Americans are increasingly declining employer offers of insurance coverage (Cooper & Vistnes, 2003; Cooper & Schone, 1997). It is this declining "take-up rate" that is largely responsible for the decline in private health insurance coverage.

---

[1] Author's calculations from the Medical Expenditure Panel Survey, 2005.

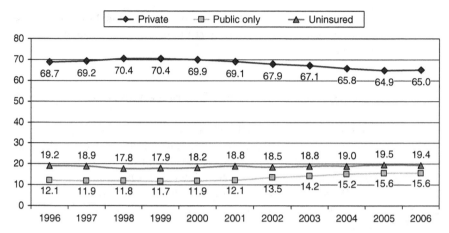

Figure 2.1 Percentage of Civilian Non-Institutionalized Population under 65, by Health Insurance Status, First Half 1996–2006. (*Source*: Medical Expenditure Panel Survey, *1996–2006*, Center for Financing, Access and Cost Trends, Agency for Healthcare Research and Quality.)

Medicaid and the State Children's Health Insurance Program (SCHIP), enacted in 1996 for uninsured children, have compensated in part for the decline in private insurance. The percentage of non-elderly Americans covered by public programs rose substantially over the last decade, from 12.1 in 1996 to 15.6 in 2006 (Figure 2.1). This growth has slowed considerably over the last several years. In part, this is because enrollment in the SCHIP program naturally slowed as the program matured, but also because some states have cut back on SCHIP and Medicaid due to recent budget difficulties. The number of uninsured individuals has begun to slowly rise again during the past decade after dipping slightly in the 1990s. Most analyses expect this trend to continue in the near term as employer-provided health insurance systems continue to strain under rising health care costs and premiums. The current state and federal budget problems reduce the possibility of further expansions of SCHIP and Medicaid and increase the likelihood of actual cuts in public health and MH/SA insurance coverage.

A number of at-risk populations are especially vulnerable to the high costs of medical care, including MH/SA services, because they lack health insurance coverage. About 20% of Blacks and one third of Hispanics are uninsured (AHRQ, 2006b). Lack of insurance is a major contributing factor (but by no means the only factor) to the well-known racial and ethnic disparities in health and health care in the United States (Lillie-Blanton & Hoffman, 2005; Kirby, Taliaferro, & Zuvekas, 2006; AHRQ, 2007). Disparities in MH/SA services are especially large (AHRQ, 2007; McGuire & Miranda, 2007; McGuire, Alegria, Cook, Wells, & Zaslavsky, 2006). Blacks and Hispanics are much more likely to have public coverage than other Americans and much less likely to have private coverage. The principal reason for this lower rate of private coverage is that Blacks and, especially, Hispanics are more likely to work for employers that do not offer health insurance coverage.

Less well-known are the low rates of health insurance coverage among young adults, which have especially important implications for mental disorders.

Thirty-five percent of those aged 19–24 are uninsured, but even 27% of 30- to 34-year-olds lack health insurance (AHRQ, 2006b). The vast majority of uninsured young adults are healthy. Yet they are also vulnerable as they transition from their parents' homes to school (for some) and into the workforce (for others). The onset of many mental disorders, such as schizophrenia and bipolar disorder, tends to occur at precisely this time. Without health insurance coverage, they may not get the early services they need. And while many employers cover dependents up to age 22 (or in rarer cases 25) as long as they are in school, if the student is forced to drop out because of mental health issues, they may lose that coverage.

Insurance, Managed Care, and Financing: Principles and Evidence

Principles of Insurance: Moral Hazard

The main function of insurance is to protect people from financial risk when a catastrophic event occurs. In this sense, health insurance is much like automobile, homeowners, or life insurance. Instead of paying a fixed amount to a family if a family member dies under a life insurance policy or paying to rebuild their house, health insurance helps pay medical bills when they are sick. When private health insurance plans first began in the 1940s and 1950s, they principally covered inpatient hospital stays. But as other medical services became increasingly important and expensive, insurance coverage has expanded substantially to cover physician expenses and, more recently, prescription drug expenses.

Health insurance contracts tend to be more open-ended than other types of insurance contracts because it is difficult to predict beforehand which of the many different types of illnesses you might get and how much health care you might need. That is, health insurance contracts are rarely written in such a way that if a person gets, say, leukemia, he or she will be paid a fixed $100,000, or if they get pneumonia, they will be paid $20,000. The open-ended nature of health insurance coverage leads to a situation that economists call **moral hazard,** where people overconsume health care. With health insurance coverage, out-of-pocket costs are generally much less than the true cost of providing health care. At some point, the benefits of additional health care services (for example, extra tests) in terms of improving one's health are not really worth their full costs, but because the insured only pay a fraction of the costs, he or she still want to use the services.

Consumer cost-sharing evolved in response to this fundamental problem of moral hazard. By shifting at least some of the costs of health care to consumers, they become more sensitive to the true costs of health care. Current health care reform discussions often refer to this idea as consumers having "skin in the game." Traditionally, health insurance plans, such as Blue Cross/Blue Shield plans, imposed a **deductible**, where the health insurance plan only paid for services after consumers had paid a certain amount out of their own pockets (typically, $250 or $500). Health plans also traditionally imposed cost-sharing in the form of **co-insurance**, where the consumer paid, for example, 20% of the cost of services (after the deductible had been met) and the plan 80%. As health insurance plans have evolved, fixed **co-payments** for particular services, for example, $20 for an office visit or $15 for a prescription drug, have become common. While consumer cost-sharing can reduce excess use of health care services, it can also reduce appropriate use of health care services. Thus, there is always a trade-off between the benefits of more generous insurance coverage and moral hazard. The goal with cost-sharing is to strike a balance in this trade-off (Zeckhauser, 1970; Besley, 1988).

The best-known evidence regarding moral hazard in health insurance coverage comes from the RAND Health Insurance Experiment (HIE), a large-scale, randomized control trial conducted from 1977 to 1982. This landmark study found that consumers' use of mental health services was twice as responsive to price as other medical services (Keeler, Manning, & Wells, 1988). Other studies during the 1970s and 1980s came to similar conclusions, but were based upon observational data and not randomized trials (Frank & McGuire, 1986). The RAND HIE results became the main justification for providing less generous coverage for mental health services on economic efficiency grounds. However, many question whether these results still hold today. The RAND HIE specifically measured consumer responsiveness to outpatient psychotherapy, which was common in the 1970s. This is far from the standard of evidence-based services today, and there is no theoretical reason to expect that consumers respond in the same way now. In fact, there are good reasons to expect that consumers are less likely to be sensitive to price if they have greater expectations that services will actually work. While the RAND HIE has not been repeated recently and will not be repeated anytime soon because of the enormous expense of running such a trial, several lines of evidence suggest that indeed consumers are no longer very sensitive to the price of outpatient mental health services (Meyerhoefer & Zuvekas, 2010).

A further problem is that the RAND HIE itself cannot justify less generous coverage for inpatient mental health services. Again, the finding of increased consumer responsiveness applied strictly to outpatient psychotherapy, so there is no basis for making this leap to inpatient services. Similarly, while greater consumer responsiveness may justify higher deductibles and cost-sharing for outpatient visits, the same efficiency argument cannot be made for capping the number of visits a consumer can receive, which is a common practice still in place today. The more likely explanation for this pattern of differential coverage of MH/SA services is adverse selection.

PRINCIPLES OF INSURANCE: ADVERSE AND FAVORABLE RISK SELECTION

Economists refer to moral hazard as a type of market failure because it leads to less than 100% insurance coverage. **Risk selection** can lead to even more severe forms of market failure. Consumers with greater anticipated health needs are naturally more motivated to seek insurance coverage to cover the costs of services, and the more generous the coverage the better. This will drive up costs in plans that attract sicker-than-average patients (**adverse selection**). Insurers can respond by raising premiums, restricting coverage so as not to attract higher risk consumers, and/or using other means to discourage higher risk consumers. If insurers raise premiums, this can lead to a situation where the healthier consumers drop coverage (because it is no longer as good a deal). This causes premiums to go still higher, in turn, causing the next-healthiest consumers to drop coverage, and so on (Rothschild & Stiglitz, 1976). In the extreme, this can lead to an insurance "death spiral," where the insurance market ceases to exist altogether, something that has been observed in the real world (Cutler & Reber 1998, Cutler & Zeckhauser, 1998).

There are good reasons to believe that adverse selection may be especially acute in the case of MH/SA disorders (Frank & McGuire, 2000; Frank, Glazer, & McGuire, 2000). Consumers with MH/SA disorders have much higher medical costs on average than consumers without MH/SA disorders and are thus unattractive risks from a health plan's perspective. For example, depression frequently co-occurs with diabetes and heart disease. The federal employee health plan program during the 1960s and 1970s provides the classic illustration of adverse selection (Frank & McGuire, 2000; Padgett, Patrick, Burns, Schlesinger, & Cohen, 1993). Federal employees have long had the choice of a number of health plans. Several of the plans in the federal program began offering generous mental health coverage, while others did not. Not surprisingly, consumers with MH/SA disorders migrated to the more generous plans, which raised costs. In response, the generous plans cut their MH/SA coverage so that coverage was low in all the plans by the late 1970s. MH/SA coverage remained low in the federal health plans until 2001, when an executive order mandating parity coverage in all plans went into effect (Goldman et al., 2006).

Regulatory actions such as parity mandates are one potential solution to adverse selection. **Risk adjustment**, where payments vary according to the risk the plan faces in their population, is another standard approach to mitigating adverse selection. Risk adjustment is used, for example, in the payments made to Medicare and Medicaid managed care plans. Much work has gone into devising better risk-adjustment methodologies over the last few decades, but they remain imperfect: predicting future medical expenditures is inherently difficult. With imperfect adjustments for risks, insurance plans have strong incentives to seek out better risks (often referred to as "cream-skimming" or "cherry picking") and avoid sicker patients.

Mechanisms to induce pooling of consumers are another potential means for mitigating adverse selection. The dominance of employment-related health insurance arose partly by accident as employers used health insurance coverage as a means to attract and retain high quality workers, much like retirement benefits. But public policy, since World War II, has also deliberately encouraged this development. Employer groups are seen as a convenient way to pool consumers that is independent of their health status. The value of health insurance benefits is not taxed, creating incentives for employers to provide, and employees to receive, compensation in the form of health insurance benefits, rather than higher wages, which are taxable. Some argue that this tax subsidy encourages too much insurance and overconsumption of medical care due to moral hazard, and many current reform proposals would eliminate the tax subsidy altogether or tax so-called Cadillac plans above a certain threshold (for example, $25,000). Others argue that it is the glue that keeps the employment-related insurance system together and that the system might fall apart altogether due to adverse selection as the healthier workers opt out without the subsidy (Bernard & Selden, 2002; Monheit & Selden, 2000).

PRINCIPLES OF INSURANCE: SOCIAL INSURANCE

The Medicare and Medicaid programs that finance much of MH/SA services and the SSDI and SSI programs that provide many with severe and persistent mental illness with income support are examples of social insurance programs. Social insurance programs serve two primary purposes: 1) they are a means of overcoming market failure in private markets, and 2) they serve a redistributive function in providing safety-net resources to vulnerable populations. The Medicare program, enacted in 1965, serves both functions. Medicare Part A, which covers hospital services, was made compulsory explicitly to overcome adverse selection problems and is funded out of general revenue. Nearly all people 65 and older are covered by Part A. Medicare, after a two-year waiting period, also covers those under the age of 65 who have qualified for the SSDI program (those with a disability who paid into the Social Security system for 40 or more quarters). The Medicare Part B program, which covers office-based and other services, while not compulsory, is funded 25% out of Medicare beneficiaries' own pockets and 75% out of general revenues. The premiums for the optional Medicare Part D drug benefit are similarly heavily subsidized, encouraging high rates of participation, as well. The large subsidy has also been effective in overcoming adverse selection: 90% of Medicare beneficiaries eligible for Part D prescription drug coverage have some form of coverage (CMS, 2008a).

The Medicaid program, unlike Medicare, was not designed to provide broad-based coverage for the population, but to be an insurer of last resort for vulnerable populations. It provides coverage to low-income children and their parents (many with Temporary Assistance to Needy Families), low-income pregnant women, low-income elderly, and people with disabilities. Eligibility varies widely by state. Medicaid is an especially important source of coverage for people with mental disorders who qualify for SSI income support (many of whom do not have enough quarters of work to qualify for SSDI and thus, Medicare). It also plays an important role in filling in gaps for Medicare, which requires significant cost-sharing and does not cover many MH/SA services. Concerns regarding the potential loss of Medicaid and Medicare coverage create strong disincentives for people with disabilities to seek work and incentives to stay on social insurance programs and have led to a number of initiatives, such as the Ticket to Work program. (U.S. Department of Labor, 2007)

PRINCIPLES OF INSURANCE: MANAGED CARE

Managed care is now ubiquitous in health care, no more so than in MH/SA treatment. But it also takes many different forms and is hard to categorize, especially with the extensive hybridization of forms in recent years. Managed care evolved as another way to control the use of health care services and restrain health care cost increases, which continued to rise rapidly in spite of the widespread use of consumer cost-sharing in health insurance plans. Traditional staff/group model Health Maintenance Organizations (HMOs), such as Kaiser Permanente of Northern California and Group Health of Puget Sound, pioneered many of the basic managed care techniques. These Staff/Group model HMOs offered substantially reduced consumer cost-sharing compared to traditional fee-for-service (FFS) plans in return for 1) restrictive provider networks, with providers either salaried directly by the HMO or members of large groups contracted principally with the HMO; 2) physician gatekeeping, that is, requiring a referral from the patient's primary care provider to see specialists; 3) extensive utilization controls, such as prior authorization for services such as inpatient hospitals stays, physical therapy, and MH/SA services; and 4) drug formularies, where HMOs frequently offered market exclusivity to manufacturers in return for price breaks on specific drugs.

Traditional indemnity insurance has all but disappeared in private health insurance markets, supplanted by HMO plans, Preferred Provider Organization (PPO) plans, and hybrid plans. PPOs consist of networks of providers who provide services to plan members at a discounted price negotiated with the PPO. Consumer cost-sharing is much lower for network ("preferred") providers, but consumers have a choice of whether to use in-network providers or pay more for out-of-network providers. In contrast, in a closed HMO, consumers must use HMO providers (the HMO may either hire the provider directly as in a staff/group model HMO or contract with individual and groups of providers). PPOs also differ from closed HMOs in that they generally do not require referrals to access physician specialists. Some insurers offer both HMO and PPO products using the exact same network of providers, differing mainly in the use of physician gatekeeping and the ability to use out-of-network providers. Point of Service (POS) plans contain elements of both HMO and PPO plans. For example, an "open-ended" HMO plan might allow consumers to see out-of-network providers (with higher cost-sharing) but still require referrals for specialists (gatekeeping).

HMOs enjoyed rapid growth into the late 1990s, doubling from 39.0 million enrollees in 1992 to a peak of 80.5 million in 1999 (Interstudy, 2002; 2003). However, HMO enrollment has since declined to 74 million in 2002 (Interstudy, 2003) and 71 million in 2006 (Interstudy, 2007), as a managed care "backlash" took place against this most restrictive form of managed care organization (MCO). PPOs and hybrid plans grew rapidly at the expense of both HMOs and traditional FFS plans in the 1990s and into the 21st century.

In contrast to private health insurance, Medicare remains largely a traditional fee-for-service program. Managed care plans were first introduced in the Medicare program in 1990. Enrollment in what are now called Medicare Advantage plans has grown unevenly over time, but accelerated recently with the introduction of new options reaching 20% of the Medicare population in 2007 (CMS, 2008a). State Medicaid programs continue to shift Medicaid recipients into managed care plans. In 1997, almost half (48%) of Medicaid recipients were enrolled in managed care plans, mostly in HMOs. By 2006, this had grown to almost two-thirds (65%) of all Medicaid recipients (CMS, 2006).

There are several competing theories about how managed care plans might allocate resources within a closed system in the absence of a formal market where consumers make the health care purchasing decisions (Frank, Glazer, & McGuire 2000; Glazer & McGuire, 2002; Baumgardner, 1991, Ramsey & Pauly, 1997). But without good measures of patient outcomes and health status, it is not clear the extent to which managed care plans are more efficient and the extent to which they are simply reducing care or engaging in favorable selection. In practice, much of the cost savings from managed care appears to come from reducing both the length and number of inpatient hospitalizations through utilization controls such as prior authorization and concurrent utilization review. The management of outpatient medical services is relatively much more costly, as the volume of services is much greater than inpatient services, but the cost per service is much lower. Inpatient controls proved easy to reproduce, and HMOs quickly lost much of their natural cost advantage as the controls came to be adopted by almost all health plans (the single biggest exception being the traditional Medicare program). Drug formularies followed a similar trajectory. PPOs came to dominate the private insurance market by adopting the lowest hanging fruit of the HMOs in terms of inpatient (and to a somewhat lesser extent drug-costs) controls, but offering greater choice than HMOs. HMOs in turn, have relaxed utilization controls on ambulatory services to some degree. However, in recent years, all types of plans have been forced to look back at consumer cost-sharing as a tool to reduce health care cost increases.

Principles of Reimbursement

Private health plans, public insurance programs, and state and local mental health authorities all face difficult decisions in choosing how to organize and pay for health care services provided to clients. A wide variety of reimbursement mechanisms has evolved over time. Each creates its own set of incentives, good and bad.

Closed systems, such as the Department of Veterans Affairs (VA), state and local psychiatric institutions, and the original staff/group HMOs typically own their own hospitals and clinics. They also typically hire providers directly, paying them a salary, or use other similar contractual methods to provide care. In principle, monitoring of provider behavior and patient outcomes is easier in a closed system, and providers can be made to follow the dictates of the organization if their salary depends on it (either explicitly or implicitly). The VA system, for example, was able to implement a wide-scale quality improvement effort based around health information technology (Health IT) simply by administrative order. After decades of complaints about inattention and poor quality, the VA system is now held up as a model of Health IT implementation, but progress has been much slower in the rest of the (fragmented) health care systems. Success depends upon the strength of internal monitoring systems and organizational dynamics. In the public sector, political considerations also have an impact. For example, it proved politically difficult to reduce unneeded beds and close public institutions altogether as deinstitutionalization progressed, in part because these institutions were often the dominant employer in the rural areas where they were located. As a result, public resources were slow to follow clients from inpatient facilities into the community. The VA system faces similar political obstacles in shifting resources around the country.

Closed systems have other problems. The large investments needed to build, maintain, and staff closed systems, even in the private sector, reduce flexibility to shift resources as circumstances change. Many consumers also dislike the restricted choice of providers in closed systems. Finally, it is not clear how resource allocation decisions should be made.

The many variants of cost-based and fee-for-service reimbursement are administratively simple alternatives to directly hiring providers. Cost-based reimbursement, where providers submit their actual costs, was once common for hospital services, but is now the exception. Medicare, for example, paid hospitals on a strictly retrospective cost-basis until 1982 (Hodgkin & McGuire, 1994). Under a fee-for-service system, providers receive a fixed amount for each service performed. This fee is administratively set in the traditional Medicare and Medicaid programs (although providers can indirectly influence fee-setting through the political process). In private plans, the fees are usually set in negotiation with providers. However, a significant percentage of MH/SA providers, especially in large metropolitan areas, have opted out of insurance-based reimbursement, focusing on clients who pay up front out of their own pockets (with some patients filing claims with health plans, and some declining to do so) at rates set by the providers (Wilk, West, Narrow, Rae, & Regier, 2005; O'Malley & Reschovsky, 2006; Mitchell & Cromwell, 1982). Other providers opt out of specific plans, most commonly Medicaid plans, because of low reimbursement rates. Low reimbursement rates were originally built into the Medicaid program on the theory that Medicaid should only cover the variable costs of a practice (mostly, the provider's time) with other sources picking up the fixed, capital costs of the practice. In practice, budget pressures and political considerations that have constrained the growth of Medicaid programs have also affected reimbursement rates. As a result, many providers do not take Medicaid patients at all (or Medicaid assignment) or restrict their numbers of new patients, often complaining that the rates do not even cover their variable costs (Zuckerman, McFeeters, Cunningham, & Nichols, 2004; Mitchell, 1991; Cunningham & May, 2006). The declining number of providers willing to treat patients with Medicaid raises concerns that access to care for individuals with low incomes and disabilities has diminished (Cohen & Cunningham, 1995; Cunningham & Hadley, 2008; Cunningham & May, 2006). Low reimbursement rates have also led to significant market segmentation, where some providers (some argue lower quality providers) specialize in Medicaid patients and others in more lucrative private insurance and self-pay patients (Cunningham & May, 2006; Fosett & Peterson, 1989).

Cost-based and fee-for-service reimbursement also create incentives to overprovide services, as providers earn more revenue the more services they perform as long as the actual reimbursement amount covers their costs. For example, there is substantial evidence that paying hospitals fixed per diem rates creates incentives for longer lengths of stay (Hodgkin & McGuire, 1994). Actual costs tend to be front-loaded, so patients become increasingly profitable the longer they stay. Perversely, cost-based and fee-for-service reimbursement can even create incentives for poor quality care, since there are no real consequences for bad outcomes and providers can earn still more revenue correcting their mistakes. Fee-for-service systems have the additional disadvantage of distorting treatment decisions, as some types of services are more profitable than others. For example, primary care providers are rarely reimbursed separately for screening for depression and MH/SA disorders, while they are routinely reimbursed for laboratory tests, a significant barrier to wide-scale MH/SA screening.

Capitation and other prospective payment systems were developed in response to the poor incentives created under fee-for-service or cost-based reimbursement systems. The basic idea is to shift some or all of the financial risk of additional services to providers, creating incentives to be as efficient as possible in providing services. Capitation to health plans and capitation to providers are commonly confused. Under provider capitation, providers receive a fixed amount per month (or quarter or year) for each patient in that provider's panel (or at least those covered by the plan), regardless of the amount of services they use or whether a particular patient uses services at all. Under plan capitation, the health plan receives a fixed amount for each patient to cover all the health care services for all the providers in the plan, essentially an insurance premium. Plan capitation is far more common than provider capitation. Even in capitated managed care plans, including carve-outs to MBHOs, the predominant form of reimbursement to providers is fee-for-service or salary (Zuvekas & Cohen, 2005; Strunk & Reschovsky, 2002). This is primarily due to the administrative complexity of determining capitation formulas and unwillingness of providers, especially in small or solo practices, to assume risk.

Medicare's Prospective Payment System, where hospitals receive a fixed payment for all patients within a Diagnosis Related Group (DRG) regardless of the services they use (with provisions for outliers), works in similar fashion to capitation. Lengths of inpatient hospital stays fell dramatically after Medicare switched to this system in 1983. Many state Medicaid programs and even private health insurance plans have adopted similar prospective payment systems.

While there is some evidence that capitation and prospective payment increase efficiency of care, they also create incentives to under-provide care (in contrast to the over-provision of care in fee-for-service systems). This is especially true where outcomes are difficult to monitor. Capitation and prospective payment reimbursement also create strong incentives for the same types of risk selection behavior (cream-skimming or cherry picking) evident in health insurance markets. Healthier patients will obviously be much more profitable than sicker patients. As a result, the same types of risk-adjustment methods are also commonly applied to capitated and prospective payment systems, again imperfectly.

There is increasing recognition that both fee-for-service and capitation are imperfect reimbursement methods if they are not linked explicitly to outcomes and/or quality. The term "pay-for-performance" has become ubiquitous in recent years to describe various attempts to create better incentives in payment systems. Results to date are mixed, but public and private payers continue to experiment with and develop these programs (Rosenthal, Landon, Normand et al., 2007; Rosenthal, Landon, Howitt et al., 2007b, Rosenthal, Frank, Li, & Epstein, 2005).

Implications for Mental Health

Closer integration with the constantly changing and evolving insurance-based and -financed systems of health care in the United States has profound implications for the way behavioral health care services are financed, organized, and delivered. In this section, we consider key current and future challenges for behavioral health arising from this integration in financing. We begin with recent efforts to mandate parity in coverage for specialty behavioral health care services in health insurance plans, and consider whether mandates can achieve true parity. We next consider the now widespread phenomenon of "carving-out" behavioral health services to specialized managed care firms by private health plans and Medicaid programs. Rapidly rising costs have similarly led insurers to seek new ways to manage prescription drug benefits. We discuss the implications of this management on access to psychopharmacological treatments in private health plans, Medicaid, and the new Medicare Part D prescription drug benefit. Rising costs for all health care services have put enormous strains on the employer-based private health insurance system. We discuss the implications of rising numbers of uninsured Americans and the implications of market-based reform efforts for the private insurance system that covers the majority of mental health service consumers. States as well must grapple with rising costs, while at the same time facing the additional pressures of diminished budgetary revenue and greater demand for Medicaid and public mental health systems during tough economic times. We consider the special challenges faced by community-based mental health service providers, who must mix a variety of sources of financing to provide services. Finally, we conclude with a discussion of the implications of the integration in financing for consumers of MH/SA treatment.

COVERAGE FOR SPECIALTY MH/SA SERVICES: PARITY AND BEYOND

Coverage for MH/SA services continues to lag behind coverage for other physical health services in private health insurance plans (Zuvekas & Meyerhoefer, 2006; Barry et al., 2003). Since the 1990s, advocates have pushed hard to improve coverage for mental health and substance abuse services, with the ultimate goal of achieving parity in coverage with physical health services. Proponents of parity advanced two main arguments. First, it is discriminatory to provide less generous coverage to those with MH/SA disorders, even if there might be economic efficiency arguments for doing so, because of the potential for moral hazard, the RAND HIE study found. Second, parity was affordable in the context of managed care, as a number of case studies by researchers strongly supported (Goldman et al., 2006; National Advisory Mental Health Council [NAMHC], 2000, 1998). The economists' argument for mitigating the effects of adverse selection through government parity mandates were used less often.

Mental health advocates successfully pushed almost every state to enact at least some legislation designed to strengthen mental health coverage in private health plans. Most of this state legislation fell well short of full parity. Even in states with fairly strong parity laws, parity failed to cover most people (Buchmueller, Cooper, Jacobsen, & Zuvekas, 2007). Under the provisions of the 1974 Employment Retirement and Security Act (ERISA), as interpreted by the courts, firms that self-insure are exempt from state health insurance regulations including parity mandates. Consequently, strong parity laws cover only 20% of working Americans with health coverage (Buchmueller et al., 2007). In addition, most of these strong laws cover only severe or "biologically based" disorders and typically do not apply to drug and alcohol services.

Parity in private plans remained an elusive goal until the end of 2008. The 1996 Federal Mental Health Parity Act, which eliminated dollar limits on coverage in private plans, was largely a symbolic victory. Insurers and employers simply rewrote policies to replace the dollar limits with limits on the number of days in the hospital or office visits. Recognizing the limits of a state-based strategy, advocates continued to push year after year for stronger legislation at the federal level. The affordability issue was largely settled in the scientific literature (Goldman et al., 2006), and the Congressional Budget Office's revised estimates suggested that full parity would increase overall health care costs by 1% or less (Bowman, Hagen, & Ahlstrom 2002). After many attempts, the "Paul Wellstone–Pete Domenici Mental Health Parity and Addiction Equity Act of 2008" was enacted as part of the Emergency Economic Stabilization Act (H.R. 1424, Sec. 512) in October 2008. This federal parity mandate eliminates differential co-payments and co-insurance, deductibles, and limits on number of visits and days for MH/SA treatment for firms that offer MH/SA coverage beginning in 2010–11. However, small employers with 50 or fewer employees are exempt, as are plans purchased in the individual market, and there is no requirement that firms must offer mental health coverage.

The push to achieve parity in the Medicare program similarly stalled for years. Currently all outpatient mental health services, except visits for medication management, are subject to 50% consumer cost-sharing. This higher cost-sharing is due to concerns that, under the traditional fee-for-service Medicare program that covers most enrollees, there would be no managed care mechanism to restrain cost-increases. However, in July 2008, Congress overrode a presidential veto and enacted legislation (HR 6331) that gradually reduces the cost-sharing requirement to 20% between 2010 and 2014.

State Medicaid programs cover MH/SA services provided by psychiatrists and psychiatric institutes with little or no cost-sharing by Medicaid recipients. However, not all states will reimburse psychologists, social workers, or other types of specialty mental health providers. This may limit access to non-medication forms of treatment. As discussed above, many psychiatrists, and many physicians in general, do not accept Medicaid because of its low reimbursement rates, creating the potential for additional access problems.

Parity does not seem to cost insurers much, but what does it mean for consumers? The available evidence suggests that parity does indeed reduce the out-of-pocket burden of MH/SA services, albeit modestly (Goldman et al., 2006). Parity's effects on access to MH/SA services are less certain (Barry & Busch, 2008; Busch et al., 2006; Pacula & Sturm, 2000). In theory, parity should increase access with reduced cost-sharing holding all else equal. But all else is not equal. Parity creates incentives to tighten the management of specialty MH/SA services to offset cost increases, the very reason it is "affordable" (NAMHC, 2000; 1998; Ridgely, Burnam, Barry, Goldman, & Hennessy, 2006). Parity may exist in the *nominal* benefits stated in policy booklets, but it is difficult to regulate the *effective* benefits that consumers actually receive in a managed care environment.

MANAGED BEHAVIORAL HEALTH CARE

The much-talked-about managed care backlash of the last decade largely bypassed MH/SA services. In part, this is because the backlash largely bypassed state

Medicaid programs, which serve many MH/SA clients and continue to expand their use of HMO and similar managed care plans. The managed behavioral health organizations (MBHOs), with which many Medicaid managed care plans and most private health plans contract, also show no signs of declining. Their growth, however, naturally reached a plateau as they came to dominate the market for specialty MH/SA services in the last decade.

MBHOs spread rapidly during the 1980s and 1990s by successfully adapting many of the techniques originally pioneered by HMOs to the management of specialty MH/SA services. MBHOs developed their own networks of MH/SA specialists, usually reimbursed on a fee-for-service basis, extensive prior authorization and utilization review systems, and employee assistance plans (EAP). Products marketed to both employers (direct carve-out) and health plans (indirect carve-out) range from EAP plans to stand-alone utilization management products to comprehensive packages providing all specialty MH/SA services (network plus utilization management). Industry sources show total enrollment in MBHO products increasing from 86 million in 1992 to an astounding 227 million in 2002 (Open Minds, 2002). These industry numbers somewhat overstate the actual reach of MBHOs because they include those enrolled in EAP programs only (76 million in 2002). In 2002, approximately 43 million were enrolled in stand-alone utilization management products, 59 million were enrolled in risk-based comprehensive plans (where the MBHO is capitated or otherwise at risk), 45 million were enrolled in non-risk-based plans (the MBHO assumes no risk), and 17 million were enrolled in integrated EAP/comprehensive plans. The MBHO industry has become highly concentrated, with the top three firms (all for-profit) having more than 50% of the share of the market.

MBHOs achieved impressive cost savings early on due primarily to dramatically reduced lengths of stays for inpatient hospitalizations (NAMHC, 2000, 1998; Ma & McGuire, 1998; Sturm, 1997). This success led more and more plans and employers to contract with MBHOs. As seen in Figure 2.2, annual growth rates for MH/SA expenditures nose-dived during the mid-1990s at the same time that MBHOs spread rapidly. However, annual growth rates have increased once again as the low-hanging fruit of long inpatient hospital stays were squeezed out early on. MBHOs also achieved cost-savings partly through negotiated discounts from network providers, and partly through what are termed "network" effects: the fear that providers will be discontinued from the network if they provide too many services to patients (Ma & McGuire, 2002).

MBHOs' effects on access and quality of MH/SA services remain ambiguous. On balance, reducing lengthy inpatient stays and shifting resources to outpatient settings has likely been beneficial to patients. There is also evidence that MBHOs accelerated the diffusion of evidence-based practices (Ling, Berndt, & Frank, 2008; see Chapter 21 in this volume for more on this). But there are also concerns that MBHOs restrict access to specialty services, so that patients must seek treatment in primary care settings. MBHOs are also rarely at risk for the costs of psychotropic medications (management of prescription medications are generally contracted to yet another third party, see below). This creates incentives for psychotropic medication interventions, at the possible expense of evidence-based behavioral therapies (the cost for which they would be responsible). Evidence of cost-shifting either to

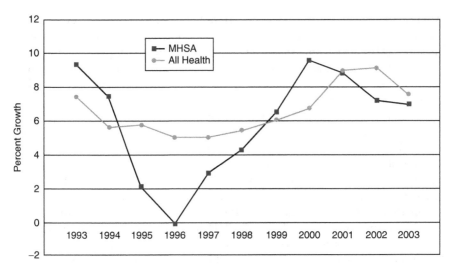

Figure 2.2 Growth of MH/SA Expenditures and All Health Expenditures, 1993–2003. (*Source*: Mark, Levit, McKusick, Harwood, Bouchery et al. (2007).)

primary care settings or to prescription drugs, however, is mixed (Zuvekas Rupp, & Norquist, 2007; Norton, Lindrooth, & Dickey, 1997; Dickey et al., 2001).

Prescription Drug Financing

Once a somewhat peripheral concern, prescription drug financing is now central to MH/SA treatment. Similar to specialty MH/SA services, management of prescription drugs in the private plans, including plans that serve Medicare and Medicaid populations, is now largely contracted out to third-party administrators called Pharmacy Benefit Managers (PBMs). Also similar to MBHOs, PBMs contract directly with employers who have carved out their prescription benefits from the rest of their health coverage. In contrast to specialty MH/SA services, psychotropic medications are generally not separated out from other medications. That is, parity by and large already exists for psychotropic medications, but important issues remain.

PBMs apply many of the basic tools of managed care to prescription medications. They develop and maintain networks of pharmacies with which they negotiate prices. They negotiate discounts and rebates from pharmaceutical manufacturers and wholesalers. Much like MBHOs, the PBM industry is highly concentrated, so PBMs are able to leverage their volume purchasing power with both pharmacies and manufacturers. Leverage with manufacturers is further increased through the use of drug *formularies*, essentially lists of approved drugs. Multi-tiered formularies are the norm and, in private plans, are closely tied to consumer cost-sharing. In a standard three-tier plan, the first tier includes inexpensive generic medications with low co-payment levels to encourage their use. The second tier includes a preferred medication(s) in a therapeutic class, with somewhat higher cost-sharing. The third tier includes non-preferred medications in a therapeutic class, with the highest cost-sharing. Not all medications in a therapeutic class will necessarily appear in a formulary; formularies vary widely in their restrictiveness. Some particularly expensive medications, such as cancer drugs and atypical antipsychotics, may be listed but require prior authorization before use. PBMs, managed care plans that manage their own pharmacy benefits and Medicaid programs use the leverage of tiers or preferred status of drugs in return for discounts and rebates from manufacturers. The treatment of psychotropic medications in drug formularies is an area of great controversy. Patients respond differently to the range of medications within therapeutic classes such as antidepressants and atypical antipsychotics. A restrictive formulary can thus create barriers to treatment for patients who do not respond to preferred drugs.

Consumer cost-sharing can also create barriers to treatment. Higher cost-sharing can lead to reduced use of medications (Hodgkin, Thomas, Simoni-Wastila, Ritter, & Lee, 2008; Wang et al., 2008; Landsman, Yu, Liu, Teutsch, & Berger, 2005; Huskamp et al., 2005; Goldman et al., 2004). In recognition of this potential problem, some employers and health plans have recently experimented with lower cost-sharing or eliminating it altogether for maintenance medications used to treat chronic conditions.

MEDICAID

State Medicaid plans have struggled in recent years with exploding drug costs. Medicaid programs also develop and maintain formularies and negotiate directly with manufacturers, achieving estimated average rebates for all medications of about 20% of the purchase price (Tepper & Lied, 2004). Forty-one states have responded by imposing nominal co-payments (Kaiser Family Foundation, 2006). About half of the states also limit the number of prescription fills covered each month or year (Kaiser Family Foundation, 2006). MH/SA service clients tend to have a lot of prescription drugs fills, not only for their MH/SA needs but the chronic conditions that often co-occur. The cumulative effect of these nominal co-payments can still be burdensome for these low-income populations and limits on fills can shift a significant amount of burden to Medicaid recipients, deterring use (Miller, Banthin, & Selden, 2008). States have also focused in particular on the management of atypical antipsychotics, the cost of which more than quintupled between 1995 and 2005 to $5.5 billion (Law, Ross-Degnan, & Soumerai, 2008). At least ten states (Law et al., 2008) have imposed prior authorization requirements for non-preferred antipsychotics, but there is evidence that these requirements are associated with increased treatment discontinuities (Soumerai et al., 2008).

MEDICARE PART D

The Medicare Part D prescription drug benefit went into effect in 2006 and was the most important expansion of public health insurance programs since the original passage of the Medicare and Medicaid programs in the mid-1960s. The Part D program also has profound implications for the MH/SA services. Part D is an optional benefit, but the premium is heavily subsidized (75%) by the federal government, and most eligible Medicare beneficiaries are enrolled in the program. Under the Part D program, consumers enroll with privately run Prescription Drug Plans (PDPs), who often then contract with PBMs for the actual administration of the plan. The Part D program set a standard benefit structure, but PDPs are free to develop any cost-sharing structure that is actuarially equivalent. The Medicare Modernization Act, which created the Part D benefit, also contains substantial subsidies to private employers to maintain prescription drug coverage for retirees, so that the Part D program did not "crowd-out" private coverage. Ninety percent of the Medicare population is now covered by at least some form of prescription drug coverage (CMS, 2008a). Early evidence shows that the program reduced out-of-pocket costs and modestly increased utilization as a result (Lichtenberg & Sun, 2007; Chen et al., 2008; Yin et al., 2008).

In implementing the Part D program, the federal government was required to develop formulary guidelines for use by all PDPs. Originally, only selected antipsychotics and antidepressants were to be included, but the final formulary guidelines required PDPs to cover "all or substantially all" medications in these classes. However, plans can still differentiate among medications in these classes by preferred and non-preferred status (with differential cost-sharing), and many plans exclude certain medications. PDPs can also require prior authorization for these medications. Benzodiazepines and barbiturates used to treat bipolar, anxiety, and other disorders are currently excluded, but legislation passed in 2008 (HR 6331) removes this restriction beginning in 2013 (Huskamp et al., 2007).

The Medicare Part D program also has significant implications for Medicare beneficiaries with Medicaid coverage. These *dually eligible* beneficiaries were required to enroll in Medicare Part D plans (with cost-sharing requirements waived) rather than have their prescription drugs paid for by Medicaid. There is evidence that this led to both medication switching (with uncertain impact on outcomes) and treatment discontinuities because of the more restrictive preferred medication lists and prior authorization requirements in some plans (West et al., 2007). The switch also has the potential to affect state Medicaid programs' ability to bargain with pharmaceutical manufacturers over prices for the remaining Medicaid population. Prior to 2006, state Medicaid programs accounted for up to 75% of the atypical antipsychotic market (Duggan, 2005). There is also evidence that the PDPs paid higher prices than the state Medicaid programs, increasing the net cost to taxpayers of providing medications to the dual eligibles (U.S. House of Representatives, 2008).

Implications of Rising Costs in Private Health Insurance Markets and Reform Efforts

Rising health care costs and premiums continue to threaten the employment-based private health insurance system that provides health insurance coverage to most Americans under the age of 65. Medicaid and SCHIP have picked up some of the slack, but the ranks of the uninsured have grown in the last few years. Many predict the employer-based insurance system will continue to slowly erode, increasing the pressure on state Medicaid budgets and public mental health systems.

Market-based reform efforts to shore up the private health insurance system also have implications for the coverage of MH/SA services. The 1993 Medicare Modernization Act contained provisions to encourage the creation of **Health Savings Accounts (HSAs)**. HSAs allow individuals to pay for health care services and save for future health expenses tax-free. However, these accounts can only be used by consumers who purchase High Deductible Health Plans (for individuals, a deductible of at least $1,000 and families $2,000). This requirement means that individuals and families pay more for health care including MH/SA services directly out of their own pockets. Legislation has also encouraged employers to offer similar types of savings accounts in combination with high-deductible health plan coverage. Not all of these high-deductible plans provide MH/SA benefits (Wildsmith, 2005). High-deductible plans have so far grown slowly, but could accelerate as cost pressures increase on employers. Other proposed market-based reforms would supplant the employment-based system altogether with vouchers for the purchase of individual health insurance plans.

The coverage of MH/SA services is an unsettled issue in these proposals, some of which would focus on "basic benefits." Adverse selection could also threaten MH/SA coverage in an individual-based private health insurance market.

BUDGETARY CHALLENGES FOR STATE MEDICAID PROGRAMS AND STATE MENTAL HEALTH AUTHORITIES

Medicaid continues to consume an ever-growing proportion of federal and state budgets. Policymakers have long looked for ways to constrain this growth, but the pressure is mounting given the large federal deficit and the severe budgetary problems facing most states. States have responded in varying degrees by cutting back eligibility requirements, cutting benefits, increasing cost-sharing, and increasing managed care enrollment. These in turn are likely to place increasing pressure on public mental health systems at a time when resources in those systems are unlikely to grow substantially (if at all).

COMMUNITY-BASED PROVIDERS

Insurance-based financing and the rise of managed care has led to substantial fragmentation in public mental health systems. State and local mental health authorities no longer have direct control over spending for substantial percentages of the severely and persistently mentally ill (SMI) populations they traditionally served (see Chapter 13 in this volume). However, they remain an important source of financing for community-based providers. Community mental health centers and other providers must blend revenue from a variety of sources including Medicaid and state and local authorities to provide comprehensive services to the SMI population. They must also now negotiate with Medicaid managed care plans and MBHOs over whether they will be included in restricted networks and the reimbursement rates they will receive. Community health centers, as primary care providers for low income populations, are increasingly becoming important for the treatment of depression, anxiety, and other disorders, but must similarly negotiate with Medicaid programs and managed care plans. State and local authorities are also increasingly using contractual mechanisms, including capitation, rather than grants for services to their clients.

Conclusion

The share of the nation's resources devoted to MH/SA services, as measured by gross domestic product (GDP), has remained level since the 1970s (Frank & Glied, 2006). This stands in marked contrast with the health care system as a whole, which has grown from 7% to 16% of GDP since 1970 (CMS, 2008b). In one sense, this represents a phenomenal success (Frank & Glied, 2006; Druss, 2006). The continued movement away from hospitals to community settings has allowed millions more Americans to be drawn into the MH/SA service systems, without increasing the share of the country's resources needed to finance these services. However, the shift to insurance-financed treatment systems has also led to a relative shift in resources away from individuals with severe and persistent mental illness toward those with other mental disorders such as anxiety, depression, and attention-deficit/ hyperactivity disorder (ADHD). Treatment has undoubtedly improved for most people with severe and persistent mental illness (SMI), but the increasingly fragmentary nature of financing still creates substantial gaps (Frank & Glied, 2006; Druss, 2006; Mechanic, 2007). Ironically, it is the *integration* with insurance-based systems that has led to *fragmentation* in financing for treatment of people with SMI, as we have seen. Overcoming this fragmentation in SMI treatment is a central goal of current mental health reform efforts as laid out in the President's New Freedom Commission report *Achieving the Promise: Transforming Mental Health Care in America* (2003). Achieving this goal of transformation so that people with SMI do not fall through the cracks of the financing system will be difficult, but important work.

References

Agency for Healthcare Research and Quality. (2006a). Private-sector data by firm size, industry group, ownership, age of firm, and other characteristics [tables from the *2006 Medical Expenditure Panel Survey Insurance Component*]. Available online at http://www.meps.ahrq.gov/mepsweb/data_stats/quick_tables.jsp. Accessed October 28, 2008.

Agency for Healthcare Research and Quality. (2006b). Table 1: Health insurance coverage of the civilian noninstitutionalized population; Percent by type of coverage and selected population characteristics, United States, first half of 2006 [tables from the *2006 Medical Expenditure Panel Survey Household Component*]. Available online at http://www.meps.ahrq.gov/mepsweb/data_stats/quick_tables.jsp. Accessed October 28, 2008.

Agency for Healthcare Research and Quality. (2007). *National Healthcare Quality & Disparities Reports*. Rockville, MD: Author.

Barry, C. L., & Busch, S. H. (2008). Caring for children with mental disorders: Do state parity laws increase access to treatment? *Journal of Mental Health Economics and Policy, 11*, 57–66.

Barry, C. L., Gabel, J. R., Frank, R. G., Hawkins, S., Whitmore, H. H., & Pickreign, J. D. (2003). Design of mental health benefits: Still unequal after all these years. *Health Affairs 22*(5), 27–137.

Baumgardner, J. (1991). The interaction between forms of insurance contract and types of technical change in medical care. *Rand Journal of Economics, 22*(1), 36–51.

Bernard, D., & Selden T. M. (2002). Employer offers, private coverage, and the tax subsidy for health insurance: 1987 and 1996. *International Journal of Health Care Finance and Economics, 2*(4), 297–318.

Berndt, E., Bhattacharjya, A., Mishol, D., Arcelus, A., & Lasky, T. (2002). An analysis of the diffusion of new antidepressants: Variety, quality, and marketing efforts. *Journal of Mental Health Policy and Economics, 5*, 3–19.

Besley, T. J. (1988). Optimal reimbursement health insurance and the theory of Ramsey taxation. *Journal of Health Economics, 4*, 321–336.

Bowman, J., Hagen, S., & Ahlstrom, A. (2002, March 26). *Preliminary Analysis of Selected Mental Health Parity Legislative Options*. Congressional Budget Office Memorandum.

Buchmueller, T. C., Cooper, P. C., Jacobsen, M., & Zuvekas, S. H. (2007). Parity for whom? Exemptions and the extent of state mental health parity legislation. *Health Affairs, 26*(4), w483–w487.

Busch, A. B., Huskamp, H. A., Normand, S.-L. T., Young, A. S., Goldman, H., & Frank, R. G. (2006). The impact of parity on major depression treatment quality in the Federal Employees' Health Benefits Program after parity implementation. *Medical Care, 44*(6), 506–512.

Cafferata, G. L., & Kasper, J. A. (1983). *Psychotropic Drugs: Use, Expenditures, and Sources of Payment. National Health Care Expenditures Study Data Preview 14*. Rockville, MD: U.S. Dept. of Health and Human Services, Public Health Service, National Center for Health Services Research.

Centers for Medicare and Medicaid Services. (2006). *Medicaid Managed Care Enrollment Report Summary Statistics as of June 30, 2006*. Baltimore, MD: Author.

Centers for Medicare and Medicaid Services. (2008a). *Medicare & Medicaid Statistical Supplement*. Baltimore, MD: Author.

Centers for Medicare and Medicaid Services. (2008b). *National Health Expenditures Web Tables*. Baltimore, MD: Author.

Chen, H., Nwangwu, A., Aparasu, R., Essien, E., Sun, S., & Lee, K. (2008). The impact of Medicare Part D on psychotropic utilization and financial burden for community-based seniors. *Psychiatric Services, 59*(10), 1191–1197.

Cohen, J. W., & Cunningham, P. J. (1995). Medicaid physician fee levels and children's access to care. *Health Affairs, 14*(1), 255–262.

Cooper, P. F., & Schone, B. S. (1997). More offers, fewer takers for employment-based health insurance: 1987 and 1996. *Health Affairs, 16*(6), 142–149.

Cooper, P. F., & Vistnes, J. P. (2003). Workers' decisions to take-up offered health insurance coverage: Assessing the importance of out-of-pocket premium costs. *Medical Care, 41*(Suppl. 7), 35–43.

Cunningham, P. J., & Hadley, J. (2008). Effects of changes in incomes and practice circumstances on physicians' decisions to treat charity and Medicaid patients. *Milbank Quarterly, 86*(1), 91–123.

Cunningham, P., & May, J. (2006). *Medicaid Patients Increasingly Concentrated among Physicians*. Tracking Report No. 16, Results from the Community Tracking Survey. Washington, DC: Center for Studying Health Systems Change.

Cunningham, R. (2003). The mental health commission tackles fragmented services: An interview with Michael Hogan. *Health Affairs*, (Suppl.), w3.440–w3.448.

Cutler, D. M., & Reber, S. J. (1998). Paying for health insurance: The tradeoff between competition and adverse selection. *Quarterly Journal of Economics, 113*(2), 433–466.

Cutler, D. M., & Zeckhauser, R. J. (1998). Adverse selection in health insurance. In A. Garber (ed.)., *Frontiers in Health Policy Research* (vol. 1). Cambridge, MA: MIT Press.

Dickey, B., Normand, S.-L., Norton, E. C., et al. (2001). Managed care and children's behavioral health services in Massachusetts. *Psychiatric Services, 52,* 183–188.

Donohue, J., Berndt, E., Rosenthal, M., Epstein, A., & R. Frank. (2004). Effects of pharmaceutical promotion on adherence to the treatment guidelines of depression. *Medical Care, 42,* 1176–1185.

Druss, B. (2006). Rising mental health costs: What are we getting for our money? *Health Affairs, 25*(3), 614–622.

Duggan, M. (2005). Do new prescription drugs pay for themselves? The case of second-generation antipsychotics. *Journal of Health Economics, 24*(1), 1–31.

Fosett, J. W., & J. A. Peterson. (1989). Physician supply and Medicaid participation: The causes of market failure. *Medical Care, 27*(4), 386–396.

Frank, R. G., Glazer, J., & McGuire, T. G. (2000). Measuring adverse selection in managed health care. *Journal of Health Economics, 19*(6), 829–854.

Frank, R. G., & Glied, S. (2006). Changes in mental health financing since 1971: Implications for policymakers and patients. *Health Affairs, 25*(3), 601–613.

Frank, R. G., & Glied, S. (2007). Mental health in the mainstream of healthcare. *Health Affairs, 26*(6), 1539–1541.

Frank, R. G., & McGuire, T. G. (1986). A review of studies of the impact of insurance on the demand and utilization of specialty mental health services. *Health Services Research, 21*(2, Pt. 2), 241–265.

Frank, R. G., & McGuire, T. G. (2000). Economics and mental health. In A. J. Culyer & J. P. Newhouse (Ed.), *Handbook of Health Economics* (vol. 1). New York: Elsevier.

Glazer, J., & McGuire, T. (2002). Setting health plan premiums to ensure efficient quality in health care: Minimum variance optimal risk adjustment. *Journal of Public Economics, 84,* 153–173.

Goldman, D. P., Joyce, G. F., Escarce, J. J., Pace, J. E., Soloman, M. D., & Laouri, M. (2004). Pharmacy benefits and the use of drugs by the chronically ill. *Journal of the American Medical Association, 291*(19), 2344–2350.

Goldman, H. H., Frank, R. G., Burnam, M. A., Huskamp, H. A., Ridgely, M. S., Normand, S. L., et al. (2006). Behavioral health insurance parity for federal employees. *New England Journal of Medicine, 354*(13), 1378–1386.

Hahn, B., & Lefkowitz, D. (1992). *Annual Expenses and Sources of Payment for Health Care Services.* National Medical Expenditure Survey Research Findings 14. Rockville, MD: U.S. Dept. of Health and Human Services, Public Health Service, Agency for Health Care Policy and Research, Center for General Health Services Intramural Research.

Hodgkin, D., & McGuire, T. (1994). Payment levels and hospital response to prospective payment. *Journal of Health Economics, 13*(1), 1–29.

Hodgkin, D., Thomas, C. P., Simoni-Wastila, L., Ritter, G. A., & Lee, S. (2008). The effect of a three-tier formulary on antidepressant utilization and expenditures. *Journal of Mental Health Policy and Economics, 11*(2), 67–78.

Huskamp, H. A., Deverka, P. A., Epstein, A. M., Epstein, R. S., McGuigan, K. A., Muriel, A. C., et al. (2005). Impact of 3-tier formularies on drug treatment of attention-deficit/hyperactivity disorder in children. *Archives of General Psychiatry, 62*(4), 435–441.

Huskamp, H. A., Stevenson, D. G., Donohue, J. M., Newhouse, J. P., & Keating, N. L. (2007). Coverage and prior authorization of psychotropic drugs under Medicare Part D. *Psychiatric Services, 58*(3), 308–310.

Interstudy. (2002). *The Interstudy Competetive Edge 12.1: Part II, HMO Industry Report.* St. Paul, MN: Interstudy Publications.

Interstudy. (2003). *The Interstudy Competetive Edge 13.1: Part II, HMO Industry Report.* St. Paul, MN: Interstudy Publications.

Interstudy. (2007). *The Interstudy Competetive Edge 17.1: Part II, HMO Industry Report.* St. Paul, MN: Interstudy Publications.

Kaiser Family Foundation. (2006, October). *Medicaid Benefits: Online Database; Benefits by Service; Prescription Drugs.*

Kasper, J. A. (1982). *Prescribed Medicines: Use, Expenditures, and Sources of Payment; National Health Care Expenditures Study Data Preview 9.* Rockville, MD: U.S. Department of Health and Human Services, Public Health Service, Office of Health Research, Statistics, and Technology, National Center for Health Services Research.

Keeler, E. B., Manning, W. G., & Wells, K. B. (1988). The demand for episodes of mental health services. *Journal of Health Economics, 7*(4), 369–392.

Kessler, R. C., Demler, O., Frank, R. G., Olfson, M., Pincus, H. A., Walters, E. E., et al. (2005). Prevalence and treatment of mental disorders, 1990 to 2003. *New England Journal of Medicine, 352*(24), 2515–2523.

Kirby, J. B., Taliaferro, G. S., & Zuvekas, S. H. (2006). Explaining racial and ethnic disparities in health care. *Medical Care, 44*(Suppl. 5), I64–I72.

Landsman, P. B., Yu, W., Liu, X., Teutsch, S. M., & Berger, M. L. (2005). Impact of 3-tier pharmacy benefit design and increased consumer cost-sharing on drug utilization. *American Journal of Managed Care, 11*(10), 621–628.

Law, M. R., Ross-Degnan, D., & Soumerai, S. B. (2008). Effect of prior authorization of second-generation antipsychotic agents on pharmacy utilization and reimbursements. *Psychiatric Services, 59*(5), 540–546.

Lichtenberg, F. R., & Sun, S. X. (2007). The impact Of Medicare Part D on prescription drug use by the elderly. *Health Affairs, 26*(6), 1735–1744.

Lillie-Blanton, M., & Hoffman, C. (2005). The role of health insurance coverage in reducing racial/ethnic disparities in health care. *Health Affairs, 24*(2), 398–408.

Ling, D. C., Berndt, E. R., & Frank, R. G. (2008). Economic incentives and contracts: The use of psychotropic medications. *Contemporary Economic Policy, 26*(1), 49–72.

Ma, C.-T A, & McGuire, T. G. (1998). Costs and incentives in a behavioral health carve-out. *Health Affairs, 17*, 53–69.

Ma, C.-T. A., & McGuire, T. G. (2002). Network incentives in managed health care. *Journal of Economics & Management Strategy, 11*(1), 1–35.

Manning, W. G., Newhouse, J. P., Duan, N., Keeler, E. B., & Leibowitz, A. (1987). Health insurance and the demand for medical care: Evidence from a randomized experiment. *American Economic Review, 77*(3), 251–277.

Mark, T. L., Levit, K. R., Coffey, R. M., McKusick, D. R., Harwood, H. J., Bouchery, E., et al. (2007). *National Expenditures for Mental Health Services and Substance Abuse Treatment 1993–2003.* Rockville, MD: Substance Abuse and Mental Health Services Administration.

McGuire, T. G., Alegria, M., Cook, B. L., Wells, K. B., & Zaslavsky, A. M. (2006). Implementing the Institute of Medicine definition of disparities: An application to mental health care. *Health Services Research, 41*(5), 1979–2005.

McGuire, T., & Miranda, J. (2007). Measuring trends in mental health care disparities, 2000–2004. *Psychiatric Services, 58*(12), 1533–1540.

Mechanic, D. (2007). Mental health services then and now. *Health Affairs, 26*(6), 1548–1550.

Meyerhoefer, C. D., & Zuvekas, S. H. (2008). The shape of demand: What does it tell us about direct-to-consumer marketing of antidepressants? *B.E. Journal of Economic Analysis & Policy, 8*(2), art. 4.

Meyerhoefer, C. D., & Zuvekas, S. H. (2010). New estimates of the demand for physical and mental health treatment. *Health Economics, 19*(3), 297–315.

Miller, G. E., Banthin, J., & Selden, T. (2008). *Prescription Drug Expenditures and Healthcare Burdens in the Medicaid Population.* Unpublished working paper, Center for Financing Access and Cost Trends, Agency for Healthcare Research and Quality.

Mitchell, J. B. (1991). Physician participation in Medicaid revisited. *Medical Care, 29*(7), 645–653.

Mitchell, J. B., & Cromwell, J. (1982). Medicaid participation by psychiatrists in private practice. *American Journal of Psychiatry, 139*(6), 810–813.

Monheit, A. C., & Selden, T. M. (2000). Cross-subsidization in the market for employment-related health insurance. *Health Economics, 9*(8), 699–714.

National Advisory Mental Health Council. (1998). *Parity in Financing Mental Health Services: Managed Care Effects on Cost, Access, and Quality; An Interim Report to Congress.* Rockville, MD: Department of Health and Human Services, National Institutes of Health, National Institute of Mental Health.

National Advisory Mental Health Council. (2000). *Insurance Parity for Mental Health: Cost, Access, and Quality; Final Report to Congress.* Bethesda, MD: Department of Health and Human Services, National Institutes of Health, National Institute of Mental Health.

New Freedom Commission on Mental Health. (2003). *Achieving the Promise: Transforming Mental Health Care in America; Final Report.* DHHS Pub. No. SMA-03-3832. Rockville, MD: Author.

Norton, E. C., Lindrooth, R. C., & Dickey, B. (1997). Cost-shifting in a mental health carve-out for the AFDC population. *Health Care Financing Review, 18*(3), 95–108.

O'Malley, A. S., & Reschovsky, J. D. (2006, May). No exodus: Physicians and managed care networks. *Tracking Report/Center for Studying Health System Change,* (14), 1–4.

Open Minds. (2002). *Open Minds Yearbook of Managed Behavioral Health & Employee Assistance Program Market Share in the United States, 2002–2003.* Gettysburg, PA: Behavioral Health Industry News.

Pacula, R. L., & Sturm, R. (2000). Mental health parity legislation: Much ado about nothing? *Health Services Research, 35*(1, Pt. 2), 263–275.

Padgett, D. K., Patrick, C., Burns, B. J., Schlesinger, H. J., & Cohen, J. (1993). The effect of insurance benefit changes and use of child and adolescent outpatient mental health services. *Medical Care, 31*(2), 96–110.

Ramsey, S., & Pauly, M. V. (1997). Structural incentives and adoption of medical technologies in HMO and fee-for-service health insurance plans. *Inquiry, 34*(3), 228–236.

Ridgely, M. S., Burnam, M. A., Barry, C. L., Goldman, H. H., & Hennessy, K. D. (2006). Health plans respond to parity: Managing behavioral health care in the Federal Employees Health Benefits Program. *Milbank Quarterly, 84*(1), 201–218.

Rosenthal, M. B., Frank, R. G., Li, Z., & Epstein, A. M. Early experience with pay-for-performance: From concept to practice. *Journal of the American Medical Association, 294*(14), 1788–1793.

Rosenthal, M. B., Landon, B. E., Howitt, K., Song, H. R., & Epstein, A. M. (2007). Climbing up the pay-for-performance learning curve: Where are the early adopters now? *Health Affairs, 26*(6), 1674–1682.

Rosenthal, M. B., Landon, B. E., Normand, S. L., Frank, R. G., Ahmad, T. S., & Epstein, A. M. (2007). Employers' use of value-based purchasing strategies. *Journal of the American Medical Association, 298*(19), 2281–2288.

Rothschild, M., & Stiglitz, J. (1976). Equilibrium in competitive insurance markets: An essay on the economics of imperfect information. *Quarterly Journal of Economics, 90*(4), 629–649.

Soumerai, S. B., Zhang, F., Ross-Degnan, D., Ball, D. E., LeCates, R. F., Law, M. R., et al. (2008). Use of atypical antipsychotic drugs for schizophrenia in Maine Medicaid following a policy change. *Health Affairs, 27*(3), w185–195.

Strunk, B. C., & Reschovsky, J. D. (2002). *Kinder and Gentler: Physicians and Managed Care, 1997–2001.* Tracking Report No. 5. Washington, DC: Center for Studying Health Systems Change.

Sturm, R. (1997). How expensive is unlimited mental health coverage under managed care? *Journal of the American Medical Association, 278*(18), 1533–1537.

Tepper, C. D., & Lied, T. R. (2004). Trends in Medicaid prescribed drug expenditures and utilization. *Health Care Financing Review, 25*(3), 69–78.

U.S. Department of Labor, Office of Disability Employment Policy. (2007). *Increasing Options: The Ticket to Work and Self Sufficiency Program* [Fact sheet]. Available online at http://www.dol.gov/odep/pubs/fact/options.htm. Accessed October 28, 2008.

U.S. House of Representatives, Committee on Oversight and Government Reform, Majority Staff. (2008). *Medicare Part D: Drug Pricing and Manufacturer Windfalls.* Washington, DC: Author.

Wang, P. S., Patrick, A. R., Dormuth, C. R., Avorn, M., Maclure, M., Canning, C. F., et al. (2008). The impact of cost sharing on antidepressant use among older adults in British Columbia. *Psychiatric Services, 59*(4), 377–383.

West, J. C., Wilk, J. E., Muszynski, I. L., Rae, D. S., Rubio-Stipec, M., Alter, C. L., et al. (2007). Medication access and continuity: The experiences of dual-eligible psychiatric patients during the first 4 months of the Medicare prescription drug benefit. *American Journal of Psychiatry, 164*(5), 789–796.

Wildsmith, T. F. (2005). *Individual Health Insurance: A Comprehensive Survey of Affordability, Access, and Benefits.* Washington, DC: America's Health Insurance Plans.

Wilk, J. E., West, J. C., Narrow, W. E., Rae, D. S., & Regier, D. A. (2005). Access to psychiatrists in the public sector and in managed health plans. *Psychiatric Services, 56*(4), 408–410.

Wosinska, M. (2005). Direct-to-consumer advertising and drug therapy compliance. *Journal of Marketing Research, 42,* 323–332.

Yin, W., Basu, A., Zhang, J. X., Rabbani, A., Meltzer, D. O., & Alexander, G. C. (2008). The effect of the Medicare Part D prescription benefit on drug utilization and expenditures. *Annals of Internal Medicine, 148*(3), 169–177.

Zeckhauser, R. (1970). Medical insurance: A case study of the tradeoff between risk spreading and appropriate incentives. *Journal of Economic Theory, 2*(1), 10–26.

Zuckerman, S., McFeeters, J., Cunningham, P., & Nichols, L. (2004, June 23). Changes in Medicaid physician fees, 1998–2003: Implications for physician participation. *Health Affairs,* (Suppl. Web Exclusives), W4.374–384.

Zuvekas, S. H. (1999). Health insurance, health reform, and outpatient mental health treatment: Who benefits? *Inquiry, 36,* 127–146.

Zuvekas, S. H. (2001). Trends in the use and expenditures for mental health services in an era of managed care: 1987–1996. *Health Affairs, 20*(2), 214–224.

Zuvekas, S. H., & Cohen, J. W. (2005). Trends in provider capitation, 1996–2000. *Journal of Economic and Social Measurement, 30,* 145–156.

Zuvekas, S. H., & Meyerhoefer, C. D. (2006). Coverage for mental health treatment: Do the gaps still persist? *Journal of Mental Health Policy and Economics, 9*(3), 155–163.

Zuvekas, S. H., Rupp, A. E., & Norquist, G. S. (2007). Cost-shifting and managed behavioral health care. *Psychiatric Services, 58*(1), 100–110.

Chapter 3

LAW, SERVICES DELIVERY, AND POLICY

John Petrila, JD, LLM; and Bruce Lubotsky Levin, DrPH, MPH

Introduction

Mental health law emerged in the 1960s from the legal foundation established by the African American civil rights movement. When the United States Supreme Court decided *Brown v. Board of Education* in 1954, the Court did more than rule that schools segregated by race violated the federal Constitution. The ruling, perhaps the single most important Supreme Court decision of the twentieth century (Klarman, 2007), also effectively established the federal courts as the forum where groups sought redress for claims that their constitutional rights had been violated.

As the civil rights movement began, state mental hospitals were the largest provider of mental health services in the United States. Individuals usually entered state hospitals through involuntary civil commitment. There were no limits on the amount of time a person might be involuntarily held. Forced medication was common. State mental institutions were overcrowded, and many were understaffed, badly maintained, and, in some instances, rife with violence (Sobel, 1981).

Beginning in the mid-1960s, civil rights attorneys began challenging the state-operated public mental health systems. Claims were filed in federal court asserting that civil commitment decisions should be made by judges rather than doctors. At the same time, lawyers challenged the often inhumane conditions that existed in many state mental hospitals, asserting that states had an obligation to keep people safe and to provide adequate care. The federal courts endorsed these claims, as well as similar claims made on behalf of people confined in state facilities for individuals with developmental disabilities and in state prisons and jails. As remedies, courts directed that civil commitment laws be more narrowly drafted, made judges rather than psychiatrists the ultimate decision makers on civil commitment decisions, assumed operating control of many state mental institutions, and granted individuals with mental disorders a "right to refuse" treatment.

The "constitutional law" era of mental health law held sway for approximately two decades. From the mid-1980s through the present, mental health law has taken on a substantially different character. There are two primary reasons for this. First, an increasingly conservative Supreme Court redefined and in many cases restricted the application of federal constitutional principles that had created the foundation for rights-based mental health law. Second, and as important, state mental hospitals became less important as a place where mental health services were delivered. Today, few people with serious mental disorders ever enter a state mental hospital. In this new environment, legal strategies that launched the mental health law movement have little applicability (Petrila in Frost & Bonnie, 2001).

The courts have had extraordinary influence over the development of mental health law, but other types of law also affect the lives of people with mental disorders and treatment providers. For example, legislation and regulation has been important in shaping policy and treatment. Important examples include the Community Mental Health Centers Act, the Americans with Disabilities Act, Social Security, Medicaid and Medicare statutes and regulations, and parity legislation. Traditional health law issues, such as malpractice and confidentiality, have influence as well.

This chapter describes the ways in which the law has influenced and in some cases defined mental health policy since the mid-1960s. It also describes how the law has been influenced by changes in judicial philosophy, political ideology, economic conditions, and service systems. The chapter has four main sections. The first describes the constitutional era of mental health law and its eventual waning. The second discusses legal issues that have emerged in the aftermath of deinstitutionalization and the end of the constitutional era, including the Americans with Disabilities Act. The third focuses on the application of health care law issues such as malpractice and confidentiality to the care of people with mental disorders. The fourth section focuses on two recent developments, research into coercion and the criminalization of mental illness, and the implications of those two developments for mental health law. The chapter concludes with a brief discussion of the current relationship between mental health law and the organization and delivery of services to people with mental disorders.

The Constitutional Era of Mental Health Law: Its Emergence and Waning

In 1960, Morton Birnbaum, a physician and attorney, argued that individuals involuntarily committed to state psychiatric institutions had a "right to treatment" based upon federal constitutional principles (Birnbaum, 1960). His argument, novel at the time, created a legal and conceptual framework for what fairly may be described as the revolution in mental health law that lasted from 1965 to 1982. During this era, the federal courts exercised wide-ranging authority over state officials, laws, and institutions; the era began to recede as a more conservative United States Supreme Court redefined the limits of federal judicial authority.

Until the mid-1960s, a discrete body of "mental health law" did not exist. There were occasional malpractice lawsuits brought in the aftermath of a patient's suicide, or in cases of blatant mistreatment of patients by therapists, but the states exercised broad power regarding the conditions under which people with mental disorders were confined and treated. Involuntary civil commitment is one of the few areas of law (other than criminal law) where the state can take away an individual's liberty. In 1960, most state civil commitment laws permitted the indefinite involuntary commitment of a person on the certification of a physician (who did not have to be a psychiatrist in many jurisdictions) that the person had a mental disorder. The process and criteria for commitment were largely medical, and there were few checks on a person's confinement (Melton, Petrila, & Poythress et al., 2007).

The Supreme Court's decision in *Brown v. Board of Education* (1954) transformed the American judicial and political landscape. The Court reaffirmed its primacy in interpreting and applying the U.S. Constitution and made clear that state laws that denied individuals their federal constitutional rights would have to give way. The decision also made the federal courts the preferred forum for claims by individuals and groups that government had denied them rights. As a result, the African American civil rights movement led to social rights movements for prisoners, for women, and for people with mental disorders.

Federal lawsuits were brought in many states challenging the treatment of people with mental disorders. These lawsuits had three primary goals. The first was to make it more difficult to impose involuntary civil commitment on a person. The second was to improve the institutional (and in some cases community) conditions in which people were confined. The third was to extend to people with mental disorders certain rights (the right to be considered competent to make decisions until proved otherwise, the right to make treatment decisions) that most citizens have. Advocates had early success in obtaining these goals, as the next sections illustrate.

INVOLUNTARY CIVIL COMMITMENT

In 1955, the number of people confined in state and county mental hospitals peaked at 558,922. That number had begun to decline by the 1960s as medications were introduced that could control some symptoms of mental disorders. However, involuntary civil commitment was still widely used, and as the number of state mental hospital beds began to decline, there was an increase in the number of people hospitalized elsewhere (often referred to as "trans-institutionalization"), for example, in nursing homes and psychiatric beds in community hospitals (Kiesler & Sibulkin, 1987).

The Fourteenth Amendment to the U.S. Constitution provides that government may not take someone's liberty without "due process" of law. Civil commitment historically had been considered a medical decision, so the first task for advocates was to persuade the courts that civil commitment was essentially a deprivation of constitutionally protected liberty. This was necessary to bring constitutional principles to bear on civil commitment law. Advocates made three arguments in support of this claim. The first was that psychiatric diagnosis was so imprecise that it could not reasonably be used to take someone's liberty away. The second was that people who were involuntarily hospitalized suffered great social stigma, as well as a collateral loss of basic civil rights. The third, and most effective, was that conditions in mental hospitals were often horrific, and that indefinite confinement in such facilities based upon imprecise medical diagnoses violated fundamental constitutional rights.

These arguments prevailed. In a seminal case, a federal court in Wisconsin held that civil commitment involved fundamental issues of individual liberty (*Lessard v. Schmidt*, 1972). The court made three findings that influenced virtually every other federal court decision on the constitutionality of a medically oriented civil commitment law. First, the court found that civil commitment had an impact on the individual worse than that associated with being convicted for a crime. The court wrote:

> It is obvious that the commitment adjudication carries with it an enormous and devastating effect on an individual's civil rights. In some respects, such as the limitation on holding a driver's license, the civil deprivations which follow civil commitment are more serious than the deprivations which accompany a criminal conviction. (*Lessard v. Schmidt*, 1972, p. 1089)

Traditionally, a criminal conviction and the subsequent risk of confinement and stripping of civil rights was considered the most significant (though justified) action the state could take against an individual. Here, a federal court concluded that civil commitment, theoretically designed for the benefit of the person, had even more negative consequences. This finding led inexorably to the second finding, and the heart of the court's opinion. A person charged with a criminal offense is given several "rights" because of the potential consequences of a guilty verdict. These include the right to counsel, the right to present testimony and to cross-examine adverse witnesses, the right against self-incrimination, and the right to judicial decision making. The court in *Lessard* ruled that individuals subject to civil commitment must be given each of these rights (noted above), with the exception of the right against self-incrimination. Finally, the court also ruled that mental illness alone was legally insufficient as a basis for commitment. Rather, a person had to be an imminent danger to self or others as evidenced by an "overt act" before commitment could occur. In addition, hospitalization could occur only after consideration of the feasibility of treating the person in the "least restrictive environment."

The *Lessard* ruling had a profound effect nationally. Within a few years, nearly all states had revised their civil commitment laws to comply with its standards. The commitment hearing itself became more legalistic, at least in theory, and the medical model of commitment was replaced by a quasi-legalistic model, in which the person's behavior was as important as the existence of a mental disorder. While there is no limit on the amount of time a person may be hospitalized after commitment, a judicial hearing is necessary after a short evaluation period (ranging from 2 to 15 days, depending upon the particular state), and judicial review is necessary at fixed intervals, for example, six months after the initial commitment.

The Right to Treatment

As noted earlier, Birnbaum (1960) first proposed that people confined in state mental hospitals had a constitutional right to treatment in exchange for deprivation of their liberty. In 1965, the Federal Court of Appeals for the District of Columbia became the first court to rule that such a right existed, finding that prisoners with mental disorders in the District had a *statutory* right to treatment (*Rouse v. Cameron*, 1966). The first recognition of a *constitutional* right to treatment came in 1974, when a federal court of appeals held that a person confined to a psychiatric facility for years with no treatment "has a constitutional right to receive such individual treatment as will give him [or her] a reasonable opportunity to improve his [or her] condition" (*Donaldson v. O'Connor*, 1974, p. 520).

Other courts also ordered states to improve conditions in state mental health facilities, state facilities for people with developmental disabilities, and prisons. In many instances, federal courts assumed operational control of these facilities and issued orders governing every area of facility operation, from the number of different types of staff that had to be employed to water temperature in showers (*Wyatt v. Stickney*, 1972). These cases undoubtedly resulted in improvements in mental health institutional conditions. In some cases, state officials, eager to have increased expenditures on mental health, voluntarily entered settlements in which they obligated the state to improve the care of people with mental disorders and other disabilities. However, in order to comply with judicial orders requiring fixed staff-to-patient ratios, some states also discharged many patients to the community without adequate community mental health services. The result, paradoxically, was improved (though hardly perfect) mental health institutional conditions for those who remained, with little treatment or support available for those who had been discharged to the community (King, 1992).

Right to treatment cases focused on mental health institutional care because that was where advocates believed the most significant maltreatment and neglect occurred. In addition, the fact that (state) government operated those institutions gave the courts a legal foundation to invoke constitutional principles, beginning with the proposition that the state may not take away liberty without due process of law. However, advocates found significant legal barriers in extending the right to treatment to community settings. While an early federal case ruled that the District of Columbia had a statutory obligation to create a community treatment capacity (*Dixon v. Weinberger*, 1975), the United States Supreme Court eventually brought the tentative development of a constitutional right to community mental health care to a halt in decisions discussed below.

THE RIGHT TO REFUSE TREATMENT

Any competent adult has a right to give or withhold consent to proposed medical treatment before it occurs. The New York Court of Appeals first articulated this principle in United States law in 1914 when it wrote:

> Every human being of adult years and sound mind has a right to determine what shall be done with his [or her] own body; and a surgeon who performs an operation without his patient's consent commits an assault for which he may be liable in damages. (*Schloendorff v. Society of New York Hospital*, p. 93)

While this is a basic individual right, people with mental disorders were often denied the right to give informed consent simply because of a diagnosis of mental illness. This illustrates a central point regarding the civil rights movement: One of its primary goals, whether for African Americans, women, individuals with mental disorders, or people of non-heterosexual orientation, is to provide equal rights to all groups, unless there is an *individual* reason why the right should not apply in a particular situation. African Americans were routinely denied basic civil liberties because of color; the civil rights movement was designed in large measure to eliminate discrimination against groups of people. In the case of people with mental disorders, one goal for advocates was to provide people with the right to refuse treatment absent a specific reason (for example, a lack of competency) why the right should be denied.

There is no single definition of competency (Berg, Appelbaum, Parker et al., 2001). The general notion is that the individual must have the cognitive functioning and intellectual maturity necessary to understand and act on information regarding the risks and benefits of a proposed treatment, of alternative treatments, and of no treatment. Although the principle that a competent individual reserves the right to make treatment decisions is long-standing, it came comparatively late to the area of mental health. In part, this delay may have been attributable to legal rules that *assumed* mental illness necessarily caused incompetence. It may also have been due in part to conceptual confusion created by the widespread use of involuntary civil commitment. Many mental health professionals struggled to understand how a person ill enough to warrant civil commitment could function well enough to refuse the treatment for which commitment was presumably intended.

The litigation over this issue was brought on behalf of people in state-operated mental health facilities where patients were routinely subject to over-drugging with disabling side effects. Advocates again relied on constitutional law. They argued that the harmful side effects of psychiatric medication warranted regulation of its use. Most federal and state courts, confronted with this issue, agreed and ruled that a person could not be forcibly medicated over his or her objections, absent an emergency or absent judicial or administrative review. For example, the New York Court of Appeals ruled that medication could be forced in only limited circumstances because while medications had some benefit, "numerous side effects are associated with their usage, including extrapyramidal symptoms, akathesia, Parkinsonisms, dystonic reactions, akinesia and dyskinesia. The most potentially devastating side effect is tardive dyskinesia" (*Rivers v. Katz*, 1986, p. 76).

As a result of these cases, all states recognize that people in state mental hospitals have a right to refuse treatment if they are competent, absent an emergency that endangers the person or others. Individuals treated in community mental health settings may exercise informed consent, which is based upon public health principles rather than constitutional law. Informed consent requires that a person's consent be voluntary, be competent, and be knowledgeable about the risks and benefits of treatment, alternative treatments, or no treatment. This has created an interesting paradox; the constitutional right to refuse treatment in government-operated institutions in some states is triggered by the patient's refusal, which means that a person may be given medication based upon the *absence* of a refusal, even though the person might be incompetent under informed consent law. Regardless, it is clear today that most adults with mental disorders are competent in most circumstances to provide informed consent (Grisso & Appelbaum, 1998).

THE SUPREME COURT AND THE END OF AN ERA

The United States Supreme Court provided leadership and the legal framework for the civil rights era that ultimately resulted in the creation of "mental health law." However, over time, as more conservative presidents took office, the membership of the Supreme Court changed, as did its judicial philosophy. A new majority on the United States Supreme Court was no longer interested in expanding constitutional law, but focused instead on recalibrating the relationship between the federal judiciary and state government. This led to several decisions that marked the effective end of the constitutional era of mental health law.

In 1979, the Court issued two rulings on civil commitment that were very different in orientation than decisions such as *Lessard*. Federal courts had insisted on the similarities between civil commitment and criminal process, but in *Addington v. Texas* (1979), the Court rejected an argument that proof that a person met civil commitment standards should be "beyond a reasonable doubt," the standard used in criminal cases. The Court made clear that it believed that civil commitment was quite different from criminal proceedings, and that requirements considered constitutionally essential in the latter were not always required in the former. In *Parham v. J.R.* (1979), the Court ruled that the judicial hearing that had become an integral part of civil commitment hearings for adults was not required for children. Rather, the Court concluded that parents, guardians, and the state (when acting as the child's custodian) could admit a child to a psychiatric facility under a state's civil commitment law as long as an independent administrative or medical review of the decision occurred. These decisions left intact the principle that civil commitment was a deprivation of constitutionally protected liberty. However, the Supreme Court also made clear that states had considerably more discretion over civil commitment than the lower federal courts had suggested.

Shortly thereafter, the Court fundamentally realigned the relationship between the federal courts and the states in its decision in *Youngberg v. Romeo* (1982). The case involved a claim by an individual who had been injured repeatedly while a resident of a Pennsylvania institution for people with mental disabilities. The Court said he and others had a right to safety and to freedom from unreasonable restraint. However, the Court went on to say that the courts must review claims that even this comparatively limited right had been denied by using a standard that presumed the correctness of the judgments made by state treatment and administrative officials. The core of the ruling announced that "in determining whether the State has met its obligations in these respects, decisions made by the appropriate professional are entitled to a presumption of correctness" (p. 324). The Court has extended the principle of the presumptive validity of the judgment of state officials far beyond treatment issues. While the decision was criticized as an unwarranted grant of authority and an abdication of responsibility by the courts (Stefan, 1992), the *Youngberg* ruling as a practical matter ended the constitutional era of mental health law.

By the mid-1980s, it had been firmly established that civil commitment was not simply a medical decision and that there were limits on its exercise. It was also clear that government could not warehouse individuals in mental health institutions with no regard for their safety. The notion that mental illness necessarily disqualified an individual from exercising basic rights had also dissipated. These all represented important gains for a large group of people who, for several decades, had been virtually invisible legally and in many cases literally. However, other trends had become plain as well. The courts had become more conservative, reflecting larger social trends. Deinstitutionalization had continued, with state mental hospitals rapidly emptying, but few communities had adequate community mental health services for these individuals. Homelessness was becoming a major phenomenon in most large cities, and debates began over whether state mental hospital discharge policies caused homelessness. And most pertinent here, the legal doctrines that had provided new rights since the mid-1960s had little utility in this new environment. The next section of this chapter will discuss mental health law in the age of deinstitutionalization and homelessness.

Deinstitutionalization and Beyond: The Search for a New Legal Framework

Mental health law took its original shape because government was the primary provider of services and because most people were treated in mental health institutions. However, that is no longer the case today. There are fewer than 50,000 people in state mental hospitals; most people with serious mental disorders are hospitalized, if at all, in psychiatric beds in general hospitals. Civil commitment is still an issue, but for many people with mental disorders, the primary issue is obtaining access to care, not being protected from inhumane care from the state. In this environment, there are three important sources of law: 1) rights enunciated in state statutes; 2) contract law; and 3) the Americans with Disabilities Act (ADA). Each source of the law is discussed briefly below.

STATE LAW

All states have statutory provisions that establish rights for people with mental disorders. For example, the state of New York provides a long list of rights for people in its psychiatric centers, including civil rights (for example, the right to vote), personal rights (for example, the right to a safe environment, the right to freedom from abuse), rights to privacy and confidentiality (topics discussed in more detail below), and the right to communicate and have visitors (New York State Office of Mental Health, 2009). States also provide statutory protections for people treated in community mental health settings. For example, Florida law provides rights to informed consent, to quality treatment, and to receive care regardless of ability to pay in any setting in which treatment occurs (Florida Statute Annotated, S.394.459).

As the federal courts became less sympathetic to the claims of people with mental disorders, advocates turned to the state courts to enforce rights granted under state law. These claims have sometimes been successful. For example, state courts have ordered reforms at juvenile detention facilities in response to inhumane conditions (Dale, 1998). At least one state Supreme Court used state statutory law to order the creation of community-based mental health services (*Arnold v. Arizona Department of Health Services*, 1989). However, for a number of reasons, including judicial wariness about intruding too far into matters falling within the province of state legislatures and governors, state law has not been effective in creating new capacity in community mental health systems (Eyer, 2003).

CONTRACT LAW

A number of people with mental disorders will need treatment only once or for a brief period of time. For these individuals, a rights-based approach to mental health law is not particularly applicable, particularly when they seek treatment voluntarily. Access to health care is not a right in the United States, which is the only westernized nation without universal health care coverage of some type. As a result, individuals require either private insurance or eligibility for public pay plans such as Medicare or Medicaid to gain access to treatment (see Chapter 2 in this volume for a discussion of the financing of and insurance for mental health services).

Individuals do have some rights under private and publicly financed insurance programs. For example, Congress enacted the Health Insurance Portability and Accountability Act (HIPAA) in 1996 in an effort to make it easier for individuals to retain health insurance when they switched jobs. Insurers were denying coverage of people with "pre-existing conditions," which created barriers to people changing jobs. Insurance contracts can be enforced through litigation if necessary. This is true in both private insurance plans and public plans such as Medicaid and Medicare, where federal and state law confer a right to certain benefits if the individual is eligible for coverage. However, litigation is ineffectual in *enlarging* benefits in either situation. For example, if a person's insurance plan provides coverage for six outpatient mental health visits and the person needs continuing care, there is no available legal theory that will force the insurer to add visits to the plan (Rich, Erb, & Gale, 2005).

AMERICANS WITH DISABILITIES ACT

The Americans with Disabilities Act (ADA) was enacted in 1990 and became effective in 1992 (U.S. Congress, 1990). The ADA bars discrimination on the basis of disability in employment, public accommodations, telecommunications, and transportation. The Fair Housing Amendments Act of 1988 (U.S. Congress, 1988) bars discrimination on the basis of disability in housing. The ADA is the most important civil rights legislation since the Civil Rights Act of 1964, which barred discrimination on the basis of race.

The statutes define "disability" broadly. The definition includes 1) a physical or mental impairment that substantially limits one or more major life activities; 2) a record of having such an impairment; or 3) being regarded as having an impairment. "Reasonable accommodation" must be provided for an individual with a disability to ameliorate the impact of the disability. For example, it is because of the ADA that lifts have been installed on city buses, ramps constructed in public buildings, and special restroom accommodations installed in buildings where the public has access.

The ADA has also been an important source of litigation in the employment context for people with physical and with mental disabilities. An individual who has a disability must meet the basic qualifications for the job and be able to perform the "essential functions" of the job with or without reasonable accommodation. An "essential job" function might be the skill at the heart of the job; for example, if the job involves welding, then the person must have the requisite skills required of a welder.

The United States Supreme Court has heard multiple cases involving the ADA. The Court interpreted the statute increasingly narrowly in employment cases, and in doing so made it more difficult for employees to successfully bring claims. In particular, the Court defined "disability" very narrowly, and as a result, individuals with serious disorders, such as major depression or epilepsy, were found not to have a disability under the ADA (Petrila, 2002). In 2008, Congress enacted the Americans with Disabilities Amendments Act (U.S. Congress, 2008), expressly reversing several Supreme Court decisions. In doing so, it made clear that the courts were to interpret "disability" broadly. As a result, increased litigation by employees is anticipated, with more cases decided in favor of employees (Petrila, 2009).

The ADA was also the basis for a Supreme Court decision in 1999 that some thought might finally create a legal theory that would support right to treatment litigation in community mental health settings. In *Olmstead v. L.C.* (1999), the Court addressed a claim by two individuals who had been confined in Georgia mental institutions despite the fact that staff thought they could be appropriately treated in the community. The Supreme Court ruled that confinement in those circumstances was discrimination within the meaning of the ADA. Two factors were important in the Court's judgment. First, institutionalization "perpetuates unwarranted assumptions that persons so isolated are incapable or unworthy of participating in community life" (*Olmstead v. L.C.*, 1999, p. 600). Second, institutionalization "severely diminishes" the individual's ability to engage in many everyday activities, including family relations, social contacts, and work (*Olmstead v. L.C.*, 1999, p. 601).

While the Court endorsed theories regarding the impact of institutionalization that had been pressed by patient advocates for years, the Court also provided the state with several defenses. The state could rely on the judgment of its own professionals regarding the most appropriate place of treatment, a patient could not be placed against her will, and the state had to be permitted to show whether making resources available to a plaintiff would strip resources from others in the state's care. Finally and most important, the state could prevail in a lawsuit like *Olmstead* if it could

> demonstrate that it had a comprehensive, effectively working plan for placing qualified persons with mental disabilities in less restrictive settings, and a waiting list that moved at a reasonable pace not controlled by the state's endeavors to keep its institutions fully populated. (*Olmstead v. L.C.*, 1999, pp. 605–606)

These defenses effectively blunt the impact of *Olmstead* in part because they mirror the "professional judgment" rule created in response to constitutional right to treatment cases (Bauman, 2000).

At the same time, the majority of states have created "*Olmstead* plans" to illustrate how they will place people in community mental health settings when clinically indicated. While these plans have been created as a defense to an *Olmstead* lawsuit, they do cause state officials to focus their attention on the myriad of issues that make creation of community mental health capacity difficult. These issues include shortages of qualified workers, financial barriers, and difficulties in finding acceptable housing sites for people with mental disorders (DiPolito, 2006). Implementation of these plans often has been slow, and while *Olmstead* has had some impact, its effect has been less than many hoped for in the aftermath of the decision.

The relationship between where services occur and legal theory is significant. Constitutional law was well suited to a public mental health system that relied heavily (and often inappropriately) on state mental institutions as the primary place of mental health care. However, it is much less important in service systems where access to community mental health care is an overarching concern. Rather, access to care ultimately depends upon legislative policies and decisions made by those who administer the private and publicly financed insurance plans that pay for much of the mental health care that is available. For the many that are uninsured, no litigation can change that status. The ultimate solution is legislative, through adoption of comprehensive health care reform that assures all individuals a minimum level of health and mental health coverage.

Practice Issues: Malpractice and Confidentiality

While much of mental health law has focused on rights issues, there are also many issues that arise in the relationship between patient/client and the mental health professional. Two of the most important, malpractice and confidentiality, are now discussed.

Mental health professionals are sued less frequently than other health care professionals, though the number of claims has increased. In the 1980s, approximately 1 in 25 psychiatrists was sued in a year; by 2000, that had increased to 1 in 12 (Tsao & Layde, 2007). There are many reasons a claim may be filed; a review (Simon, 1998) of malpractice claims against psychiatrists found these were the most frequently filed claims:

- Suicide or attempted suicide (33% of claims);
- Incorrect diagnosis (11%);
- Improper civil commitment (5%);
- Breach of confidentiality (4%);
- Unnecessary hospitalization (4%);
- Undue familiarity (3%);
- Libel/slander (2%); and
- Other (improper use of electroconvulsive therapy, abandonment of the therapeutic relationship, etc.) (4%).

Of course, not all claims lead to judgments against a mental health professional and in fact, financial judgments paid on behalf of psychiatrists on average were 35% lower than for all medical specialties (Tsao & Layde, 2007).

As the types of claims enumerated above suggest, there are two broad categories of cases that are brought. One is for errors in practice (for example, a wrong diagnosis or for suicide resulting from clinical decisions), and the other is for violations of boundaries that are essential to the therapeutic relationship. It is both legally and ethically wrong, for example, for a mental health professional to engage in a sexual relationship with a client because of the lack of equity in the relationship. The professional is treating someone who is in a vulnerable state; for a caregiver (or, e.g., an attorney, or teacher, or scout leader) to take advantage of that vulnerability and exploit the power differential in the relationship is simply wrong. All licensed professions have adopted codes of ethics, and any practitioner or administrator should be familiar with the one applicable to his or her profession. There is also a significant literature discussing specific malpractice and ethical issues (see for example, Bersoff, 2003).

While most mental health professionals will never face a malpractice claim, it is useful to understand what a plaintiff must prove to prevail. There are four elements to any claim, including 1) the existence of a duty on the part of the treatment professional to the person claiming harm; 2) a breach of that duty; and 3) damages 4) caused by the breach.

Duty

The general duty of any health or mental health professional is to practice in accordance with generally accepted professional standards. A duty does not exist until the therapeutic relationship is established. The professional standards that govern practice come from a variety of sources. For example, the insert in a medication detailing circumstances for its use would be viewed in a legal setting as evidence of the standard to which a prescribing physician must adhere. A commonly used textbook might also be a source for practice standards, as are guidelines developed by professional associations. Courts can also create new legal duties. An illustration is provided in the section on confidentiality in the discussion of a decision by the California Supreme Court that imposed, on mental health professionals, a duty to protect third parties in some situations.

Breach of Duty

Once it is established that a treating professional (or treatment organization) has a sufficient relationship with the person to establish a duty of care, the plaintiff must show that the defendant has breached (or violated) his or her duty. For example, if a plaintiff claims that she was released inappropriately from inpatient care and as a result of untreated problems attempted suicide, the plaintiff would have to show that staff was negligent in deciding to discharge the person and/or that the arrangements for after-care were inadequate. In most malpractice cases, much of the evidence on the question of breach comes from expert witnesses.

CAUSATION

A breach of duty is not legally significant unless it also causes damages to the plaintiff. Law has a somewhat different paradigm in considering causation than psychology. Law has a more linear view, attempting to decide what, in an often complex and overlapping series of events, "caused" the negative outcome. In contrast, the field of psychology sees causation in a more nuanced way, attempting to consider the possible effects of multiple variables. In a legal setting, however, the law's more linear view prevails, though not without confusion in some circumstances. For example, if an individual is discharged from inpatient care and is referred to after-care, but then misses an appointment, is the causative event the release? The patient's own behavior, if the patient has not kept an appointment after discharge? The community provider's failure to call the patient to find out why the appointment was missed? Each of these events has some causative effect, and the task in a malpractice case is to sort out relative causation so that liability can be assigned, if appropriate (Appelbaum, 2000).

DAMAGES

Finally, the plaintiff must show that the defendant's breach of duty has caused damages of some type. Damages are awarded monetarily and so must be quantified. This can be done easily in some circumstances. For example, if a plaintiff suffered physical injuries during a suicide attempt that require ongoing medical care, the cost of that care can be estimated. If the injury forces the person to miss time at work, lost wages can be calculated. Other types of damages are more difficult to quantify, and jurors often view these with suspicion. These include damages for "pain and suffering" and in some cases for emotional injury. There is no question that people can suffer emotional injury and can also endure great physical pain as a result of an injury or misdiagnosed illness. However, quantifying the monetary value of such damages is much more difficult. As a result, state legislatures increasingly have placed caps on such damages (Avraham, 2006).

CONFIDENTIALITY AND PRIVACY

Confidentiality is a core ethical and legal principle. Communications between therapist and patient generally are confidential, absent an explicit exception created by law. As a principle, confidentiality rests on three assumptions. First, confidentiality promotes trust in the therapeutic relationship. The United States Supreme Court endorsed the importance of trust as a cornerstone of treatment in a decision in which it created a psychotherapist privilege in the federal courts. A "privilege" is a legal rule that permits information to be ruled confidential by a judge when it would otherwise be available to the parties in a legal proceeding. The Court wrote:

> Effective psychotherapy . . . depends upon an atmosphere of confidence and trust in which the patient is willing to make a frank and complete disclosure of facts, emotions, memories, and fears. Because of the sensitive nature of the problems for which individuals consult psychotherapists, disclosure of confidential communications made during counseling sessions may cause embarrassment or disgrace. For this reason, the mere possibility of disclosure may impede development of the confidential relationship necessary for successful treatment. (*Jaffee v. Redmond*, 1996)

The Court's ruling had significant impact in a variety of areas, including a greater willingness on the part of state courts to recognize a similar privilege under state law (Daly, 2006). Second, confidentiality may lessen the chance that a person will face discrimination or prejudice because of knowledge that the person has a mental illness. While the Americans with Disabilities Act provides formal protection against discrimination based upon disability, public attitudes regarding mental illness have softened but continue to suggest wariness, antipathy, and in some cases fear about people with mental disorders (Link, Phelan, Bresnahan, Stueve, & Pescosolido, 1999; Bhugra, 2007). Given that discrimination in the workplace and elsewhere remains an issue, the ability of a person to seek treatment in confidence provides a protective factor. Finally, there is evidence that a person's perception of the relative privacy of treatment may affect the decision to seek mental health care (Mermelstein & Wallack, 2008; Alpert, 1998).

Confidentiality can be a confusing subject because there are several sources of sometimes conflicting law that define confidentiality. These include state and federal statutory law, as well as judicial decisions such as the *Jaffee* case.

Judicially Created Law

The courts can sometimes expand confidentiality as was the case in *Jaffee*. The courts can also create exceptions to confidentiality through rulings in malpractice cases. Perhaps the most famous case in mental health practice is the case of *Tarasoff v. Regents of University of California* (1976). In *Tarasoff*, the California Supreme Court first ruled that a mental health professional with reason to believe that his or her client presented a threat to an identifiable third party had to warn that person of the potential danger. The Court later ruled that there was a duty to protect identifiable third parties. The Court issued its rulings despite claims by the American Psychiatric Association and the American Psychological Association that this would irreparably harm the clinical relationship, since ethically a clinician must tell a client of the limits of confidentiality. The ruling was quite controversial, though over time virtually every state has addressed the issue either legislatively or judicially. It is important for a clinician or administrator to recognize that application of the principle announced in *Tarasoff* varies by state, so it cannot be assumed that such a duty exists in the state in which an issue of danger to a third party arises. Some states make taking steps to protect a third party entirely discretionary on the part of the treatment staff; others impose a more affirmative obligation. Because of these differences, practitioners and administrators must understand the specific legal rule in the jurisdiction in question.

State Statutory Law

Each state has statutes that define confidentiality and create exceptions to it. There may be multiple statutes in the same state. For example, one statute may define confidentiality for public health purposes. These statutes usually set rules for hospitals, health care professionals, and others. There may also be a separate statutory provision establishing procedures for breaching the confidentiality of information related to a person's HIV status. Finally, most states have separate statutory sections establishing the rules for confidentiality of mental health and substance abuse information.

Federal Statutory and Regulatory Law

Traditionally, the confidentiality of health information and records was a matter of state law. However, there are three sources of federal statutory and regulatory law pertinent here. First, the privacy of educational records is addressed by the Family Educational Right to Privacy Act (or FERPA, U.S. Congress, 1974). Second, the confidentiality of information held by a program providing substance abuse and alcohol treatment is defined by a federal regulation enacted in 1975 and commonly known as 42 CFR Part 2 (U.S. Department of Health and Human Services, 2002). These regulations are extraordinarily strict in the protection they provide. They were enacted in an effort to increase treatment use by veterans returning from the Vietnam War. Any disclosure of the use of illegal substances in treatment created potential criminal liability, so stringent rules were created to protect the confidentiality of such treatment. The third source of federal statutory and regulatory law is the regulations that implement the Health Insurance Portability and Accountability Act of 1996. These regulations, commonly known as the HIPAA regulations, create a federal standard for the confidentiality of "protected health information" (45 CFR 160, 45 CFR 165, U.S. Department of Health and Human Services, 2002).

Application of these different sources of law to practice can be confusing because of differences between state and federal law and between HIPAA and 42 CFR Part 2. While a full discussion of the nuances of confidentiality law is beyond the scope of this chapter, understanding several points is essential to any clinician, administrator, or policymaker.

First, HIPAA establishes a baseline for protecting the privacy of protected health information (PHI). The definition of PHI is quite broad. It includes "any oral or recorded information relating to the past, present, or future physical or mental health of an individual; the provision of health care to the individual; or payment for health care" (45 CFR 160.103, U.S. Department of Health and Human Services, 2002). However, HIPAA only applies to "covered entities," which are health plans (essentially payers of health care, such as insurers), health care clear-inghouses (entities that process claims information), and health care providers who transmit health information in electronic form. HIPAA does *not* require patient consent for transmitting information for purposes of further health care, payment of claims, or "health care operations" (which include a broad array of activities such as quality assurance, evaluating performance, and staff training). HIPAA also provides for dissemination of information, with particular rules for some types of dissemination to public health officials, the courts, law enforcement, and others.

Second, if a state law provides stricter protection of confidentiality than HIPAA, then the state law applies. For example, state laws usually require a patient's consent before health care information is made available to another health care provider. HIPAA does not require consent in this situation. Therefore, the state law would govern, because it is more protective of confidentiality than the comparable provision in HIPAA. Similarly, in cases involving substance abuse or alcohol treatment, the federal rules on the confidentiality of substance abuse treatment (42 CFR Part 2, U.S. Department of Health and Human Services, 2002) would apply because they have more stringent rules for disclosing information than does HIPAA.

Third, in devising solutions to problems faced by people with mental disorders who find themselves in multiple systems over time, information sharing is essential. For example, a person with a mental illness may find herself arrested for trespassing, have her case heard by a mental health court, and be directed into treatment and placed on probation. Multiple parties (the judge, the arresting officer, the treatment staff, and the probation officer) may have an interest in information regarding her mental state. There are ways to share information that respect the essential values that underlie confidentiality, while permitting these various decision makers to play their roles. However, concerns over HIPAA can sometimes create barriers to these legitimate exchanges of information (Petrila, 2007).

Confidentiality is an important legal and ethical principle, but it is not an absolute value. In the interest of the client's autonomy, obtaining consent before releasing information about the person's health or mental health status is preferred. However, there are situations in which it is legally and ethically appropriate to release information absent consent, and the administrator and health care professional should have a good understanding of the basic rules regarding confidentiality in his or her jurisdiction.

Criminalization of Mental Illness

There are approximately 15 million arrests in the United States each year. The prevalence of acute mental illnesses among arrestees is estimated conservatively to be about 8%, with estimates of all mental and substance use disorders among individuals in jails and prisons running as high as 70% to 80% (James & Glaze, 2006; Lamb & Weinberger, 1998; U.S. Department of Justice, 1997). Estimates are similar (or higher) for juveniles in detention (Teplin, Abram, McClelland, Dulcan, & Mericle, 2002). Many of those who are most ill have been arrested repeatedly for nonviolent misdemeanors. They often face a cycle of arrest, brief jail time, release, and re-arrest. The volume of individuals that come into the criminal justice system with serious mental disorders or substance use disorders has become overwhelming in many jurisdictions, creating significant burdens for law enforcement, the courts, and jails. As a result, diverting people with mental disorders from further involvement with the criminal justice system has become a major priority among mental health and criminal justice policymakers.

Diversion efforts take a number of forms and can occur at a number of points in the criminal process. For example, some communities have created the capacity to assess individuals who may have a mental illness *before* they are arrested, and this enables the responding law enforcement officer to take the person to a treatment facility in lieu of arrest (Lattimore, Broner, Sherman, Frisman, & Shafer, 2003). Other communities divert people after arrest, for example at booking, if a person is identified as having a mental illness, or from the jail after booking but before court proceedings begin (Draine & Solomon, 1999).

Many communities also use special jurisdiction courts, such as drug courts and mental health courts, to divert people to treatment. These courts have grown increasingly popular, and at the time of this writing, there were approximately 2,000 drug courts and nearly 200 mental health courts in the United States with similar courts emerging in Australia and Canada (Schneider, Bloom, & Heerema, 2007). Drug courts and mental health courts have common features but also important differences (Petrila, 2003). For example, both drug and mental health courts typically consolidate cases meeting the court's jurisdictional requirements before a specially designated judge. Both types of courts attempt to divert their target population into treatment. These courts typically do not use a strict due process, adversarial model. Instead, all parties, including the judge, prosecutor, and defense attorney attempt to resolve both legal and non-legal issues presented by the defendant. A traditional criminal court is concerned primarily with the issue of the defendant's guilt or innocence and then sentencing the defendant accordingly. In contrast, drug and mental health courts focus on treatment and social welfare issues such as sobriety and housing (Denckla, 2003). There are also differences between drug and mental health courts. For example, the former routinely use punishment, principally jail, in response to a defendant who does not comply with treatment, while the use of such sanctions among mental health courts is more variable (Redlich, Steadman, Monahan, Robbins, & Petrila, 2006).

There is an emerging research base on the effectiveness of various diversion efforts. One multi-site study comparing participants in three pre-booking and three post-booking diversion programs to non-diverted individuals concluded that diversion reduced time in jail without increasing public safety risks, and also increased access to treatment (Steadman & Naples, 2005). Multiple studies suggest that drug courts can reduce recidivism and increase treatment adherence (King & Pasquarella, 2009), though at least one study found that DUI offenders did not experience reduced recidivism (Bouffard & Richardson, 2007). Single-site studies of mental health courts indicate that they may increase access to treatment (Boothroyd, Poythress, McGaha, & Petrila, 2003; Cosden, Ellens, Schnell, & Yamini-Diouf, 2005). While this evidence is suggestive, it is not conclusive. Continuing research is needed to address whether diversion efforts work, not just in general, but for whom and why. In addition, diversion to treatment may "work" in the sense that people spend less time in jail (an undeniably important outcome), but whether treatment has an impact on mental health status and functioning is a separate question, as is the potential impact of treatment on recidivism and public risk.

The issue of criminalization will continue to be a major policy issue for the criminal justice, social welfare, and treatment systems. The volume of arrests in the United States combined with high prevalence of mental disorders and the lack of integrated mental health systems in most communities makes this inevitable. The question is whether interventions designed to divert people into treatment can have enough of an impact to become part of a permanent solution to such issues or whether resolution must await the development of more effective community based care systems (for additional discussion of the issues emerging from the interface between the criminal justice and treatment systems, see Chapter 18 in this volume).

Coercion

The use of coercion is one of the distinguishing features of mental health treatment. Discussion of coercion historically has focused on the use of involuntary inpatient civil commitment. Early litigation challenged the standards and processes used to commit a person to inpatient care. In recent years, debate has turned to the use of outpatient civil commitment. However, it is increasingly apparent that coercion (and other types of leverage) is used in a variety of situations in community mental health care.

Nearly all states have some form of involuntary outpatient commitment (IOC). Outpatient commitment statutes permit an individual to be involuntarily committed to outpatient care as an alternative to inpatient commitment. While criteria vary from state to state, New York's law (called "Kendra's law" after the woman who was pushed to her death in the subway by a person with a mental illness) is typical of more recently enacted IOC statutes. The New York law permits commitment if a judge finds that the person:

1. is 18 years or older;
2. has a mental illness;
3. is unlikely to survive safely in the community without supervision, based upon a clinical determination;
4. has a history of lack of compliance with treatment for mental illness;
5. as a result of his or her mental illness, is unlikely to participate in voluntary treatment or with conscientious explanation and disclosure of the purpose of the placement is not able to determine if placement is necessary;
6. requires IOC to prevent a relapse or deterioration that would result in serious bodily harm to self or others;
7. is likely to benefit from IOC;
8. all available, less restrictive alternatives that would offer an opportunity for improvement of his or her condition have been judged to be inappropriate or unavailable; and
9. the person has a) at least twice in the past 36 months been involuntarily admitted as the result of an emergency commitment or received mental health

services in a forensic correctional facility or b) engaged in one or more acts of serious violent behavior towards self or others, or attempts at serious bodily harm to self or others within the preceding 36 months. (Laws of New York, 1999, Chapter 408)

A treatment plan must be submitted with the petition for IOC, and the services specified in the treatment plan must be available.

Use of IOC statutes in the United States varies considerably. For example, the New York law has been used several thousand times since its passage, while the California and Florida laws have been used very infrequently (Appelbaum, 2003; Petrila & Christy, 2008). Part of the reason is access to services. In New York, a person committed to outpatient care receives preferential access to intensive case management and in some cases to housing. In contrast, Florida, like many other states, did not allocate new resources when it enacted its IOC law.

The lack of available treatment is an important factor, since a study conducted of IOC in the United States concluded that an outpatient commitment order of more than six months duration, combined with treatment over that period, was effective in reducing hospitalizations, jail days, and violence among people with psychotic (but not affective) disorders (Swartz, et al. 1999). In other countries, IOC is referred to more commonly as "community treatment orders." A recent meta-review of 72 studies from 6 countries on community treatment orders and IOC concluded that it was not yet clear that IOC was beneficial or harmful to patients; the review also found that similar types of patients, regardless of the jurisdiction, were ordered into care (Churchill, 2007). As Dawson (2005) found in a study of treatment orders in several jurisdictions, those ordered into care were more likely to be men (60%) than women (40%), often with schizophrenia, and with histories of multiple hospitalizations and forensic involvement.

While IOC has commanded significant attention, efforts to induce individuals to adhere to treatment occur in many other settings. Monahan and colleagues (2005) asked more than 1,000 individuals in five sites across the United States who were currently receiving mental health treatment in the community about their past experiences with the use of leverage by treatment staff, judges, probation officers, and others in four situations, including money, housing, criminal justice, and outpatient commitment. The percentage of patients who reported that they had experienced at least one of these types of leverage ranged from 44 to 59 percent across sites. Generally, leverage was used more frequently with individuals who were younger; who had more disabling, severe, and longer-lasting illnesses; who had been hospitalized multiple times; and who used outpatient services intensively. Use of the various forms of leverage varied from 7 to 19 percent of patients with the use of money; 12 to 20 percent reporting some type of outpatient commitment; 15 to 30 percent reporting experience with the use of a criminal sanction (for example, receiving probation with a condition of treatment instead of incarceration); and 23 to 40 percent reporting that housing had been conditioned on treatment compliance.

This study and subsequent studies raise three interesting points. First, the use of leverage (or coercion) in community mental health treatment goes far beyond outpatient commitment. In fact, respondents reported that housing was most often conditioned on treatment adherence. Second, the use of leverage (or coercion) is not reserved for a small minority of people in care. More than one half of the respondents in five sites reported experience with at least one form of leverage during their lives. Third, not all forms of leverage or efforts to induce someone to adhere to treatment are necessarily coercive. Debates over civil commitment, whether inpatient or outpatient, were usually contested in ideological terms, with proponents of commitment characterized as paternalistic and opponents characterized as willing to let people with mental illnesses "die with their rights on" (Treffert, 1974). In the view of some commentators, these debates reached an intellectual dead end because of the predictable nature of the discourse. Bonnie and Monahan (2005) have suggested reframing the debate by focusing on whether the proposed action (outpatient commitment, offering mental health court rather than traditional criminal court) improves or worsens the person's "baseline" if the person accepts the offer. They would consider offers that worsened the person's "baseline" to be coercive and those that would improve it non-coercive. Applying their analysis, outpatient commitment typically would be coercive, since the alternative might be inpatient commitment while a mental health court would be non-coercive if it offered an alternative to incarceration. Their argument has been criticized on the ground that individuals faced with options offered by the government, for example in criminal court, have no real choice, and so a framework based on offer and acceptance is inapplicable. However, the strength of their assertion is that it does permit a more nuanced and non-judgmental examination of the myriad ways decision makers in various systems attempt to induce people with mental illnesses to accept and adhere to treatment.

Implications for Mental Health

Mental health law emerged in response to the inhumane conditions in state-operated mental hospitals. In its original incarnation, it was primarily anchored in the civil rights movement. Lawyers sought to narrow civil commitment statutes, improve institutional conditions, and expand individual autonomy over treatment decisions. However, service conditions today are dramatically different. The role of state hospitals has been substantially reduced, and the vast majority of people with mental disorders reside permanently in community mental health settings. In this environment, the dominant issue is access to care. Given this, mental health law has become much more closely aligned with general health care law. Rights issues continue to exist, but for most people they are less important than finding access to care.

The fundamental difference between the United States and other westernized countries is that the United States alone does not provide universal health care coverage. A guarantee of universal health care is not a panacea. However, in its absence, individuals in need of care must rely on their eligibility for private or public insurance, or use hospital emergency rooms as a primary venue for care. Individuals inappropriately denied care guaranteed by their insurance plan can bring a breach of contract claim in response. However, neither contract law nor civil rights law has any theory under which a court could be persuaded to force a payer to *expand* benefits beyond those provided in an insurance contract or in

Medicare or Medicaid plans. Only the legislature can provide universal coverage, and to date Congress and most state legislatures have shown little appetite for this challenge.

There are three areas in which the law will be intertwined with the delivery of mental health services in the foreseeable future, beyond practice issues such as confidentiality and malpractice. The first is in challenges to alleged discrimination on the basis of disability, using the Americans with Disabilities Act as a tool. As noted above, Congress in 2008 overturned a string of United States Supreme Court decisions that had tilted enforcement of the ADA toward employers. One can anticipate increased ADA claims, particularly in the workplace, based upon claims of discrimination because of mental or physical disability. The second is in continuing efforts to divert people with mental disorders from the criminal and juvenile justice systems into treatment. There is no evidence that the volume of people with mental disorders entering the justice system is abating significantly. Therefore, one can anticipate continued growth in the use of pre-booking and post-booking diversion programs and drug and mental health courts. Finally, coercion and leverage will remain as common features of the mental health system. However, continuing research will provide greater understanding of the relationship between coercion, leverage, and the therapeutic relationship. Such research, if translated into practice, may lessen the use of explicit coercion, while enabling treatment providers to use leverage in ways that are more consistent with individual autonomy while increasing treatment adherence.

References

Addington v. Texas, 441 U.S. 418 (1979).

Alpert, S. (1998). Health care information: Access, confidentiality, and good practice. In K. W. Goodman (ed.), *Ethics, Computing, and Medicine: Informatics and the Transformation of Health Care* (pp. 75–101). Cambridge, UK: Cambridge University Press.

Appelbaum, P. S. (2000). Patients' responsibility for their suicidal behavior. *Psychiatric Services*, *51*(1), 15–16.

Appelbaum, P. S. (2003). Ambivalence codified: California's new outpatient commitment statute. *Psychiatric Services*, *54*(1), 26–28.

Arnold v. Arizona Department of Health Services, 160 Ariz. 593, 775 P. 2nd 521 (1989).

Avraham, R. (2006). Putting a price on pain-and-suffering damages: A critique of the current approaches and a preliminary proposal for change. *Northwestern University Law Review*, *100*(1), 87–119.

Bauman, R. L. (2000). Needless institutionalization of individuals with mental disabilities as discrimination under the ADA: Olmstead v. L.C. *New Mexico Law Review*, *30*, 287–306.

Berg, J. W., Appelbaum, P. S., Parker L. S., et al. (2001). *Informed Consent: Legal Theory and Clinical Practice* (2nd ed.). Oxford and New York: Oxford University Press.

Bersoff, D. N. (2003). *Ethical Conflicts in Psychology* (2nd ed.). Washington, DC: American Psychological Association.

Bhugra, D. (2007). *A Select Annotated Bibliography of Public Attitudes toward Mental Illness, 1975–2005*. Lewiston, NY: Edwin Mellen Press.

Birnbaum, M. (1960). The right to treatment. *American Bar Association Journal*, *46*(5), 499–505.

Bonnie, R. J., & Monahan, J. (2005). From coercion to contract: Reframing the debate on mandated community treatment for people with mental disorders. *Law and Human Behavior*, *29*(4), 485–503.

Boothroyd, R. A., Poythress, N. G., McGaha, A. C., & Petrila, J. (2003). The Broward County mental health court: Process, outcomes, and service utilization. *International Journal of Law and Psychiatry*, *26*(1), 55–71.

Bouffard, J. A., & Richardson, K. A. (2007). The effectiveness of drug court programming for specific kinds of offenders: Methamphetamine and DWI offenders versus other drug-involved offenders. *Criminal Justice Policy Review*, *18*(3), 274–293.

Brown v. Board of Education, 347 U.S. 483 (1954).

Churchill, R. (2007). *International Experiences of Using Community Treatment Orders*. London: Institute of Psychiatry.

Confidentiality of alcohol and drug abuse patient records. (2002). Title 42 Code of Federal Regulations, Part 2. Sections 2.1-2.67.

Cosden, M., Ellens, J., Schnell, J., & Yamini-Diouf, Y. (2005). Efficacy of a mental health treatment court with assertive community treatment. *Behavioral Sciences & the Law*, *23*(2), 199–214.

Dale, M. (1998). Lawsuits and public policy: The role of litigation in correcting conditions in juvenile detention centers. *University of San Francisco Law Review*, *32*(4), 675–733.

Daly, R. (2006). Too early to judge impact of precedent-setting ruling. *Psychiatric News*, *41*(12), 13–35.

Dawson, J. (2005). *Community Treatment Orders: International Comparisons*. Dunedin, New Zealand: Faculty of Law, University of Otago.

Denckla, D. A. (2003). Essay: Forgiveness as a problem-solving tool in the courts; A brief response to the panel on forgiveness in criminal law. *Fordham Urban Law Journal*, *27*, 1613–1619.

DiPolito, S. A. (2006). Olmstead v. L.C.: Deinstitutionalization and community integration; An awakening of the nation's conscience? *Mercer Law Review*, *58*, 1381–1409.

Dixon v. Weinberger, 405 F., Supp. 974, D.D.C. (1975).

Donaldson v. O'Connor, 493 F., 2d 507, 5th Cir. (1974).

Draine, J., & Solomon, P. (1999). Describing and evaluating jail diversion services for persons with serious mental illness. *Psychiatric Services*, *50*(1), 56–61.

Eyer, K. (2003). Litigating for treatment: The use of state laws and constitutions in obtaining treatment rights for individuals with mental illness. *Review of Law and Social Change*, *28*(1), 1–67.

Florida Statutes Annotated (2009), Section 394.459.

Goodman, K. W. (1998). *Ethics, Computing, and Medicine Informatics and the Transformation of Health Care*. Cambridge, UK, and New York: Cambridge University Press.

Grisso, T., & Appelbaum, P. S. (1998). *Assessing Competence to Consent to Treatment: A Guide for Physicians and Other Health Professionals*. New York: Oxford University Press.

Jaffee v. Redmond, 518 U.S. 1 (1996).

James, D. J., & Glaze, L. E. (2006). Mental health problems of prison and jail inmates. *Bureau of Justice Statistics Special Report*. Available online at http://www.ojp.usdoj.gov/bjs/pub/pdf/mhppji.pdf. Accessed May 7, 2009.

Kiesler, C. A., & Sibulkin, A. E. (1987). *Mental Hospitalization: Myths and Facts about a National Crisis*. Newbury Park, CA: Sage Publications.

King, P. (1992). Rights within the therapeutic relationship. *Journal of Law and Health*, *6*(1), 31–60.

King, R. S., & Pasquarella, J. (2009). *Drug Courts: A Review of the Evidence*. Washington, DC: Sentencing Project.

Klarman, M. J. (2007). *Brown v. Board of Education and the Civil Rights Movement: Abridged Edition of "From Jim Crow to Civil Rights: The Supreme Court and the Struggle for Racial Equality."* New York: Oxford University Press.

Lamb, H. R., & Weinberger, L. E. (1998). Persons with severe mental illness in jails and prisons: A review. *Psychiatric Services*, *49*(4), 483–492.

Lattimore, P. K., Broner, N., Sherman, R., Frisman, L., & Shafer, M. S. (2003). A comparison of prebooking and postbooking diversion programs for mentally ill substance-using individuals with justice involvement. *Journal of Contemporary Criminal Justice*, *19*(1), 30–64.

Laws of New York, 1999, Chapter 408, Appendix 1.

Lessard v. Schmidt, 349 Suppl. 1078 (1972).

Link, B. G., Phelan, J. C., Bresnahan, M., Stueve, A., & Pescosolido, B. A. (1999). Public conceptions of mental illness: Labels, causes, dangerousness, and social distance. *American Journal of Public Health, 89*(9), 1328–1333.

Melton, G. B. (2007). *Psychological Evaluations for the Courts: A Handbook for Mental Health Professionals and Lawyers* (3rd ed.). New York: Guilford Press.

Melton G., Petrila J., Poythress N., et al. (2007). *Psychological Evaluation for the Courts: A Handbook for Mental Health Professionals and Lawyers.* (3rd ed.) New York: Guilford Press.

Mermelstein, H. T., & Wallack, J. J. (2008). Confidentiality in the age of HIPAA: A challenge for psychosomatic medicine. *Psychosomatics, 49*(2), 97–103.

Monahan, J., Redlich, A. D., Swanson, J., Robbins, P. C., Appelbaum, P. S., Petrila, J., et al. (2005). Use of leverage to improve adherence to psychiatric treatment in the community. *Psychiatric Services, 56*(1), 37–44.

Moore, K. A., Harrison, M., Young, S. M., & Ochshorn, E. (2008). A cognitive therapy treatment program for repeat DUI offenders. *Journal of Criminal Justice, 36*(6), 539–545.

Moore, K., Young, M. S., Barrett, B., & Ochshorn, E. (2009). Twelve-month outcome findings from a residential facility serving homeless clients with co-occurring disorders. *Journal of Social Sciences Review, 35*(4): 322–335.

New York State Office of Mental Health. (2009). *Rights of Inpatients in Psychiatric Centers of the New York State Office of Mental Health.* Albany: New York State Office of Mental Health. Available online at http://www.omh.state.ny.us/omhweb/patientrights/inpatient_rts.htm.

Olmstead v. L.C., 527 U.S. 581 (1999).

Parham v. J. R., 440 U.S. 584 (1979).

Petrila, J. (2001). From constitution to contracts: Mental health law at the turn of the century. In L. E. Frost & R. J. Bonnie (eds.), *The Evolution of Mental Health Law* (1st ed., pp. 75–100). Washington, DC: American Psychological Association.

Petrila, J. (2002). The US Supreme Court narrows the definition of disability under the Americans With Disabilities Act. *Psychiatric Services, 53*(7), 797–798.

Petrila, J. (2003). An introduction to special jurisdiction courts. *International Journal of Law and Psychiatry, 26*(1), 3–12.

Petrila, J. (2007). *Dispelling the Myths about Information Sharing between the Mental Health and Criminal Justice Systems.* Delmar, NY: CMHS National GAINS Center for Systemic Change for Justice-Involved People with Mental Illness. Available online at http://gainscenter. samhsa.gov/text/integrated/Dispelling_Myths.asp.

Petrila, J. (2009). Congress restores the Americans With Disabilities Act to its original intent. *Psychiatric Services, 60*(7), 878–879.

Petrila, J., & Christy, A. (2008). Florida's outpatient commitment law: A lesson in failed reform. *Psychiatric Services, 59*, 21–23.

Redlich, A. D., Steadman, H. J., Monahan, J., Robbins, P. C., & Petrila, J. (2006). Patterns of practice in mental health courts: A national survey. *Law and Human Behavior, 30*(3), 347–362.

Rich, R. F., Erb, C. T., & Gale, L. J. (2005). Judicial interpretation of managed care policy. *Elder Law Journal, 13*, 85–89.

Rivers v. Katz, 67 NY 485, 495 N.E. 2d 337 (1986).

Rouse v. Cameron, 373 F. 2d 451 D.C.C. (1966).

Schloendorff v. Society of New York Hospital, 211 N.Y. 2nd 125; 105 N.E. 2d 92 (1914).

Schneider, R. D., Bloom, H., & Heerema, M. (2007). *Mental Health Courts: Decriminalizing the Mentally Ill.* Toronto, Ontario: Irwin Law.

Simon, R.I. (1998). *A Concise Guide to Psychiatry and Law for Clinicians.* Washington, DC: American Psychiatric Association Press.

Sobel, D. (1981, February 10). State psychiatric hospitals forced to change or close. *New York Times*.

Steadman, H. J., & Naples, M. (2005). Assessing the effectiveness of jail diversion programs for persons with serious mental illness and co-occurring substance use disorders. *Behavioral Sciences & the Law*, *23*(2), 163–170.

Stefan, S. (1992). Leaving civil rights to the "experts": From deference to abdication under the professional judgment standard. *Yale Law Journal*, *102*, 639–752.

Swartz, M. S., Swanson, J. W., Wagner, H. R., Burns, B. J., Hiday, V. A., & Borum, R. (1999). Can involuntary outpatient commitment reduce hospital recidivism? Findings from a randomized trial with severely mentally ill individuals. *American Journal of Psychiatry*, *156*(12), 1968–1975.

Tarasoff v. Regents of the University of California, 17 Cal. 3d 425, 551 P. 2d 334 (1976).

Teplin, L. A., Abram, K. M., McClelland, G. M., Dulcan, M. K., & Mericle, A. A. (2002). Psychiatric disorders in youth in juvenile detention. *Archives of General Psychiatry*, *59*(12), 1133–1143.

Treffert, D. A. (1974). Dying with their rights on. *Prism*, *2*, 47–52.

Tsao, C. I., & Layde, J. B. (2007). A basic review of psychiatric medical malpractice law in the United States. *Comprehensive Psychiatry*, *48*(4), 309–312.

U.S. Bureau of Justice Statistics. (1997). *Correctional Populations in the United States*. Washington, DC: Author.

U.S. Congress. (1974). Federal Educational Right to Privacy. Public Law 93–579.

U.S. Congress. (1988). Fair Housing Amendments Act. Public Law 100–430.

U.S. Congress. (1990). Americans with Disabilities Act. Public Law 101–336.

U.S. Congress. (2008). Americans with Disabilities Amendments Act. Public Law 110–135.

U.S. Department of Health and Human Services (2002). *Confidentiality of Alcohol and Drug Abuse Patient Records*. 42 Code of Federal Regulations (CFR) Part 2.

Wyatt v. Stickney, 344 F. Suppl. 373 M.D. Ala. (1972).

Youngberg v. Romeo, 457 U.S. 302 (1982).

Chapter 4

QUALITY IMPROVEMENT

Kevin D. Hennessy, PhD

Between the health care we have and the care we could have lies not just a gap, but a chasm.

Institute of Medicine, 2001

THE "CHASM" noted in this seminal Institute of Medicine (IOM) report is one of quality, where health care systems and providers too often fall short in delivering to patients and their families anticipated benefits of recovery, improved functioning, or even symptom relief or reduction. As a result, patients and families are frequently left frustrated, angry, and with diminished hope for the future. While this phenomenon is recognized throughout our health care system, it may be particularly relevant to those seeking mental health services (McGlynn et al., 2003; Wang, Demler, & Kessler, 2002).

This chapter provides an overview of efforts to address this phenomenon—namely efforts both to identify and improve the quality of care and services received by individuals with mental disorders in the United States. These efforts have taken many forms and appear to be accelerating in recent years (Institute of Medicine [IOM], 2006). The promotion of evidence-based practices and other empirically supported treatments (Beutler & Castonguay, 2005; Nathan & Gorman, 2002), the development and nurturing of a quality measurement and reporting infrastructure (IOM, 2006; Herman, 2005), the movement toward broader adoption of electronic health records (Trabin & Maloney, 2003), the advancement of models of care

---

Disclaimer: The views expressed in this chapter are those of the author and not necessarily those of the Substance Abuse and Mental Health Services Administration or the U.S. Department of Health and Human Services.

coordination (Gilbody, Whitty, Grimshaw, & Thomas, 2003; Unutzer, Katon, Williams Jr. et al., 2001; Weisner, Mertens, Parthasarathy et al. 2001), and the promotion of workforce development initiatives (IOM, 2006; O'Connell, Morris, & Hoge, 2004) all represent important components of an emerging quality improvement agenda in mental health and health care more generally. While the literature in each of these areas is extensive, the current chapter seeks to describe and highlight key activities and issues in all of these areas relevant to both informing and contributing to a broader agenda of mental health quality improvement.

Background and Rationale

Quality of care has been defined as "the degree to which health services for individuals and populations increase the likelihood of desired health outcomes and are consistent with current professional knowledge" (IOM, 1990, p. 21). Yet, a number of recent studies clearly document that a discrepancy exists between the mental health care that research has demonstrated to be effective and the care that is typically or routinely delivered in most practice settings (Bauer, 2002; Buchanan, Kreyenbuhl, Zito, & Lehman, 2002; Druss, Miller, Rosenheck, Shih, & Bost, 2002; Lehman, 1999; Roy-Byrne, Katon, Cowley et al., 2001; Unutzer, Simon, Pabiniak et al., 2000; Wang, Demler, & Kessler, 2002; Watkins, Burnam, Kung, & Paddock, 2001; Wells, Schoenbaum, Unutzer et al., 1999). Results of these studies have consistently found that many individuals receiving mental health services (i.e., pharmacological and/or psychosocial interventions) do not receive care that is consistent or conforms with current scientific knowledge and/or accepted practice guidelines. The consequences of these discrepancies—in terms of disability, impaired or lost functioning, and premature death—can be both wide-ranging and far-reaching.

Increasing awareness of the negative consequences associated with inadequate or poor quality mental health treatment has led decision makers in both government and the private sector to formulate and advance a wide range of quality improvement activities. Some of the activities are stimulated by health care purchasers, employers, and government entities, who are interested in holding providers and health systems more accountable for the outcomes of the services they deliver. The growing emphasis on evidence-based practices (Goodheart, Kazdin, & Sternberg, 2006; Wampold, 2001) and the increased use of process assessment and outcomes measurement tools (Herman, 2005) can, in part, be seen as responses to the greater accountability now expected by health plans and other service purchasers. Other activities, such as movement toward broader adoption of electronic health records, are perceived by many as critical to improving both the safety and efficiency of the health care delivery system and integral to achieving the overarching goal of consumer-driven or patient-centered care (IOM, 2006). Still other quality improvement activities, including care coordination efforts and growing attention to workforce development issues, have been advanced by clinicians and administrators who recognize that a trained and competent workforce and improved coordination and care integration are essential to ensuring that the mental health care delivered meets adequate standards of quality (Daniels & Walter, 2002; Hoge, 2002; Pincus, 2003).

A number of recent, high-profile reports focused on the overall health care system (IOM, 2001, 2002, 2003), as well as the mental health system specifically (U.S. Department of Health and Human Services, 1999; IOM, 1997, 2006; New Freedom Commission on Mental Health, 2003), have further accelerated efforts to advance the quality of mental health care in this country. These reports have been instrumental in raising awareness and galvanizing energy and resources to pursue the various quality improvement activities described in the remainder of this chapter.

Evidence-Based Practices

Entire volumes as well as hundreds of journal articles describe and document both research and informed opinion about evidence-based mental health practices: what they are (and are not); how and why they developed; how (and by whom) they should be used; and whether or not their use really improves the quality of services delivered by mental health professionals (Barlow, 1996; Goodheart et al., 2006; Hayes, Barlow, & Nelson-Gray, 1999; Tanenbaum, 2005; Westen, Novotny, & Thompson-Brenner, 2004). It is also probably accurate to assert that, within the mental health field, one's perspective on what qualifies as "evidence-based," and under what circumstances such a practice should be used, depends in part on one's professional role and/or affiliation as a policymaker, service purchaser, program administrator, health services researcher, clinical provider, or consumer/family member.

A basic premise cited by supporters of evidence-based practices is that those needing mental health care are served best by receiving treatments that have been demonstrated through rigorous research and evaluation to consistently produce positive outcomes. Proponents of evidence-based practices further contend that the broader use of these practices by skilled clinicians who are cognizant and incorporate consumer/patient service preferences is a key to improving the overall quality of mental health care in this country (IOM, 2001, 2006; New Freedom Commission on Mental Health, 2003).

While the concept of evidence-based medicine has existed since the middle of the twentieth century, the last two decades have led to enhanced efforts both to synthesize and apply the results of research (i.e., the evidence) in ways that make it more accessible, understood, and utilized by practitioners and the general public. These efforts include the production of systematic reviews (both qualitative and quantitative—or meta-analytic—reviews) and the development of evidence-based practice guidelines and registries of evidence-based programs. Table 4.1 provides a list of some of the most recognized web-based resources for systematic reviews and evidence-based practice guidelines and registries of mental health services.

Despite these and other organized and formal efforts to consolidate, synthesize, review, and rate the quality of evidence for various mental health services, numerous challenges remain in broadly and successfully implementing evidence-based guidelines and treatments into routine clinical and community-based practice settings. Inadequate organizational and/or administrative commitment, limited or insufficient training and/or supervision, lack of attention to implementation with

Table 4.1   Selected Web-Based Resources for Evidence-Based Reviews, Practice Guidelines, and/or Mental Health Services

Resource	Sponsor	Internet Address/URL
Blueprints for Violence Prevention	Department of Justice's (DOJ's) Center for the Study and Prevention of Violence	www.colorado.edu/cspv/ blueprints
Campbell Collaboration	Campbell Collaboration	www.campbellcollaboration. org
Cochrane Collaborative	Cochrane Collaborative	www.cochrane.org
Evidence-Based Practices Implementation Resource Kits	Substance Abuse and Mental Health Services Administration's (SAMHSA's) Center for Mental Health Services	www.mentalhealth.samhsa. gov/cmhs/ CommunitySupport/
Evidence-Based Treatment for Children and Adolescents	American Psychological Association, Division 53	www.effectivechildtherapy. com
Helping America's Youth	Office of the President	http://www.findyouthinfo. gov/
National GAINS Center	Substance Abuse and Mental Health Services Administration's (SAMHSA's) Center for Mental Health Services	www.gainscenter.samhsa.gov/ html/ebps/
National Guideline Clearinghouse	Agency for Healthcare Research and Quality (AHRQ)	www.guideline.gov
National Implementation Research Network	University of North Carolina	http://www.fpg.unc. edu/~nirn/
National Registry of Evidence-based Programs and Practices	Substance Abuse and Mental Health Services Administration (SAMHSA)	www.nrepp.samhsa.gov
Suicide Prevention Resource Center	Substance Abuse and Mental Health Services Administration's (SAMHSA's) Center for Mental Health Services	www.sprc.org Best Practices Registry

fidelity, failure to adapt practices to align and support cultural norms, and general resistance by clinical and support staff have all been cited as factors that can impede or undermine the adoption of evidence-based practices in "real-world" service settings (Aarons, 2006; Fixen, Naoon, Blasé et al., 2005; Isett, Burnam, Coleman-Beattie et al., 2007; McHugo, Drake, Whitley et al., 2007; Nelson & Steele, 2008; Osher & Steadman, 2007; Pazano & Roth, 2006; Torrey, Drake, Dixon et al., 2001). If sustained progress in implementing these practices is to be achieved, it is imperative that both service purchasers and program administrators identify and direct resources to support ongoing efforts to address and overcome these implementation obstacles.

Although inadequate efforts to apply the existing mental health knowledge base are notable and well documented, of equal and perhaps greater concern is the lack of research, or gaps in the evidence-base, in many areas. Limited knowledge is available regarding efficacious and effective treatments for a number of important subpopulations, including children and adolescents, older adults, individuals with co-morbidities, trauma survivors, and various ethnic and cultural minorities (IOM, 2006). These knowledge gaps present significant challenges to the broader adoption of evidence-based practices and arguably support calls to expand research efforts in these areas, as well as expand our collective understanding of what may be acceptable evidence in the absence of formal and/or rigorous studies (Essock, Drake, Frank, & McGuire, 2003; Sternberg, 2006; Tanenbaum, 2006).

As both public and private payers examine mental health service expenditures and attempt to manage and control projected cost increases, it is likely that additional expectations, and perhaps requirements, for the use of evidence-based practices will emerge. To the extent that broader use of these practices is both supported consistently and reimbursed adequately, such efforts may lead to substantial improvements in the overall quality of mental health services available to those in need. However, if efforts by insurers and other purchasers to implement evidence-based practices are overly prescriptive toward clinicians, supported with poor or inconsistent training, and/or reimbursed inadequately, the promise of improved quality through the use of evidence-based practices will remain largely unrealized (see Chapter 2 in this volume for additional information on insurance and financing mental health services).

Quality Measurement and Reporting Infrastructure

The ability to accurately and consistently measure and report changes in health care processes, health outcomes, or both would seem a prerequisite for determining whether quality of care is indeed improving within particular populations and/or settings. In particular, the past two decades have witnessed a great deal of activity among myriad stakeholder groups in the development and promotion of various quality assessment tools and performance measures for both physical and mental health (see Hermann, 2005, for a more detailed description of these activities). However, the lack of coordinated and collaborative efforts to create a quality measurement and reporting infrastructure, particularly within the mental health and substance use fields, has substantially limited progress in the quality improvement arena (Agency for Healthcare Research and Quality [AHRQ], 2003; IOM, 2006). Although a thorough discussion of the factors contributing to the current piecemeal approach to quality measurement and reporting is beyond the scope of this chapter, several issues and related promising activities in this area are noteworthy.

First, a recent Institute of Medicine report, *Improving the Quality of Health Care for Mental and Substance Use Conditions*, describes the necessary components of a measurement and reporting infrastructure and offers recommendations to advance the development and adoption of such a system. The report specifically emphasizes the need to convene relevant stakeholders for the purpose of "reaching consensus on and implementing a common, continuously improving set of mental and substance use health care quality measures for providers, organizations, and systems of care." (IOM, 2006, p. 195). As an influential and authoritative source, the Institute of Medicine recommendations may provide important leverage to organize heretofore disparate and uncoordinated efforts in quality assessment within the mental health and substance abuse fields.

In addition, the federal government has increasingly supported efforts to measure performance and improve organizational and administrative processes that are likely to enhance the quality of care received by individuals with mental and/or substance use disorders. For example, the Substance Abuse and Mental Health Services Administration (SAMHSA) has developed and promoted a core set of National Outcome Measures that are practical in nature (e.g., access to services, retention in treatment, employment, stable housing, social connectedness) and that states and other funding recipients are required to report (Substance Abuse and Mental Health Services Administration [SAMHSA], 2008a). SAMHSA also has partnered with the Robert Wood Johnson Foundation to create the Network for the Improvement of Addiction Treatment (or NIATx) to assist frontline providers in the identification and implementation of process improvements that will increase access to and retention in addiction treatment (Capoccia, Cotter, Gustafson et al., 2007; McCarty, Gustafson, Wisdom et al. 2007). These and other federally sponsored efforts provide an important foundation upon which to further design and build a quality measurement and reporting infrastructure that, while coordinated with the general health care system, will also create learning collaboratives and address the needs of specialty stakeholders within mental health and substance abuse.

Moreover, there is growing recognition of the need to create incentives, particularly financial ones, to assess and reward performance in delivering quality care and achieving desired outcomes (Clarke, Lynch, Spofford, & DeBar; 2006; Patel, Butler, & Wells, 2006). Initial findings from broader "pay-for-performance" initiatives in the general health care sector have been mixed, with some suggesting that they facilitate improvement in one or more quality indicators (Christianson, Leatherman, & Sutherland, 2007), and others purporting that they have not demonstrated measurable quality improvement and may not improve care or contain costs any more effectively than fee-for-service systems (Frieden & Mostashari, 2008). While concerns exist that these pay-for-performance experiments could limit or undermine quality improvement efforts in behavioral health by narrowing the focus of such efforts to only those activities where incentives exist, this remains largely an empirical question to date. Nevertheless, the broader concept of using incentives to leverage quality improvement and other positive changes appears sufficiently promising that the Institute of Medicine report previously noted also included recommendations that government and private purchasers should use mental and substance use quality measures in procurement and accountability processes, as well as "increase the use of funding mechanisms that link some funds to measures of quality" (IOM, 2006, p. 346).

Electronic Health Records

Many experts believe that information technology (IT), and more specifically the widespread adoption of automated medical records, will play an essential role in improving the quality of health care for future generations (IOM, 2001). Despite several decades of attention to developing and promoting the use of electronic health records (IOM, 1991), concerns by consumers and policymakers regarding the privacy and confidentiality of data in these records, the costs to providers for capital investments in IT systems, and the nature of organizational and clinical changes that will be required by these systems have all limited progress in attaining broader use of electronic health records, particularly among mental health and substance abuse providers (IOM, 2001, 2006; Trabin & Maloney, 2003).

Recently, the federal government established an Office (and staff) of the National Coordinator for Health Information Technology within the U.S. Department of Health and Human Services (DHHS) to facilitate coordination and progress in the development of a national health information infrastructure, a foundational component for a system of interoperable electronic health records. Much more information on the mission and work of the Office of the National Coordinator (ONC) is available through the DHHS health information technology Web site at http://healthit.hhs.gov/portal/server.pt. As a major public health and services agency within DHHS, SAMHSA has worked, and will continue to work, closely with both the ONC and a broad group of stakeholders in the mental health and substance abuse fields to ensure that behavioral health needs and priorities are reflected in both the design and functioning of the evolving national health information infrastructure (SAMHSA, 2006).

The degree to which the vision of a national health information infrastructure that contains a dynamic and interoperable system of electronic health records becomes reality will depend largely on the adequate resolution of a number of important policy issues and barriers, including the nature of data standards and reporting requirements; privacy and confidentiality provisions; financial and technical support for adopting organizations and providers; and service and system reimbursement policies and procedures. While many of these issues and barriers are common to both physical and behavioral health practitioners, some of the challenges, as well as some of the potential solutions, are unique to mental health and substance abuse systems and personnel. Thus, it is critical that mental health and substance abuse specialty providers and organizations become involved in major national committees and initiatives seeking to set standards and develop policy in these areas (IOM, 2006). For additional information on mental health informatics, see Chapter 22 in this volume.

Care Coordination

Unfortunately, coordination between mental health and physical health care is more often the exception than the rule within the current health care environment (IOM, 2006). As research has demonstrated, individuals with a mental illness often experience co-occurring substance abuse as well as other co-occurring physical illnesses (Henningsen, Zimmerman, & Sattel, 2003; Katon, 2003; Kroenke, 2003; Mertens, Lu, Parthasarathy, Moore, & Weisner, 2003; Sokol, Messias, Dickerson et al., 2004). Yet, in most cases, different delivery systems exist for addressing these different illnesses, and these systems, and the providers within them, do little to communicate or coordinate with each other regarding the care of particular patients (Friedmann, McCulloch, Chin, & Saitz, 2000; Graber, Bergus, Dawson et al., 2000; Miller, Druss, Dombrowski, & Rosenheck, 2003). At best, this lack of coordination can impede the delivery of appropriate, high quality care; at worst, poor or inadequate coordination contributes to medical errors that can result in disability or even death (IOM, 2006).

The fact that many individuals with mental illness receive treatment in non–health care settings (e.g., schools, human services agencies, jails, and prisons) creates additional challenges regarding appropriate care delivery and coordination (see Chapters 17 and 18 in this volume on school mental health and mental health treatment in criminal justice settings, respectively). Moreover, existing federal and state regulations governing the sharing and/or release of medical information, while important in protecting such sensitive information, may be perceived by providers, accurately or not, as barriers to more effective communication and care coordination.

To date, the most extensive research on collaborative care has focused on the treatment of depression in primary care settings (Bower, Gilbody, Richards, Fletcher, & Sutton, 2006; Gilbody, Bower, Fletcher, Richards, & Sutton, 2006). A meta-analysis of 37 randomized studies including over 12,000 patients by Gilbody and his colleagues documented improvements in depression outcomes through collaborative care relative to standard care that were sustained over a period of several years (Gilbody et al., 2006). Key factors contributing to positive depression outcomes included the use of case managers with a specific mental health background and the provision of regular supervision to these case managers (Bower, Gilbody et al., 2006). Of note, some of these quality improvement interventions (Wells, Sherbourne, Schoenbaum et al., 2000, 2004) have been adapted and proven effective with other conditions including anxiety disorders and bipolar disorder (Roy-Byrne, Craske, Stein et al., 2005; Simon, Ludman, Unutzer et al., 2005). However, given that most of these initiatives occurred within highly organized, well-established, and "resource-rich" care settings, the challenge, and ultimate proof, will be translating these results into more routine (and fragmented) practice environments (Patel et al., 2006).

Realizing the benefits of care coordination for individuals with co-occurring or multiple disorders requires commitment to quality improvement by both organizational leaders and frontline clinicians. Factors that promote care coordination, such as collocation and clinical integration of services, shared medical records, case management, and formal interagency agreements, are often necessary but not sufficient to achieve improved care quality for individuals with complex health needs. Ultimately, the leadership and dedication of both administrative and clinical personnel to greater collaboration and more effective communication on behalf of the patients they jointly serve may prove to be the key ingredient to promoting demonstrable and sustained quality improvement (Pincus, 2003). For additional information on co-occurring addictive and mental disorders, see Chapter 12 in this volume.

Workforce Development

The continued development and maintenance of a well-trained and highly skilled cadre of professionals able to competently and compassionately care for individuals with mental and/or addictive disorders may provide the greatest opportunity, and pose the greatest set of challenges, to improving the overall quality of mental health services in this country. While the tremendous variability in education, training, and practical experience among those providing mental health and substance use services is an asset to addressing the range and nature of the problems of those seeking services, this variability also poses substantial challenges to the development and advancement of core competencies among professionals in the field (Hoge, 2002; Hoge, Tondora, & Marrelli, 2005; Hoge, Paris, Adger, et al., 2005). Moreover, the emergence of consumers and family members into professional roles within the mental health and addictions workforce offers exciting new prospects for enhancing and expanding the array and quality of existing service models, while simultaneously challenging both current professional identities and established patterns of service delivery (Morris & Stuart, 2004).

In general, there is criticism that the education and training of health professionals lags behind advances in the scientific knowledge base and changes in health care delivery (IOM, 2001, 2003). Deficiencies in professional education programs in mental health specifically have been noted, particularly in preparing graduates to understand and employ evidence-based practices and practice guidelines; utilize appropriate quality improvement strategies; and advance multidisciplinary approaches to patient care (Hays, Rardin, Jarvis et al., 2002; Hoge, Jacobs, Belitsky, & Migdole, 2002; Weissman, Verdeli, Gameroff et al., 2006). Moreover, there is inadequate assurance across most disciplinary training programs that students have obtained competencies in specific treatments or select advanced skills (Hoge, Morris, Daniels et al., 2000c). Too often, employers lament that new graduates arrive with limited knowledge and skills and must then learn and apply these missing competencies while on the job.

Similar concerns have been expressed about continuing education. The content of what providers choose to study is often idiosyncratic and usually not subject to oversight or approval by licensing or regulatory bodies (Daniels & Walter, 2002). Moreover, research suggests that the methods commonly used to teach continuing education have little effect on changing clinical practice and appear inconsistent with more successful models of adult learning (Davis, O'Brien, Freemantle et al., 1999; Mazmanian & Davis, 2002). Further, the organizations in which professionals work may encourage the possession of particular competencies, but may lack sufficient resources and capacity to support the actual performance of these competencies in ways that promote meaningful improvements among service recipients (Hoge, Tondora, & Marrelli, 2005; Stuart, Tondora, & Hoge, 2004).

Given the history of "well-intentioned but short-lived workforce initiatives" (IOM, 2006, p. 312) in mental health over the past several decades, it is understandable that those committed to workforce development are cautious in their optimism regarding new efforts in this area. Nevertheless, two hopeful signs are the recent contributions of the Annapolis Coalition and the SAMHSA support for creation of a workforce development resource center Web portal. The Annapolis

Coalition has leveraged initial funding from SAMHSA to develop an organization and infrastructure that is partnering with others to provide technical assistance to state and regional authorities in developing competency standards, career initiatives, and behavioral health workforce strategic plans (Annapolis Coalition, 2008). Similarly, SAMHSA has supported the development of a Workforce Development Resource Center (http://www.workforce.samhsa.gov) to provide a centralized Web site to access 1) an array of workforce development training and technical assistance documents; 2) customized, searchable information on formal and informal education and training opportunities; 3) descriptions of state licensing and continuing educational requirements; and 4) a customized, searchable job registry (with links to other registries) for both existing professionals and individuals interested in entering the mental health and/or substance use fields (SAMHSA, 2008b).

Given the current challenges, it is clear that progress in developing and maintaining an adequate supply of competent, committed, and compassionate behavioral health professionals will require pursuing new strategies for educating and training a range of individuals, including consumers and their family members, as well as the design of new models for organizing, delivering, and financing services that meet or exceed the public's growing expectations for quality care. Individuals and organizations working in isolation are unlikely to make much progress on these issues. Meaningful and sustained solutions to the current workforce challenges facing mental health and substance abuse will require coordinated efforts and shared responsibility (for more information on workforce development in mental health services, see Chapter 5 in this volume).

Implications for Mental Health

As the efforts noted in this chapter suggest, at least several dozen steps have already been taken in the journey toward improving the quality of mental health services in this country. Recent reflections on the progress that has been made over the past 25 years cite greater use of mental health services, shifts toward community-based care, and more understanding, and less stigmatization, of mental illness. However, also noted are challenges that remain, including greater use of evidence-based practices, more progress in integrating mental health with primary health and other sectors, and maximizing the recovery of those with mental illness (Mechanic, 2007) (for additional information on the integration of primary care services with mental health services, see Chapter 16 in this volume).

There is no doubt that our capacity for further advancing on this journey, and the direction in which we travel, will be influenced substantially by economic and political forces that are largely beyond the control of individual stakeholders in mental health or health care in general. At the time of this writing, both a new President and different members of Congress are proposing various approaches to expanding and improving health care. How various political and economic factors will influence the nature and extent of health care reform efforts and how such reform will address quality improvement remains to be seen.

Nevertheless, a key to improving quality lies in the ability of everyone in the mental health field to renew their efforts to publicly emphasize the importance and value of effective mental health services. Interestingly, a recent national survey revealed that two-thirds of Americans reported a basic lack of understanding about the mental health treatment process itself, including a lack of confidence in the outcome(s), a lack of knowledge about how to find the right professional, or not knowing if it is appropriate to even seek help (American Psychological Association, 2008). While potentially discouraging, such results also point to the critical need to disseminate more effectively the existing knowledge about the value and quality of mental health services and the potential that such services have for positively transforming the lives of those with mental illness. Hopefully, the information conveyed in this and other chapters in this volume is sufficient to convince readers of the necessity of taking up this challenge.

Efforts to advance the quality of mental health services are, relatively speaking, quite nascent and fairly circumscribed, so it is difficult at this point to assess their implications for promoting broader systemic changes in our nation's approach to public health or health care delivery. Nevertheless, a few observations are worth sharing.

First, renewed attention to quality improvement in health care generally, and mental health specifically, provides a strong conceptual and organizational framework to what otherwise might be perceived as disparate and possibly resource competitive efforts to advance evidence-based practices, quality measurement, electronic health records, care coordination, and workforce development. While these issues can be pursued as part of a larger and well-coordinated quality improvement agenda in mental health, it is possible and indeed likely that additional progress in these areas, over and above that which might be realized singularly, can be achieved.

Second, it also appears that the limited progress in improving the quality of mental health services in this country is attributable less to a lack of good ideas than to the capacity, determination, and resources to take good ideas to scale. All of the recent high-profile mental health reports previously cited in this chapter are replete with examples of how individuals and organizations have successfully improved services and/or achieved targeted outcomes. However, what largely remains a mystery is how best to translate, adapt, or otherwise transfer (and in some cases, reimburse) these isolated efforts so that similar success can be achieved across broad populations and service settings.

Third, the expansion of mental health services into more general settings such as schools, correctional institutions, social service agencies, and primary care clinics offers additional opportunities to engage those in need of, but who might otherwise not receive, mental health services. If efforts to improve the quality of mental health promotion and treatment in these nontraditional settings are successful, the public health impact of mental disorders in this country could be substantially reduced.

Lastly, while progress in improving the quality and outcomes of mental health services is likely to promote the sustainability (and perhaps the growth) of these services, it is also possible that such efforts may lead to continued reductions in the stigma often associated with receiving mental health services, as well as a greater sense of optimism and hope for recovery among future service recipients.

References

Aarons G. A. (2006). Transformational and transactional leadership: Association with attitudes toward evidence-based practice. *Psychiatric Services*, *57*(8), 1162–1169.

Agency for Healthcare Research and Quality. (2003). *National Healthcare Quality Report*. Rockville, MD: U.S. Department of Health and Human Services.

American Psychological Association. (2008). *Mental Health Treatment: It's Commonly Accepted Yet Not So Easy to Obtain or Understand*. Available online at http://www.medicalnewstoday.com/articles/113905.php. Accessed July 7, 2009.

Annapolis Coalition on the Behavioral Health Workforce. (2008). Available online at http://www.annapoliscoalition.org. Accessed July 17, 2009.

Barlow, D. H. (1996). Health care policy, psychotherapy research, and the future of psychotherapy. *American Psychologist*, *51*, 1050–1058.

Bauer, M. S. (2002). A review of quantitative studies of adherence to mental health clinical practice guidelines. *Harvard Review of Psychiatry*, *10*(3), 138–153.

Beutler, L. E., & Castonguay L. G. (Eds.). (2005). *What Works in Psychology, and Why*. New York: Oxford University Press.

Bower, P., Gilbody, S., Richards, D., Fletcher, J., & Sutton, A. (2006). Collaborative care for depression in primary care. *British Journal of Psychiatry*, *189*, 484–493.

Buchanan, R. W., Kreyenbuhl, J., Zito, J. M., & Lehman, A. (2002). The schizophrenia PORT pharamacological treatment recommendations: Conformance and implications for symptoms and functional outcome. *Schizophrenia Bulletin*, *28*(1), 63–73.

Capoccia, V. A., Cotter, F., Gustafson, D. H., et al. (2007). Making "stone soup": Improvements in clinic access and retention in addiction treatment. *Joint Commission Journal of Quality and Safety*, *33*(2), 95–103.

Christianson, J. B., Leatherman, S., & Sutherland, K. (2007). Paying for quality: Understanding and assessing physician pay-for-performance initiatives. In *The Synthesis Project Policy Brief No. 13*. Princeton, NJ: Robert Wood Johnson Foundation.

Clarke, G., Lynch, F., Spofford, M., & DeBar, L. (2006). Trends influencing future delivery of mental health services in large healthcare settings. *Clinical Psychology: Science and Practice*, *13*(3), 287–292.

Daniels, A. S., & Walter, D. A. (2002). Current issues in continuing education for contemporary behavioral health practices. *Administration and Policy in Mental Health*, *29*(4/5), 359–376.

Davis, D., O'Brien, M., Freemantle, N., et al. (1999). Impact of formal continuing medical education: Do conferences, workshops, rounds, and other traditional continuing education activities change physician behavior or health care outcomes? *Journal of the American Medical Association*, *282*(9), 867–874.

Druss, B. G., Miller, C. L., Rosenheck, R. A., Shih, S. C., & Bost, J. E. (2002). Mental health care quality under managed care in the United States: A view from the Health Employer Data and Information Set (HEDIS). *American Journal of Psychiatry*, *159*(5), 860–862.

Essock, S. M., Drake, R. E., Frank, R. G., & McGuire, T. G. (2003). Randomized controlled trials in evidence-based mental health care: Getting the right answer to the right question. *Schizophrenia Bulletin*, *29*(1), 115–123.

Fixen, D. L., Naoon, S. F., Blasé, K. A., et al. (2005). *Implementation Research: A Synthesis of the Literature*. FMHI pub no. 231. Tampa: University of South Florida, Louis de la Parte Florida Mental Health Institute, National Implementation Research Network.

Frieden, T. R., & Mostashari, F. (2008). Health care as if health mattered. *Journal of the American Medical Association*, *299*(8), 950–952.

Friedmann, P. D., McCulloch, D., Chin, M. H., & Saitz, R. (2000). Screening and intervention for alcohol problems: A national survey of primary care physicians and psychiatrists. *Journal of General Internal Medicine*, *15*(2), 84–91.

Gilbody, S., Bower, P., Fletcher, J., Richards, D., & Sutton, A. (2006). Collaborative care for depression: A cumulative meta-analysis and review of longer-term outcomes. *Archives of Internal Medicine, 166*, 2314–2321.

Gilbody, S., Whitty, P., Grimshaw, J., & Thomas, R. (2003). Educational and organizational interventions to improve the management of depression in primary care: A systematic review. *Journal of the American Medical Association, 289*(23), 3145–3151.

Goodheart, C. D., Kazdin, A. E., & Sternberg, R. J. (Eds.). (2006). *Evidence-Based Psychotherapy: Where Practice and Research Meet.* Washington, DC: American Psychological Association.

Graber, M., Bergus, G., Dawson, J., et al. (2000). Effect of a patient's psychiatric history on physicians' estimation of probability of disease. *Journal of General Internal Medicine, 15*(3), 204–206.

Hayes, S. C., Barlow, D. H., & Nelson-Gray, R. O. (1999). *The Scientist Practitioner: Research and Accountability in the Age of Managed Care* (2nd ed.). Boston: Allyn & Bacon.

Hays, K. A., Rardin, D. K., Jarvis, P. A., et al. (2002). An exploratory survey on empirically supported treatments: Implications for internship training. *Professional Psychology: Research and Practice, 33*(2), 207–211.

Henningsen, P., Zimmerman, T., & Sattel, H. (2003). Medically unexplained physical symptoms, anxiety, and depression: A meta-analytic review. *Psychosomatic Medicine, 65*(4), 528–533.

Hermann, R. C. (2005). *Improving Mental Healthcare: A Guide to Measurement-Based Quality Improvement.* Washington, DC: American Psychiatric Publishing.

Hoge, M. A. (2002). The training gap: An acute crisis in behavioral health education. *Administration and Policy in Mental Health, 29*(4/5), 305–317.

Hoge, M. A., Jacobs, S., Belitsky, R., & Migdole, S. (2002). Graduate education and training for contemporary behavioral health practice. *Administration and Policy in Mental Health, 29*(4/5), 335–357.

Hoge, M. A., Morris, J. A., Daniels, A. S., et al. (2005). Report of recommendations: The *Annapolis Coalition* conference on behavioral health workforce competencies. *Administration and Policy in Behavioral Health, 32*(5/6), 651–663.

Hoge, M. A., Paris, M., Adger, H., et al. (2005). Workforce competencies in behavioral health: An overview. *Administration and Policy in Behavioral Health, 32*(5/6), 593–632.

Hoge, M. A., Tondora, J., & Marrelli, A. F. (2005). The fundamentals of workforce competency: Implications for behavioral health. *Administration and Policy in Behavioral Health, 32*(5/6), 509–532.

Institute of Medicine. (1990). *Medicare: A Strategy for Quality Assurance.* Washington, DC: National Academy Press.

Institute of Medicine (with R. S. Dick & E. B. Steen [Eds.]). (1991). *The Computer-Based Patient Record: An Essential Technology for Health Care.* Washington, DC: National Academy Press.

Institute of Medicine (with M. Edmunds, R. Frank, M. Hogan, D. McCarty, R. Robinson-Beale, & C. Weisner [Eds.]). (1997). *Managing Managed Care: Quality Improvement in Behavioral Healthcare.* Washington, DC: National Academy Press.

Institute of Medicine. (2001). *Crossing the Quality Chasm: A New Health System for the 21st Century.* Washington, DC: National Academy Press.

Institute of Medicine (with J. Eden & B. M. Smith [Eds.]). (2002). *Leadership by Example: Coordinating Government Roles in Improving Health Care Quality.* Washington, DC: National Academy Press.

Institute of Medicine (with J. M. Corrigan & K. Adams [Eds.]). (2003). *Priority Areas for National Attention: Transforming Health Care Quality.* Washington, DC: National Academy Press.

Institute of Medicine. (2006). *Improving the Quality of Health Care for Mental and Substance-Use Conditions.* Washington, DC: National Academy Press.

Isett, K. R., Burnam, M. A., Coleman-Beattie, B., et al. (2007). The state policy context of implementation issues for evidence-based practices in mental health. *Psychiatric Services, 58*(7), 914–921.

Katon, W. (2003). Clinical and health services relationships between major depression, depressive symptoms, and general medical illness. *Biological Psychiatry, 54*(3), 216–226.

Kroenke, K. (2003). Patients presenting with somatic complaints: Epidemiology, psychiatric co-morbidity and management. *International Journal of Methods in Psychiatric Research, 12*(1), 34–43.

Lehman, A. (1999). Quality of care in mental health: The case of schizophrenia. *Health Affairs, 18*(1), 52–65.

Mazmanian, P. E., & Davis, D. A. (2002). Continuing medical education and the physician as learner: Guide to the evidence. *Journal of the American Medical Association, 288*(9), 1057–1060.

McCarty, D., Gustafson, D., Wisdom, J., et al. (2007). The network for the improvement of addiction treatment (NIATx): Strategies to enhance access and retention. *Drug and Alcohol Dependence,* 88(2–3), 138–145.

McGlynn, E. A., Asch, S. M., Adams, J., et al. (2003). The quality of health care delivered to adults in the United States. *New England Journal of Medicine, 348,* 2635–2645.

McHugo, G. J., Drake, R. E., Whitley, R., et al. (2007). Fidelity outcomes in the national implementing evidence-based practices project. *Psychiatric Services, 58*(10), 1279–1284.

Mechanic, D. (2007). Mental health services then and now. *Health Affairs, 26*(6), 1548–1550.

Mertens, J. R., Lu, Y. W., Parthasarathy, S., Moore, C., & Weisner, C. M. (2003). Medical and psychiatric conditions of alcohol and drug treatment patients in an HMO: Comparison with matched controls. *Archives of Internal Medicine, 163*(20), 2511–2517.

Miller, C. L., Druss, B. G., Dombrowski, E. A., & Rosenheck, R. A. (2003). Barriers to primary medical care at a community mental health center. *Psychiatric Services, 54*(8), 1158–1160.

Morris, J. A., & Stuart, G. W. (2004). Training and education needs of consumers, families, and front-line staff in behavioral health practice. *Administration and Policy in Mental Health, 29*(4/5), 377–402.

Nathan, P. E., & Gorman, J. M. (2002). *A Guide to Treatments that Work* (2nd ed.). New York: Oxford University Press.

Nelson, T. D., & Steele, R. G. (2008). Influences on practitioner treatment selection: Best research evidence and other considerations. *The Journal of Behavioral Health Services and Research, 35*(2), 170–178.

New Freedom Commission on Mental Health. (2003). *Achieving the Promise: Transforming Mental Health Care in America; Final Report.* U.S. DHHS Pub. No. SMA-03-3832. Rockville, MD: President's New Freedom Commission on Mental Health.

O'Connell, M. J., Morris, J. A., & Hoge, M. A. (2004). Innovation in behavioral health workforce education. *Administration and Policy in Mental Health, 32*(2), 131–165.

Osher, F. C, & Steadman, H. J. (2007). Adapting evidence-based practices for persons with mental illness involved with the criminal justice system. *Psychiatric Services, 58*(11), 1472–1478.

Patel, K. K., Butler, B., & Wells, K. B. (2006). What is necessary to transform the quality of mental health care. *Health Affairs, 25*(3), 681–693.

Pazano, P. C., & Roth, D. (2006). The decision to adopt evidence-based and other innovative mental health practices: Risky business? *Psychiatric Services, 57*(8), 1153–1161.

Pincus, H. A. (2003). The future of behavioral health and primary care: Drowning in the mainstream or left on the bank? *Psychosomatics, 44*(1), 1–11.

Roy-Byrne, P. P., Katon, W., Cowley, D. S., et al. (2001). A randomized effectiveness trial of collaborative care for patients with panic disorder in primary care. *Archives of General Psychiatry, 58,* 869–876.

Roy-Byrne, P. P., Craske, M. G., Stein, M. B., et al. (2005). A randomized effectiveness trial of cognitive-behavioral therapy and medication for primary care panic disorder. *Archives of General Psychiatry, 62*(3), 290–298.

Simon, G. E., Ludman, E. J., Unutzer, J., et al. (2005). Randomized trial of a population-based care program for people with bipolar disorder. *Psychological Medicine, 35*(1), 13–24.

Sokol, J., Messias, E., Dickerson, F. B., et al. (2004). Comorbidity of medical illnesses among adults with serious mental illness who are receiving community psychiatric services. *Journal of Nervous and Mental Diseases, 192*(6), 421–427.

Sternberg, R. J. (2006). Evidence-based practice: Gold standard, gold plated, or fool's gold? In C. D. Goodheart, A. E. Kazdin, & R. J. Sternberg (Eds.), *Evidence-Based Psychotherapy: Where Practice and Research Meet*. Washington, DC: American Psychological Association.

Stuart, G. W., Tondora, J., & Hoge, M. A. (2004). Evidence-based teaching practice: Implications for behavioral health. *Administration and Policy in Mental Health*, 32(2), 107–130.

Substance Abuse and Mental Health Services Administration. (2006). Electronic records: Health care in the 21st century. *SAMHSA News*, 14(6), 1–4.

Substance Abuse and Mental Health Services Administration. (2008b). *Workforce Development Resource Center*. Available online at http://www.workforce.samhsa.gov. Accessed July 17, 2009.

Substance Abuse and Mental Health Services Administration. (2008a). *National Outcome Measures*. Available online at http://www.nationaloutcomemeasures.samhsa.gov. Accessed July 17, 2009.

Tanenbaum, S. J. (2005). Evidence-based practice as mental health policy: Three controversies and a caveat. *Health Affairs*, 24, 163–173.

Tanenbaum, S. J. (2006). Expanding the terms of the debate: Evidence-based practice and public policy. In C. D. Goodheart, A. E. Kazdin, & R. J. Sternberg (Eds.), *Evidence-Based Psychotherapy: Where Practice and Research Meet*. Washington, DC: American Psychological Association.

Torrey, W. C., Drake, R. E., Dixon, L., et al. (2001). Implementing evidence-based practices for persons with severe mental illnesses. *Psychiatric Services*, 52(1), 45–50.

Trabin, T., & Maloney, W. (2003). Information systems. In S. Feldman (Ed.), *Managed Behavioral Health Services: Perspectives and Practices* (pp. 326–370). Springfield, IL: Charles C. Thomas Publishers.

Unutzer, J., Simon, G., Pabiniak, C., et al. (2000). The use of administrative data to assess quality of care for bipolar disorder in a large staff model HMO. *General Hospital Psychiatry*, 22, 1–10.

Unutzer, J., Katon, W., Williams, J. W., Jr., et al. (2001). Improving primary care for depression in late life. *Medical Care*, 39(8), 785–799.

U.S. Department of Health and Human Services. (1999). *Mental Health: A Report of the Surgeon General*. Rockville, MD: U.S. Department of Health and Human Services, Substance Abuse and Mental Health Services Administration, Center for Mental Health Services, National Institutes of Health, National Institute of Mental Health.

Wampold, B. E. (2001). *The Great Psychotherapy Debate: Models, Methods, and Findings*. Mahwah, NJ: Erlbaum.

Wang, P., Demler, O., & Kessler, R. (2002). Adequacy of treatment for serious mental illness in the United States. *American Journal of Public Health*, 92, 92–98.

Watkins, K. E., Burnam, A., Kung, F-Y, & Paddock, S. (2001). A national survey of care for persons with co-occurring mental and substance use disorders. *Psychiatric Services*, 52(8), 1062–1068.

Weisner, C., Mertens, J., Parthasarathy, S., et al. (2001). Integrating primary medical care with addiction treatment: A randomized controlled trial. *Journal of the American Medical Association*, 286(14), 1715–1723.

Weissman, M. M., Verdeli, H., Gameroff, M. J., et al. (2006). National survey of psychotherapy training in psychiatry, psychology, and social work. *Archives of General Psychiatry*, 63(8), 925–934.

Wells, K., Schoenbaum, M., Unutzer, J., et al. (1999). Quality of care for primary care patients with depression in managed care. *Archives of Family Medicine*, 8, 529–536.

Wells, K. B., Sherbourne, C., Schoenbaum, M., et al. (2000). Impact of disseminating quality improvement programs for depression in managed primary care: A randomized controlled trial. *Journal of the American Medical Association*, 283(2), 212–220.

Wells, K. B., Sherbourne, C., Schoenbaum, M., et al. (2004). Five-year impact of quality improvement for depression: Results of a group-level randomized controlled trial. *Archives of General Psychiatry*, 61(4), 378–386.

Westen, D., Novotny, C. M., & Thompson-Brenner, H. (2004). Empirical status of empirically-supported psychotherapies: Assumptions, findings, and reporting in controlled clinical trials. *Psychological Bulletin*, 130, 631–663.

Chapter 5

WORKFORCE

Rebecca Morris, MPA; and Anne Lezak, MPA

Introduction

There is a widely acknowledged and severe workforce crisis in mental health that is limiting the availability of treatment and undermining the quality and appropriateness of the treatment that is available. Although other health disciplines share some of the same problems, such as an insufficient number of providers, inadequate compensation, an aging workforce and leadership cadre, and inadequate provider diversity, many aspects of the crisis in mental health are unique or unusually widespread (Annapolis Coalition on Behavioral Health Workforce, 2007; Institute of Medicine [IOM], 2006, 2008; Whittier et al., 2006).

Primary among these challenges is a fragmented system of care. Only for behavioral health disorders are there specialty, disorder-specific treatment systems with separate treatment infrastructures and separate financing, despite the fact that most people initially seek treatment outside the specialty system. Numerous efforts have been made to link in various ways the physical health, mental health, and addictions treatment systems, but this triumvirate system of care remains firmly institutionalized (IOM, 2006) (see Chapter 16 in this volume for an additional discussion of integrating primary care with specialty mental health care).

The fragmentation is reflected in the current workforce: trained and inculcated in up to 20 different disciplines, including psychiatry, clinical psychology, clinical social work, counseling, marriage and family therapy, psychiatric nursing, psychosocial rehabilitation, school psychology, applied and clinical sociology, pastoral counseling, and art, music, and dance therapy, among others; with different histories, curricula, competencies, and expectations; with overlapping scopes of practice, but little and often no cross-training; and with a generation of leaders who are being challenged to go beyond their original education and early work histories to move the field in a new direction. This extraordinary degree of fragmentation undermines the ability to meet demands for a transformed mental health system that is consumer centered, grounded in the expectation of recovery, and built on a foundation of evidence-based best practices that generate measurable, quality outcomes. Such efforts are occurring in the face of severe budget cutbacks in many states, high annual turnover rates, and a crisis mentality in many organizations (Annapolis Coalition, 2007; IOM, 2006; Robiner, 2006; Whittier et al., 2006).

In the last decade, a significant number of national, regional, and state surveys; environmental scans; and other reports and studies have defined the nature of the workforce crisis and its implications (see, for example, Annapolis Coalition, 2007; Broadus, Brosh, Hartje, & Roget, 2008; Duffy et al., 2004; Hanrahan, 2004; Hoge, 2002; Hoge & Morris, 2002; Hoge et al., 2005; IOM, 2006; Kaplan, 2003; Landis, Earp, & Libretto, 2002; National Alliance on Mental Illness [NAMI], 2006; National Association of State Mental Health Program Directors [NASMHPD], 2005; President's New Freedom Commission on Mental Health, 2003; Robiner, 2006; U.S. Department of Health and Human Services [USDHHS], 1999; Whittier et al., 2006). These efforts have succeeded, first, in identifying the characteristics of the workforce; second, in defining the nature of the challenges it faces; and third, in reporting the widespread consensus that has emerged about the solutions that are required.

The challenge now is to expand the existing infrastructure so it can support coordination of consistent efforts to implement these solutions among a wide array of institutions over a significant period of time. As the IOM noted in its 2006 study of the mental health and substance abuse workforce:

> Sustained multiyear attention and resources have been applied successfully to the education and training of physicians and nurses . . . A similar sustained, multiyear strategy as well as action by institutions of higher education, licensing boards, accrediting bodies, the federal government, and purchasers, is needed to increase the mental health/substance use disorders workforce's competencies to deliver high-quality care. (IOM, 2006, pp. 287–288)

This chapter provides an overview of the characteristics of the mental health workforce crisis and of efforts to develop such an infrastructure and strategy. It defines the mental health workforce, identifies the challenges in measuring it, and discusses recent trends in its composition. The authors also discuss the challenges in expanding the workforce even as "baby boomers" are beginning to retire, while also improving education and training for provision of consumer-centered, recovery-based systems of care. Finally, this chapter identifies federal, state, and private-sector initiatives that are under way and discusses emerging challenges and implications for mental health policy.

Defining the Mental Health Workforce

Precise definitions of the mental health workforce have been elusive because there is no agreed methodology or consistent infrastructure for collecting consistent data across jurisdictional and disciplinary boundaries, and there are few mechanisms for linking the various data collection initiatives of state agencies, educational institutions, licensing and certification boards, and professional associations, especially on an ongoing basis (Substance Abuse and Mental Health Services Administration [SAMHSA], 2004; Leff et al., 2007; Robiner, 2006). The workforce, as Robiner (2006) noted, is "a chaotic amalgam of separate disciplines with ambiguous boundaries, and overlapping roles and scopes of practice, whose practitioners both collaborate and compete with each other" (p. 603). Even determining the occupations that make up the workforce "is confounded by the fact that differing sources group jobs by differing criteria and descriptions, and use differing occupational names . . . no one source appears to include all of the occupations" (Leff et al., 2007, p. 7).

Estimates of the size of the workforce generally range between 500,000 and 550,000. The most recent definitive estimate was developed for the 2004 edition of *Mental Health, United States,* a comprehensive compendium of data and other information about the mental health field, usually published biennially by the Center for Mental Health Services (CMHS) within SAMHSA and generated by CMHS's mental health statistics program. In that publication, Duffy et al. (2004) drew on a wide array of data sources, including professional associations and licensing and credentialing boards, to estimate conservatively the total number of mental health professionals at 537,857. Differing methodologies and time frames for developing disciplinary data may have resulted in underestimates (Duffy et al., 2004; Robiner, 2006).

At least 20 disciplines have been identified as contributing to the mental health workforce. Five core disciplines are identified by the National Institute of Mental Health and the Health Resources Services Administration (HRSA): psychiatrists; clinical psychologists; clinical social workers; psychiatric nursing specialists; and marriage and family therapists. The study by Duffy et al. (2004) included five additional disciplines: counselors; psychosocial rehabilitation specialists; school psychologists; applied and clinical sociologists; and pastoral counselors. Robiner (2006) identified an additional 10 "related disciplines" that provide a variety of mental health and mental health–related services: art therapists; music therapists; dance therapists; creative arts therapists; occupational therapists; psychiatric aides; recreational therapists; genetics counselors; applied philosophers; and clinical pharmacists. Missing from most surveys is the category of "peer specialists" and other designations for consumers who provide a variety of peer-to-peer specialized services.

In the early to middle part of the 2000s, clinical social workers and counselors were, by far, the two largest clinically trained professional groups providing mental health services (103,128 and 100,533, respectively), followed by psychologists (84,883) and marriage and family therapists (50,158). Some analysts argue that the number of social workers is substantially understated (Scheffler & Kirby, 2003). The last two decades have been marked by a considerable slowing in the growth of the number of psychiatrists and sizable increases in the numbers of social workers, psychologists, and especially direct-service workers. These trends partly reflect the penetration of managed-care systems, which have encouraged increasing reliance on lower-cost professions and an expansion in their scopes of practice, as well as a response to urgent demands for more mental health workers of all types.

The category of "counseling" is often disaggregated to reflect different areas of focus, training, practice settings, professional affiliation, licensing, and certification. For example, the Bureau of Labor Statistics within the U.S. Department of Labor publishes data for counselors in mental health, substance abuse and behavioral disorders, and marriage and family therapy, as well as rehabilitation; educational, vocational, and school; and a miscellaneous category of "other," which includes a significant number of counselors with various types of credentials who address mental health disorders and issues (U.S. Department of Labor, n.d.). Each of these categories includes professionals who are identified in one or more of the categories identified by Duffy et al. (2004) and Robiner (2006), depending upon who is doing the counting.

Often overlooked in the mental health workforce are the estimated 145,000 members of the workforce who have bachelor's degrees or less education and provide support services. They make up an estimated 40–50% of the workforce in many public-sector settings and often are left out of discussions not only about specific needs for education, specialized training, and the application of evidence-based practices, but also discussions about ways to expand the workforce in order to alleviate critical shortages (Annapolis Coalition, 2007; Morris & Stuart, 2002; Robiner, 2006). "The most intensive workforce training is directed at occupations that comprise professional practitioners . . . whereas the least intensive training is given to direct care, non-professional occupations" (Leff et al., 2007, p. 7).

There are no reliable national estimates of the number of consumers and family members in the workforce, whether or not they are formally certified, but widespread efforts are under way to expand consumer roles in mental health systems. One recent and extensive study (National Association of State Mental Health Program Directors [NASMHPD], 2008) highlighted several of these initiatives, including one of the largest, in Arizona, that reflects recent growth across the country. In that state, META Services (now called Recovery Innovations) trained recipients of mental health services to work as peer support providers and graduated 15 peer support specialists in 2000. Today, more than 225 specialists work there in a range of recovery programs, providing more than $6 million of Medicaid-reimbursable services. The expansion of consumer roles reflects ongoing advocacy by consumer organizations as well as federal and state policy and funding of expanded peer services.

As shown in Table 5.1, mental health–related occupations are expected to be among the 20 fastest-growing occupations during the next decade (U.S. Department of Labor, 2008).

However, there still will not be a workforce large enough to meet the general demand for services or sufficiently trained and appropriately located to meet the demand for specialized, research-based services to a variety of populations, including women, members of ethnic minority groups, children, older adults, veterans, rural residents, immigrants, and others (Annapolis Coalition, 2007; Duffy et al., 2004; IOM, 2008; Koppelman, 2004; Mohatt, 2006; Robiner, 2006; Rosen, 2005).

Rural Americans are among the most underserved. More than 60% live in areas designated as mental health professional shortage areas, and more than 65% get their mental health care from physical health providers. Slightly more than 55% of the 3,075 rural counties have *no* practicing psychiatrists, psychologists, or social

Table 5.1 Occupational Outlook for Mental Health Disciplines, 2006–2016

Discipline	2006* Number	Projected 2016* Number	Increase
Mental Health and Substance Abuse Social Workers	122,000	159,000	30,000 24%
Mental Health Counselors	100,000	130,000	30,000 30%
Substance Abuse and Behavioral Disorder Counselors	83,000	112,000	29,000 34%
Counselors, all other	27,000	32,000	4,500 17%
Psychologists (clinical, counseling, and school)	152,000	176,000	24,000 16%
Marriage and Family Therapists	25,000	32,000	7,000 30%

Source: U.S. Department of Labor, Bureau of Labor Statistics. (2008). *Occupational Outlook Handbook (OOH), 2008–09 Edition.* Available from http://www.bls.gov/oco.
* Numbers rounded.

workers (Annapolis Coalition, 2007; Hartley, Hart, Hanrahan, & Loux, 2004; Mohatt, 2006). Historically, there has been a widespread perception that mental health and substance use disorders are less prevalent in rural than in urban and suburban areas, and thus there is less demand for mental health treatment, but several studies have established that these disorders are at least as prevalent; there is, however, less capacity to address them. For example, a 2000 study of substance abuse in midsize cities and rural areas, commissioned by the U.S. Conference of Mayors, produced this very telling set of numbers: Eighth-graders in rural America, compared with those in urban centers, are 83% more likely to use crack cocaine, 50% more likely to use cocaine, 34% more likely to smoke marijuana, 29% more likely to drink alcohol, and 70% more likely to get drunk (National Center on Addiction and Substance Abuse, 2000).

Demographics of the Workforce

As shown in Tables 5.2 and 5.3, the mental health workforce is predominantly White, female, and aging, at a time when the client base is increasingly diverse. Psychiatrists and pastoral counselors are 72% and 68% male, respectively, and only a slight majority of psychologists overall are female (51%), but all other workforce disciplines are predominantly female; the percentages range generally from 70% to more than 90% (Duffy et al., 2004; Robiner, 2006).

A number of studies demonstrate that racial and ethnic minorities achieve better health outcomes when treated by minority providers in race-concordant relationships (and that in many therapeutic situations, women achieve better outcomes when treated by female providers) (Bach, Pham, Schrag, Tate, & Hargraves, 2004; Cooper & Powe, 2004; IOM, 2001). The mental health workforce, however, is overwhelmingly White. Social workers, for example, are 87% White; in clinical counseling, the percentage is 78%; and among marriage and family therapists, the percentage is 92% (Duffy et al., 2004).

Table 5.2 Age Distribution for Selected Mental Health Disciplines, by Sex, for Specified Years

Age	Social Work (2004)		Psychology (2004)		Marriage & Family Therapy (2004)		Counseling (2004)		Psychiatry (2002)		Advanced Practice Psychiatric Nursing (2003)*	
	Female	Male	Female	Male	Female	Male	Female	Male	Female	Male	Female	Male
% under 35	13.7	23.5	8.9	2.8	6.1	6.2	18.2	11.1	3.8	1.5	2.9	4.0
% 45 and older	65.3	76.5	67.0	84.7	79.3	81.2	69.3	76.6	66.5	83.6	65.6	60.2
% 55 and older	26.4	30.1	36.7	57.0	47.0	47.0	45.8	53.0	30.2	57.8	31.6	15.3

Adapted from Duffy et al. (2004), Table 22.2.
* Age unknown: female, 22.8 percent; male, 21.2 percent.

Table 5.3 Race and Ethnicity Distribution for Selected Mental Health Disciplines, by Sex, for Specified Years

Race and Ethnicity	Social Work (2004)		Psychology (2004)		Marriage & Family Therapy (2004)		Counseling (2004)		Psychiatry (2002)		Advanced Practice Psychiatric Nursing (2003)	
	Female	Male	Female	Male	Female	Male	Female	Male	Female	Male	Female	Male
White (not Hispanic)	89.3	85.1	91.8	94.4	92.5	91.3	82.6	80.0	73.8	75.6	80.5	82.4
Black (not Hispanic)	4.2	6.4	2.7	1.6	1.6	2.2	4.2	3.8	4.0	1.9	3.2	2.5
Hispanic	2.6	4.3	2.9	2.2	2.7	2.5	2.1	1.9	4.3	4.5	2.6	1.5
Asian/Pacific Islander	1.1	1.5	2.0	1.4	1.5	1.5	0.8	0.7	13.2	8.8	1.0	1.3

Adapted from Duffy et al. (2004), Table 22.2.

Providing Appropriate, Consumer-Centered, Culturally Competent Treatment

The mental health workforce not only must have sufficient numbers of workers who are appropriately located, but also must be capable of delivering research-based treatments that match the needs of diverse clients. In the last two decades, however, the ability of the workforce to meet those needs has been challenged as the mental health field and its best practices have been redefined, with a resulting need for corresponding shifts in education, training, treatment protocols, and organizational practices.

The research agenda has broadened the frame for examining mental health disorders, demographically and systematically, to identify how different population groups define and respond to mental health disorders, the need for treatment, and types of treatment. The literature now includes a much greater recognition of co-morbidity, mental health, substance abuse, and physical health disorders, and the implications for the primary and specialty health care systems that provide treatment through multiple doors (see Chapter 12 in this volume for more information on co-occurring disorders; see Chapter 9 in this volume on mental disorders in adults; and see Chapter 11 in this volume for more information on alcohol and drug use disorders). Most fundamentally, the literature has established the reality of recovery from mental health disorders and the importance of consumer-centered treatment systems and has defined the practices that support recovery among different population groups (see Chapter 20 in this volume on recovery).

The report of the President's New Freedom Commission on Mental Health in 2003 reflected this expanded research base. In defining a new consensus for the field, it placed consumers at the center of decision making, confirmed a new paradigm for defining best practices, and challenged the workforce to facilitate "transformation" of an existing "patchwork relic" of a system (President's New Freedom Commission, 2003).

While the field has continued to develop the understanding of transformational practices, the development of the workforce to implement them has lagged. For example, in children's mental health, "there is a growing body of knowledge that illuminates which medications and which types of psycho- and behavioral therapies yield the best outcomes for children with a range of mental disorders. Best practices are even being developed for public systems of care that treat children with serious emotional disturbances" (Koppelman, 2004, p. 3). At the same time, there is an acute shortage of "providers trained with the skills necessary to work effectively in a family-centered, community-based, culturally and linguistically competent, and collaborative service delivery model" (National Technical Assistance Center for Children's Mental Health, 2005).

As Koppelman (2004) notes, "it is widely acknowledged that much of how providers are being trained, how they practice, and what is being reimbursed by public and private insurers does not match the strategies that have been found to work" (p. 3). Nearly identical statements about gaps between research and practice can be found in the literature of virtually every specialty in mental health.

Another dramatic shift has been the beginning of efforts to incorporate consumers into the workforce as professionals at all organizational levels: as peer counselors, educators, and advocates; and as independent providers of peer services, in both inpatient and outpatient settings, in order to help ensure consumer-centered care (Chinman et al., 2008; Davidson et al., 1999; Dubois, 2007; NASMHPD, 2008; National Association of Peer Specialists, 2007; Resnick, Armstrong, Sperazza, Harkness, & Rosenheck, 2004). Formal mental health peer specialist training and/or certification programs now operate in most states (NASMHPD, 2008). "Peer Specialist" is the most common title; other titles include Peer Mentor, Peer Counselor, Peer Advocate, Consumer Advocate, Recovery Support Specialist, Recovery Aide, and Peer Bridger.

As former consumers and professional staff members increasingly work side-by-side as colleagues, many in the field are exploring ways to redefine professional–consumer relationships. This announcement for a continuing education course in Pennsylvania reflects some of these issues:

> Whether provider as employer, or peer or non-peer professional as practitioner, all are increasingly aware of the need to evaluate the nature of these newly defined relationships. As peers move from the role of recipient to the role of colleague, as practitioners move from providers of service to colleague, or in some cases supervisor, professional boundaries are an issue that peer specialists and providers will need to address together. ("Professional Boundaries," 2008)

Because the roles and underlying assumptions about consumers in the workforce historically have been very different in the fields of mental health and substance use disorders, these issues can be especially challenging for organizations that provide both types of services and for those addressing co-occurring disorders. See Chapter 19 in this volume for more information on disparities, and see Chapter 12 in this volume for additional discussion on co-occurring addictive and mental disorders.

Aspects of the Workforce Crisis

In the last two decades, general agreement has developed about the central issues that must be addressed in order to develop a mental health workforce capable of meeting emerging needs.

Ongoing Collection of Quality Data

Every researcher who examines the mental health workforce encounters the absence of reliable, high-quality data, comparable across disciplines and geographic boundaries, and collected on an ongoing basis (Annapolis Coalition, 2007; IOM, 2006; Moskowitz, 2007; President's New Freedom Commission, 2003; Robiner, 2006). Despite a number of efforts to improve the capability for data collection, "this information deficit plagues all mental health professions" (Duffy et al., 2004; see further discussion in Robiner, 2006). Snapshots of different parts of the workforce have been assembled by SAMHSA and SAMHSA-funded studies, many states, the

Addiction Technology Transfer Centers, a number of university centers, and several professional associations (for example, SAMHSA, 2002, 2004; Gallon, Gabriel, & Knudsen, 2003; Hogg Foundation for Mental Health, 2007; Iowa Department of Public Health, 2006; Kaplan, 2003; Landis et al., 2002; McRee et al., 2003; North Carolina Department of Health and Human Services, 2008; TriWest Group, 2003; Whitaker, Weismiller, Clark, & Wilson, 2006).

However, each of these studies and others rely primarily on state-level data collection systems that vary tremendously in methodology, degree of consistency, and quality. The lack of mental health data is part of a larger problem regarding general health workforce data. In one study of eight states, selected to represent different population sizes and geographic locations, the author found that "states vary tremendously in the health professions information systems, and responsibility for data collection and analysis typically is divided among various state agencies and organizations . . . Licensing data may be only voluntarily reported, and not all licensing boards collect demographic data" (Moskowitz, 2007, p. 9). Most workforce analyses provide a snapshot of only one moment in time and are project driven, often intended to address current political or budgetary interests. Federally designated Centers for Health Workforce Studies have experienced significant budget cuts and also vary widely in their areas of focus (Moskowitz, 2007).

Missing is an integrated infrastructure that can support ongoing collection of data rigorously and consistently defined. Such efforts have encountered significant difficulties in measuring outcomes in behavioral health, as well as disagreements among disciplines about what should be measured and how. Nevertheless, the absence of these data is a central limiting factor in developing the ability to identify and assess workforce needs and to develop sustained collaborations among relevant stakeholders for addressing workforce challenges (see Chapter 22 in this volume for further discussion on problems associated with data collection and access to national mental health data).

AGING OF THE WORKFORCE AND THE POPULATION

Twin drivers of the workforce crisis are the aging of the workforce, including its leadership cadre, and the aging of the population. Baby-boomer mental health professionals are beginning to retire at the same time that demand for mental services, especially those targeted to the needs of older adults, is beginning an anticipated sharp increase. This is due, in part, to the fact that as the population ages, the incidence and acuity of mental health disorders also increase (about 20% of older adults suffer from one or more mental health disorders [USDHHS, 1999; IOM, 2008]). The aging of the population will cut across all other demographic categories. Between 2005 and 2030, the number of adults age 65 and older will almost double, from 37 million to more than 70 million, and from 12% of the population to more than 20%. It is difficult to foresee any circumstances in which the needs of older adults will not increase substantially. As SAMHSA reported in 2002 for just one mental health indicator, "even if the incidence rate of substance abuse among the elderly in 1995 is assumed to drop by half in 2030, there will be increased demand for treatment" (Korper & Raskin, 2002, p. 8.). Already there is an acute lack of behavioral health professionals trained to address the needs of older adults; the effects can be seen especially in areas of the country with larger older populations (IOM, 2008; Rosen, 2005; President's New Freedom Commission, 2003).

The associated rise in health care expenditures is likely to place additional cost pressures on both private and public health insurers, which in turn will create disincentives for prospective mental health professionals to enter the field. Those already in the workforce may face financial disincentives to geriatric specialization, including a lack of scholarships and other financial support for degree programs and for continuing education. A historic disincentive, a disparity in reimbursement policies, in which Medicare has required a 50% copayment for outpatient mental health services compared with 20% for most other medical services, will be phased out by 2014 (Health Resources and Services Administration [HRSA], 2003; IOM, 2006, 2008; Rosen, 2005; Whittier et al., 2006).

Table 5.2 shows how much the age of the mental health workforce is skewed toward the retirement end of the spectrum. The median age of social workers, the largest single group in the mental health workforce, is 50.5 years (Center for Health Workforce Studies, 2006). At mid-decade, 65.3% of clinically trained female social workers were age 45 or older, and more than a quarter were age 55 or older. In the other major mental health disciplines, the percentages of workers age 45 or older were even higher, up to 79.3%, in the fields of marriage and family therapy. The age distribution is skewed even more significantly for men than for women. The declining proportion of the population between ages 18 and 30 raises concerns about the ability to attract a sufficient number of new workers (HRSA, 2003).

In a major study, IOM (2008) recommended a three-pronged approach to improve health care generally for older adults:

- Enhance the competence of all individuals in the delivery of geriatric care;
- Increase the recruitment and retention of geriatric specialists and caregivers; and
- Redesign models of care and broaden provider and patient roles to achieve greater flexibility (see Chapter 10 in this volume for more information on older adults).

LACK OF EVIDENCE-BASED TEACHING METHODS, TRAINING IN EVIDENCE-BASED PRACTICES, AND CROSS-TRAINING ACROSS DISCIPLINES IN A FRAGMENTED SYSTEM

There is a significant gap between research evidence, training, and clinical practice in mental health. Teaching methods used in schools where behavioral health professionals are trained reflect "little cognizance of the advance that has been made in evidence-based teaching methods and lifelong learning" (IOM, 2006, p. 287). Similarly, Weissman et al. (2006) found that in clinical training programs for psychiatrists, psychologists, and social workers, most required training in new treatments did not meet the "gold standard" of evidence-based teaching methods for learning a new treatment (a combination of didactic program plus clinical supervision), and that the two disciplines with the largest number of students and emphasis on clinical training, professional clinical psychology (PsyD) and social work, had the largest percentage of programs not requiring such methods in any evidence-based therapy.

Available education and training programs generally are not well connected to professional associations, licensing and certification boards, and state mental health departments, and there are few systematic mechanisms for planning and coordinating programs and curricula to identify and meet needs in the field. Such connections could help overcome the traditional segregation among mental health disciplines and facilitate agreements regarding competencies required for practice and identification of what constitutes appropriate evidence in "evidence-based practices." Without such agreements, it is difficult to develop standardized training and especially cross-training in an environment in which people requiring mental health services are more likely to present in physical health care settings than in specialty mental health settings, and the health workforce increasingly is called upon to treat co-occurring physical, mental, and substance use disorders.

The lack of these connections more generally reflects the fragmented system of care for physical and mental health services disorders. Between 50% and 85% of the care for common mental disorders is provided in general medical settings, despite the fact that physical health care providers typically lack specialized training in mental health diagnosis and treatment (SAMHSA, 2008). Individuals with drug use disorders typically are treated in the offices of private physicians or other health care professionals rather than specialty providers (Compton, Thomas, Stinson, & Grant, 2007).

Among the conservatively estimated 5.2 million adults with co-occurring mental health and substance use disorders, only 8.5% receive treatment for both disorders; 38.4% receive treatment for one or the other disorder; and 53% receive no treatment at all (SAMHSA, 2007). Even though they are connected under the general rubric of "behavioral health," few mental health and addictions treatment professionals receive cross-training or have ongoing opportunities to collaborate, and there are different fundamental assumptions within the two sets of disciplines about professional vs. experiential training, evidence-based practices, required competencies, and appropriate approaches to the treatment of co-occurring disorders. One recent study provided a stark example of the clinical impact of this fragmentation. Women with co-occurring depression and addictions told researchers that those who treated them for substance abuse assumed their depression would diminish once they were sober for a long enough period, while those who treated them for depression assumed their drinking would stop once the depression was treated. During the study, only two women received concurrent treatment, and then only after multiple hospitalizations for suicide attempts (Ambrogne, 2007).

Even when professionals do receive appropriate training, "the adoption of best practices [in a clinical environment] requires a stable infrastructure, organizational commitment and staff development" (Whittier et al., 2006), difficult attributes to sustain in an environment of budget cutbacks and understaffed organizations. Indeed, all of these challenges are exacerbated by an extraordinarily complex web of funding streams that make it more difficult to plan effective services and develop the workforce based on need rather than funding availability. Figure 5.1,

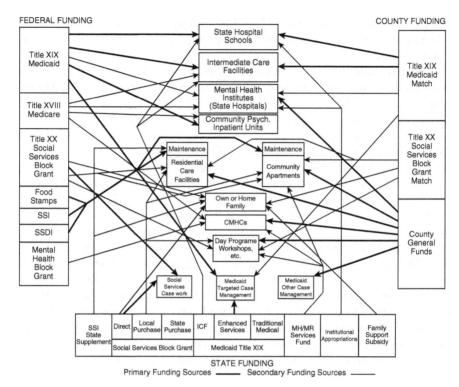

FEDERAL FUNDING

COUNTY FUNDING

STATE FUNDING

Primary Funding Sources ———— Secondary Funding Sources ————

Figure 5.1   Funding Sources for Mental Health Programs in Iowa. (Torrey, E. F. (1996). *Out of the Shadows: Confronting America's Mental Illness Crisis.* New York: John Wiley and Sons. Reprinted with permission from the publisher.)

"Funding sources for mental health programs in Iowa," shows the daunting situation facing program and organizational leaders in just one state.

Recruitment and Retention of Quality Personnel

Recruitment and retention challenges in mental health are similar to those in other health fields but are more acute and broad based. Stigma, low compensation, poorly defined career ladders and lattices, mismatches between demand and supply, inadequate professional development opportunities, and confusion about the roles and responsibilities of the multiple mental health disciplines all combine to deter potential entrants to the field and to generate high rates of frustration, burnout, and turnover. Although the category of "mental health counselors" is among the 10 fastest growing, mental health organizations frequently cite difficulties in finding and keeping qualified counselors and supervisors with the appropriate training in evidence-based, recovery-driven practices. Available data suggest that turnover in behavioral health is more than double the rates in other public health fields, and in some organizations it is as high as 50% (Annapolis Coalition, 2007; Center for Health Workforce Studies, 2006; U.S. Department of Labor, 2008; Whittier et al., 2006).

Public mental health systems for children are just one example of mental health systems experiencing severe workforce shortages. "There's a cry from the children's mental health directors in the states. They're having a terrible time getting qualified people to come and work within the public sector," says Joan Dodge, with the National Technical Assistance Center for Children's Mental Health at Georgetown University (Koppelman, 2004). Ninety percent of states have reported difficulty in recruiting and retaining child welfare case workers (see Chapter 8 in this volume for more information on children and adolescent mental health).

Those who are attracted to mental health and addiction treatment careers often are seeking careers in which they can be of service, and expectations of monetary rewards are relatively modest. Nevertheless, low compensation has been cited repeatedly in various forums and literature as a primary deterrent to new entrants and as a cause of high turnover, especially among those in lower-paying positions (Annapolis Coalition, 2007).

For example, in a 2004 survey of social workers, 71% cited "higher salary" as a factor that might cause them to consider changing jobs, more than any other factor (Center for Health Workforce Studies, 2006). A Texas review of that state's mental health system reported extensive difficulties in recruiting mental health professionals, especially in rural areas. "Social work positions in the mental health area are more difficult to fill than vacancies in other areas of social work. It has been suggested that the problem, at least in urban areas, is not so much a shortage of professionals as having professionals who are willing to work for the salaries offered" (Hogg Foundation for Mental Health, 2007). Especially in the publicly funded state systems, recent budget cuts mean even fewer available resources and an unlikely reduction in salary scale disparities between mental health and other health professions (see Chapter 13 in this volume on state mental health services).

Other financial incentives, such as scholarships, fellowships, and other forms of tuition assistance; loan forgiveness; training stipends; and paid internships, have dropped sharply in the last 25 years. Federal support for professional training in mental health has fallen from a high of $117 million in 1972 to about $1 million in 2007 (Annapolis Coalition, 2007).

Virtually all surveys of recruitment and retention challenges have recommended similar sets of strategies to bring qualified people to the field and reduce turnover rates. These include expansion of evidence-based training in community and four-year colleges; financial incentives for both initial and continuing education; development of new curricula and degree programs and use of technology to deliver training; expansion of the candidate pool to include nontraditional sources, such as paraprofessionals, veterans, and others; recruiting consumers and family members to the workforce; developing early pipelines among younger students and explicit career pathways; using marketing campaigns to highlight career opportunities in mental health and to counteract stigma; clarifying the competencies, skills, and attitudes required for particular positions; ameliorating stress and burnout; streamlining administrative duties so professionals can focus on service; and expanding mentoring and appropriate supervision to enhance performance and opportunities for advancement (see, for example, Annapolis Coalition, 2007; Center for Health Statistics, 2006; Hogg Foundation for Mental Health, 2007; North Carolina Department of Health and Human Services, 2008; Northeast Addiction Technology

Transfer Center, 2004; Taylor, Larson, Hewitt, McCulloh, & Sauer, 2007; TriWest Group, 2003; Whittier et al., 2006).

Initiatives are hampered by the fragmented system of care, which is characterized by multiple competing disciplines and an absence of well-established connections among higher-education institutions, professional associations, and licensing boards that can pursue joint strategies. A recent IOM report recommends establishment of a Council on the Mental and Substance Use Health Care Workforce to, among other priorities, develop national competency and licensing standards to be adopted by licensing boards, accrediting bodies, and purchasers (IOM, 2006).

In one example of a coordinated state recruitment initiative, California academic and professional groups collaborated to devise a "Ladder of Learning" for social work education, which "systemically demonstrates how one could move through community college certificates or degrees, to baccalaureate education and on to graduate education, including post graduate certificates, licensure, and attainment of a doctoral degree" (Black, Buckles, & Ryan, 2006, p. 14). The group recommends that the "Ladder of Learning" be incorporated into workforce development as early as high school, along with the various levels of higher education in California.

Similarly, several reports recommend that marketing campaigns be extended throughout the educational system in order to combat stigma and prepare students to hear messages about potential careers in mental health. "It is also important to give students early, positive and clear images of the field to counter negative stereotypes and misperceptions they may have developed or encountered. Educational efforts should begin as early as elementary school, continuing through middle school and high school" (Whittier et al., 2006).

Stress, burnout, and compassion fatigue routinely rank high among reasons for leaving the workforce. Retention strategies have incorporated expanded opportunities for training and professional development—especially for direct-care staff, who often lack specialized education—and encouragement of strong staff support networks, opportunities for recognition, and celebrations of excellence (Annapolis Coalition, 2007; Skinner and Roche, 2005). Improved training and support for new supervisors also can reduce turnover, which often is attributed to poor relations with existing supervisors (North Carolina Department of Health and Human Services, 2008).

CULTURALLY COMPETENT CARE

There is growing recognition of the need to increase the cultural diversity of the mental health workforce and to ensure that all its members understand and can address the needs of various populations (HRSA, 2006). Table 5.3 shows that the mental health workforce is overwhelmingly White. Only among female psychiatrists does the percentage of White workers fall below 75% (73.8%). In counseling and advanced-practice psychiatric nursing, the percentage of White workers is in the lower 80s, but in the remaining disciplines, it is above 90%. There remains an acute lack of behavioral health professionals among minority groups, including among Hispanics in areas with fast-growing Hispanic populations.

Ethnic minorities typically have received less care, poorer care, and care that is not culturally competent (USDHHS, 2001). Although the research base showing best practices for different populations has expanded dramatically in recent years, there is a significant lag in translating research to practice (IOM, 2006; Balas & Boren, 2000).

Increasing the number of minority mental health providers is key to improving access to quality mental health care for consumers from ethnic minority groups. In both physical and mental health care, race-concordant relationships between provider and consumer tend to result in better care (Saha & Shipman, 2006). "Because of the greater need for cultural sensitivity in dealing with mental health issues, extensive issues of trust, and the increasing language barrier between provider and patients, disparities in the workforce may count for more disparities in mental health than general health care" (Miranda, McGuire, Williams, & Wang, 2008, p. 1105).

In 2007, SAMHSA asked the National Alliance of Multi-Ethnic Behavioral Health Associations (NAMBHA) to coordinate development of a National Network to Eliminate Disparities in Behavioral Health (NNED). After extensive discussions among stakeholders, the resulting "Blueprint" document for the Network (National Alliance of Multi-Ethnic Behavioral Health Associations [NAMBHA], 2008) identified priority areas and strategies. Many recommendations apply broadly to the workforce and reflect priorities among most stakeholders addressing workforce development. For example, the plan recommends significantly expanding "the number of competent and diverse individuals within all levels of the behavioral health workforce"; developing early pipelines, especially in minority communities; expanding the use of technology in training; improving compensation; increasing financial incentives for training; and highlighting "current career ladder initiatives for natural leaders (natural helpers, promotora/es, etc.) that are funded and built into the structure of state and local behavioral health authorities, colleges and universities, etc." (NAMBHA, 2008, p. 19).

Additionally, the following initiatives and strategies are among those in the plan:

- Expand the capacity of the workforce within communities by developing cultural broker, promotoras/es, cultural case management, and other liaison models, and develop career development and permanent funding streams for these workers.
- Aggressively collect, analyze, and disseminate data profiling problems and challenges that groups of color face in entering behavioral health professions and training.
- Require licensure and certification competencies in cultural and linguistic competencies for all sectors of the workforce. Support generalist training that includes broad characteristics of shared experiences of underserved populations (racism, oppression, poverty, and relation to behavioral health problems and well-being, etc.) for all behavioral health professionals and those studying to enter the field.
- Create culture-specific training programs.
- Accumulate, promote, and disseminate approaches to recruitment and retention of groups of color into behavioral health professions in higher education and entry/retention in the behavioral health workforce.

- Create recognition, awards, and other incentives for public, non-profit, and private-sector innovators who increase workforce diversity and develop effective training programs.
- Develop pathways for those who have been trained in their countries of origin in behavioral health but who cannot practice in this country due to certification and licensure restrictions (see Chapter 19 in this volume on mental health disparities).

"Cultural competency" also refers to an understanding of the wide variety of cultural factors that influence consumer needs and help determine effective treatment. An aging workforce with inadequate opportunities for continuing education, strained professional development budgets, and lags in effectively translating research to clinical best practices has resulted in ineffective, irrelevant, or mismatched treatment for older adults; children; people from rural areas; women, especially those with histories of trauma; people who are homeless; veterans; and others. In the face of such barriers, many people go untreated.

For example, civilian mental health providers generally are unfamiliar with military culture and experience but are being asked to treat large numbers of veterans returning from wars in Afghanistan and Iraq, especially those from National Guard units who often lack realistic access to military care. Providers may, for the first time, have caseloads that include a number of individuals with post-traumatic stress disorder that has resulted from combat, rather than from sexual assault or other traumas with which civilian providers may be more familiar, and they often lack training to understand the special needs of veterans. Although there is widespread recognition of the problem and initiatives by some professional associations and colleges, the scope of these effort's initiatives has not been large enough to match the problem.

CONSUMERS IN THE WORKFORCE

Consumers have an enormous role to play, both in expanding the size of the available workforce and in providing services that they are uniquely qualified to provide. Experience as a person in recovery has long been respected in substance use disorders practices, but inclusion of former or current consumers as program staff is a more recent development in mental health. A growing number of state and local mental health authorities are recognizing the tremendous potential of peer support and realizing that consumers and family members are an undertapped resource.

In a number of states, peer training programs have become well-respected avenues to employment in community-based and inpatient mental health programs. Consumers often work in designated peer support positions, providing consumers with support, advocacy, and counseling. However, peers can be found in nearly every capacity: as organizational leaders, crisis intervention specialists, case managers, educators, and transition specialists, or "Peer Bridgers," helping people leaving hospitals to become established in the communities (Bluebird, 2008).

Also important are efforts to ensure that supervisors, non-consumer professional staff, and consumers can transition from previous relationships to accept each other as colleagues. Increasingly, consumers and family members are providing training to the mental health workforce, both as part of professionals' academic curricula and through ongoing professional development efforts at the state and agency levels. Including people in recovery in the role of trainers and educators is an important step in building a more recovery-oriented workforce, while enhancing the recovery orientation of organizations enhances the ability of traditional staff to value the role of peer providers. Additionally, more mental health professionals are revealing that they are former consumers.

Consumers increasingly are operating stand-alone consumer-run services, which many consumers see as valuable resources. Some use them as adjuncts to traditional mental health services, whereas others prefer to rely exclusively on self-help centers. They range from informal drop-in centers to comprehensive programs providing employment and housing services, recreational facilities, and a range of classes and workshops. Although rigorous evaluations are just now being undertaken, early assessments indicate that consumer-operated programs contribute to participants' recovery and sense of well-being (Campbell et al., 2006) (see Chapter 20 in this volume on recovery).

Service Delivery Impacts

The continuing workforce shortage is reflected in the national figures of mental health service use. Similar to past findings, the 2007 National Survey on Drug Use and Health (SAMHSA, 2007) reported that less than half of the 24.3 million adults experiencing serious psychological stress, including 2 million adults with diagnosable serious mental illnesses, received mental health services. Least likely to access mental health services were young adults age 18 to 25 with serious psychological distress, only 29.4% of whom received services.

Of this number, 10.9 million reported unmet needs for mental health care, with nearly half of those, 5.4 million, receiving no services at all. An estimated 1 in 10 persons with substance use disorders receives specialty treatment, and only one in four receives some type of treatment or assistance.

The unavailability of treatment is due to several factors. In many cases, the problem is financial; even when care is available, insurance coverage for care is limited. This results in part from the historic lack of insurance parity between mental and physical health conditions (due to end in January 2010), but also from the patchwork of funding mechanisms that providers must use to fund their services; these sources and mechanisms determine what conditions are covered, which people can be treated, and by which providers. In the National Survey on Drug Use and Health, more than half (54.5%) of those not receiving needed mental health care said they could not afford the cost or that their insurance coverage was insufficient (SAMHSA, 2007).

The uneven distribution of mental health professionals among geographic areas (IOM, 2006) contributes to lengthy delays in treatment, especially in rural and semirural areas. Half of rural counties have no mental health professionals at all (Annapolis Coalition, 2007), and states and organizations have faced significant barriers in attempting to recruit even some of the providers necessary to fill the needs.

The number of minority providers in rural areas is especially low, and continuing education and professional development in culturally competent practices may be even less available than in more urban areas with greater concentrations of academic facilities. In certain practice areas, acute shortages are a problem nearly everywhere in the country. This includes geriatric practitioners; child, youth, and family specialists, especially those versed in treating adolescents with substance use disorders; and professionals trained in addressing co-occurring mental health and substance abuse issues.

Consumers are ill served by this combination of unavailable or limited services, uneven geographic coverage, and limited funding mechanisms, and there are frequent mismatches between what agencies provide and what consumers need. For example, too many agencies are limited to providing acute treatment; they are unable to serve those with moderate needs—people who, untreated, may end up in crisis. Agencies deliver services and hire providers that their funding streams support, which does not always match community needs. Consumers often receive uncoordinated, inefficient care; for example, individuals with co-occurring mental health, substance abuse, and/or physical health needs are treated by two or more systems, by providers versed only in single specialties, often with little coordination or even communication among providers (IOM, 2006).

The results are long waiting lists, treatment that is inappropriate for a consumer's condition, or care that is lacking in cultural competence. In the face of all these barriers, individuals who initially reach out for help often retreat back into the ranks of the untreated. (SAMHSA, 2007) (see Chapter 7 in this volume on the epidemiology of mental disorders and Chapter 14 in this volume on community mental health).

Policy Issues

Mental health financing policies and the lack of rigorous standards and training requirements across mental health-related disciplines are the two main sets of constraints limiting the ability to create an adequately staffed, well-prepared, and responsive mental health workforce.

The financing policy issues fall into two broad areas. First, funding streams tend to reflect their political roots and bureaucracies of origin more than carefully planned, well-coordinated strategies that focus on identified needs. Providers then are left to sort through the resulting maze and cobble together treatment resources that make sense for their communities. Second, infusion of more resources into workforce development is desperately needed on the front end of the pipeline so that these resources provide incentives for people to enter the field, especially in areas of acute need, and in order to strengthen the capabilities of the current workforce.

Multiple unconnected funding streams, such as the situation in Iowa pictured in Figure 5.1, are typical. Although mental health leaders recognize the imminent need to strengthen the workforce, reimbursement is overwhelmingly directed at services, not service improvement. The services that can be offered, the providers who can provide them, and the consumers who can receive them are all dictated by often conflicting regulations, limitations, and requirements. A significant amount of the typical publicly funded agency's budget is spent dealing with "administrivia": determining and proving eligibility, submitting reimbursement forms, and myriad other record-keeping tasks.

Publicly funded entities are assembling multiple funding sources simply to stay afloat and are looking for ways to reduce all but the most essential expenditures. Rather than comprehensive staff development programs, mental health authorities and agencies look for opportunities to do training on the cheap, such as one-shot workshops: practices that do not reflect the research on effective evidence-based training methods. Few resources are devoted to the vital issue of building skills in supervisors and agency leaders. Quality improvement programs tend to be scattershot and symbolic. As the Annapolis Coalition reported in 2007, there exists "a propensity to do what is affordable, not what is effective" (p. 68) (see Chapter 2 in this volume on financing mental health services).

Increasing the quantity and improving the quality of the workforce mostly depends upon developing vibrant pipelines that attract new people to the field and offer substantial financial support for professional training. Although current federally funded programs such as minority fellowships and loan forgiveness programs do make a difference, they address only a fraction of the need. Experts have identified the general areas of acute need (recognizing that there are regional and even local variations): more minority providers and those who can speak a second language; more rural providers, particularly in specialty areas; more staff trained to work with children and adolescents, older persons, and those with dual diagnoses of mental illness and substance use disorders; and more general practitioners with training in screening and identification of mental health and substance use problems (IOM, 2006). A concerted public/private initiative is needed to strengthen the pipelines and ensure that funding is available for the many potential providers whose ability to complete training significantly hinges on the availability of loan forgiveness programs, grants, or scholarships. These newly minted professionals then can be deployed in the areas where they are most needed, as payback for their publicly supported education.

Workforce development is also hampered by the multiple approaches to training, certification, and licensing used by the numerous mental health and substance use treatment disciplines, and they vary by jurisdiction. The great number of disciplines, the disparate training programs with great variation from state to state and even institution to institution, and the lack of national standards for training, licensing, and accreditation make it difficult, if not impossible, to assess and improve the quality of mental health and substance use services and to undertake efforts to match the appropriate providers with recognized needs. As recommended in the 2006 IOM study, national leadership is needed to identify clinical competencies, develop national standards for credentialing and licensing, and ensure close coordination between education programs and the professional disciplines in mental health and substance use treatment. Key to this effort will be incorporating evidence-based practices throughout training programs, so that research is effectively translated into practice throughout all disciplines.

Recognizing the tremendous benefits to be gained, some states are moving ahead with ambitious efforts to develop statewide standards and bolster educational requirements. A key feature of Connecticut's Workforce Development Plan is curriculum, faculty, and individual course development based upon collaboration between higher education, the state mental health agency, and professional and consumer stakeholders. Ohio has created 10 Coordinating Centers of Excellence, which are training, technical assistance, consultation, and research partnerships between the state mental health agency and universities. Among the Centers are "Integrated Dual Disorder Treatment," "Illness Management and Recovery," and "Center for Learning Excellence." (California Social Work Education Center, 2005; Ganju, 2008). Federal policy makers can draw from these and other efforts across the country to develop rational and robust policies and funding mechanisms.

Federal, State, and Provider Initiatives

The federal government, primarily SAMHSA, the states, and the professional associations, have major initiatives under way to expand and enhance the mental health workforce, but these initiatives are often not well coordinated.

Since the early 2000s, SAMHSA has funded a series of workforce surveys and special studies that together have provided the primary basis for understanding the characteristics of the workforce and the scope of the crisis (Annapolis Coalition, 2007; Duffy et al., 2004; Kaplan, 2003; Landis et al., 2002; Whittier et al., 2006). In 2006, SAMHSA launched the Behavioral Health Workforce Development Initiative to coordinate a wide array of activities aimed at further expanding the knowledge base regarding workforce development activities throughout the country, enhancing recruitment and retention, developing and disseminating workforce competencies, and assembling and disseminating information and resources that have been scattered and not easily accessible. Central to the initiative is the planned development of a Workforce Development Resource Center Web Portal (http://www.samhsa.gov/matrix2/matrix_workforce.aspx), a national clearinghouse of behavioral health workforce information and the hub of an information infrastructure to support stakeholders and professionals in the field as they pursue workforce development at the individual, organizational, state, and regional levels.

In collaboration with the National Institute of Mental Health, HRSA, and professional associations, SAMHSA has an ongoing program to expand the scope and quality of workforce data collection and publishes such data biennially (Duffy et al., 2004).

SAMHSA has also funded a series of grants and special programs, especially the Transformation State Incentive Grant Program and various leadership development programs, designed to help states transform their mental health systems; most programs involve some evaluation of the mental health workforce and/or workforce development activity. SAMHSA also funds a significant number of technical assistance centers that often are housed at and/or affiliated with universities and draw on their resources; the National Technical Assistance Center for Children's Mental Health at Georgetown University and several of the 14 regional Addiction Technology Transfer Centers are examples. These centers are a primary locus of national research-to-practice initiatives and often serve as conveners of stakeholders to develop regional workforce development collaborations.

With or without federal funding, a significant number of states, for example, California, Colorado, Connecticut, Iowa, Maryland, North Carolina, and Texas, have conducted surveys of their mental health workforces and identified central issues that need to be addressed. Several have adopted special incentives, such as scholarships and loan repayment programs, to encourage more people to enter the field. Others have developed ongoing collaborations with universities, new certifications for specialized mental health practitioners, training and certification programs for peer specialists, and other initiatives (see, for example, Bacon & Stallings, 2003; Eisenberg, Bellows, & Brown, 2005; Flaum, 2006; Hogg Foundation for Mental Health, 2007; Iowa Department of Human Services, 2008; Iowa Department of Public Health, 2006; National Alliance on Mental Illness, 2006; North Carolina Department of Health and Human Services, 2008; TriWest Group, 2003; University of California, 2003; Workgroup on Cultural Competency and Workforce Development for Mental Health Professionals Act, 2007). By most accounts, however, these efforts are often hampered by restricted funding and especially by recent budget cutbacks.

Since the early part of this decade, the overwhelming majority of states have initiated efforts to assess, analyze, and respond to general health care workforce shortages, typically in response to acute shortages of physicians and/or nurses. As a result, there is a developing infrastructure and capability at the state level to address workforce development in health care, especially in the areas of data collection, pipeline development, retention, licensing and credentialing, and educational capacity building. Although this infrastructure can be applied to the mental health field, only a few states have funded active, ongoing mental health programs; instead, most such programs are funded by SAMHSA (Moskowitz, 2007).

In his 2007 examination of state activities, Moskowitz found a lack of comprehensive planning, divided responsibility for workforce activities, a frequent absence of political leadership, and diffuse areas of focus, with most activities designed to respond to immediate crises. Nevertheless, he concluded that "new cross-professions approaches to the health workforce are emerging, which will enable states to look beyond current crises and address broader emerging trends and concerns" (Moskowitz, 2007, p. 15).

Some state-level activity has focused on the roles of licensing and certification boards, especially in expanding the scope of practice for certain disciplines in order to increase overall capacity (Duffy et al., 2004; Moskowitz, 2007; National Alliance on Mental Illness, 2006). However, most states have few relationships among licensing boards, higher education, state agencies, and professional associations to align strategies across platforms for establishing competencies in evidence-based practices and expanding the workforce (Weissman, et al., 2006) (see Chapter 13 in this volume on state mental health agencies).

Provider associations have conducted surveys of their members and have been a primary medium for disseminating evidence-based practices to the field and for providing continuing education and training to their members. The National Council for Community Behavioral Healthcare; The National Association of Social Workers; NAADAC, the Association for Addiction Professionals; and others have developed an array of initiatives that include certification programs, several types of leadership training and development, mentoring, e-learning, Listservs, publications, and other initiatives. Provider associations have also been key advocates of additional federal and state funding for workforce development.

Future Challenges

QUALITY DATA

Every significant investigation of the mental health workforce dilemma has concluded that, whatever the specific course of future initiatives, they must be sustained at a high level in a consistent manner over a significant period of at least a decade, and very likely longer (for example, Duffy et al., 2004; Hogg Foundation for Mental Health, 2007; IOM, 2006; Moskowitz, 2007). At the root of these initiatives must be a significantly enhanced system for collecting, analyzing, and disseminating comparable quality data about the workforce, and, most importantly, on an ongoing basis (Duffy et al., 2004; IOM, 2006, Moskowitz, 2007; Robiner, 2006).

After presenting the most comprehensive picture of the mental health professions then available, and surveying significant efforts since at least 1998 to upgrade the workforce data, Duffy et al. (2004) noted that:

> Given the severe consequences of psychiatric disability, it is essential that relevant policy makers work together to improve the quality of information available on human resources in mental health . . . Since definitive information about the availability of clinically active providers in local communities and the forces contributing to their locations is not identifiable from State data, policy makers cannot ascertain from the present data the information they need to determine the amount and kinds of service they must provide to consumers in local areas. (p. 298)

Following a survey of the Texas mental health workforce in 2007, the Hogg Foundation identified the five types of information required

> to undertake effective workforce development in the state, including 1) standardized and reliable supply and demand data for each professional type; 2) an examination of the potential functions that consumers and family members can provide within the workforce; 3) an inventory and analysis of existing community and state recruitment and retention activities, including those targeting different cultural groups; 4) an evaluation of higher education and continuing education content and teaching methods and their relationship to state licensing standards in light of the evidence on effective practices provided by recent research; and 5) an analysis of higher education's capacity within the mental health professions to increase the supply of graduates. (p. 17)

Moskowitz (2007) called for "a comprehensive, up-to-date repository of health workforce data that compiles information from all relevant agencies" (p. 9) and is available to federal and state policymakers, researchers, local planning agencies, mental health organizational leaders, consumers, and other stakeholders.

Among the areas of need he cited are the number, demographics, and geographic distribution of licensed professionals; vacancy rates; retention and turnover rates; compensation trends; inter- and intrastate migration; availability of education programs in states and regions; enrollment and graduation rates in general education and training programs; enrollment and graduation rates in programs that train for specialized services; special populations; and employment of consumers in both inpatient and outpatient settings and the services they provide.

Although data on these issues are available from snapshot surveys, there is no infrastructure to establish a consistent set of well-defined data that can be collected on an ongoing basis. One initiative in that direction is a planned national survey by the national office of the Addiction Technology Transfer Centers that is intended to provide the foundation for ongoing data collection from multiple sources in the addictions treatment field.

PARITY

In late 2008, the Paul Wellstone and Pete Domenici Mental Health and Addiction Equity Act of 2008 was passed by the U. S. Congress. This "Parity Act" came into effect on January 1, 2010, and will help equalize insurance coverage of physical, mental health, and addiction disorders. It will also have far-reaching implications for provider organizations and individual professionals as they seek to realize the benefits of parity in the context of a health care market dominated by managed-care systems, one in which the majority of individuals seek mental health care from physical health care providers rather than in the specialty treatment systems (SAMHSA, 2004).

One possible outcome of the Parity Act that is being discussed informally, but with some urgency, within provider groups is an acceleration of efforts to integrate physical health, mental health, and substance abuse treatment systems, perhaps driven by a desire by health insurance plans to rationalize and minimize their costs in administering a parity system. Such a market outcome not only would put new demands on the workforce but would also run headlong into the long-standing, widely recognized challenges associated with integration, including distinctive philosophies and approaches to treating mental health and substance use disorders in different settings; separate education and training systems; separate revenue streams and financing mechanisms; an absence of provider cross-training; and poorly developed care structures to support treatment of co-occurring disorders (see, for example, Kautz, Mauch, & Smith, 2008; National Council for Community Behavioral Healthcare [NCCBH], 2002) (see Chapter 2 in this volume on insurance for mental health services).

CONTINUING ACUTE SHORTAGES

At a time of growing demands to transform mental health systems by doing more and doing it better, there are not enough mental health professionals to do it, period, and the shortages are likely to get worse in the near term. Mental health professionals have sought to adopt recruitment and retention strategies from other fields that have faced shortages, such as nursing and teaching, as well as to identify solutions to meet the specific needs of mental health practitioners. Policy makers seeking to invest in the best strategies have a wealth of options, but few of them to date have been well funded, and mental health organizations and practices routinely identify lack of funding as a primary barrier to expansion of the workforce.

Especially instructive may be an examination of strategies developed in rural settings, where shortages of mental health professionals are especially acute and individuals therefore must seek treatment predominantly from physical health care systems and from hospital-based providers. Mohatt (2006) identified the following strategies to enhance rural capacity: improved supervision to nurture existing staff and promote retention, distance learning targeted at enabling rural residents to learn from providers in rural settings, developing a formal mid-level provider strategy to extend a limited doctoral-level workforce, enhanced access to telehealth technology to support training and care delivery, and new reimbursement models to enhance the marketplace.

Diversity of the Workforce

The growing demographic mismatch between the mental health workforce and people in need is likely to be exacerbated by the aging of the population (see Chapter 10 in this volume on older adults) and growing ethnic diversity. There is in particular a growing gap between the number of Hispanic consumers and providers (IOM, 2004). Every major report on workforce development highlights the importance of recruiting more people who share the ethnic and cultural background of the people being served. Language is a continuing barrier, and finding providers who are bilingual, as well as interpreters for those individuals who speak languages that are not common in their communities, is a key requirement for a workforce that can respond effectively to population diversity.

Increasingly, policy makers understand that diversity extends beyond race and ethnicity. Congruency between service provider and recipient means increasing the number of providers with rural backgrounds in rural settings; those who identify themselves as lesbian, gay, bisexual, or transgendered to work with clients similarly identified; seasoned older practitioners to whom elderly consumers can readily relate, and so on.

Promoting a diverse workforce requires devoting energy and resources to the issue. Pipelines for ethnic and cultural minorities need to be developed and nurtured, starting as early as middle school, with marketing, mentoring, and financial support, all of which are important strategies. Recognizing this, a number of state mental health authorities have invested in minority recruitment. As of 2004, 21 states had initiatives to recruit and train members of minority groups, ethnic groups, or other special populations to work in public mental health. Ten states had staff recruitment initiatives for Blacks/African Americans, seven for Hispanics, six for Asians, five for Native Americans, and four for Pacific Islanders. Additionally, a number of states had implemented staff training programs directed at minority staff (Lutterman, Mayberg, & Emmett, 2004).

Leadership development efforts within federal and state agencies and local provider organizations can help to ensure that organizational decision makers reflect increasing ethnic and cultural diversity. Thoughtful recruitment and retention strategies can attract and keep staff who represent and are sensitive to "diversity" in the broadest sense. Building a diverse workforce is congruent with another important workforce goal: increasing the role of consumers. Training and hiring people who have "been there" and can readily relate to the experiences and backgrounds of service recipients is another strategy to ensure a workforce that is able to relate and respond to the needs of consumers from diverse backgrounds (see Chapter 19 in this volume on mental health disparities).

Research to Practice: Adoption of Evidence-Based Practices

The well-documented lag between development of evidence-based practices and widespread teaching and use of these practices (Balas & Boren, 2000) is exacerbated by several factors. One of the primary barriers is training at every level, which is "too often governed by traditions and intuitive beliefs that are neither grounded in theory nor empirically justified" (Stuart, Tondora, & Hoge, 2004, p. 108). A particular challenge is that those in the front lines, who generally have the least education, also tend to receive the least amount of in-service training resources. Without effective channels to get current best practices into the hands of those carrying out the direct services, it is unrealistic to expect that evidence-based practices will become the norm.

Institutional habits are hard to break, and academia, government, and the professional disciplines must collaborate to ensure that training curricula and practice change to reflect current research. A recent report reviewed the findings on effective workforce development strategies to promote evidence-based practices in mental health and concluded, "Moving to evidenced-based training for evidence-based practices will take careful planning, changes in policy, and resources to implement those changes" (Leff et al., 2007, p. 49). The authors offered six key recommendations that could help guide this effort nationally. These include, in brief:

1. A study that identifies a taxonomy of mental health occupations, the number of workers in each of them, and their workforce development needs;
2. A comprehensive review of mental health occupational competencies, including an assessment of the extent to which competencies cover the requirements for implementing evidence-based practices; this should be followed by competency revisions by multi-stakeholder groups as called for;
3. Development of research protocols that can be used to identify the most effective and efficient training strategies;
4. Increased resources devoted to evaluating workforce development strategies, coordinated with SAMHSA's evaluation of implementation of the SAMHSA Evidence-Based Practice KITS, national workforce development plans, and federal and state mental health transformation efforts;

5. A review of workforce development evaluations that expand focus on study methods and outcomes, with the results disseminated nationally (perhaps through the National Registry of Evidence-Based Programs and Practices); and

6. Partnerships of a broad range of consumer, provider, and academic stakeholders at the federal, state, and local levels to collaborate on development and implementation of evidence-based training strategies (see Chapter 15 in this volume for more information on evidence-based practice and evidence-based medicine).

Implications for Mental Health

The mental health field has been redefined in the last two decades. A new consensus has identified and characterized the consumer-centered, recovery-based systems of care that can provide the most effective support and treatment for mental health consumers. The research base has expanded beyond the historic use of middle-class White males as proxies and identified the strengths and needs of various populations. Federal and state agencies, professional associations, researchers, and other stakeholders have identified the ways in which the workforce at all levels must be transformed and expanded in order to meet consumer needs, as well as the barriers that undermine the recruitment, training, retention, and professional development of such a workforce. Federal, state, and private-sector initiatives not only have made strides in improving the workforce, but also have helped to highlight the philosophical frictions, absence of institutional connections, and inadequate policies that limit the success of these initiatives.

As IOM and numerous researchers have noted, the challenge now for all stakeholders is to sustain a consistent, multiyear effort across geographical, organizational, and disciplinary boundaries so that these widespread activities do not merely reflect the political and budgetary opportunities of the moment but succeed in achieving a lasting transformation of the workforce.

References

Ambrogne, J. A. (2007). Managing depressive symptoms in the context of abstinence: Findings from a qualitative study of women. *Perspectives in Psychiatric Care, 43*(2), 84–92.

Annapolis Coalition on Behavioral Health Workforce. (2007). *An Action Plan For Behavioral Health Workforce Development: A Framework for Discussion*. Rockville, MD: Substance Abuse and Mental Health Services Administration.

Bach, P. B., Pham, H. H., Schrag, D., Tate, R. C., & Hargraves, J. L. (2004). Primary care physicians who treat blacks and whites. *New England Journal of Medicine, 351*, 575–584.

Bacon, T. J., & Stallings, K. D. (2003). Workforce demands of mental health reform. *North Carolina Medical Journal, 64*(5), 231–232.

Balas, E. A., & Boren, S. A. (2000). Managing clinical knowledge for health care improvement. In J. Bemmel & A. McCray (Eds.), *Yearbook of Medical Informatics* (pp. 65–70). Stuttgart, Germany: Schattauer Publishing Company.

Black, J., Buckles, B., & Ryan, J. (2006). *Partners in Transformation: Innovative Solutions to the Mental Health Workforce Crisis*. Available online at http://www.llu.edu/pages/grad/socialwork/documents/mhincswepres2006.pdf. Accessed March 2, 2009.

Bluebird, G. (2008). *Paving New Ground: Peers Working in In-Patient Settings*. Alexandria, VA: National Association of State Mental Health Program Directors.

Broadus, A., Brosh, J., Hartje, J., & Roget, N. (2008). *Workforce Annotated Bibliography*. Reno, NV: Center for the Applications of Substance Abuse Technologies.

California Social Work Education Center Mental Health Initiative. (2005). *Development of the Mental Health Competency Document*. Available online at http://calswec.berkeley.edu/CalSWEC/MH_Competency_develop.pdf. Accessed March 2, 2009.

Campbell, J., Lichtenstein, C., Teague, G., Johnsen, M., Yates, B., Sonnefeld, J., et al. (2006). *The Consumer-Operated Services Program (COSP) Multisite Research Initiative Final Report*. Saint Louis, MO: Coordinating Center at the Missouri Institute of Mental Health.

Center for Health Statistics. (2006). *Recruitment and Retention of Health Care Providers in Underserved Communities in Texas*. Austin: Texas Department of State Health Services, Health Professions Resource Center.

Center for Health Workforce Studies. (2006). *Licensed Social Workers in Behavioral Health, 2004*. Washington, DC: Author.

Chinman, M., Hamilton, A., Butler, B., Knight, E., Murray, S., & Young, A. (2008). *Mental Health Consumer Providers: A Guide for Clinical Staff*. Santa Monica, CA: Rand Corporation.

Compton, W. M., Thomas, Y. F., Stinson, F. S., & Grant, B. F. (2007). Prevalence, correlates, disability, and co-morbidity of DSM-IV drug abuse and dependence in the United States: Results from the national epidemiologic survey on alcohol and related conditions. *Archives of General Psychiatry, 64*, 566–576.

Cooper, L. A., & Powe, N. R. (2004). *Disparities in Patient Experiences, Health Care Processes, and Outcomes: The Role of Patient-Provider Racial, Ethnic, and Language Concordance*. New York: The Commonwealth Fund.

Davidson, L., Chinman, M., Kloos, B., Weingarten, R., Stayner, D., & Tebes, J. K. (1999). Peer support among individuals with severe mental illness: A review of the evidence. *Clinical Psychology, 6*(2), 165–187.

Dubois, J. (2007). Hands Across Long Island, Inc. opens the first peer run clinic in the nation. Available online at http://www.hali8.org/?c=128&a=1176. Accessed October 1, 2009.

Duffy, F. F., West, J. C., Wilk, J., Narrow, W. E., Hales, D., Thompson, J., et al. (2004). Mental health practitioners and trainees. In R. W. Manderscheid & J. T. Berry (Eds.), *Mental Health, United States, 2004*. DHHS Publication No. SMA 06-4195. Rockville, MD: Substance Abuse and Mental Health Services Administration.

Eisenberg, D., Bellows, N., & Brown, N. (2005). *Measuring Mental Health in California's Counties: What Can We Learn*. Berkeley: University of California, Berkeley School of Public Health.

Flaum, M. (2006). *Iowa's Mental Health System*. Available online at http://www.medicine.uiowa.edu/icmh/archives/documents/Consumerempowermentconference.pdf. Accessed March 2, 2009.

Gallon, S., Gabriel, R., & Knudsen, J. (2003). The toughest job you'll ever love: A Pacific Northwest treatment workforce survey. *Journal of Substance Abuse Treatment, 24*(3), 83–196.

Ganju, V. J. (2008). *Mental Health Workforce Development Initiatives: Models for Future Action*. Paper presented at the meeting of the Dialogues on Behavioral Health Conference, New Orleans, LA.

Hanrahan, N. (2004). *Crisis in the Mental Health Workforce: The State of the Advanced Practice Nurse Workforce*. Abstract No. 2094. Available online at http://gateway.nlm.nih.gov/MeetingAbstracts/ma?f=103625128.html. Accessed March 2, 2009.

Hartley, D., Hart, V., Hanrahan, N., & Loux, S. (2004). *Are Advanced Practice Psychiatric Nurses a Solution to Rural Mental Health Workforce Shortages?* Working Paper No. 31. Portland: University of Maine, Edmund S. Muskie School of Public Service, Maine Rural Health Research Center Institute for Health Policy.

Health Resources and Services Administration. (2003). *Changing Demographics and the Implications for Physicians, Nurses, and Other Health Workers*. Rockville, MD: Author. Available online at http://bhpr.hrsa.gov/healthworkforce/reports/changedemo/default.htm. Accessed March 2, 2009.

Health Resources and Services Administration. (2006). *The Rationale for Diversity in the Health Professions: A Review of the Evidence*. Rockville, MD: U.S. Department of Health and Human Services.

Hoge, M. A. (2002). The training gap: An acute crisis in behavioral health education. *Administration & Policy in Mental Health, 29*(4/5), 305–317.

Hoge, M. A., & Morris, J. A. (2002). Guest editors' introduction. *Administration & Policy in Mental Health, 29*(4/5), 297–303.

Hoge, M. A., Paris, M., Adger, H., Collins, F. L., Finn, C. V., Fricks, L., et al. (2005). Workforce competencies in behavioral health: An overview. *Administration and Policy in Mental Health, 32*(5/6), 593–631.

Hogg Foundation for Mental Health. (2007). *The Mental Health Workforce in Texas: A Snapshot of the Issues*. Available online at http://www.hogg.utexas.edu/PDF/TxMHworkforce.pdf. Accessed March 2, 2009.

Institute of Medicine. (2001). *Crossing the Quality Chasm*. Washington, DC: National Academy Press.

Institute of Medicine. (2004). *In the Nation's Compelling Interest: Ensuring Diversity in the Health Care Workforce*. Washington, DC: National Academy Press.

Institute of Medicine. (2006). *Improving the Quality of Health Care for Mental Health and Substance-Use Conditions*. Washington, DC: National Academy Press.

Institute of Medicine. (2008). *Retooling for an Aging America: Building the Health Care Workforce*. Washington, DC: National Academy Press.

Iowa Department of Human Services. (2008). *Strengthening Iowa's Mental Health and Disability Services: Building and Sustaining Competencies*. Available online at http://www.dhs.state.ia.us/mhdd/docs/MHDSCenterforClinicalCompetenceSUMMARY.pdf. Accessed March 2, 2009.

Iowa Department of Public Health, Center for Health Workforce Planning Bureau. (2006). *Iowa's Mental Health Workforce*. Available online at http://www.idph.state.ia.us/hpcdp/common/pdf/workforce/mentalhealth_0306.pdf. Accessed March 2, 2009.

Kaplan, L. (2003). *Substance Abuse Treatment Workforce Environmental Scan*. Cambridge, MA: Abt Associates.

Kautz, C., Mauch, D., & Smith, S. A. (2008). *Reimbursement of Mental Health Services in Primary Care Settings*. DHHS Publication No. SMA-08-4324. Rockville, MD: Substance Abuse and Mental Health Services Administration, Center for Mental Health Services.

Koppelman, J. (2004, October 26). *The Provider System for Children's Mental Health: Workforce Capacity and Effective Treatment*. Issue Brief No. 801. Washington, DC: The George Washington University, National Health Policy Forum.

Korper, S. P., & Raskin, I. E. (2002). The impact of substance use and abuse by the elderly: The next 20–30 years. In S. Korper & L. Carol (Eds.), *Substance Use by Older Adults: Estimates of Future Impact on the Treatment System* (p. 8). Rockville, MD: Substance Abuse and Mental Health Services Administration, Office of Applied Studies.

Landis, R., Earp, B., & Libretto, S. (2002). *Report on the State of the Substance Abuse Treatment Workforce in 2002: Priorities and Possibilities*. (Available from Danya International, Inc., 8737 Colesville Road, Suite 1100, Silver Spring, MD 20910)

Leff, H. S., Leff, J. A., Chow, C., Cichocki, B., Phillips, D., & Joseph, T. (2007). *Evidence-Based Workforce Development Strategies for Evidence-Based Practices in Mental Health*. Cambridge, MA: Abt Associates.

Lutterman, T., Mayberg, S., & Emmet, W. (2004). State mental health agency implementation of the New Freedom Commission on Mental Health goals: 2004. In Substance Abuse and Mental Health Services Administration, *Mental Health, United States, 2004*. DHHS Publication No. SMA 06-4195. Rockville, MD: Substance Abuse and Mental Health Services Administration.

McRee, T., Dower, C., Briggance, B., Vance, J., Keane, D., & O'Neil, E. H. (2003). *The Mental Health Workforce: Who's Meeting California's Needs?* San Francisco: University of California, San Francisco, Center for the Health Professions, California Workforce Initiative.

Miranda, J., McGuire, T. G., Williams, D. R., & Wang, P. (2008). Mental health in the context of health disparities. *American Journal of Psychiatry, 165,* 1102–1108.

Mohatt, D. (2006). *Rural and Frontier Children's Mental Health Workforce Development.* Paper presented at the meeting of the National Association of State Mental Health Program Directors, Children, Youth and Families Division, Subcommittee on Leadership and Workforce. Available from the Western Interstate Commission for Higher Education by contacting Dennis Mohatt at dmohatt@wiche.edu.

Morris, J. A., & Stuart, G. W. (2002). Training and education needs of consumers, families and front-line staff in behavioral health practice. *Administration and Policy in Mental Health, 29*(4/5), 359–376.

Moskowitz, M. C. (2007). *State Actions and the Health Workforce Crisis.* Washington, DC: Association of Academic Health Centers.

National Alliance on Mental Illness. (2006). *Grading the States: A Report on America's Health Care System for Serious Mental Illness.* Available online at http://www.nami.org/content/navigation menu/grading_the_states/full_report/full_report.htm.

National Alliance of Multi-Ethnic Behavioral Health Associations. (2008). *Blueprint for the National Network to Eliminate Disparities in Mental Health.* Washington, DC: Author.

National Association of Peer Specialists. (2007). Peer specialist compensation/satisfaction: 2007 survey report. Available online at http://www.naops.org/id22.html. Accessed March 2, 2009.

National Association of State Mental Health Program Directors. (2005). *Mental Health Transformation Survey* [Data file]. Available online at http://www.nasmhpd.org/general_files/publications/tta_pubs/QuarterlyTransformationreport042605.pdf.

National Association of State Mental Health Program Directors, Office of Technical Assistance. (2008). *Paving New Ground: Peers Working in In-Patient Settings.* Available online at http://www.nasmhpd.org/general_files/publications/ntac_pubs/BluebirdGuidebookFINAL041508.pdf. Accessed March 2, 2009.

National Center on Addiction and Substance Abuse. (2000). *No Place to Hide: Substance Abuse in Mid-Size Cities and Rural America.* New York: Author.

National Council for Community Behavioral Healthcare. (2002). *Behavioral Health/Primary Care Integration: The Four-Quadrant Model and Evidence-Based Practices.* Rockville, MD: Author.

National Technical Assistance Center for Children's Mental Health. (2005, February). *Transforming the Workforce in Children's Mental Health.* Washington, DC: Georgetown University Center for Child and Human Development. Available online at http://www.annapoliscoalition.org/pages/images/Transforming_the_Workforce_in_Childrens_Mental_Health.pdf.Accessed March 2, 2009.

North Carolina Department of Health and Human Services. (2008). *Workforce Development Initiative.* Available online at http://www.ncdhhs.gov/mhddsas/statspublications/reports/workforcedevelopment-4-15-08-initiative.pdf. Accessed March 2, 2009.

Northeast Addiction Technology Transfer Center. (2004, January). *Workforce Development Summit: Taking Action to Build a Stronger Addiction Workforce.* Pittsburgh, PA: Author.

President's New Freedom Commission on Mental Health. (2003). *Achieving the Promise: Transforming Mental Health Care in America.* DHHS Publication No. SMA-03-3832. Rockville, MD: U.S. Department of Health and Human Services.

Professional boundaries in the peer specialist/provider relationship: Identifying challenges and finding solutions. (2008, October 24). Continuing Education program sponsored by the University of Pittsburgh Presbyterian-Shadyside, Western Psychiatric Institute and Clinic, Office of Education and Regional Programming, and the Mercer County Behavioral Health

Commission. Available from the University of Pittsburgh by contacting Joanne Slappo at slappojm@upmc.edu

Resnick, S. G., Armstrong, M., Sperazza, M., Harkness, L., & Rosenheck, R. A. (2004). A model of consumer-provider partnership: Vet-to-vet. *Psychiatric Rehabilitation Journal*, *28*(2), 185–187.

Robiner, W. N. (2006). The mental health professions: Workforce supply and demand, issues, and challenges. *Clinical Psychology Review*, *26*, 600–625.

Rosen, A. L. (2005, January 24). *Testimony to the Policy Committee of the White House Conference on Aging: The Shortage of an Adequately Trained Geriatric Mental Health Workforce.* Available online at http://www.whcoa.gov/about/policy/meetings/summary/rosenwhcoa testimony.pdf. Accessed March 2, 2009.

Saha, S., & Shipman, S. A. (2006). *The Rationale for Diversity in the Health Professions: A Review of the Evidence.* Rockville, MD: Health Resources and Services Administration, Bureau of Health Professions.

Scheffler, R. M., & Kirby, P. B. (2003). The occupational transformation of the mental health system. *Health Affairs*, *22*(5), 177–188.

Skinner, N., & Roche, A. M. (2005). *Stress and Burnout: A Prevention Handbook for the Alcohol and Other Drugs Workforce.* Adelaide, Australia: National Centre for Education and Training on Addiction.

Stuart, G. W., Tondora, J., & Hoge, M. A. (2004). Evidence-based teaching practice: Implications for behavioral health. *Administration and Policy in Mental Health*, *32*(2), 107–130.

Substance Abuse and Mental Health Services Administration (SAMHSA). (2002). *Mental Health, United States, 2002.* DHHS Publication No. SMA04-3938. Rockville, MD: U.S. Department of Health and Human Services.

Substance Abuse and Mental Health Services Administration. (2004). *Mental Health, United States, 2004.* DHHS Publication No. SMA 06-4195. Rockville, MD: U.S. Department of Health and Human Services.

Substance Abuse and Mental Health Services Administration, Office of Applied Studies. (2007). *Results from the 2007 National Survey on Drug Use and Health: National Findings.* DHHS Publication No. SMA 08-4343, NSDUH Series H-34. Rockville, MD: Author. Available online at http://www.oas.samhsa.gov/NSDUH/2k7NSDUH/2k7results.cfm.

Substance Abuse and Mental Health Services Administration, Office of Applied Studies. (2008). *The 2007 National Survey on Drug Use and Health.* Rockville, MD: Author.

Taylor, M., Larson, S., Hewitt, A., McCulloh, N., & Sauer, J. (2007). *National Training Institute for Frontline Supervisors (NTIFFS): Final Report.* Minneapolis: University of Minnesota, Research and Training Center on Community Living, Institute on Community Integration.

TriWest Group. (2003). *The Status of Mental Health Care in Colorado.* Denver, CO: Mental Health Funders Collaborative.

University of California, San Francisco, the Center for the Health Professions. (2003). *Demand Likely to Outstrip Available Mental Health Workforce in California, UCSF Researchers Find.* Available online at http://www.futurehealth.ucsf.edu/press_releases/CWImental.html. Accessed March 2, 2009.

U.S. Department of Health and Human Services (USDHHS). (1999). *Mental Health: A Report of the Surgeon General.* Rockville, MD: Substance Abuse and Mental Health Services Administration & National Institutes of Health, National Institute of Mental Health.

U.S. Department of Health and Human Services. (2001). *Mental Health: Culture, Race, Ethnicity Supplement to "Mental Health; A Report of the Surgeon General."* Rockville, MD: Substance Abuse and Mental Health Services Administration & Office of the Surgeon General.

U.S. Department of Labor, Bureau of Labor Statistics. (2008). *Occupational Outlook Handbook (OOH), 2008–09 Edition.* Available online at http://www.bls.gov/oco

U.S. Department of Labor, Bureau of Labor Statistics. (n.d.). Occupational employment statistics. Available online at http://www.bls.gov/OES

Weissman, M. M., Verdeli, H., Gameroff, M. J., Bledsoe, S. E., Betts, K., & Mufson, L., et al. (2006). National survey of psychotherapy training in psychiatry, psychology, and social work. *Archives of General Psychiatry, 63,* 925–934.

Whitaker, T., Weismiller, T., Clark, E., & Wilson, M. (2006). *Assuring the Sufficiency of a Frontline Workforce: A National Study of Licensed Social Workers; Special Report; Social Work Services in Behavioral Health Care Settings.* Washington, DC: National Association of Social Workers.

Whittier, M., Bell, E. L., Gaumond, P., Gwaltney, M., Magana, C. A., & Moreaux, M. (2006). *Strengthening Professional Identity: Challenges of the Addictions Treatment Workforce.* Cambridge, MA: Abt Associates.

Workgroup on Cultural Competency and Workforce Development for Mental Health Professionals Act, Maryland H.B. 524, 7lr2400, Regular Session (2007). Available online at http://mlis. state.md.us/2009rs/bills/hb/hb0524f.pdf. Accessed March 2, 2009.

PART II

SELECTED POPULATIONS AND TREATMENT SETTINGS

Section A

At-Risk Populations

Chapter 6

ADDRESSING THE GLOBAL BURDEN OF MENTAL DISORDERS: THE WHO WORLD MENTAL HEALTH SURVEY INITIATIVE

Philip S. Wang, MD, DrPH; Sergio Aguilar-Gaxiola, MD, PhD;
Jordi Alonso, MD, PhD; Sing Lee, MB, BS, FRCPsych; Tevfik Bedirhan
Üstün, MD; Ronald C. Kessler, PhD; for the
WHO World Mental Health Survey Consortium

Introduction

Surveys of mental disorders have been conducted within countries since the end of World War II (Hagnell, 1966; Langner & Michael, 1963; Leighton, 1959). However, conducting such efforts cross-nationally has been a more difficult task due to the inconsistent application of methods for making diagnoses. The development in the 1980s of the first psychiatric diagnostic interview designed for use by lay interviewers, the landmark Diagnostic Interview Schedule (DIS), dramatically changed this situation (Bland, Orn, & Newman, 1988). The advent of the DIS allowed psychiatric epidemiologists to conduct a series of parallel surveys in a number of countries (Bland et al., 1988; Hwu, Yeh, & Chang, 1989; Lépine et al., 1989; Robins & Regier, 1991). These, in turn, provided the opportunity to conduct among the first comparative analyses of results across nations that are a central focus of the present day World Health Organization (WHO) World Mental Health (WMH) Survey Initiative (Weissman et al., 1997; Weissman, Bland, Canino, Faravelli et al., 1996; Weissman et al., 1994; Weissman, Bland, Canino, Greenwald et al., 1996). The DIS also gave rise to the subsequent Composite International Diagnostic Interview (CIDI) and other methodologic developments now employed in surveys throughout the world (Andrade, de Lolio, Gentil, Laurenti, & Werebe, 1996; Andrade, Walters, Gentil, & Laurenti, 2002; Bijl, van Zessen, Ravelli, de Rijk, & Langendoen, 1998; Caraveo, Martinez, & Rivera, 1998; Kessler et al., 1994; Kýlýç, 1998; Vega et al., 1998; Wittchen, 1998) (see Chapter 7 in this volume on the epidemiology of mental disorders).

These earlier cross-national comparisons, based upon the DIS and CIDI, first revealed important findings that have since been confirmed in the WMH surveys, including that over one-third of respondents typically meet criteria for a lifetime mental disorder (WHO International Consortium of Psychiatric Epidemiology, 2000) and that most respondents with mental disorders failed to receive treatment (Alegria, Bijl, Lin, Walters, & Kessler, 2000; Bijl et al., 2003). However, legitimate concerns have been raised with such results, including that many mental disorders may be self-limited or mild and that treating them would not be possible in even the most economically advantaged countries (Regier et al., 1998; Regier, Narrow, Rupp, Rae, & Kaelber, 2000). Unfortunately, the initial DIS and CIDI surveys were primarily designed to estimate the prevalence rather than the seriousness of disorders, and investigators have had to create post-hoc measures of disorder severity. Secondary analyses of early surveys using such measures have found that while as many as one-half of mental disorders were mild, use of mental health services was consistently correlated with the severity of and disability from disorders. Furthermore, between one-third to two-thirds of the most serious cases failed to receive treatment (Bijl et al., 2003; Narrow, Rae, Robins, & Regier, 2002).

The ongoing WMH Survey Initiative represents a major expansion of these earlier cross-national efforts, which were typically limited to a few developed countries. WMH surveys are being carried out within countries in every geographic region of the world, as well as at every level of economic development, markedly increasing the proportion of the world's population on which the Initiative can shed new light. The WMH Survey Initiative was explicitly designed to provide a high degree of coordination and therefore improve the validity of cross-national comparisons. WMH surveys also improve upon other limitations in earlier cross-national DIS and CIDI efforts. Specifically, they have addressed the lack of rigorous measurement of disorder severity, and they distinguish between disorder severity, and the related construct of disability (i.e., the negative consequences of a disorder on one's daily life). Unlike earlier DIS and CIDI efforts, the WMH surveys also contain standardized questions about treatment and allow for the assessment of the adequacy of treatments received.

In the remainder of this chapter, the authors will first discuss some of these overarching issues in the Methodologic Considerations section. The authors then present readers with major findings to date from the WMH surveys in the Emerging Results section. A final important goal of the WMH Survey Initiative is to provide some of the first available data for policymakers on both the mental health needs of their citizenry as well as how to successfully address them. So throughout this chapter and particularly in the final sections on Implications and Future Directions, the authors consider how the WMH Survey Initiative can be used by a variety of stakeholders to help inform their decisions regarding mental health policy, financing, resource allocation, treatment programs, and other services.

Methodologic Considerations

General Design Issues

One overarching purpose of the WMH surveys is to describe patterns in the occurrence of mental disorders and service use over a period of time. The choice of the length of period over which to make assessments involves several considerations. Respondents' recent experiences (e.g., within the past 30 days) have been one focus, in part to minimize biased retrospective recall of events (Jenkins et al., 1997; Shiffman, Stone, & Hufford, 2008; Stone & Broderick, 2007). However WMH surveys also assess respondents' experiences over longer periods (e.g., the prior year and one's lifetime) even though the ability to accurately recall generally decreases with the length of the recall interval. This has been possible because some types of assessments may be less vulnerable to biased recall than others when made over longer periods. For example, respondents may be more able to recall lifetime hospitalizations for depression or lifetime suicide attempts than more numerous or less vividly recalled events such as the number of days over a lifetime that a particular symptom of depression was present. Therefore, the general approach for minimizing recall bias used in the WMH surveys has been to include detailed questions about experiences in the past 30 days, less detailed questions about experiences in the past 12 months, and even less detailed questions about experiences occurring over an entire lifetime.

Another important feature of the WMH Surveys is that they are, for the most part, cross-sectional and, as such, not ideal for studying changes over time. Yet how things are changing over time is often of particular interest and relevance to policymakers. To meet these challenges, the cross-sectional WMH surveys can be expanded to include new samples for monitoring aggregate population changes (i.e., trend surveys), repeated surveys on the same respondents to study within-person changes (i.e., panel surveys), or both (i.e., mixed panel–trend surveys). Country-specific WMH efforts, such as the National Comorbidity Survey (NCS) in the United States, are being expanded in one or more of these ways. The longitudinal nature of these expanded WMH surveys will provide stakeholders the prospective data needed to make inferences. However, even in WMH countries limited to baseline cross-sectional data collections, additional methodologic features should make it possible to draw inferences from retrospective reports about temporal patterns. For example, special question wording sequences and memory-priming probes were developed to facilitate complete recall and accurate dating of events. These made it possible to conduct the analyses of lifetime prevalences, age-of-disorder-onset, and delays in initial treatment seeking presented in the Emerging Results section of this chapter.

A final issue to keep in mind about the WMH Surveys is that they are naturalistic (observed phenomena) rather than experimental. For this reason, they may not be optimal for answering questions about cause-and-effect relationships that, again, are often asked by policymakers. As a result, WMH survey results should be carefully interpreted, and any relationships observed in the analyses should be treated as descriptive associations rather than causal. Nonetheless, WMH survey findings can identify promising targets for both further study and more definitive intervention studies. An example of how such an association in the first wave of the United States WMH survey (the original NCS) between major depression and impaired work performance spurred the design and testing of a highly successful enhanced care intervention for depressed workers is presented in the Future Directions section of this chapter.

Assessing Mental Disorders across Countries

It is important to consider several issues when making assessments of mental disorders across countries (Haro et al., in press; Kessler et al., in press). One fundamental question is whether the DSM and ICD nosologic systems that were developed for use in largely Western and developed nations are also pertinent for the forms of psychopathology in other countries. It is certainly conceivable that the occurrence of disorders and their symptom expression might be different in some parts of the world. In the extreme, this could result in either disorders currently assessed by the CIDI not existing in certain countries or commonly occurring culture-bound syndromes in some countries not being captured by CIDI diagnoses. In terms of the first possibility, it is worth pointing out that each collaborating country's WMH Survey Initiative team contains culturally competent mental health professionals, none of whom have indicated that the ICD or DSM disorders being assessed by the WMH CIDI fail to exist in their country. On the other hand, interesting questions are being raised about whether some disorders captured by the CIDI are expressed differently cross-nationally. An example of such a line of inquiry is looking at whether social anxiety disorder may be expressed differently in Asian countries where a high value is placed on not offending others (Choy, Schneier, Heimberg, Oh, & Liebowitz, 2008). Intriguing questions are also being raised about some culture-related specific syndromes, which may be variants of the disorders assessed in the CIDI but which may not be adequately captured in WMH surveys (Tseng, 2006).

A second and related issue to consider is whether the reliability and validity of the diagnoses made in WMH surveys might vary across countries. On one hand, good concordance has been observed between CIDI diagnoses and diagnoses made during blind clinical re-interviews in the countries that participated in coordinated WMH CIDI clinical reappraisal studies. However, it is worth pointing out that these clinical reappraisal studies were only conducted in developed Western countries. The accuracy of CIDI diagnoses could be worse in other countries where different concepts and phrases may be used to describe mental disorders. In addition, respondents may be more reluctant to endorse emotional problems in countries that have less of a tradition of free speech and anonymous public opinion surveying. Finally, differences in the rigor with which surveys were implemented (e.g., in translation, monitoring for quality control in the field, data cleaning, and coding) could also have affected the accuracy of diagnoses. Some indirect evidence that these issues may have contributed to the underestimation of disorders in countries with the lowest prevalence rates includes the observation that these countries had the highest proportions of treated respondents who were classified as subthreshold cases. Clinical reappraisal studies are currently under way in both developed and less developed WMH countries in all major regions of the world to evaluate the issue of cross-national differences in CIDI diagnostic validity and to make revisions to the WMH study protocol in ways appropriate to address the problems found in these methodological studies.

As noted above in the discussion of earlier DIS/CIDI cross-national surveys, it is critical to assess not just the occurrence but also the severity of mental disorders, in part to be able to know how many of the large number of individuals receiving no services are indeed in need of treatment. For this reason, all WMH surveys include explicit measures of the severity of specific mental disorders. Furthermore, the WMH CIDI contains separate measures of the related but distinct construct of disability, including both global measures of functioning (e.g., the WHO Disability Assessment Schedule, or WHO-DAS) (World Health Organization, 1998) as well as disorder-specific measures of disability (e.g., the Sheehan Disability Scales [SDS]) (Leon, Olfson, Portera, Farber, & Sheehan, 1997).

Assessments of Treatment and Treatment Adequacy

Making cross-national assessments of the mental health services that are being used requires careful consideration of some additional issues. Most importantly, it is necessary to recognize the highly variable nature of mental health treatments, both within as well as potentially between countries. For example, patients can receive mental health treatments from a broad range of physicians, such as general medical doctors (e.g., internal medicine, family practice), mental health specialists (e.g., psychiatrists, behavioral neurologists), and other medical specialty doctors (e.g., ob-gyn). The specific treatments received from these physicians (e.g., medications, psychotherapies) may also differ depending upon their specialization and training. However, what makes the treatment of mental disorders considerably more variable than the treatment of most general medical conditions is that a wide range of other personnel offer services for emotional problems, including mental health specialists (e.g., psychologists, marriage and family counselors, psychiatric social workers), human services professionals (e.g., human services caseworkers, religious and spiritual advisors), and complementary-alternative medicine (CAM) providers (e.g., traditional healers, acupuncturists, self-help group moderators). To truly understand the mental health services used nationally and cross-nationally, WMH surveys had to systematically capture this breadth of information on potential treatments for mental disorders from respondents.

In addition to assessing respondents' use of a wide range of services, the WMH surveys contain sufficient detail to begin comparing respondents' actual treatment regimens to those recommended in evidence-based practice guidelines. Such information is crucial to begin breaking down the problem of unmet need for effective treatment into its component parts, such as failure to receive any treatment, receiving treatment but only after long delays, or receiving treatment that is inadequate in relation to published treatment guidelines and therefore unlikely to be effective. As covered in the Implications section of this chapter, WMH survey information on the magnitude and potentially modifiable determinants of these component problems is a necessary cornerstone in designing, targeting, and testing future interventions to improve the mental health care that patients receive and the outcomes they can achieve.

Emerging Results from the WMH Surveys

As mentioned above, it is essential to consider whether methodologic reasons underlie any cross-national differences in the prevalence of mental disorders observed in the WMH surveys (Chang et al., 2008; Cooke, Hart, & Michie, 2004;

Simon, Goldberg, Von Korff, & Ustun, 2002), and follow-up studies investigating these possibilities are currently under way (Haro et al., 2008; Kessler et al., 2008). For this reason, our focus in this section will largely be on highlighting important similarities that have emerged to date from the WMH Survey Initiative. Likewise, we caution readers that restraint is required when offering substantive interpretations for any cross-national differences that have been observed in WMH surveys.

The WHO WMH Survey Initiative is the largest coordinated series of cross-national psychiatric epidemiological surveys undertaken to date. Results were gathered from discrete surveys of seventeen different countries on four continents, many of which had never before collected data on the prevalence or correlates of mental disorders in their country, and other countries had information on mental disorders only from small regional studies prior to the WMH surveys (see Table 6.1 for a complete list of the participating countries.)

The Occurrence of Mental Disorders over Respondents' Lifetimes

Lifetime Prevalence of Mental Disorders

One important similarity to have emerged from the WMH surveys is that the experience of mental disorders during respondents' lifetimes was quite common in all countries studied. The inter-quartile range (i.e., 25th–75th percentiles across countries; IQR) of lifetime prevalence for any disorder was 18.1–36.1%. Over one-third of respondents had at least one lifetime CIDI disorder in five countries (Colombia, France, New Zealand, Ukraine, United States), over one-quarter had at least one lifetime disorder in six countries (Belgium, Germany, Lebanon, Mexico, Netherlands, South Africa), and over one-sixth had at least one disorder in four countries (Israel, Italy, Japan, Spain). (Table 6.1) Two remaining countries, China (13.2%) and Nigeria (12.0%), had much lower prevalence estimates that were likely to have been downwardly biased (Gureje, Lasebikan, Kola, & Makanjuola, 2006; Shen et al., 2006). Taken together, the WMH data on the lifetime prevalence of mental disorders indicate that mental disorders are a major public health problem throughout the globe.

The WMH surveys also reveal that all four of the classes of diagnoses assessed by the WMH CIDI are important components of overall burden from mental disorders in most countries. Anxiety disorders were the most prevalent class in ten countries (4.8–31.0%, IQR: 9.9–16.7%) and mood disorders in all of the remaining countries but one (3.3–21.4%, IQR: 9.8–15.8%). Impulse-control disorders were the least prevalent in most of the countries that conducted a relatively full assessment of these disorders (0.3–25.0%, IQR: 3.1–5.7%). Substance use disorders were generally the least prevalent among the remaining countries (1.3–15.0%, IQR: 4.8–9.6). It is worth pointing out, however, that illicit drug abuse-dependence was not assessed in Western European countries, leading to artificially low prevalence estimates of substance use disorders in those countries (1.3–8.9%) compared to other countries (2.2–15.0%). The prevalence of substance use disorders may also have been reduced because substance dependence was assessed only in the presence of abuse (Hasin & Grant, 2004).

The co-occurrence of lifetime disorders was also quite common in most countries. This can be illustrated by the finding that the sum of the prevalence estimates for the four separate disorder classes is generally between 30% and 50% higher than the prevalence estimates of having any lifetime disorder.

Ages of Onset for Mental Disorders

Another important similarity to emerge from the WMH surveys is the consistency in standardized age-of-onset distributions across countries. The earliest median ages of onset (AOO) were for impulse-control disorders, including 7–9 years of age for attention-deficit/hyperactivity disorder, 7–15 for oppositional-defiant disorder, 9–14 for conduct disorder, and 13–21 for intermittent explosive disorder. The AOOs for anxiety disorders fall into two sets, with very early ones for phobias and separation anxiety disorder (median 7–14, IQR: 8–11) and much later ones for generalized anxiety disorder, panic disorder, and post-traumatic stress disorder (median 24–50, IQR: 31–41). The AOOs for mood disorders also range between the late 20s and the early 40s (median 29–43, IQR: 35–40). Although there is considerable cross-national variation in AOO distributions for substance disorders, results across countries consistently show that few onsets occur prior to the mid-teens but rapidly increase in adolescence and early adulthood.

Cohort Effects

Earlier research has suggested that the lifetime risk for mental disorders may be greater in more recent cohorts (WHO International Consortium of Psychiatric Epidemiology, 2000). While prospective tracking studies are necessary to definitively answer whether such cohort effects are occurring, the cross-sectional WMH surveys can nevertheless provide some indirect evidence based upon the available retrospective age-of-onset reports. This has been done by predicting the onset of disorders across age groups (e.g., 18–34, 35–49, 50–64, and 65+) using discrete-time survival analysis. Because the first round of WMH surveys was completed between 2002 and 2005, the most recent cohorts (18–34 at interview) correspond to those born in the years from approximately 1968 and later. Cohorts with ages 35–49 at interview correspond roughly to respondents born in 1953–1970, those ages 50–64 were born in 1938–1955, and those ages 65+ were born before 1938. Results from these survival analyses have shown that the relative risks for anxiety, mood, and substance use disorders are generally higher in more recent cohorts compared to older ones. However for impulse control disorders, such cohort effects have generally not been found (Tables 6.2–6.5).

DELAY AND FAILURE IN TREATMENT SEEKING AFTER FIRST ONSET OF MENTAL DISORDERS

Although effective treatments for mental disorders are available, few nations seem either willing or able to pay for their widespread use (Saxena, Sharan, & Saraceno, 2003).

Table 6.1 Lifetime Prevalence and Projected Lifetime Risk as of Age 75 of DSM-IV/CIDI Disorders[1]

	Any anxiety disorder				Any mood disorder				
	Previous			Proj. LT risk		Previous			Proj. LT risk	
	%	n	(se)	%	(se)	%	n	(se)	%	(se)
WHO: Regional Office for the Americas (AMRO)										
Colombia	25.3	948	(1.4)	30.9	(2.5)	14.6	666	(0.7)	27.2	(2.0)
Mexico	14.3	684	(0.9)	17.8	(1.6)	9.2	598	(0.5)	20.4	(1.7)
United States[3]	31.0	2692	(1.0)	36.0	(1.4)	21.4	2024	(0.6)	31.4	(0.9)
WHO: Regional Office for Africa (AFRO)										
Nigeria	6.5	169	(0.9)	7.1	(0.9)	3.3	236	(0.3)	8.9	(1.2)
South Africa	15.8	695	(0.8)	30.1	(4.4)	9.8	439	(0.7)	20.0	(2.4)
WHO: Regional Office for the Eastern Mediterranean (EMRO)										
Lebanon	16.7	282	(1.6)	20.2	(1.8)	12.6	352	(0.9)	20.1	(1.2)
WHO: Regional Office for Europe (EURO)										
Belgium	13.1	219	(1.9)	15.7	(2.5)	14.1	367	(1.0)	22.8	(1.7)
France	22.3	445	(1.4)	26.0	(1.6)	21.0	648	(1.1)	30.5	(1.4)
Germany	14.6	314	(1.5)	16.9	(1.7)	9.9	372	(0.6)	16.2	(1.3)
Israel	5.2	252	(0.3)	10.1	(0.9)	10.7	524	(0.5)	21.2	(1.6)
Italy	11.0	328	(0.9)	13.7	(1.2)	9.9	452	(0.5)	17.3	(1.2)
Netherlands	15.9	320	(1.1)	21.4	(1.8)	17.9	476	(1.0)	28.9	(1.9)
Spain	9.9	375	(1.1)	13.3	(1.4)	10.6	672	(0.5)	20.8	(1.2)
Ukraine	10.9	371	(0.8)	17.3	(2.0)	15.8	814	(0.8)	25.9	(1.5)
WHO: Regional Office for the Western Pacific (WPRO)										
People's Republic of China	4.8	159	(0.7)	6.0	(0.8)	3.6	185	(0.4)	7.3	(0.9)
Japan	6.9	155	(0.6)	9.2	(1.2)	7.6	183	(0.5)	14.1	(1.7)
NewZealand	24.6	3171	(0.7)	30.3	(1.5)	20.4	2755	(0.5)	29.8	(0.7)

[1] See the text for a discussion of between-country differences in the disorders included in each of the diagnostic groups.
[2] Projected lifetime risk to age 65 due to the sample including only respondents up to age 65.
[3] The results reported here for the United States differ somewhat from those in Chapter 7 as a result of updates in the coding scheme implemented in the analyses reported here compared to the analyses reported in Chapter 7.
[4] Cell size was too small to be included in analysis.
[5] Impulse disorders not assessed.

Any impulse-control disorder					Any substance disorder					Any disorder				
Previous			Proj. LT risk		Previous			Proj. LT risk		Previous			Proj. LT risk	
%	n	(se)	%	(se)	%	n	(se)	%	(se)	%	n	(se)	%	(se)
9.6	273	(0.8)	10.3	(0.9)	9.6	345	(0.6)	12.8	(1.0)	39.1	1432	(1.3)	55.2[2]	(6.0)
5.7	152	(0.6)	5.7	(0.6)	7.8	378	(0.5)	11.9	(1.0)	26.1	1148	(1.4)	36.4[2]	(2.1)
25.0	1051	(1.1)	25.6	(1.1)	14.6	1144	(0.6)	17.4	(0.6)	47.4	3929	(1.1)	55.3	(1.2)
0.3	9	(0.1)	−[4]	−	3.7	119	(0.4)	6.4	(1.0)	12.0	440	(1.0)	19.5	(1.9)
−[5]	−	−	−	−	13.3	505	(0.9)	17.5	(1.2)	30.3	1290	(1.1)	47.5	(3.7)
4.4	53	(0.9)	4.6	(1.0)	2.2	27	(0.8)	−	−[4]	25.8	491	(1.9)	32.9	(2.1)
5.2	31	(1.4)	5.2	(1.4)	8.3	195	(0.9)	10.5	(1.1)	29.1	519	(2.3)	37.1	(3.0)
7.6	71	(1.3)	7.6	(1.3)	7.1	202	(0.5)	8.8	(0.6)	37.9	847	(1.7)	47.2	(1.6)
3.1	31	(0.8)	3.1	(0.8)	6.5	228	(0.6)	8.7	(0.9)	25.2	573	(1.9)	33.0	(2.5)
−[5]	−	−	−	−	5.3	261	(0.3)	6.3	(0.4)	17.6	860	(0.6)	29.7	(1.5)
1.7	27	(0.4)	−[4]	−	1.3	56	(0.2)	1.6	(0.3)	18.1	612	(1.1)	26.0	(1.9)
4.7	37	(1.1)	4.8	(1.1)	8.9	210	(0.9)	11.4	(1.2)	31.7	633	(2.0)	42.9	(2.5)
2.3	40	(0.8)	2.3	(0.8)	3.6	180	(0.4)	4.6	(0.5)	19.4	842	(1.4)	29.0	(1.8)
8.7	91	(1.1)	9.7	(1.3)	15.0	293	(1.3)	18.8	(1.7)	36.1	1074	(1.5)	48.9	(2.5)
4.3	37	(0.9)	4.9	(0.9)	4.9	128	(0.7)	6.1	(0.8)	13.2	419	(1.3)	18.0	(1.5)
2.8	11	(1.0)	−[4]	−	4.8	69	(0.5)	6.2	(0.7)	18.0	343	(1.1)	24.4	(1.8)
−[5]	−	−	−	−	12.4	1767	(0.4)	14.6	(0.5)	39.3	4815	(0.9)	48.6	(1.5)

Table 6.2 Intercohort Differences in Lifetime Risk of Any DSM-IV/CIDI Anxiety Disorder[1]

	18–34			35–49			50–64			65+[2]					
	OR	(95% CI)	n	OR	(95% CI)	n	OR	(95% CI)	n	OR	(95% CI)	n	χ²	df	n
WHO: Regional Office for the Americas (AMRO)															
Colombia	1.6*	(1.2–2.1)	825	1.3	(0.9–1.8)	906	1.0	—	379	—	—	271	10.0*	2	2381
Mexico	2.4*	(1.6–3.4)	896	1.6*	(1.1–2.4)	840	1.0	—	359	—	—	267	25.3*	2	2362
United States[3]	3.5*	(2.8–4.4)	1939	3.4*	(2.7–4.1)	1831	2.5*	(2.0–3.0)	1213	1.0	—	709	159.2*	3	5692
WHO: Regional Office for Africa (AFRO)															
Nigeria	3.1*	(1.4–6.9)	971	2.3*	(1.1–4.9)	549	2.8*	(1.5–5.4)	369	1.0	—	254	11.1*	3	2143
South Africa	2.3*	(1.3–4.0)	2172	1.8*	(1.1–3.1)	1264	1.3	(0.8–2.1)	638	1.0	—	241	16.5*	3	4315
WHO: Regional Office for the Eastern Mediterranean (EMRO)															
Lebanon	3.2*	(1.6–6.2)	349	2.5*	(1.2–5.1)	348	1.0	(0.5–2.1)	199	1.0	—	135	24.1*	3	1031

WHO: Regional Office for Europe (EURO)

Belgium	2.6*	(1.3–5.0)	254	1.6	(0.8–3.2)	331	1.3	(0.6–2.6)	278	1.0	–	180	14.2*	3	1043
France	3.1*	(1.5–6.4)	388	3.2*	(1.5–6.7)	472	1.6	(0.8–3.3)	362	1.0	–	214	21.3*	3	1436
Germany	3.1*	(1.9–5.1)	316	2.3*	(1.4–3.9)	436	2.3*	(1.3–4.1)	345	1.0	–	226	21.8*	3	1323
Israel	4.7*	(2.6–8.3)	1627	2.7*	(1.6–4.4)	1302	2.1*	(1.4–3.3)	1069	1.0	–	861	27.3*	3	4859
Italy	1.5	(0.7–3.0)	496	1.6	(0.9–2.8)	516	1.3	(0.8–2.2)	454	1.0	–	313	3.3	3	1779
Netherlands	3.6*	(2.1–6.1)	264	4.5*	(3.0–6.8)	358	3.0*	(2.0–4.6)	302	1.0	–	170	60.6*	3	1094
Spain	3.8*	(2.2–6.5)	545	2.8*	(1.5–5.2)	556	1.3	(0.8–2.2)	456	1.0	–	564	28.7*	3	2121
Ukraine	1.7*	(1.1–2.6)	420	1.0	(0.6–1.6)	434	1.0	(0.7–1.6)	412	1.0	–	454	6.5	3	1720

WHO: Regional Office for the Western Pacific (WPRO)

People's Republic of China	1.7	(0.6–4.4)	379	1.1	(0.5–2.5)	726	1.6	(0.7–3.9)	357	1.0	–	166	3.3	3	1628
Japan	5.6*	(2.2–13.8)	155	2.8*	(1.3–6.1)	219	2.6*	(1.2–5.6)	295	1.0	–	218	14.9*	3	887
New Zealand	3.4*	(2.7–4.2)	2517	2.6*	(2.1–3.1)	2474	2.1*	(1.7–2.7)	1517	1.0	–	927	126.3*	3	7435

* Significant at the .05 level, two-sided test.
[1] Based on discrete-time survival models with person-year as the unit of analysis; controls are time intervals.
[2] Referent category unless otherwise noted.
[3] The results reported here for the United States differ somewhat from those in Chapter 7 as a result of updates in the coding scheme implemented in the analyses reported here compared to the analyses reported in Chapter 7, this volume .

Table 6.3 Intercohort Differences in Lifetime Risk of any DSM-IV/CIDI Mood Disorder[1]

	18–34			35–49			50–64			65+			χ^2	df	n
	OR	(95% CI)	n	OR	(95% CI)	n	OR	(95% CI)	n	OR	(95% CI)	n			
WHO: Regional Office for the Americas (AMRO)															
Colombia	6.3*	(4.2–9.3)	1431	2.3*	(1.6–3.1)	1735	1.0	–	730	–	–	530	92.7*	2	4426
Mexico	4.0*	(2.6–6.1)	2060	1.6*	(1.1–2.3)	2236	1.0	–	840	–	–	646	65.0*	2	5782
United States[3]	9.5*	(7.3–12.4)	3034	5.0*	(3.7–6.6)	2865	3.0*	(2.3–3.9)	1922	1.0	–	1461	383.6*	3	9282
WHO: Regional Office for Africa (AFRO)															
Nigeria	3.7*	(1.8–7.6)	3175	1.8	(0.9–3.6)	1631	1.2	(0.7–2.1)	1104	1.0	–	842	19.4*	3	6752
South Africa	9.6*	(5.5–16.7)	2172	5.5*	(3.1–9.9)	1264	2.5*	(1.4–4.4)	638	1.0	–	241	95.6	3	4315
WHO: Regional Office for the Eastern Mediterranean (EMRO)															
Lebanon	6.2*	(3.0–12.8)	965	3.1*	(1.4–6.7)	931	1.7	(0.8–3.2)	553	1.0	–	408	60.5*	3	2857

WHO: Regional Office for Europe (EURO)

Belgium	11.3*	(6.1–20.9)	573	4.9*	(3.2–7.5)	775	3.6*	(2.0–6.4)	570	1.0	—	501	87.3*	3	2419
France	9.0*	(6.0–13.5)	743	3.0*	(2.2–4.2)	942	1.8*	(1.2–2.6)	719	1.0	—	490	146.4*	3	2894
Germany	12.2*	(7.1–21.0)	815	5.2*	(3.5–7.7)	1180	2.4*	(1.6–3.4)	893	1.0	—	667	94.4*	3	3555
Israel	6.5*	(4.5–9.4)	1627	2.8*	(2.0–4.0)	1302	1.8*	(1.3–2.5)	1069	1.0	—	861	118.4*	3	4859
Italy	5.7*	(3.8–8.4)	1326	3.6*	(2.6–5.0)	1393	2.3*	(1.6–3.3)	1153	1.0	—	840	91.3*	3	4712
Netherlands	11.7*	(6.6–20.8)	564	6.4*	(4.0–10.2)	729	2.9*	(1.7–4.8)	627	1.0	—	452	115.7*	3	2372
Spain	9.6*	(6.6–13.9)	1567	4.2*	(3.0–5.9)	1431	2.2*	(1.6–3.0)	1024	1.0	—	1451	176.3*	3	5473
Ukraine	1.9*	(1.4–2.4)	1194	1.0	(0.8–1.3)	1225	0.9	(0.8–1.1)	1180	1.0	—	1126	38.2*	3	4725

WHO: Regional Office for the Western Pacific (WPRO)

People's Republic of China	20.8*	(9.4–45.8)	1209	4.4*	(2.3–8.4)	2261	2.5*	(1.4–4.4)	1184	1.0	—	547	76.5*	3	5201
Japan	23.7*	(13.4–42.0)	410	7.7*	(4.5–13.2)	571	3.8*	(2.4–5.8)	764	1.0	—	691	146.2*	3	2436
New Zealand	10.0*	(8.2–12.2)	3949	5.0*	(4.1–6.0)	4102	2.9*	(2.4–3.6)	2697	1.0	—	2244	653.9*	3	12992

*Significant at the .05 level, two-sided test.

1 Based on discrete-time survival models with person–year as the unit of analysis; controls are time intervals.

2 Referent category unless otherwise noted.

3 The results reported here for the United States differ somewhat from those in Chapter 7 as a result of updates in the coding scheme implemented in the analyses reported here compared to the analyses reported in Chapter 7.

Table 6.4 Intercohort Differences in Lifetime Risk of Any DSM-IV/CIDI Impulse Disorders[1]

	18–34		35–49[2]		50–64[3]		65+[3]			
	OR	(95% CI)	OR	(95% CI)	OR	(95% CI)	OR	(95% CI)	χ^2	df
WHO: Regional Office for the Americas (AMRO)										
Colombia	1.4	(0.9–2.0)	1.0	–	–	–	–	–	2.4	1
Mexico	1.8*	(1.2–2.9)	1.0	–	–	–	–	–	7.8*	1
United States[4]	1.2	(1.0–1.4)	1.0	–	–	–	–	–	4.0*	1
WHO: Regional Office for Africa (AFRO)										
Nigeria[5]	–	–	–	–	–	–	–	–	–	–
South Africa[6]	–	–	–	–	–	–	–	–	–	–
WHO: Regional Office for the Eastern Mediterranean (EMRO)										
Lebanon	1.4	(0.6–3.3)	1.0	–	–	–	–	–	0.8	1
WHO: Regional Office for Europe (EURO)										
Belgium	1.4	(0.6–3.4)	1.0	–	–	–	–	–	0.6	1
France	1.5	(0.7–3.2)	1.0	–	–	–	–	–	1.3	1
Germany	1.1	(0.3–4.1)	1.0	–	–	–	–	–	0.0	1
Israel[6]	–	–	–	–	–	–	–	–	–	–
Italy[5]	–	–	–	–	–	–	–	–	–	–
Netherlands	1.3	(0.4–4.1)	1.0	–	–	–	–	–	0.2	1
Spain	1.5	(0.5–5.3)	1.0	–	–	–	–	–	0.5	1
Ukraine	1.4	(0.6–3.2)	1.0	–	–	–	–	–	0.8	1
WHO: Regional Office for the Western Pacific (WPRO)										
People's Republic of China	0.5	(0.2–1.3)	1.0	–	–	–	–	–	1.9	1
Japan[5]	–	–	–	–	–	–	–	–	–	–
New Zealand[6]	–	–	–	–	–	–	–	–	–	–

*Significant at the .05 level, two-sided test.
[1] Based on discrete-time survival models with person-year as the unit of analysis; controls are time intervals.
[2] Referent category unless otherwise noted.
[3] There was no data for these age ranges as impulse disorders were estimated among Part 2 respondents in the age range 18–39/44. All countries, with the exception of Nigeria, People's Republic of China, and Ukraine (which were age restricted to ≤ 39) were age restricted to ≤ 44.
[4] The results reported here for the United States differ somewhat from those in Chapter 7 as a result of updates in the coding scheme implemented in the analyses reported here compared to the analyses reported in Chapter 7.
[5] Cell size was too small to be included in analysis.
[6] Impulse disorder was not assessed.

Table 6.5 Intercohort Differences in Lifetime Risk of Any DSM-IV/CIDI Substance Disorders[1]

	18–34			35–49			50–64			65+[2]			χ^2	df	n
	OR	(95% CI)	n	OR	(95% CI)	n	OR	(95% CI)	n	OR	(95% CI)	n			
WHO: Regional Office for the Americas (AMRO)															
Colombia	2.3*	(1.6–3.3)	1431	1.1	(0.7–1.6)	1735	1.0	—	730	—	—	530	39.3*	2	4426
Mexico	1.7*	(1.3–2.4)	2060	1.2	(0.9–1.7)	2236	1.0	—	840	—	—	646	12.8*	2	5782
United States[3]	6.7*	(4.6–10.0)	1939	4.9*	(3.5–7.0)	1831	3.5*	(2.4–5.3)	1213	1.0	—	709	111.0*	3	5692
WHO: Regional Office for Africa (AFRO)															
Nigeria	3.4*	(1.1–10.1)	971	4.9*	(1.8–13.3)	549	2.9	(1.0–8.7)	369	1.0	—	254	11.8*	3	2143
South Africa	2.6*	(1.3–5.4)	2172	1.5	(0.8–2.9)	1264	1.0	(0.6–1.9)	638	1.0	—	241	29.1	3	4315
WHO: Regional Office for the Eastern Mediterranean (EMRO)															
Lebanon[4]	—	—	—	—	—	—	—	—	—	—	—	—	—	—	—
WHO: Regional Office for Europe (EURO)															
Belgium	5.0*	(2.6–9.8)	254	3.6*	(1.7–7.3)	331	2.6*	(1.2–5.4)	278	1.0	—	180	26.7*	3	1043
France	5.8*	(3.3–10.0)	388	3.3*	(2.0–5.7)	472	2.5*	(1.4–4.2)	362	1.0	—	214	44.1*	3	1436
Germany	5.6*	(2.9–10.7)	316	3.7*	(2.0–6.8)	436	3.9*	(2.1–7.1)	345	1.0	—	226	35.0*	3	1323
Israel	11.3*	(5.9–21.6)	1627	4.6*	(2.4–9.0)	1302	2.5*	(1.2–5.1)	1069	1.0	—	861	119.9*	3	4859
Italy	2.6*	(1.0–6.7)	496	1.8	(0.8–4.1)	516	1.6	(0.6–3.9)	454	1.0	—	313	5.5	3	1779
Netherlands	12.4*	(7.0–21.8)	264	7.0*	(3.8–13.1)	358	6.8*	(3.4–13.9)	302	1.0	—	170	85.3*	3	1094
Spain	9.3*	(3.6–24.2)	545	5.0*	(1.8–13.7)	556	1.5	(0.6–4.2)	456	1.0	—	564	38.1*	3	2121
Ukraine	10.8*	(5.8–20.1)	420	5.0*	(2.4–10.4)	434	2.8*	(1.3–5.8)	412	1.0	—	454	116.4*	3	1720

(Continued)

Table 6.5 Intercohort Differences in Lifetime Risk of Any DSM-IV/CIDI Substance Disorders[1] *(Continued)*

	18–34			35–49			50–64			65+[2]			χ²	df	n
	OR	(95% CI)	n	OR	(95% CI)	n	OR	(95% CI)	n	OR	(95% CI)	n			
WHO: Regional Office for the Western Pacific (WPRO)															
People's Republic of China	8.2*	(1.0–67.2)	379	4.0	(0.6–28.2)	726	1.5	(0.2–11.2)	357	1.0	–	166	31.9*	3	1628
Japan	1.9	(0.6–6.0)	155	2.3*	(1.1–4.9)	219	2.5*	(1.1–5.7)	295	1.0	–	218	6.7	3	887
New Zealand	8.1*	(6.1–10.7)	3949	3.5*	(2.7–4.7)	4102	2.5*	(1.9–3.3)	2697	1.0	–	2244	283.7*	3	12992

*Significant at the .05 level, two-sided test.

[1] Based on discrete-time survival models with person-year as the unit of analysis; controls are time intervals.

[2] Referent category unless otherwise noted.

[3] The results reported here for the United States differ somewhat from those in Chapter 7 due to updates in the coding scheme implemented in the analyses reported here compared to the analyses reported in Chapter 7.

[4] Cell size too small to be included in analysis

This has left many nations seeking strategies to efficiently use what limited resources they have to address mental health burdens (World Health Organization, 2001). One promising strategy may be to use treatment resources earlier in the disease courses of affected individuals, before many negative sequelae from mental illnesses develop (Kohn, Saxena, Levav, & Saraceno, 2004). To help inform decision making in this area, WMH surveys have sought to shed light on the treatment-seeking process that respondents typically follow after the first onset of mental disorders.

Cumulative Probabilities and Median Delays in Treatment Contact

The proportions of lifetime cases with anxiety disorders making treatment contact in the year of disorder onset is shown in Table 6.6. It ranges from a low of 0.8% in Nigeria to a high of 36.4% in Israel (IQR: 3.6–19.8). By 50 years of age, the proportions of lifetime cases with anxiety disorders making treatment contact range from 15.2% in Nigeria to 95.0% in Germany (IQR: 44.7–90.7). Among cases that eventually made treatment contact, the duration of delays was shortest in Israel (median 3.0 years) and longest in Mexico (median 30.0 years). Delays were generally longer in developing than developed countries.

The proportions of lifetime cases with mood disorders that made treatment contact in the year of disorder onset ranged from 6.0% in Nigeria and China to 52.1% in Netherlands (IQR: 16.0–42.7) (see Table 6.7). The proportions of cases with mood disorders making treatment contact by 50 years ranged from 7.9% in China to 98.6% in France (IQR: 56.8–96.4%). Among cases of mood disorders eventually making treatment contact, the median duration of delay was the shortest in five countries (Belgium, the Netherlands, Spain, China, and Japan; median delay 1.0 year) and longest in Mexico (median delay 14.0 years).

Among lifetime cases of substance use disorders, the proportions making treatment contact in the year of disorder onset ranged from 0.9% in Mexico to 18.6% in Spain (IQR: 2.8–13.2%) (Table 6.8). By 50 years, 19.8% of cases in Nigeria to 86.1% in Germany with substance use disorders made treatment contact (IQR: 25.7–66.6%). The shortest delays among cases eventually making treatment contact occurred in Spain (median 6.0 years) and the longest in Belgium (median 18.0 years).

Correlates of Lifetime Treatment Contact

In discrete-time survival models of lifetime treatment contact for anxiety disorders, females were significantly more likely to make initial treatment contact in four countries (see Table 6.9). Significant, monotonic relationships between being in younger cohorts and higher probabilities of treatment contact exist in 13 countries. Cases with earlier ages of onset of their anxiety disorders were significantly less likely to make treatment contact in 14 countries.

For mood disorders, females were significantly associated with higher likelihoods of treatment contact in three countries (see Table 6.10). Younger cohorts had

Table 6.6 Proportional Treatment Contact in the Year of Onset of Any Anxiety Disorder and Median Duration of Delay among Cases That Subsequently Made Treatment Contact

	Making treatment contact in year of onset % (SE)	Making treatment contact by 50 years % (SE)	Median duration of delay in years % (SE)
WHO: Regional Office for the Americas (AMRO)			
Colombia	2.9 (0.6)	41.6 (3.9)	26.0 (1.5)
Mexico	3.6 (1.1)	53.2 (18.2)	30.0 (5.1)
United States	11.3 (0.7)	87.0 (2.4)	23.0 (0.6)
WHO: Regional Office for Africa (AFRO)			
Nigeria	0.8 (0.5)	15.2 (2.6)	16.0 (4.2)
WHO: Regional Office for the Eastern Mediterranean (EMRO)			
Lebanon	3.2 (1.1)	37.3 (11.5)	28.0 (3.9)
WHO: Regional Office for Europe (EURO)			
Belgium	19.8 (2.8)	84.5 (4.9)	16.0 (3.5)
France	16.1 (1.8)	93.3 (1.9)	18.0 (1.8)
Germany	13.7 (1.8)	95.0 (2.3)	23.0 (2.3)
Israel	36.4 (0.9)	90.7 (1.3)	3.0 (0.1)
Italy	17.1 (2.1)	87.3 (8.5)	28.0 (2.2)
Netherlands	28.0 (3.7)	91.1 (2.8)	10.0 (1.6)
Spain	23.2 (2.0)	86.6 (5.2)	17.0 (3.2)
WHO: Regional Office for the Western Pacific (WPRO)			
People's Republic of China	4.2 (2.0)	44.7 (7.2)	21.0 (3.1)
Japan	11.2 (2.4)	63.1 (6.2)	20.0 (2.4)
New Zealand	12.5 (0.8)	84.2 (2.5)	21.0 (0.8)

higher probabilities of treatment contact in 10 countries. Earlier ages of onset were significantly associated with lower likelihoods of treatment contact in 13 countries.

For substance use disorders, females were significantly more likely to make initial treatment contact in one country (see Table 6.11). Younger cohorts had higher probabilities of initial treatment contact in eight countries. Having an earlier age-of-onset was significantly associated with lower likelihoods of initial treatment contact in eight countries.

PREVALENCE AND SEVERITY OF MENTAL DISORDERS
IN THE YEAR PRIOR TO INTERVIEW

12-Month Prevalence

The 12-month prevalence of any mental disorder ranged between 27.0% in the United States to 6.0% in Nigeria (IQR: 9.8–19.1%; see Table 6.12). Between one-fifth and one-quarter of the population in five countries (Colombia, France, New Zealand, Ukraine, United States) met criteria for one of the 12-month disorders

Table 6.7 Proportional Treatment Contact in the Year of Onset of Any Mood Disorder and Median Duration of Delay Among Cases That Subsequently Made Treatment Contact

	Making treatment contact in year of onset % (SE)	*Making treatment contact by 50 years % (SE)*	*Median duration of delay in years % (SE)*
WHO: Regional Office for the Americas (AMRO)			
Colombia	18.7 (2.7)	66.6 (3.7)	9.0 (1.6)
Mexico	16.0 (2.2)	69.9 (8.5)	14.0 (3.1)
United States	35.4 (1.2)	94.8 (2.5)	4.0 (0.2)
WHO: Regional Office for Africa (AFRO)			
Nigeria	6.0 (1.7)	33.3 (7.2)	6.0 (3.3)
WHO: Regional Office for the Eastern Mediterranean (EMRO)			
Lebanon	12.3 (2.0)	49.2 (5.2)	6.0 (2.1)
WHO: Regional Office for Europe (EURO)			
Belgium[1]	47.8 (2.7)	93.7 (2.5)	1.0 (0.3)
France[1]	42.7 (2.1)	98.6 (1.4)	3.0 (0.3)
Germany[1]	40.4 (3.8)	89.1 (5.0)	2.0 (0.4)
Israel[1]	31.9 (0.8)	92.7 (0.5)	6.0 (0.3)
Italy[1]	28.8 (3.0)	63.5 (5.9)	2.0 (0.5)
Netherlands[1]	52.1 (2.9)	96.9 (1.7)	1.0 (0.3)
Spain[1]	48.5 (2.3)	96.4 (3.1)	1.0 (0.3)
WHO: Regional Office for the Western Pacific (WPRO)			
People's Republic of China	6.0 (2.2)	7.9 (2.6)	1.0 (2.0)
Japan	29.6 (4.0)	56.8 (7.3)	1.0 (0.7)
New Zealand	41.4 (1.3)	97.5 (1.0)	3.0 (0.2)

[1] Used major depressive episode instead of any mood disorder.

assessed in the surveys. Between one-eighth and one-sixth of the population in another five countries (Belgium, Lebanon, Mexico, Netherlands, South Africa) had one or more of these 12-month disorders.

Anxiety disorders were the most common disorders in all but three countries (prevalences of mood disorders were higher in Israel and Ukraine, while impulse-control disorders had a higher prevalence in China), ranging between 3.0–19.0% (IQR: 6.5–12.2%). Mood disorders were the next most common in all but three countries (with higher prevalences of substance disorders in South Africa and of impulse-control disorders in the United States and China), ranging between 1.1–9.7% (IQR: 3.4–6.8%). Substance disorders (0.2–6.4%; IQR: 1.2–2.8%) and impulse-control disorders (0.1–10.5%; IQR: 0.6–2.6%) were less prevalent across most countries.

Severity

The proportions of cases with serious disorders ranged between 12.8% and 36.8% (IQR: 18.5–25.7%; see Table 6.13). Cases classified as moderate ranged between 12.5% and 47.6% (IQR: 33.9–42.6%). The proportion of disorders classified as

Table 6.8 Proportional Treatment Contact in the Year of Onset of Any Substance Use Disorder and Median Duration of Delay among Cases That Subsequently Made Treatment Contact

	Making treatment contact in year of onset % (SE)	Making treatment contact by 50 years % (SE)	Median duration of delay in years % (SE)
WHO: Regional Office for the Americas (AMRO)			
Colombia	3.6 (0.8)	23.1 (7.1)	11.0 (5.0)
Mexico	0.9 (0.5)	22.1 (4.8)	10.0 (3.3)
United States[1]	10.0 (0.8)	75.5 (3.8)	13.0 (1.2)
WHO: Regional Office for Africa (AFRO)			
Nigeria[1]	2.8 (1.7)	19.8 (7.2)	8.0 (1.8)
WHO: Regional Office for the Eastern Mediterranean (EMRO)			
Lebanon[1]	—[2]	—[2]	—[2]
WHO: Regional Office for Europe (EURO)			
Belgium	12.8 (4.8)	61.2 (17.7)	18.0 (5.8)
France	15.7 (5.4)	66.5 (14.1)	13.0 (3.7)
Germany	13.2 (5.7)	86.1 (8.6)	9.0 (3.9)
Israel	2.0 (0.5)	48.0 (2.4)	12.0 (0.5)
Italy[1]	—[2]	—[2]	—[2]
Netherlands	15.5 (5.4)	66.6 (7.9)	9.0 (3.1)
Spain	18.6 (7.6)	40.1 (14.1)	6.0 (4.9)
WHO: Regional Office for the Western Pacific (WPRO)			
People's Republic of China[1]	2.8 (1.8)	25.7 (9.0)	17.0 (3.7)
Japan[1]	9.2 (5.1)	31.0 (7.8)	8.0 (4.6)
New Zealand	6.3 (0.8)	84.8 (15.4)	17.0 (1.3)

[1] Assessed in the Part 2 sample.
[2] Disorder was omitted as a result of insufficient cases ($n < 30$).

mild ranged from 28.0% to 74.7% (IQR: 35.7–40.5%). There were positive associations between overall prevalence of any disorder and both the proportion of cases classified as serious (Pearson $r = .46$, $p < .001$) and the proportion of cases classified as either serious or moderate (Pearson $r = .77$, $p < .001$).

Severity and Impairment

To validate the severity classification used in the WMH surveys, its relationship with mean number of days out of role due to mental disorders was examined. As shown in Table 6.14, statistically significant monotonic associations between reported disorder severity and days out of role existed in all but four surveys. Serious disorders were typically associated with at least 40 days in the past year when respondents were totally unable to carry out usual activities because of their disorders (IQR: 56.7–135.9 days). By comparison, moderate cases were associated with

Table 6.9 Socio-demographic Predictors of Lifetime Treatment Contact of Any Anxiety Disorder

	Sex			Cohort (age at interview)							Age of onset						
	Female			Age 18–34		Age 35–49		Age 50–64			Early		Early-average		Late-average		
	OR	(95% CI)	χ^2	OR	(95% CI)	OR	(95% CI)	OR	(95% CI)	χ^2	OR	(95% CI)	OR	(95% CI)	OR	(95% CI)	χ^2
WHO: Regional Office for the Americas (AMRO)																	
Colombia	1.1	(0.7–1.8)	0.1	3.4*	(1.4–8.2)	1.6	(0.8–3.3)	1.0	—	9.6*	0.2*	(0.1–0.3)	0.3*	(0.2–0.6)	0.3*	(0.1–0.5)	33.4*
Mexico	1.1	(0.6–1.8)	0.1	2.3	(0.8–6.4)	2.3	(0.8–6.4)	1.0	—	2.6	0.2*	(0.1–0.3)	0.2*	(0.1–0.3)	0.2*	(0.1–0.3)	59.1*
United States	1.3*	(1.0–1.6)	5.4*	2.5*	(1.9–3.3)	1.4*	(1.1–1.8)	1.2	(0.9–1.6)	62.6*	0.2*	(0.2–0.2)	0.2*	(0.2–0.3)	0.2*	(0.2–0.3)	326.4*
WHO: Regional Office for Africa (AFRO)																	
Nigeria	1.1	(0.4–3.3)	0.0	0.6	(0.1–3.0)	0.1*	(0.0–0.7)	0.3	(0.1–1.9)	7.9*	0.3*	(0.2–0.7)	0.6	(0.2–2.0)	0.5	(0.2–1.5)	10.1*
WHO: Regional Office for the Eastern Mediterranean (EMRO)																	
Lebanon	0.5	(0.2–1.2)	2.5	1.9	(0.2–20.0)	1.3	(0.1–11.3)	0.8	(0.1–6.9)	2.6	0.1*	(0.0–0.3)	0.2*	(0.1–0.4)	0.7	(0.3–1.5)	28.7*

(Continued)

Table 6.9 Sociodemographic Predictors of Lifetime Treatment Contact of Any Anxiety Disorder (*Continued*)

| | Sex | | | Cohort (age at interview) | | | | | | | Age of onset | | | | | | |
| | Female | | | Age 18–34 | | Age 35–49 | | Age 50–64 | | | Early | | Early-average | | Late-average | | |
	OR	(95% CI)	χ²	OR	(95% CI)	OR	(95% CI)	OR	(95% CI)	χ²	OR	(95% CI)	OR	(95% CI)	OR	(95% CI)	χ²
WHO: Regional Office for Europe (EURO)																	
Belgium	1.2	(0.7–2.1)	0.4	4.7*	(1.6–13.6)	3.0*	(1.2–7.5)	1.3	(0.6–2.8)	14.8*	0.1*	(0.1–0.3)	0.1*	(0.0–0.3)	0.2*	(0.1–0.5)	63.5*
France	1.5*	(1.1–2.1)	8.8*	4.5*	(2.5–8.1)	2.3*	(1.3–4.2)	1.3	(0.7–2.5)	52.2*	0.2*	(0.1–0.3)	0.2*	(0.1–0.3)	0.3*	(0.2–0.5)	82.4*
Germany	1.5*	(1.1–2.1)	6.6*	4.5*	(2.7–7.5)	2.3*	(1.5–3.7)	1.5	(0.8–2.9)	59.8*	0.2*	(0.1–0.3)	0.2*	(0.1–0.3)	0.2*	(0.1–0.5)	43.5*
Israel	1.0	(0.6–1.5)	0.0	5.0*	(1.8–13.9)	3.2*	(1.4–7.4)	1.9	(0.9–4.0)	10.0*	0.4	(0.2–1.0)	0.5	(0.3–1.1)	0.6	(0.3–1.2)	3.7
Italy	1.1	(0.7–1.5)	0.1	2.6*	(1.3–5.2)	2.1*	(1.2–3.7)	1.4	(0.7–2.9)	16.0*	0.1*	(0.1–0.2)	0.1*	(0.1–0.2)	0.3*	(0.2–0.5)	101.8*
Netherlands	1.1	(0.7–1.6)	0.2	3.0*	(1.8–5.1)	2.5*	(1.6–3.7)	1.0	—	26.8*	0.1*	(0.0–0.2)	0.1*	(0.1–0.3)	0.4*	(0.2–0.7)	52.0*
Spain	1.0	(0.7–1.6)	0.0	3.3*	(1.9–5.7)	2.0*	(1.1–3.7)	0.8	(0.5–1.3)	38.5*	0.1*	(0.0–0.1)	0.1*	(0.0–0.2)	0.2*	(0.1–0.4)	96.2*
WHO: Regional Office for the Western Pacific (WPRO)																	
People's Republic of China	1.0	(0.4–2.3)	0.0	4.6*	(1.4–15.6)	2.1	(0.9–5.0)	1.0	—	6.7*	0.3*	(0.1–0.9)	0.2*	(0.0–1.0)	0.7	(0.2–2.4)	8.3*
Japan	0.9	(0.5–1.6)	0.3	5.6*	(1.8–17.2)	1.7	(0.8–3.7)	1.3	(0.5–3.3)	14.1*	0.1*	(0.0–0.1)	0.1*	(0.1–0.2)	0.4	(0.2–1.0)	63.5*
New Zealand	1.3*	(1.1–1.5)	8.6*	4.3*	(2.9–6.3)	2.4*	(1.7–3.4)	1.7*	(1.3–2.4)	68.8*	0.1*	(0.1–0.1)	0.1*	(0.1–0.2)	0.2*	(0.2–0.2)	461.0*

*Significant at the .05 level, two-sided test.

Table 6.10 Sociodemographic Predictors of Lifetime Treatment Contact of Any Mood Disorder

	Sex			Cohort (age at interview)							Age of onset						
	Female			Age 18–34		Age 35–49		Age 50–64			Early		Early-average		Late-average		
	OR	(95% CI)	χ²	OR	(95% CI)	OR	(95% CI)	OR	(95% CI)	χ²	OR	(95% CI)	OR	(95% CI)	OR	(95% CI)	χ²
WHO: Regional Office for the Americas (AMRO)																	
Colombia	1.5	(0.9–2.3)	2.7	3.2*	(1.3–7.7)	1.7	(1.0–3.2)	1.0	—	6.7*	0.2*	(0.1–0.4)	0.3*	(0.2–0.7)	0.8	(0.5–1.3)	33.6*
Mexico	1.6*	(1.0–2.4)	4.6*	2.1	(0.9–4.9)	1.7	(0.8–3.3)	1.0	—	3.1	0.3*	(0.2–0.6)	0.5*	(0.2–0.9)	0.8	(0.4–1.6)	25.1*
United States	1.3*	(1.1–1.5)	10.2*	4.4*	(3.2–6.1)	3.1*	(2.3–4.1)	1.9*	(1.4–2.6)	115.5*	0.2*	(0.1–0.3)	0.3*	(0.2–0.3)	0.4*	(0.3–0.6)	176.7*
WHO: Regional Office for Africa (AFRO)																	
Nigeria	1.4	(0.5–3.6)	0.5	2.7	(0.3–22.4)	0.5	(0.1–3.7)	1.0	—	6.8*	2.6	(0.2–33.6)	1.2	(0.0–31.2)	3.3	(0.3–41.1)	3.0
WHO Region: Eastern Mediterranean Regional Office (EMRO)																	
Lebanon	1.1	(0.7–1.8)	0.2	13.8*	(2.3–83.0)	8.8*	(1.5–51.1)	5.0	(0.8–30.8)	13.4*	0.4*	(0.2–0.8)	0.2*	(0.1–0.7)	0.7	(0.3–1.4)	10.6*

(Continued)

Table 6.10 Sociodemographic Predictors of Lifetime Treatment Contact of Any Mood Disorder (*Continued*)

| | Sex | | | Cohort (age at interview) | | | | | | Age of onset | | | | | |
	OR	(95% CI)	χ²	Age 18–34 OR	(95% CI)	Age 35–49 OR	(95% CI)	Age 50–64 OR	(95% CI)	χ²	Early OR	(95% CI)	Early-average OR	(95% CI)	Late-average OR	(95% CI)	χ²
WHO Region: European Regional Office (EURO)																	
Belgium[1]	1.4	(0.9–2.1)	2.5	3.9*	(1.2–12.5)	3.9*	(1.5–10.5)	1.7	(0.7–4.0)	14.5*	0.2*	(0.1–0.6)	0.4*	(0.2–0.9)	0.6*	(0.4–0.9)	14.2*
France[1]	1.3	(0.9–1.8)	2.9	5.7*	(3.1–10.5)	4.4*	(2.4–8.0)	2.0*	(1.1–3.5)	44.3*	0.2*	(0.1–0.4)	0.4*	(0.2–0.8)	0.6	(0.3–1.2)	54.9*
Germany[1]	1.2	(0.8–2.0)	0.9	1.9	(0.7–5.1)	1.2	(0.6–2.8)	1.2	(0.5–2.5)	6.3	0.3*	(0.1–0.6)	0.5	(0.2–1.0)	1.1	(0.5–2.1)	22.5*
Israel	1.1	(0.9–1.5)	0.7	5.4*	(2.9–10.0)	4.0*	(2.3–6.8)	2.3*	(1.4–3.7)	30.9*	0.3*	(0.2–0.6)	0.4*	(0.2–0.6)	0.6	(0.4–1.0)	20.8*
Italy[1]	1.4	(0.9–2.0)	2.6	1.4	(0.7–2.8)	1.6	(0.8–2.9)	1.1	(0.6–2.1)	2.8	0.4*	(0.2–0.8)	0.8	(0.4–1.6)	0.8	(0.4–1.4)	15.7*
Netherlands[1]	0.9	(0.7–1.3)	0.1	3.9*	(1.7–8.9)	2.7*	(1.6–44)	1.0	–	18.5*	0.1*	(0.0–0.3)	0.3*	(0.1–0.6)	0.5*	(0.3–0.8)	27.1*
Spain[1]	1.2	(0.8–1.8)	1.1	1.9	(0.9–3.8)	2.7*	(1.4–5.1)	1.3	(0.8–2.1)	11.3*	0.4*	(0.2–0.8)	0.4*	(0.2–0.9)	0.7	(0.4–1.2)	8.3*
WHO Region: Western Pacific Regional Office (WPRO)																	
People's Republic of China	0.8	(0.2–3.6)	0.1	0.7	(0.2–2.9)	0.4	(0.1–1.3)	1.0	–	2.4	0.5	(0.1–3.3)	0.4	(0.1–1.7)	0.5	(0.1–1.9)	2.3
Japan	1.6	(0.8–3.5)	1.7	3.9*	(1.1–13.4)	2.0	(0.7–6.2)	1.5	(0.6–4.2)	5.0	0.2*	(0.0–0.6)	0.5	(0.2–1.3)	0.8	(0.4–1.9)	9.8*
New Zealand	1.4*	(1.2–1.6)	16.9*	3.7*	(2.7–5.2)	2.3*	(1.7–3.1)	1.6*	(1.2–2.2)	84.1*	0.2*	(0.2–0.3)	0.3*	(0.3–0.4)	0.6*	(0.5–0.8)	205.6*

*Significant at the .05 level, two-sided test.

[1] Used major depressive episode instead of any mood disorder.

Table 6.11 Sociodemographic Predictors of Lifetime Treatment Contact of Any Substance Use Disorder

	Sex			Cohort (age at interview)						Age of onset					
	Female			Age 18–34		Age 35–49		Age 50–64			Early		Early-average		Late-average		
	OR	(95% CI)	χ^2	OR	(95% CI)	OR	(95% CI)	OR	(95% CI)	χ^2	OR	(95% CI)	OR	(95% CI)	OR	(95% CI)	χ^2
WHO: Regional Office for the Americas (AMRO)																
Colombia	0.8	(0.3–2.5)	0.1	9.1*	(1.6–51.0)	5.3*	(1.0–28.2)	1.0	—	6.7*	0.2*	(0.0–0.9)	0.4	(0.1–2.1)	0.2*	(0.0–0.9)	7.9*
Mexico	2.8	(0.8–9.5)	2.9	3.6	(0.7–18.1)	0.8	(0.2–2.9)	1.0	—	8.0*	0.8	(0.2–3.6)	1.3	(0.3–5.7)	1.7	(0.5–5.5)	2.0
United States[1]	1.2	(0.8–1.6)	1.0	3.4*	(1.7–6.8)	1.7	(0.9–3.1)	1.3	(0.7–2.3)	18.2*	0.6*	(0.4–0.8)	0.6*	(0.4–0.8)	0.6*	(0.4–0.8)	14.4*
WHO: Regional Office for Africa (AFRO)																
Nigeria[1]	—[2]	—[2]	—[2]	4.7	(0.6–34.6)	2.3	(0.7–7.9)	1.0	—	3.5	0.1	(0.0–1.7)	0.5	(0.1–3.0)	0.2	(0.0–2.8)	3.1
WHO: Regional Office for the Eastern Mediterranean (EMRO)																
Lebanon[1]	—[2]	—[2]	—[2]	—[2]		—[2]		—[2]			—[2]		—[2]		—[2]		

(Continued)

143

Table 6.11 Sociodemographic Predictors of Lifetime Treatment Contact of Any Substance Use Disorder (Continued)

| | Sex | | | Cohort (age at interview) | | | | | | Age of onset | | | | | | |
| | Female | | | Age 18–34 | | Age 35–49 | | Age 50–64 | | | Early | | Early-average | | Late-average | |
	OR	(95% CI)	χ²	OR	(95% CI)	OR	(95% CI)	OR	(95% CI)	χ²	OR	(95% CI)	OR	(95% CI)	OR	(95% CI)	χ²
WHO: Regional Office for Europe (EURO)																	
Belgium	0.7	(0.1–8.3)	0.1	35.9*	(1.1–1163.4)	35.9*	(1.1–1163.4)	35.9*	(1.1–1163.4)	4.5*	0.1*	(0.0–0.2)	0.1*	(0.0–0.2)	0.1*	(0.0–0.2)	25.7*
France	0.8	(0.2–3.2)	0.2	0.2	(0.0–3.2)	0.7	(0.1–4.8)	1.0	—	2.1	0.4	(0.1–2.6)	0.4	(0.1–2.6)	0.4	(0.1–2.6)	1.0
Germany	1.4	(0.4–5.3)	0.2	4.3	(0.5–37.5)	4.3	(0.5–37.5)	1.0	—	1.9	0.2	(0.0–1.2)	0.1*	(0.0–0.3)	1.0	(0.3–3.1)	12.6*
Israel	0.2	(0.0–1.3)	2.8	9.5*	(1.8–49.7)	3.8*	(1.0–14.7)	1.0	—	7.3*	0.7	(0.2–2.8)	0.3	(0.1–1.5)	2.2	(0.7–7.6)	8.5*
Italy	—[2]		—[2]	—[2]		—[2]		—[2]		—[2]	—[2]		—[2]		—[2]		—[2]
Netherlands	0.6	(0.1–2.9)	0.4	1.4	(0.1–24.1)	1.7	(0.1–19.6)	0.4	(0.0–5.1)	2.1	0.0*	(0.0–0.7)	0.2*	(0.0–1.1)	0.1*	(0.0–0.3)	18.3*
Spain	1.5	(0.1–41.2)	0.1	8.1*	(1.4–46.8)	1.0	—	1.0	—	5.8*	0.0*	(0.0–0.1)	0.0*	(0.0–0.7)	0.2	(0.0–1.7)	16.0*
WHO: Regional Office for the Western Pacific (WPRO)																	
People's Republic of China[1]	0.4	(0.0–6.4)	0.5	1.8	(0.2–20.1)	0.5	(0.1–2.0)	1.0	—	3.0	0.5	(0.1–3.1)	0.5	(0.1–3.1)	0.8	(0.1–5.9)	0.6
Japan[1]	0.4	(0.1–3.3)	0.7	3.6	(0.1–203.0)	0.3*	(0.1–0.7)	0.3*	(0.1–0.7)	9.5*	0.2	(0.0–5.3)	0.4	(0.0–3.1)	1.3	(0.3–5.2)	2.5
New Zealand	1.3*	(1.0–1.7)	4.6*	5.6*	(2.8–11.0)	3.1*	(1.6–5.9)	1.8	(0.9–3.5)	47.1*	0.4*	(0.3–0.6)	0.3*	(0.2–0.4)	0.4*	(0.3–0.5)	63.2*

*Significant at the .05 level, two-sided test.

[1] Assessed in the Part 2 sample.

[2] Disorder was omitted as a result of insufficient lifetime cases (n < 30).

Table 6.12   12-Month Prevalence of CIDI/DSM-IV Disorders[1]

	Anxiety		Mood		Impulse[*]		Substance		Any	
	%	(se)	%	(se)	%	(se)	%	(se)	%	(se)
WHO: Regional Office for the Americas (AMRO)										
Colombia	14.4	(1.0)	7.0	(0.5)	4.4	(0.4)	2.8	(0.4)	21.0	(1.0)
Mexico	8.4	(0.6)	4.7	(0.3)	1.6	(0.3)[5]	2.3	(0.3)	13.4	(0.9)
United States	19.0	(0.7)	9.7	(0.4)	10.5	(0.7)	3.8	(0.4)	27.0	(0.9)
WHO: Regional Office for Africa (AFRO)										
Nigeria	4.2	(0.5)	1.1	(0.1)	0.1	(0.0)[6,8]	0.9	(0.2)	6.0	(0.6)
South Africa	8.2	(0.6)[2,3]	4.9	(0.4)[4]	1.9	(0.3)[6,7,8]	5.8	(0.5)	16.7	(1.0)
WHO: Regional Office for the Eastern Mediterranean (EMRO)										
Lebanon	12.2	(1.2)	6.8	(0.7)	2.6	(0.7)[8]	1.3	(0.8)	17.9	(1.7)
WHO: Regional Office for Europe (EURO)										
Belgium	8.4	(1.4)	5.4	(0.5)[4]	1.7	(1.0)[5]	1.8	(0.4)[9]	13.2	(1.5)
France	13.7	(1.1)	6.5	(0.6)[4]	2.4	(0.6)[5]	1.3	(0.3)[9]	18.9	(1.4)
Germany	8.3	(1.1)	3.3	(0.3)[4]	0.6	(0.3)[5]	1.2	(0.2)[9]	11.0	(1.3)
Israel	3.6	(0.3)[2,3]	6.4	(0.4)	–	[5,6,7,8]	1.3	(0.2)	10.0	(0.5)
Italy	6.5	(0.6)	3.4	(0.3)[4]	0.4	(0.2)[5]	0.2	(0.1)[9]	8.8	(0.7)
Netherlands	8.9	(1.0)	5.1	(0.5)[4]	1.9	(0.7)[5]	1.9	(0.3)[9]	13.6	(1.0)
Spain	6.6	(0.9)	4.4	(0.3)[4]	0.5	(0.2)[5]	0.7	(0.2)[9]	9.7	(0.8)
Ukraine	6.8	(0.7)[2,3]	9.0	(0.6)[4]	5.7	(1.0)[6,8]	6.4	(0.8)	21.4	(1.3)
WHO: Regional Office for the Western Pacific (WPRO)										
People's Republic of China	3.0	(0.5)	1.9	(0.3)	3.1	(0.7)[6,8]	1.6	(0.4)	7.1	(0.9)
Japan	4.2	(0.6)[2]	2.5	(0.4)	0.2	(0.1)[6,7,8]	1.2	(0.4)	7.4	(0.9)
New Zealand	15.0	(0.5)[2]	8.0	(0.4)	–	[5,6,7,8]	3.5	(0.2)	20.7	(0.6)

[*]Impulse disorders restricted to age ≤ 39 (China, Ukraine, Nigeria) or to age ≤ 44 (all other countries).

[1] Anxiety disorders include agoraphobia, adult separation anxiety disorder, generalized anxiety disorder, panic disorder, posttraumatic stress-disorder, social phobia, and specific phobia. Mood disorders include bipolar disorders, dysthymia, and major depressive disorder. Impulse-control disorders include intermittent explosive disorder, and reported persistence in the past 12 months of symptoms of three child-adolescent disorders (attention-deficit/hyperactivity disorder, conduct disorder, and oppositional-defiant disorder). Substance disorders include alcohol or drug abuse with or without dependence. In the case of substance dependence, respondents who met full criteria at some time in their life and who continue to have any symptoms are considered to have 12-month dependence even if they currently do not meet full criteria for the disorder. Organic exclusions were made as specified in the DSM-IV.

[2] Adult separation anxiety disorder was not assessed.

[3] Specific phobia was not assessed.

[4] Bipolar disorders were not assessed.

[5] Intermittent explosive disorder was not assessed.

[6] Attention-deficit/hyperactivity disorder was not assessed.

[7] Conduct disorder was not assessed.

[8] Oppositional-defiant disorder was not assessed.

[9] Only alcohol abuse with or without dependence was assessed. No assessment was made of other drug abuse with or without dependence.

Table 6.13   Prevalence of 12-Month CIDI/DSM-IV Disorders by Severity across Countries[1]

	Serious		Moderate		Mild	
	%	(se)	%	(se)	%	(se)
WHO: Regional Office for the Americas (AMRO)						
Colombia	23.1	(2.1)	41.0	(2.6)	35.9	(2.1)
Mexico	25.7	(2.4)	33.9	(2.2)	40.5	(2.6)
United States	25.2	(1.4)	39.2	(1.2)	35.7	(1.4)
WHO: Regional Office for Africa (AFRO)						
Nigeria	12.8	(3.8)	12.5	(2.6)	74.7	(4.2)
South Africa	25.7	(1.8)	31.5	(2.2)	42.8	(2.2)
WHO: Regional Office for the Eastern Mediterranean (EMRO)						
Lebanon	22.4	(3.1)	42.6	(4.7)	35.0	(5.5)
WHO: Regional Office for Europe (EURO)						
Belgium	31.8	(4.2)	37.8	(3.3)	30.4	(4.8)
France	18.5	(2.5)	42.7	(3.0)	38.8	(3.6)
Germany	21.3	(2.5)	42.6	(4.6)	36.1	(4.3)
Israel	36.8	(2.4)	35.2	(2.3)	28.0	(2.1)
Italy	15.9	(2.7)	47.6	(3.8)	36.5	(3.9)
Netherlands	30.7	(3.4)	31.0	(3.7)	38.3	(4.6)
Spain	19.3	(2.4)	42.3	(4.0)	38.4	(4.7)
Ukraine	22.9	(1.8)	39.4	(2.9)	37.7	(3.5)
WHO: Regional Office for the Western Pacific (WPRO)						
People's Republic of China	13.8	(3.7)	32.2	(4.9)	54.0	(4.6)
Japan	13.2	(3.1)	45.5	(5.3)	41.3	(4.6)
New Zealand	25.3	(1.0)	40.8	(1.4)	33.9	(1.2)

[1] See the text for a description of the coding rules used to define the severity levels.

an intermediate number of such days (mean 21.1–109.4; IQR: 39.3–65.3 days) and mild disorders with fewer (mean 11.7–68.9 days). Again, there were positive associations between prevalence and this indicator of role impairment. To illustrate this, in the three countries with the highest estimated overall 12-month prevalence (United States, Ukraine, New Zealand), the mean number of days out of role associated with disorders classified "severe" is in the range 98.1–142.5 compared to means in the range 48.7–56.7 in the three countries with the lowest 12-month prevalence estimates (Nigeria, China, Japan).

RECENT TREATMENT OF MENTAL DISORDERS

Even in developed countries, competing priorities and budgetary constraints make it imperative for countries to obtain information to be able to rationally design their mental health care systems and optimally allocate treatment resources. Documenting the extent and nature of unmet needs for treatment in countries with

Table 6.14 Association between Severity of 12-Month CIDI/DSM-IV Disorders and Days out of Role

	Serious		*Moderate*		*Mild*			
	Mean	*(se)*	*Mean*	*(se)*	*Mean*	*(se)*	*Wald F[1]*	*(p-value)*
WHO: Regional Office for the Americas (AMRO)								
Colombia	53.0	(8.9)	33.7	(6.7)	15.6	(3.0)	10.8*	(<.001)
Mexico	42.8	(6.9)	26.3	(5.3)	11.7	(2.7)	11.7*	(<.001)
United States	135.9	(6.9)	65.3	(4.6)	35.7	(2.7)	126.1*	(<.001)
WHO: Regional Office for Africa (AFRO)								
Nigeria	56.7	(22.3)	51.5	(18.8)	25.9	(7.4)	1.6	(.20)
South Africa	73.1	(9.7)	49.3	(6.5)	32.5	(4.8)	9.1*	(<.001)
WHO: Regional Office for the Eastern Mediterranean (EMRO)								
Lebanon	81.4	(10.6)	42.0	(9.5)	13.6	(5.4)	14.4*	(<.001)
WHO: Regional Office for Europe (EURO)								
Belgium	96.1	(26.0)	59.9	(11.6)	42.5	(9.6)	3.7*	(.025)
France	105.7	(14.3)	71.8	(16.5)	67.6	(17.3)	2.7	(.07)
Germany	77.8	(18.1)	33.2	(8.2)	45.7	(12.1)	2.2	(.12)
Israel	184.6	(12.5)	109.4	(10.1)	44.6	(9.1)	41.8*	(<.001)
Italy	178.5	(25.6)	55.6	(10.9)	41.7	(11.2)	11.7*	(<.001)
Netherlands	140.7	(19.9)	87.1	(17.1)	68.9	(22.7)	4.0*	(.018)
Spain	131.5	(15.8)	56.6	(10.0)	57.4	(22.0)	8.1*	(<.001)
Ukraine	142.5	(14.5)	103.2	(9.2)	51.6	(9.9)	13.9*	(<.001)
WHO: Regional Office for the Western Pacific (WPRO)								
People's Republic of China	48.7	(18.4)	21.1	(5.2)	21.3	(7.2)	1.5	(.23)
Japan	51.0	(17.3)	39.3	(10.6)	22.5	(6.4)	3.7*	(.024)
New Zealand	98.1	(5.9)	54.6	(3.4)	36.4	(3.6)	40.7*	(<.001)

* Significant association between severity and days out of role at the .05 level.
[1] No demographic controls were used.

different delivery systems, means of financing mental health care, and mental health policies is one way to begin generating this kind of data. For this reason, our focus in this section will depart somewhat from the overall focus of this chapter on high-lighting important similarities between WMH countries.

Use of Mental Health Services in the Prior Year

The prevalence of using any mental health services in the year prior to survey varied significantly, ranging from 1.6% in Nigeria to 17.9% in the United States (χ^2 16=764.6, p<.0001). In general, lower proportions of respondents used treatments in developing than developed countries (Table 6.15) and in countries spending less on health care than more (Table 6.16). Larger proportions used general medical (GM) than mental health specialty (MHS) sectors in most countries,

Table 6.15 12-Month Service Use by Sectors in the WMH Surveys

Country income level	Among respondents*															Among respondents using services[1]												
	Any treatment			Mental health specialty			General medical			Human services			CAM[2]			Mental health specialty			General medical			Human services			CAM[2]		
	n	%	se	n	%	se	n	%	se	n	%	se	N	%	se	n	%	se	n	%	se	n	%	se	n	%	se
WHO: Regional Office for the Americas (AMRO)																											
Colombia	217	5.5	0.6	126	3.0	0.4	82	2.3	0.4	19	0.5	0.2	10	0.2	0.1	126	53.4	4.8	82	41.7	5.1	19	9.2	2.8	10	3.7	1.4
Mexico	240	5.1	0.5	121	2.8	0.3	92	1.7	0.3	15	0.3	0.1	45	1.0	0.2	121	53.6	4.2	92	33.1	4.0	15	6.2	2.0	45	20.0	3.4
United States	1477	17.9	0.7	738	8.8	0.5	773	9.3	0.4	266	3.4	0.3	247	2.8	0.2	738	48.8	1.7	773	51.8	1.3	266	18.8	1.1	247	15.6	1.0
WHO: Regional Office for Africa (AFRO)																											
Nigeria	57	1.6	0.3	5	0.1	0.1	42	1.1	0.2	14	0.5	0.2	1	0.0	0.0	5	8.3	3.7	42	66.6	10.1	14	30.9	10.2	1	1.1	1.1
South Africa	675	15.4	1.0	108	2.5	0.4	440	10.2	0.8	169	3.7	0.4	161	3.7	0.3	108	16.3	2.2	440	66.4	2.5	169	24.0	1.9	161	23.8	2.1
WHO: Regional Office for the Eastern Mediterranean (EMRO)																											
Lebanon	77	4.4	0.6	18	1.0	0.3	53	2.9	0.5	11	0.8	0.3	0	0.0	0.0	18	22.3	5.7	53	66.6	7.4	11	17.5	6.1	0	0.0	0.0

WHO: Regional Office for Europe (EURO)

Belgium	187	10.9	1.4	96	5.2	0.7	147	8.2	1.3	6	0.4	0.2	12	0.7	0.3	96	47.9	4.4	147	75.5	3.8	6	3.7	1.8	12	6.5	2.9
France	272	11.3	1.0	111	4.4	0.5	214	8.8	0.9	10	0.4	0.2	9	0.5	0.3	111	39.4	3.6	214	78.4	3.3	10	3.4	1.2	9	4.3	2.1
Germany	183	8.1	0.8	100	3.9	0.6	102	4.2	0.6	16	1.0	0.4	15	0.6	0.2	100	48.5	4.8	102	51.7	5.1	16	12.2	4.5	15	7.4	2.5
Israel	421	8.8	0.4	215	4.4	0.3	169	3.6	0.3	71	1.6	0.2	42	0.8	0.1	215	50.5	2.6	169	40.4	2.6	71	18.0	2.0	42	9.6	1.5
Italy	141	4.3	0.4	55	2.0	0.3	107	3.0	0.3	15	0.4	0.1	4	0.1	0.0	55	47.1	5.1	107	70.9	4.8	15	9.1	2.4	4	1.5	0.7
Netherlands	202	10.9	1.2	105	5.5	1.0	141	7.7	1.1	14	0.6	0.2	27	1.5	0.4	105	51.0	6.0	141	71.2	6.1	14	5.4	1.6	27	13.5	3.8
Spain	375	6.8	0.5	200	3.6	0.4	249	4.4	0.4	11	0.1	0.1	20	0.2	0.1	200	52.2	3.6	249	64.9	3.4	11	2.1	0.8	20	3.5	1.0
Ukraine	212	7.2	0.8	39	1.2	0.3	135	4.0	0.7	47	1.7	0.4	29	1.0	0.3	39	17.2	3.8	135	55.4	7.1	47	24.1	5.1	29	14.4	4.0

WHO: Regional Office for the Western Pacific (WPRO)

People's Republic of China	74	3.4	0.6	19	0.6	0.2	41	2.3	0.5	6	0.3	0.1	18	0.7	0.3	19	18.0	5.9	41	68.5	6.8	6	7.4	3.8	18	21.2	7.3
Japan	92	5.6	0.9	43	2.4	0.5	47	2.8	0.5	8	0.8	0.5	13	0.6	0.2	43	42.5	5.5	47	50.2	8.2	8	15.0	6.7	13	11.1	4.7
New Zealand	1592	13.8	0.5	585	5.2	0.3	1122	9.2	0.4	203	1.6	0.2	265	2.6	0.3	585	37.6	1.8	1122	66.5	1.8	203	11.5	1.1	265	19.0	1.7
χ_{16}	764.6* (<.001)			679.6* (<.001)			732.2* (<.001)			262.9* (<.001)			388.0* (<.001)			232.4* (<.001)			207.3* (<.001)			201.8* (<.001)			223.1* (<.001)		

* Percentages among respondents are based on entire Part 2 samples.
[1] Percentages are based on respondents using any 12-month services.
[2] CAM: Complementary and alternative medicine.

Table 6.16 Health Care Spending and Level of Economic Development of Each WMH Country

Country	National health care budget as a percentage of total GDP*	Level of economic development
Nigeria	3.4	Low
PRC[1] Beijing	5.5	Low-middle
PRC[1] Shanghai	5.5	Low-middle
Colombia	5.5	Low-middle
South Africa	8.6	Low-middle
Ukraine	4.3	Low-middle
Lebanon	12.2	High-middle
Mexico	6.1	High-middle
Belgium	8.9	High
France	9.6	High
Germany	10.8	High
Italy	8.4	High
Israel	8.7	High
Japan	8.0	High
Netherlands	8.9	High
New Zealand	8.3	High
Spain	7.5	High
United States	13.9	High

*World Health Organization. *Project Atlas: Resources for Mental Health and Neurological Disorders.* Available at http://www.who.int/globalatlas/dataQuery/default.asp.
[1] People's Republic of China.

although this situation was reversed in Mexico, Colombia, and Israel. The human services (HS) and complementary-alternative medical (CAM) sectors were used by smaller proportions. Similar patterns of sector use were also observed among respondents receiving any 12-month services.

DISORDER SEVERITY AND USE OF SERVICES

Statistically significant relationships existed between disorder severity and service use in all WMH countries with the exception of China (Table 6.17). Lower service use was generally observed for developing vs. developed countries in all severity categories. Although this could be interpreted to mean that mental health care is being allocated rationally in most countries based on the availability of resources, it is important to point out that only between 11.0% (in China) and 62.1% (in Belgium) of serious cases received any 12-month services. In general, lower proportions of moderate and mild cases received services. Although only small proportions (between 1.0% in Nigeria to 9.7% in the United States) of respondents that did not meet criteria for 12-month disorders used treatments, these could still be potentially meaningful given that people without disorders make up the large majority of the general population. However, further analysis of these respondents who did not meet criteria for disorders, but were using services, revealed that many

Table 6.17 Percentages Using 12-Month Services by Severity of Mental Disorders in the WMH Surveys[1]

Country	Severe			Moderate			Mild			None			Test of difference in probability of treatment by severity	
	n	%[2]	se	n	%[2]	se	n	%[2]	se	n	%[2]	se	χ^2_3	(p-value)
WHO: Regional Office for the Americas (AMRO)														
Colombia	54	27.8	4.8	47	10.3	2.0	30	7.8	1.6	86	3.4	0.6	96.1*	(<.001)
Mexico	52	25.8	4.3	53	17.9	2.9	33	11.9	2.3	102	3.2	0.4	132.9*	(<.001)
United States	385	59.7	2.4	394	39.9	1.3	219	26.2	1.7	479	9.7	0.6	668.5*	(<.001)
WHO: Regional Office for Africa (AFRO)														
Nigeria	8	21.3	11.9	6	13.8	7.4	14	10.0	3.0	29	1.0	0.3	27.7*	(<.001)
South Africa	45	26.2	3.6	66	26.6	3.9	67	23.1	3.2	497	13.4	0.9	41.0*	(<.001)
WHO: Regional Office for the Eastern Mediterranean (EMRO)														
Lebanon	22	20.1	5.2	19	11.6	3.1	7	4.0	1.6	29	3.0	0.7	34.9*	(<.001)

(Continued)

Table 6.17 Percentages Using 12-Month Services by Severity of Mental Disorders in the WMH Surveys[1] *(Continued)*

	Severe			Moderate			Mild			None			Test of difference in probability of treatment by severity	
Country	n	%[2]	se	n	%[2]	se	n	%[2]	se	n	%[2]	se	χ^2_3	(p-value)
WHO: Regional Office for Europe (EURO)														
Belgium	46	62.1	9.2	30	38.4	8.3	13	12.7	4.6	98	6.8	1.1	227.1*	(<.001)
France	56	48.0	6.4	70	29.4	4.0	43	22.4	3.4	103	7.0	1.1	82.6*	(<.001)
Germany	30	40.6	8.9	39	23.9	4.7	27	20.5	5.2	87	5.9	0.9	54.5*	(<.001)
Israel	81	53.9	4.0	54	32.6	3.7	19	14.4	3.2	267	6.0	0.4	368.1*	(<.001)
Italy	29	51.6	6.5	38	25.9	4.2	21	17.8	4.5	53	2.2	0.4	192.7*	(<.001)
Netherlands	57	49.2	6.6	36	31.3	7.2	15	16.1	6.0	94	7.7	1.3	66.8*	(<.001)
Spain	79	58.7	4.9	93	37.4	5.0	35	17.3	4.3	168	3.9	0.5	446.1*	(<.001)
Ukraine	49	25.7	3.2	68	21.2	3.6	19	7.6	2.6	76	4.4	0.8	81.2*	(<.001)
WHO: Regional Office for the Western Pacific (WPRO)														
People's Republic of China	5	11.0	5.4	11	23.5	10.9	3	1.7	1.2	55	2.9	0.6	16.1*	(.001)
Japan[3]	10	24.2	5.0	16	24.2	5.0	9	12.8	4.4	57	4.5	0.9	44.5*[3]	(<.001)
New Zealand	458	56.6	2.2	421	39.8	1.9	184	22.2	1.9	529	7.3	0.5	644.8*	(<.001)
χ^2_{16}[4]	186.9* (<.001)			145.6* (<.001)			104.1* (<.001)			330.0* (<.001)				

*Significant at the .05 level, two-sided test.

[1] Percentages are based on entire Part 2 samples.

[2] Percentages are based on respondents using any services within each level of severity.

[3] Severe and moderate cases were combined into one category for Japan and the percentage using services was displayed in both columns. The χ^2 test was two degrees of freedom for this country.

[4] χ^2_{16} is from a model predicting any 12-month service use among respondents within each level of severity.

had lifetime disorders in partial remission or sub-threshold syndromes associated with meaningful role impairment and were probably using treatments appropriately (Druss et al., 2007).

Severity of Disorders and Mental Health Specialty Care

Additional evidence that treatment resources may not be optimally allocated comes from analyses examining the relationship between disorder severity and use of the mental health specialty (MHS) sector among respondents receiving services (see Table 6.18). In only six of 17 WMH countries were there significant relationships between severity and use of MHS sectors; even in countries where such relationships existed, meaningful proportions of mild and non-cases were observed to use MHS sectors.

Adequacy of Treatments

The proportion of respondents starting treatments who received any follow-up care ranged between 70.2% (Germany) and 94.5% (Italy; see Table 6.19). With a few notable exceptions, the proportions receiving any follow-up care were generally smaller in low- and middle- than in high-income countries. The relationships between disorder severity and the probability of receiving follow-up care were statistically significant in only seven countries; again, there were meaningful proportions of both severe cases who did not receive at least some follow-up care and apparent non-cases who did.

The proportions of respondents using services who received treatments that met the definition for being potentially minimally adequate ranged between 10.4% (Nigeria) and 42.3% (France; see Table 6.20). Lower income countries generally had smaller proportions, although the small proportion observed in the United States (18.1%) was a notable exception. The relationships between disorder severity and probability of receiving minimally adequate treatment were significant in only five countries. Again, there were meaningful proportions of both severe cases using services that did not receive minimally adequate treatment and apparent non-cases using services that did.

Implications for Mental Health

Even the basic descriptive information on the lifetime prevalence of mental disorders emerging from the WMH surveys has been of enormous value. For many participating countries, they provide the first representative general population data on the enormous burdens from mental disorders that are crucial for policymakers in those countries to make truly informed decisions regarding their nations' health and mental health policies, delivery systems, and resource allocation. Even this basic information from WMH surveys will be critical for comparing the worldwide disability from mental disorders to commonly occurring physical illnesses as

Table 6.18 Percentages Using Mental Health Specialty Sectors among Respondents Using Any Services in the WMH Surveys[1]

Country	Severe			Moderate			Mild			None			Test of difference in probability of treatment by severity	
	n	%[2]	se	n	%[2]	se	n	%[2]	se	n	%[2]	se	χ² (1 or 3 df)[+]	(p-value)[+]
WHO: Regional Office for the Americas (AMRO)														
Colombia	30	62.9	8.3	28	47.1	8.0	19	62.2	10.3	49	48.8	8.3	1.9	(.60)
Mexico	26	60.3	8.0	30	59.1	6.8	15	51.0	11.2	50	50.4	7.0	1.1	(.78)
United States	250	66.0	2.4	182	45.0	3.3	91	41.5	3.1	215	43.8	2.6	59.6*	(<.001)
WHO: Regional Office for Africa (AFRO)														
Nigeria	1	—[3]	—[3]	0	—[3]	—[3]	3	9.5	4.5	1	9.5	4.5	1.4	(.24)
South Africa	14	35.9	7.6	13	19.7	5.9	12	15.5	5.6	69	14.1	2.0	15.4*	(.002)
WHO: Regional Office for the Eastern Mediterranean (EMRO)														
Lebanon	7	35.6	9.2	5	35.6	9.2	1	14.0	7.3	5	14.0	7.3	3.1	(.08)

154

WHO: Regional Office for Europe (EURO)

Belgium	25	58.6	9.8	17	48.6	10.9	6	-3	-3	48	43.4	7.0	1.5	(.68)
France	27	49.7	8.6	26	33.8	8.3	13	34.1	7.0	45	40.1	6.9	2.4	(.50)
Germany	17	46.4	12.1	27	68.9	8.9	12	-3	-3	44	47.4	6.2	9.8*	(.020)
Israel	39	47.4	5.7	31	55.7	7.1	10	-3	-3	135	50.0	3.3	1.1	(.76)
Italy	10	-3	-3	11	33.8	10.6	7	-3	-3	27	63.6	7.5	7.0	(.07)
Netherlands	34	66.9	7.3	22	45.2	15.5	7	-3	-3	42	47.5	9.2	2.5	(.48)
Spain	52	65.4	7.3	55	61.3	5.5	19	41.2	10.4	74	45.8	6.5	5.6	(.13)
Ukraine	15	34.8	6.8	9	16.2	8.2	3	-3	-3	12	12.5	5.3	8.6*	(.035)

WHO: Regional Office for the Western Pacific (WPRO)

People's Republic of China	3	-3	-3	2	-3	-3	3	16.7	6.8	11	16.7	6.8	0.2	(.64)
Japan	7	-3	-3	13	-3	-3	5	34.2	6.0	18	34.2	6.0	12.0*	(<.001)
New Zealand	232	57.4	2.9	140	34.7	3.4	49	26.3	4.3	164	32.0	2.9	63.1*	(<.001)

*Significant at the .05 level, two-sided test.

[1] Percentages are based on entire Part 2 samples.

[2] Percentages are those in any mental health treatment among respondents using any services within each level of severity.

[3] Percentages not reported if the number of respondents using any services in a level of severity <30.

[4] One degree of freedom χ^2 tests were performed for Nigeria, Lebanon, Japan and People's Republic of China, where combined severe and moderate was compared against combined mild and none category. Three degree of freedom tests were performed for all other countries.

Table 6.19 Percentages Receiving Follow-up Treatment[1] Among Respondents Using Services in the WMH Surveys

Country	Any severity			Severe			Moderate			Mild			None			Test of difference in probability of follow-up treatment by severity	
	n	%[2]	se	n	%[3]	se	n	%[3]	se	n	%[3]	se	n	%[3]	se	χ^2 (1 or 3 df)[5]	(p-value)[5]
WHO: Regional Office for the Americas (AMRO)																	
Colombia	158	72.0	4.3	49	92.6	3.5	31	73.1	7.9	20	61.7	11.3	58	63.6	7.9	12.3*	(.006)
Mexico	180	74.5	4.4	40	85.5	4.2	41	76.6	6.7	25	84.3	6.9	74	67.8	7.7	6.0	(.11)
United States	1313	86.8	1.4	362	93.2	1.7	354	88.4	2.0	187	83.0	2.9	410	83.3	2.6	17.2*	(.001)
WHO: Regional Office for Africa (AFRO)																	
Nigeria	47	76.3	8.7	6	—[4]	—[4]	6	—[4]	—[4]	13	74.6	9.2	22	74.6	9.2	0.4	(.51)
South Africa	601	89.1	1.7	42	93.9	3.9	63	95.7	3.0	58	87.4	3.7	438	88.0	2.2	3.0	(.39)
WHO: Regional Office for the Eastern Mediterranean (EMRO)																	
Lebanon	62	78.9	6.9	17	84.1	4.4	15	84.1	4.4	7	75.7	10.2	23	75.7	10.2	0.8	(.37)

WHO: Regional Office for Europe (EURO)

	n	%		n	%		n	%		n	%		n	%		χ^2	
Belgium	165	84.3	3.9	42	84.4	9.5	27	84.3	10.4	12	—[4]	—[4]	84	83.1	5.1	3.1	(.38)
France	235	86.0	3.9	49	87.5	4.7	65	97.3	1.6	35	89.7	4.4	86	80.0	6.9	7.8	(.05)
Germany	152	70.2	5.1	28	89.2	8.5	37	97.1	0.7	23	—[4]	—[4]	64	61.1	7.4	66.4*	(<.001)
Israel	364	86.1	1.8	73	90.7	3.2	48	89.2	4.2	17	—[4]	—[4]	226	83.6	2.4	3.3	(.34)
Italy	129	94.5	1.5	28	—[4]	—[4]	34	93.1	3.7	19	—[4]	—[4]	48	94.4	2.4	1.3	(.73)
Netherlands	183	85.9	4.3	53	96.4	2.1	35	98.9	1.2	15	—[4]	—[4]	80	78.5	7.2	10.0*	(.007)
Spain	341	88.8	2.6	73	95.3	1.9	86	92.6	3.0	33	90.8	6.2	149	84.7	4.7	5.8	(.12)
Ukraine	167	79.1	3.8	44	92.3	3.6	51	82.3	4.5	14	—[4]	—[4]	58	71.8	7.0	12.5*	(.006)

WHO: Regional Office for the Western Pacific (WPRO)

	n	%		n	%		n	%		n	%		n	%		χ^2	
People's Republic of China	56	77.6	6.0	4	—[4]	—[4]	6	—[4]	—[4]	3	80.8	6.8	43	80.8	6.8	1.0	(.33)
Japan	83	89.8	2.6	9	—[4]	—[4]	13	—[4]	—[4]	9	91.2	3.3	52	91.2	3.3	0.9	(.33)
New Zealand	1394	85.7	1.3	421	92.5	1.4	368	88.7	1.8	151	83.5	3.2	454	81.0	2.8	15.1*	(.002)
χ^2_{16}[6]		67.1* (<.001)			25.4 (.06)			71.5* (<.001)			21.3 (.13)			47.9* (<.001)			

*Significant at the .05 level, two-sided test.

[1] Follow-up treatment was defined as receiving two or more visits to any service sector, or being in ongoing treatment at interview.

[2] Percentages are based on entire Part 2 samples.

[3] Percentages are those receiving follow-up treatment among those in treatment within each level of severity.

[4] Percentages not reported if the number of cases with any treatment in a level of severity < 30.

[5] One degree of freedom chi-square tests were performed for Nigeria, Lebanon, Japan, and People's Republic of China, where combined severe and moderate was compared against combined mild and none category. Three degree of freedom tests were performed for all other countries.

[6] χ^2_{16} is from a model predicting follow-up treatment among respondents that used any 12-month services.

Table 6.20 Percentages Receiving Minimally Adequate Treatment[1] among Respondents Using Services in the WMH Surveys

Country	Any severity			Severe			Moderate			Mild			None			Test of difference in probability of minimally adequate treatment by severity	
	n	%[2]	se	n	%[3]	se	n	%[3]	se	n	%[3]	se	n	%[3]	se	χ² (1, 2, or 3 df)[5]	(p-value)[5]
WHO: Regional Office for the Americas (AMRO)																	
Colombia	33	14.7	3.4	11	23.1	8.5	7	21.7	10.5	3	6.3	4.6	12	10.1	3.5	4.7	(.20)
Mexico	42	15.2	2.7	8	11.3	4.5	13	28.6	6.3	6	19.8	5.8	15	11.3	4.0	10.5*	(.014)
United States	302	18.1	1.1	160	41.8	3.2	101	24.8	2.1	41	4.9	0.8	—	—	—	114.0*	(<.001)
WHO: Regional Office for Africa (AFRO)																	
Nigeria	1	10.4	9.8	0	—[4]	—[4]	0	—[4]	—[4]	0	12.4	11.8	1	12.4	11.8		
South Africa	0	—[7]	—[7]	0	—[7]	—[7]	0	—[7]	—[7]	0	—[7]	—[7]	0	—[7]	—[7]		
WHO: Regional Office for the Eastern Mediterranean (EMRO)																	
Lebanon	18	24.5	7.1	5	24.0	6.2	3	24.0	6.2	3	24.8	10.7	7	24.8	10.7	0.0	(.95)

WHO: Regional Office for Europe (EURO)

Country	N	%	SE	N	%	SE	N	%	SE	N	%	SE	N	%	SE	χ^2_{13}	(p)
Belgium	78	33.6	5.2	23	42.5	8.5	12	35.5	12.6	5	—[4]	—[4]	38	29.4	6.2	1.7	(.63)
France	113	42.3	5.4	29	57.9	8.5	28	36.5	6.6	15	41.5	9.7	41	40.2	8.3	3.4	(.34)
Germany	91	42.0	6.1	21	67.3	10.7	21	53.3	8.4	14	—[4]	—[4]	35	35.4	8.8	6.1	(.11)
Israel	148	35.1	2.5	28	34.4	5.4	21	40.3	6.8	6	—[4]	—[4]	93	34.3	3.1	0.7	(.87)
Italy	45	33.0	5.1	12	—[4]	—[4]	11	35.7	9.4	6	—[4]	—[4]	16	29.9	7.4	3.5	(.32)
Netherlands	98	34.4	5.0	37	65.7	9.2	19	34.1	10.2	10	—[4]	—[4]	32	21.9	5.2	23.2*	(<.001)
Spain	152	37.3	3.3	41	47.5	7.5	37	43.6	5.6	20	44.8	9.9	54	30.1	4.4	8.5*	(.037)
Ukraine	0	—[7]	—[7]	0	—[7]	—[7]	0	—[7]	—[7]	0	—[7]	—[7]	0	—[7]	—[7]	—[7]	—[7]
χ^2_6	117.0* (<.001)			41.0* (<.001)			31.2* (.002)			25.9* (.011)			96.7* (<.001)				

WHO: Regional Office for the Western Pacific (WPRO)

Country	N	%	SE	N	%	SE	N	%	SE	N	%	SE	N	%	SE	χ^2_{13}	(p)
People's Republic of China	19	24.1	7.0	0	—[4]	—[4]	3	—[4]	—[4]	2	20.1	5.9	14	20.1	5.9	0.8	(.36)
Japan	35	31.8	6.8	6	—[4]	—[4]	6	—[4]	—[4]	5	27.9	7.0	18	27.9	7.0	4.4*	(.037)
New Zealand	0	—[7]	—[7]	0	—[7]	—[7]	0	—[7]	—[7]	0	—[7]	—[7]	0	—[7]	—[7]	—[7]	—[7]
χ^2_{13}	41.0* (<.001)			31.2* (.002)			25.9* (.011)			96.7* (<.001)							

*Significant at the .05 level, two-sided test.

[1] Minimally adequate treatment was defined as receiving eight or more visits to any service sector, or four or more visits and at least one month of medication, or being in ongoing treatment at interview.

[2] Percentages based on entire Part 2 samples.

[3] Percentages are those receiving minimally adequate treatment among those in treatment within each level of severity.

[4] Percentages not reported if the number of cases with any treatment in a level of severity < 30.

[5] The test was not performed for Nigeria because there was only one (unweighted) case with adequate treatment. One degree of freedom chi-square tests were performed for Lebanon, Japan, and People's Republic of China, where combined severe and moderate was compared against combined mild and none category. Two degree of freedom test was performed for the United States, where the mild and none categories were collapsed. Three degree of freedom tests were performed for all other countries.

[6] χ^2_{13} is from a model predicting minimally adequate treatment among respondents in each level of severity that used any 12-month services.

[7] The questions on pharmacoepidemiology were not asked in Ukraine, South Africa, or New Zealand.

part of ongoing efforts to document the relative sources of total global disease burden.

The consistent finding across WMH surveys that many lifetime cases of mental disorders have early ages of onset will be useful for designing and targeting public health interventions. It suggests that focusing on intervening earlier in childhood may be a prudent way to reduce the persistence or severity of primary disorders and possibly even prevent the onset of secondary disorders. Interventions at the local level could be applied in schools, clinics, or health care systems to reduce long periods of untreated mental illness. Components of such interventions might consist of public awareness, screening, aggressive outreach, and prompt initiation of or referral to treatment (Aseltine & DeMartino, 2004; Beidel, Turner, & Morris, 2000; Carleton et al., 1996; Connors, 1994; Jacobs, 1995; Morrissey-Kane & Prinz, 1999; MTA Cooperative Group, 1999; Regier et al., 1988; Velicer, Hughes, Fava, Prochaska, & DiClemente, 1995; Weaver, 1995). At the national level, programs and policies that support earlier help-seeking are also needed to help minimize failure and delay in initial treatment contact.

The WMH results regarding 12-month prevalences of mental disorders confirm earlier surveys in showing that recent mental disorders are highly prevalent and associated with substantial role impairment (Cross National Collaborative Group, 1994; Kessler & Frank, 1997; Ormel et al., 1994; Weissman et al., 1997; Weissman, Bland, Canino, Faravelli et al., 1996; Weissman, Bland, Canino, Greenwald et al., 1996; Wells, Bushnell, Hornblow, Joyce, & Oakley-Browne, 1989). Implications for policymakers, that mental disorders represent a serious public health problem in need of urgent attention, are only strengthened by the likelihood that these prevalence and severity estimates are conservative. As discussed above, survey non-respondents tend to have significantly higher rates as well as severity of mental illness than respondents. Furthermore, even respondents may have had greater reluctance in some WMH countries to admit to emotional problems (Allgulander, 1989; Eaton, Anthony, Tepper, & Dryman, 1992; Kessler et al., 1994; Kessler & Merikangas, 2004).

The results concerning the services received in the prior year by 12-month cases reveal that there are very high levels of unmet need for mental health treatment worldwide, including among those with the most serious disorders. Roughly half of severe cases receive no services in economically advantaged nations, and the problem is much worse in developing countries. Again, the most plausible study limitations, such as sample bias or response bias, would lead these estimates of unmet need for treatment to be conservative. Furthermore, even among the minority of cases receiving some services, far fewer are likely to have been *effectively* treated. Some treatments consisted of non-health care from CAM and human services sectors, for which little is known concerning efficacy and safety (Niggemann & Gruber, 2003). Nearly one-quarter of those initiating treatments failed to receive any follow-up care, and only a minority of treatments were observed to meet minimal standards for adequacy (Agency for Health Care Policy and Research, 1993; American Psychiatric Association, 2006; Lehman & Steinwachs, 1998; Wang et al., 2005).

Such high levels of unmet need worldwide may not be surprising given the low level of expenditures by most countries for mental health services, both in absolute terms as well as relative to the magnitude of the societal burdens posed by mental disorders (Lopez, Mathers, Ezzati, Jamison, & Murray, 2006; Saxena et al., 2003). For example, low- and middle-income countries often spend less than 1% of their already constrained health care budgets on mental health care, in spite of the enormous burdens that the WMH Surveys have shown such countries bear from mental disorders (Saxena et al., 2003). Yet beyond indicating that additional treatment resources are needed, the WMH results also reveal some strategies for countries to optimally allocate the limited mental health resources that are available. The consistent observation that so many serious cases are untreated suggests that there should be conscious and concerted attempts to meet the needs of society's most vulnerable patients. Likewise, optimal use of a country's health care sectors, perhaps with the general medical sector being used to broaden access to treatments and the mental health specialty sector being used to intensify and focus care on the most serious cases, also seems indicated (Rosenheck et al., 1998).

Finally, regardless of how treatment resources are allocated, the WMH results concerning 12-month services suggest that broad improvements are needed in the continuity and quality of the mental health treatments that are being delivered. Fortunately, a variety of successful interventions have been developed, which can improve treatment initiation, dropout, and adequacy through application of such techniques as motivational interviewing, ongoing symptom monitoring, and "academic detailing" of clinicians to promote best-practices care. An example of one such intervention, which developed out of the WMH initiative, is covered below (Wang, Aguilar-Gaxiola et al., 2007). Again, at the national level, general and mental health care policies, delivery system designs, and levels or mechanisms of financing are crucial to promote uptake of such interventions and ultimately improve the access to, quality of, and outcomes from mental health treatments.

Future Directions

The WMH Survey Initiative continues to expand, both in the number of participating countries and the scientific agendas that it can address. In terms of participating countries, national surveys in Iraq and India and a regional survey in Brazil have recently been added. Meanwhile, analyses of WMH survey data have moved beyond generating the basic descriptive information presented in the current chapter to answering a wider range of questions. For example, WMH Workgroups are currently examining important sociodemographic correlates of mental disorders, such as gender and social class, using a cross-national framework. Other WMH investigators are exploring substantive risk factors for mental disorders, such as the experience of childhood adversities and traumatic events. Another WMH Workgroup is examining the reasons for failing to receive treatment as well as for dropping out prematurely.

A large WMH effort is under way to provide a comprehensive accounting of the societal costs from mental disorders, including the impacts of early-onset disorders on reduced educational attainment, early marriage, marital instability, and low earnings, as well as the effects of recent disorders on current role functioning. A related set of analyses is employing the standard measures of health preferences contained in WMH surveys (e.g., visual analog, time trade-off, and willingness to pay) to assess the utilities associated with a wide variety of mental and general medical conditions (Gyrd-Hansen, 2005; Torrance, 2006). These results, and as well those on the epidemiology of mental disorders from WMH surveys, will help inform the update of the Global Burden of Disease initiative that is currently being undertaken (Murray et al., 2007).

Another focus of interest for the WMH investigators is shedding light on the co-morbidity between mental disorders and general medical conditions (Demyttenaere et al., 2007; Gureje et al., 2008; Ormel et al., 2007; Scott et al., 2008; Scott et al., 2007). The information gathered in the WMH surveys has also allowed collaborators to provide a truly global understanding of the phenomenon of suicidality, including ideation, plans, gestures, and attempts (Borges et al., 2006; Nock et al., 2008; Nock & Kessler, 2006). A more detailed description of the work being generated as a result of the WMH Initiative is beyond the scope of this chapter but can be found on the WMH Web site at www.hcp.med.harvard.edu/wmh.

As mentioned in the Methodologic Considerations section of this chapter, even though data from the WMH Surveys are naturalistic, they can nevertheless be critically important for informing the design, targeting, and testing of successful interventions that address unmet needs for cost-effective mental health care. An example of the process through which this may be possible starts with the critical observation in the first wave of the U.S. WMH survey (the original NCS) that major depression was associated with substantially impaired work performance among employed people (Kessler & Frank, 1997). Although these results required cautious interpretation due to the inability to rule out alternative explanations (e.g., reverse causation), they did suggest that further observational as well as experimental study was needed of whether enhanced detection and treatment of workers with depression might lead to positive returns-on-investment for employers (Kessler et al., 1999). These early findings directly led to simulation modeling that made use of both available epidemiological data to estimate the prevalence of depression and its impact on work performance as well as available treatment trial data to estimate the likely impact of screening, outreach, and expanded treatment on workers' performances (Wang et al., 2006). This program of research, built upon a foundation of observational WMH findings, led to the launch of a major experimental workplace treatment effectiveness trial. Recent results have shown that expanded detection, outreach, and treatment of depressed workers can, in fact, have a positive return on investment from the employer perspective (Wang, Simon et al., 2007).

Finally, even if the opportunities or resources to conduct true experimental intervention trials are not available, it may still be possible to make provisional causal inferences based upon descriptive WMH epidemiological data. Methodologic developments in quasi-experimental methods and analytic techniques, such as the econometric technique known as instrumental variables analysis, may make it possible in the future to produce unbiased estimates of the effect of exposures on outcomes using observational WMH survey information (e.g., Brookhart et al., 2007; Lu, 1999; Schneeweiss, Setoguchi, Brookhart, Dormuth, & Wang, 2007). Toward these ends, individual-level WMH data could be linked with those of the WHO Project Atlas (http://apps.who.int/globalatlas/default.asp) as well as the WHO Assessment Instrument for Mental Health (http://www.who.int/mental_health/evidence/WHO-AIMS/en/) on existing policies, delivery systems, and financing of mental health care (Mezzich, 2003; Saxena et al., 2003). Such linked datasets could become among the first tools for shedding light on the impacts of general and mental health care policies, delivery system designs, and levels or mechanisms of financing mental health services on the timely receipt and continuity of high quality treatment. In this way, WMH survey data could provide a wide variety of stakeholders with invaluable information to guide their future decision-making and ultimately improve both the care and the outcomes experienced by people with mental disorders worldwide.

Acknowledgments

The tables in this chapter have appeared previously in: Kessler, R. C., & Üstün, T. B. (Eds.). (2008). *The WHO World Mental Health Surveys Global Perspective on the Epidemiology of Mental Disorders*. New York: Cambridge University Press and the World Health Organization. Copyright © World Health Organization 2008. Reprinted with permission. The views and opinions expressed are those of the authors and should not be construed to represent the views of any sponsoring organization, agencies, or the U.S. Government.

References

Agency for Health Care Policy and Research. (1993). *Depression Guideline Panel: Vol 2, Treatment of Major Depression, Clinical Practice Guideline, No 5*. Rockville, MD: U.S. Department of Health and Human Services, Public Health Service, Agency for Health Care Policy and Research.

Alegria, M., Bijl, R. V., Lin, E., Walters, E. E., & Kessler, R. C. (2000). Income differences in persons seeking outpatient treatment for mental disorders: A comparison of the US with Ontario and the Netherlands. *Archives of General Psychiatry, 57*, 383–391.

Allgulander, C. (1989). Psychoactive drug use in a general population sample, Sweden: correlates with perceived health, psychiatric diagnoses, and mortality in an automated record-linkage study. *American Journal of Public Health, 79*, 1006–1010.

American Psychiatric Association. (2006). *Practice Guidelines for Treatment of Psychiatric Disorders: Compendium 2006*. Arlington, VA: American Psychiatric Association Press.

Andrade, L., de Lolio, C., Gentil, V., Laurenti, R., & Werebe, D. (1996, August). *Lifetime Prevalence of Mental Disorders in a Catchment Area in Sao Paulo, Brazil*. Paper presented at the VII Congress of the International Federation of Psychiatric Epidemiology, Santiago, Chile.

Andrade, L., Walters, E. E., Gentil, V., & Laurenti, R. (2002). Prevalence of ICD-10 mental disorders in a catchment area in the city of Sao Paulo, Brazil. *Social Psychiatry and Psychiatric Epidemiology, 37*, 316–325.

Aseltine, R. H., Jr., & DeMartino, R. (2004). An outcome evaluation of the SOS Suicide Prevention Program. *American Journal of Public Health, 94*, 446–451.

Beidel, D. C., Turner, S. M., & Morris, T. L. (2000). Behavioral treatment of childhood social phobia. *Journal of Consulting and Clinical Psychology, 68*, 1072–1080.

Bijl, R. V., de Graaf, R., Hiripi, E., Kessler, R. C., Kohn, R., Offord, D. R., et al. (2003). The prevalence of treated and untreated mental disorders in five countries. *Health Affairs (Millwood), 22*, 122–133.

Bijl, R. V., van Zessen, G., Ravelli, A., de Rijk, C., & Langendoen, Y. (1998). The Netherlands Mental Health Survey and Incidence Study (NEMESIS): Objectives and design. *Social Psychiatry and Psychiatric Epidemiology, 33*, 581–586.

Bland, R. C., Orn, H., & Newman, S. C. (1988). Lifetime prevalence of psychiatric disorders in Edmonton. *Acta Psychiatrica Scandinavica Supplement, 338*, 24–32.

Borges, G., Angst, J., Nock, M. K., Ruscio, A. M., Walters, E. E., & Kessler, R. C. (2006). A risk index for 12-month suicide attempts in the National Comorbidity Survey Replication (NCS-R). *Psychological Medicine, 36*, 1747–1757.

Brookhart, M. A., Rassen, J. A., Wang, P. S., Dormuth, C., Mogun, H., & Schneeweiss, S. (2007). Evaluating the validity of an instrumental variable study of neuroleptics: Can between-physician differences in prescribing patterns be used to estimate treatment effects? *Medical Care, 45*, S116–122.

Caraveo, J., Martinez, J., & Rivera, B. (1998). A model for epidemiological studies on mental health and psychiatric morbidity. *Salud Mental, 21*, 48–57.

Carleton, R. A., Bazzarre, T., Drake, J., Dunn, A., Fisher, E. B., Jr., Grundy, S. M., et al. (1996). Report of the Expert Panel on Awareness and Behavior Change to the Board of Directors, American Heart Association. *Circulation, 93*, 1768–1772.

Chang, S. M., Hahm, B. J., Lee, J. Y., Shin, M. S., Jeon, H. J., Hong, J. P., et al. (2008). Cross-national difference in the prevalence of depression caused by the diagnostic threshold. *Journal of Affective Disorders, 106*, 159–167.

Choy, Y., Schneier, F. R., Heimberg, R. G., Oh, K. S., & Liebowitz, M. R. (2008). Features of the offensive subtype of Taijin-Kyofu-Sho in US and Korean patients with DSM-IV social anxiety disorder. *Depression Anxiety, 25*, 230–240.

Connors, C. K. (1994). The Connors Rating Scales: Use in clinical assessment, treatment planning, and research. In M. Maruish (Ed.), *Use of Psychological Testing for Treatment Planning and Outcome Assessment.* Hillsdale, NJ: Lawrence Erlbaum Associates.

Cooke, D. J., Hart, S. D., & Michie, C. (2004). Cross-national differences in the assessment of psychopathy: Do they reflect variations in raters' perceptions of symptoms? *Psychological Assessment, 16*, 335–339.

Cross National Collaborative Group. (1994). The cross national epidemiology of obsessive compulsive disorder. *Journal of Clinical Psychiatry, 55*(Suppl.), 5–10.

Demyttenaere, K., Bruffaerts, R., Lee, S., Posada-Villa, J., Kovess, V., Angermeyer, M. C., et al. (2007). Mental disorders among persons with chronic back or neck pain: Results from the World Mental Health Surveys. *Pain, 129*, 332–342.

Druss, B. G., Wang, P. S., Sampson, N. A., Olfson, M., Pincus, H. A., Wells, K. B., et al. (2007). Understanding mental health treatment in persons without mental diagnoses: Results from the National Comorbidity Survey Replication. *Archives of General Psychiatry, 64*, 1196–1203.

Eaton, W. W., Anthony, J. C., Tepper, S., & Dryman, A. (1992). Psychopathology and attrition in the epidemiologic catchment area surveys. *American Journal of Epidemiology, 135*, 1051–1059.

Gureje, O., Lasebikan, V. O., Kola, L., & Makanjuola, V. A. (2006). Lifetime and 12-month prevalence of mental disorders in the Nigerian Survey of Mental Health and Well-Being. *British Journal of Psychiatry, 188*, 465–471.

Gureje, O., Von Korff, M., Kola, L., Demyttenaere, K., He, Y., Posada-Villa, J., et al. (2008). The relation between multiple pains and mental disorders: Results from the World Mental Health Surveys. *Pain, 135*, 82–91.

Gyrd-Hansen, D. (2005). Willingness to pay for a QALY: Theoretical and methodological issues. *Pharmacoeconomics, 23*, 423–432.

Hagnell, O. (1966). *A Prospective Study of the Incidence of Mental Disorder: A Study Based on 24,000 Person Years of the Incidence of Mental Disorders in a Swedish Population together with an Evaluation of the Aetiological Significance of Medical, Social, and Personality Factors.* Lund: Svenska Bokforlaget.

Haro, J.M., Arbabzadeh-Bouchez, S., Brugha, T. S., de Girolamo, G., Guyer, M. E., Jin, R., Lépine, J.-P., Mazzi, F., Reneses, B., Vilagut, G., Sampson, N. A., Kessler, R. C. (2006).

Concordance of the Composite International Diagnostic Interview Version 3.0 (CIDI 3.0) with standardized clinical assessments in the WHO World Mental Health Surveys. *International Journal of Methods in Psychiatric Research, 15*(4), 167–180.

Haro, J. M., Arbabzadeh-Bouchez, S., Brugha, T. S., de Girolamo, G., Guyer, M. E., Jin, R., et al. (2008). Concordance of the Composite International Diagnostic Interview Version 3.0 (CIDI 3.0) with standardized clinical assessments in the WHO World Mental Health Surveys. In R. C. Kessler & T. B. Üstün (Eds.), *The WHO World Mental Health Surveys: Global Perspectives on the Epidemiology of Mental Disorders*. New York: Cambridge University Press pp 114–127.

Hasin, D. S., & Grant, B. F. (2004). The co-occurrence of DSM-IV alcohol abuse in DSM-IV alcohol dependence: Results of the National Epidemiologic Survey on Alcohol and Related Conditions on heterogeneity that differ by population subgroup. *Archives of General Psychiatry, 61*, 891–896.

Hwu, H. G., Yeh, E. K., & Chang, L. Y. (1989). Prevalence of psychiatric disorders in Taiwan defined by the Chinese Diagnostic Interview Schedule. *Acta Psychiatrica Scandinavica, 79*, 136–147.

Jacobs, D. G. (1995). National depression screening day: Educating the public, reaching those in need of treatment and broadening professional understanding. *Harvard Review of Psychiatry, 3*, 156–159.

Jenkins, R., Bebbington, P., Brugha, T., Farrell, M., Gill, B., Lewis, G., et al. (1997). The National Psychiatric Morbidity surveys of Great Britain: Strategy and methods. *Psychological Medicine, 27*, 765–774.

Kessler, R. C., Aguilar-Gaxiola, S., Alonso, J., Angermeyer, M. C., Anthony, J. C., Brugha, T. S., et al. (2008). Prevalence and severity of mental disorders in the WMH Surveys. In R. C. Kessler & T. B. Üstün (Eds.), *The WHO World Mental Health Surveys: Global Perspectives on the Epidemiology of Mental Disorders*. New York: Cambridge University Press, pp. 534–540.

Kessler, R. C., Barber, C., Birnbaum, H. G., Frank, R. G., Greenberg, P. E., Rose, R. M., et al. (1999). Depression in the workplace: Effects on short-term disability. *Health Affairs (Millwood), 18*, 163–171.

Kessler, R. C., & Frank, R. G. (1997). The impact of psychiatric disorders on work loss days. *Psychological Medicine, 27*, 861–873.

Kessler, R. C., McGonagle, K. A., Zhao, S., Nelson, C. B., Hughes, M., Eshleman, S., et al. (1994). Lifetime and 12-month prevalence of DSM-III-R psychiatric disorders in the United States: Results from the National Comorbidity Survey. *Archives of General Psychiatry, 51*, 8–19.

Kessler, R. C., & Merikangas, K. R. (2004). The National Comorbidity Survey Replication (NCS-R): Background and aims. *International Journal of Methods in Psychiatric Research, 13*, 60–68.

Kohn, R., Saxena, S., Levav, I., & Saraceno, B. (2004). The treatment gap in mental health care. *Bulletin of the World Health Organization, 82*, 858–866.

Kýlýç, C. (1998). *Mental Health Profile of Turkey: Main Report*. Ankara, Turkey: Ministry of Health Publications.

Langner, T. S., & Michael, S. T. (1963). *Life Stress and Mental Health: The Midtown Manhattan Study*. London: Collier-MacMillan.

Lehman, A. F., & Steinwachs, D. M. (1998). Translating research into practice: The Schizophrenia Patient Outcomes Research Team (PORT) treatment recommendations. *Schizophrenia Bulletin, 24*, 1–10.

Leighton, A. H. (1959). *My Name Is Legion: Volume 1 of the Stirling County Study*. New York: Basic Books.

Leon, A. C., Olfson, M., Portera, L., Farber, L., & Sheehan, D. V. (1997). Assessing psychiatric impairment in primary care with the Sheehan Disability Scale. *International Journal Psychiatry in Medicine, 27*, 93–105.

Lépine, J. P., Lellouch, J., Lovell, A., Teherani, M., Ha, C., Verdier-Taillefer, M. G., et al. (1989). Anxiety and depressive disorders in a French population: Methodology and preliminary results. *Psychiatric Psychobiology, 4*, 267–274.

Lopez, A. D., Mathers, C. D., Ezzati, M., Jamison, D. T., & Murray, C. J. L. (Eds.). (2006). *Global Burden of Disease and Risk Factors.* New York: Oxford University Press/World Bank.

Lu, M. (1999). The productivity of mental health care: An instrumental variable approach. *Journal of Mental Health Policy Economics, 2*, 59–71.

Mezzich, J. E. (2003). From financial analysis to policy development in mental health care: The need for broader conceptual models and partnerships. *Journal of Mental Health Policy Economics, 6*, 149–150.

Morrissey-Kane, E., & Prinz, R. J. (1999). Engagement in child and adolescent treatment: The role of parental cognitions and attributions. *Clinical Child and Family Psychology Review, 2*, 183–198.

MTA Cooperative Group. (1999). A 14-month randomized clinical trial of treatment strategies for attention-deficit/hyperactivity disorder: Multimodal Treatment Study of Children with ADHD. *Archives of General Psychiatry, 56*, 1073–1086.

Murray, C. J., Lopez, A. D., Black, R., Mathers, C. D., Shibuya, K., Ezzati, M., et al. (2007). Global burden of disease 2005: Call for collaborators. *Lancet, 370*, 109–110.

Narrow, W. E., Rae, D. S., Robins, L. N., & Regier, D. A. (2002). Revised prevalence estimates of mental disorders in the United States: Using a clinical significance criterion to reconcile 2 surveys' estimates. *Archives of General Psychiatry, 59*, 115–123.

Niggemann, B., & Gruber, C. (2003). Side-effects of complementary and alternative medicine. *Allergy, 58*, 707–716.

Nock, M. K., Borges, G., Bromet, E. J., Alonso, J., Angermeyer, M., Beautrais, A., et al. (2008). Cross-national prevalence and risk factors for suicidal ideation, plans, and attempts. *British Journal of Psychiatry, 192*, 98–105.

Nock, M. K., & Kessler, R. C. (2006). Prevalence of and risk factors for suicide attempts versus suicide gestures: Analysis of the National Comorbidity Survey. *Journal of Abnormal Psychology, 115*, 616–623.

Ormel, J., Von Korff, M., Burger, H., Scott, K., Demyttenaere, K., Huang, Y. Q., et al. (2007). Mental disorders among persons with heart disease: Results from World Mental Health surveys. *General Hospital Psychiatry, 29*, 325–334.

Ormel, J., Von Korff, N., Ustun, T. B., Pini, S., Korten, A., & Oldehinkel, T. (1994). Common mental disorders and disability across cultures: Results from the WHO collaborative study on psychological problems in general health care. *Journal of the American Medical Association, 272*, 1741–1748.

Regier, D. A., Hirschfeld, R. M., Goodwin, F. K., Burke, J. D., Jr., Lazar, J. B., & Judd, L. L. (1988). The NIMH Depression Awareness, Recognition, and Treatment Program: Structure, aims, and scientific basis. *American Journal of Psychiatry, 145*, 1351–1357.

Regier, D. A., Kaelber, C. T., Rae, D. S., Farmer, M. E., Knauper, B., Kessler, R. C., et al. (1998). Limitations of diagnostic criteria and assessment instruments for mental disorders: Implications for research and policy. *Archives of General Psychiatry, 55*, 109–115.

Regier, D. A., Narrow, W. E., Rupp, A., Rae, D. S., & Kaelber, C. T. (2000). The epidemiology of mental disorder treatment need: Community estimates of medical necessity. In G. Andrews & S. Henderson (Eds.), *Unmet Need in Psychiatry* (pp. 41–58). Cambridge, UK: Cambridge University Press.

Robins, L. N., & Regier, D. A. (Eds.). (1991). *Psychiatric Disorders in America: The Epidemiologic Catchment Area Study.* New York: The Free Press.

Rosenheck, R., Armstrong, M., Callahan, D., Dea, R., Del Vecchio, P., Flynn, L., et al. (1998). Obligation to the least well off in setting mental health service priorities: A consensus statement. *Psychiatric Services, 49*, 1273–1274, 1290.

Saxena, S., Sharan, P., & Saraceno, B. (2003). Budget and financing of mental health services: Baseline information on 89 countries from WHO's project atlas. *Journal of Mental Health Policy Economics, 6*, 135–143.

Schneeweiss, S., Setoguchi, S., Brookhart, A., Dormuth, C., & Wang, P. S. (2007). Risk of death associated with the use of conventional versus atypical antipsychotic drugs among elderly patients. *Canadian Medical Association Journal, 176*, 627–632.

Scott, K. M., Bruffaerts, R., Simon, G. E., Alonso, J., Angermeyer, M., de Girolamo, G., et al. (2008). Obesity and mental disorders in the general population: Results from the World Mental Health Surveys. *International Journal of Obesity, 32*, 192–200.

Scott, K. M., Von Korff, M., Ormel, J., Zhang, M. Y., Bruffaerts, R., Alonso, J., et al. (2007). Mental disorders among adults with asthma: Results from the World Mental Health Survey. *General Hospital Psychiatry, 29*, 123–133.

Shen, Y. C., Zhang, M. Y., Huang, Y. Q., He, Y. L., Liu, Z. R., Cheng, H., et al. (2006). Twelve-month prevalence, severity, and unmet need for treatment of mental disorders in metropolitan China. *Psychological Medicine, 36*, 257–267.

Shiffman, S., Stone, A. A., & Hufford, M. R. (2008). Ecological momentary assessment. *Annual Review of Clinical Psychology, 4*, 1–32.

Simon, G. E., Goldberg, D. P., Von Korff, M., & Ustun, T. B. (2002). Understanding cross-national differences in depression prevalence. *Psychological Medicine, 32*, 585–594.

Stone, A. A., & Broderick, J. E. (2007). Real-time data collection for pain: Appraisal and current status. *Pain Medicine, 8*(Suppl. 3), S85–93.

Torrance, G. W. (2006). Utility measurement in healthcare: The things I never got to. *Pharmacoeconomics, 24*, 1069–1078.

Tseng, W. S. (2006). From peculiar psychiatric disorders through culture-bound syndromes to culture-related specific syndromes. *Transcultural Psychiatry, 43*, 554–576.

Vega, W. A., Kolody, B., Aguilar-Gaxiola, S., Alderete, E., Catalano, R., & Caraveo-Anduaga, J. J. (1998). Lifetime prevalence of DSM-III-R psychiatric disorders among urban and rural Mexican Americans in California. *Archives of General Psychiatry, 55*, 771–778.

Velicer, W. F., Hughes, S. L., Fava, J. L., Prochaska, J. O., & DiClemente, C. C. (1995). An empirical typology of subjects within stage of change. *Addictive Behaviors, 20*, 299–320.

Wang, P. S., Aguilar-Gaxiola, S., Alonso, J., Angermeyer, M. C., Borges, G., Bromet, E. J., et al. (2007). Use of mental health services for anxiety, mood, and substance disorders in 17 countries in the WHO world mental health surveys. *Lancet, 370*, 841–850.

Wang, P. S., Lane, M., Olfson, M., Pincus, H. A., Wells, K. B., & Kessler, R. C. (2005). Twelve-month use of mental health services in the United States: Results from the National Comorbidity Survey Replication. *Archives of General Psychiatry, 62*, 629–640.

Wang, P. S., Patrick, A., Avorn, J., Azocar, F., Ludman, E., McCulloch, J., et al. (2006). The costs and benefits of enhanced depression care to employers. *Archives of General Psychiatry, 63*, 1345–1353.

Wang, P. S., Simon, G. E., Avorn, J., Azocar, F., Ludman, E. J., McCulloch, J., et al. (2007). Telephone screening, outreach, and care management for depressed workers and impact on clinical and work productivity outcomes: A randomized controlled trial. *Journal of the American Medical Association, 298*, 1401–1411.

Weaver, A. J. (1995). Has there been a failure to prepare and support parish-based clergy in their role as frontline community mental health workers: A review. *Journal of Pastoral Care, 49*, 129–147.

Weissman, M. M., Bland, R. C., Canino, G. J., Faravelli, C., Greenwald, S., Hwu, H. G., et al. (1997). The cross-national epidemiology of panic disorder. *Archives of General Psychiatry, 54*, 305–309.

Weissman, M. M., Bland, R. C., Canino, G. J., Faravelli, C., Greenwald, S., Hwu, H. G., et al. (1996). Cross-national epidemiology of major depression and bipolar disorder. *Journal of the American Medical Association, 276*, 293–299.

Weissman, M. M., Bland, R. C., Canino, G. J., Greenwald, S., Hwu, H. G., Lee, C. K., et al. (1994). The cross national epidemiology of obsessive compulsive disorder: The Cross National Collaborative Group. *Journal of Clinical Psychiatry, 55*(Suppl.), 5–10.

Weissman, M. M., Bland, R. C., Canino, G. J., Greenwald, S., Lee, C. K., Newman, S. C., et al. (1996). The cross-national epidemiology of social phobia: A preliminary report. *International Clinical Psychopharmacology, 11*(Suppl. 3), 9–14.

Wells, J. E., Bushnell, J. A., Hornblow, A. R., Joyce, P. R., & Oakley-Browne, M. A. (1989). Christchurch Psychiatric Epidemiology Study, part I: Methodology and lifetime prevalence for specific psychiatric disorders. *Australian and New Zealand Journal of Psychiatry, 23*, 315–326.

WHO International Consortium of Psychiatric Epidemiology. (2000). Cross-national comparisons of the prevalences and correlates of mental disorders: An ICPE study. *Bulletin of the World Health Organization, 78*, 413–426.

Wittchen, H.-U. (1998). Early developmental stages of psychopathology study (EDSP): Objectives and design. *European Addiction Research, 4*, 18–27.

World Health Organization. (1998). *The WHO Disability Assessment Schedule II (WHO-DAS II)*. Geneva, Switzerland: World Health Organization.

World Health Organization. (2001). *The World Health Report 2001: Mental Health; New Understanding, New Hope*. Available online at http://www.who.int/whr2.

Chapter 7

THE EPIDEMIOLOGY OF
MENTAL DISORDERS

Ronald C. Kessler, PhD; Kathleen Ries Merikangas, PhD; and
Philip S. Wang, MD, DrPH

Introduction

Nearly one out of every five Americans lacks health insurance, and the proportion is growing due to reductions in employer-sponsored coverage (Holahan & Cook, 2005). Roughly three-fourths of the uninsured are working poor and disproportionately racial or ethnic minorities with limited financial means (Kaiser Commission on Medicaid and the Uninsured, 2006). Even for the insured, fragmentation of care occurs across disparate systems and funding streams (Mark et al., 2005). Approximately two-thirds of mental health care is covered by already strained public sectors (compared to less than half for health care generally), leading to particularly strong pressures on governmental agencies to contain mental health care utilization and costs (Mark et al., 2005). Furthermore, many of the people with mental health insurance coverage are underinsured, perhaps explaining the widespread low intensity, poor quality, and sub-optimal allocation of mental health treatments observed previously in the United States (Kessler, Frank et al., 1997; Wang, Berglund, & Kessler, 2000; Wang, Demler, & Kessler, 2002).

Based upon these problems, leading health care policy groups, including the President's New Freedom Commission on Mental Health (2003) and the Institute of Medicine's Crossing the Quality Chasm Committee (2006), have called for reform that would address unmet need for effective treatment, eliminate disparities in mental health and services, efficiently allocate resources, and guide future research efforts. Achieving each of these important goals requires population-based data that identify the current nature and reasons for burdens as well as potential ways to improve care and outcomes.

Data of this sort are collected in general population surveys. These surveys are a fairly recent phenomenon in the United States. The first such survey employing modern methods, the Epidemiologic Catchment Area (ECA) study, occurred in the 1980s (Robins & Regier, 1991). The second, the National Comorbidity Survey (NCS), took place in the 1990s (Kessler et al., 1994). Both surveys documented high lifetime and 12-month prevalence of mental disorders as well as widespread unmet need for treatment of these disorders.

However, the rapid pace of change in American mental health care systems has made it imperative to re-examine the burdens of mental disorders. Although new forms of treatment have been introduced and promoted, their efficacy and safety have been questioned (Eisenberg et al., 1998; Eisenberg et al., 1993; Food and Drug Administration, 2004; Leucht, Pitschel-Walz, Abraham, & Kissling, 1999; Olfson et al., 2002; Rosenthal, Berndt, Donohue, Frank, & Epstein, 2002; Schatzberg & Nemeroff, 2004). Initiatives promoting awareness, detection, help-seeking, and best-practices treatment have been launched, but little is known concerning their impacts on health outcomes (Agency for Health Care Policy and Research, 1993; American Psychiatric Association, 1998, 2000, 2002, 2004; Hirschfeld et al., 1997; Jacobs, 1995; Katon, Roy-Byrne, Russo, & Cowley, 2002; Katon et al., 1995; Lehman & Steinwachs, 1998; National Committee for Quality Assurance, 1997; Wells et al., 2000). Likewise, effects of the many delivery systems, financing, and mental health policy redesigns that have taken place are unclear (Bender, 2002; Mechanic & McAlpine, 1999; Sturm & Klap, 1999; Weissman, Pettigrew, Sotsky, & Regier, 2000; Williams, 1998; Williams et al., 1999).

To shed light on these impacts and to provide up-to-date data on the current burdens from and care of mental disorders in the United States, the National Comorbidity Survey Replication (NCS-R) was undertaken between 2001 and 2003 as part of the larger World Health Organization (WHO) World Mental Health (WMH) Survey Initiative (Kessler, Haro, Heeringa, Pennell, & Üstün, 2006) (see Chapter 6 in this volume for more information). This chapter presents basic descriptive data on trends in prevalence and treatment of mental disorders from the NCS and NCS-R as well as NCS-R data regarding lifetime prevalence of mental disorders, delay in initial treatment seeking, 12-month prevalence of disorders, and 12-month treatment use and adequacy. The authors close with a review of the implications of these findings and promising future directions for research in this area of investigation.

Methods

Samples

The NCS and NCS-R were nationally representative face-to-face household surveys of respondents ages 15–54 (NCS) or 18+ (NCS-R). Response rates and total number of completed interviews were 82.4% (NCS, n = 8098) and 70.9% NCS-R, n = 9282) (Kessler et al., 2004; Kessler et al., 1994). All respondents received a Part I interview about mental disorders. All respondents with a Part I diagnosis and a sub-sample of others were administered a Part II assessment of risk factors, treatment, and consequences of mental disorders. Weights were adjusted for biases due to differential non-response and probability of selection and residual discrepancies with Census demographic-geographic distributions. More details about samples and weights are presented elsewhere (Kessler et al., 2004; Kessler et al., 1994). The trend data presented here are from Part II in the overlapping age range of the two samples (18–54; NCS n = 5388; NCS-R n = 4319), while the separate NCS-R data presented here are from the full sample (n = 9282).

DIAGNOSTIC ASSESSMENT

Diagnoses were based upon the WHO Composite International Diagnostic Interview (CIDI) for DSM-III-R (NCS) (Robins et al., 1988) or DSM-IV (NCS-R) (Kessler & Üstün, 2004). Diagnoses included anxiety disorders (panic disorder, generalized anxiety disorder, phobias, post-traumatic stress disorder), mood disorders (major depression, dysthymic disorder, bipolar disorder), substance disorders (alcohol and drug abuse and dependence) and, in the NCS-R, externalizing disorders (attention-deficit/hyperactivity disorder, conduct disorder, oppositional-defiant disorder, intermittent explosive disorder). Clinical reappraisal interviews documented good concordance and conservative prevalence estimates compared with diagnoses based upon blinded clinician interviews (Kessler, Berglund et al., 2005; Kessler, Wittchen et al., 1998). Twelve-month disorders were considered present if they occurred at any time in the 12 months before interview, even if they subsequently remitted with treatment.

Because DSM-III-R and DSM-IV criteria differ too greatly to justify direct comparisons of prevalence, trend analysis was based upon a re-calibration of both surveys to a common summary severity rating developed in the NCS-R and then imputed to the NCS. The severity rating and imputation method are described in detail elsewhere (Kessler, Chiu, Demler, Merikangas, & Walters, 2005). In brief, serious disorder was defined as meeting 12-month criteria for schizophrenia, any other non-affective psychosis, bipolar I disorder, or substance dependence with a physiological dependence syndrome; making a suicide attempt or having a suicide plan in conjunction with any NCS-R/DSM-IV disorder; reporting two or more areas of role functioning with self-described "severe" role impairment due to a mental disorder; or reporting functional impairment associated with a mental disorder at a level consistent with a Global Assessment of Functioning (GAF) (Endicott, Spitzer, Fleiss, & Cohen, 1976) score of 50 or less. Respondents whose disorder did not meet criteria for being serious were classified as moderate or mild based upon responses to the disorder-specific Sheehan Disability Scales (Leon, Olfson, Portera, Farber, & Sheehan, 1997).

TREATMENT

All Part II respondents in both surveys were asked questions about whether they sought treatment for emotional problems in the past 12 months from a list of providers and settings. Responses were classified by sector: psychiatrist (PSY);

other mental health specialist (OMH); general medical (GM); human services (HS); and complementary-alternative medical (CAM). The more detailed information in the NCS-R compared to the NCS on processes of treatment allowed us to create a category in the NCS-R data of minimally adequate treatment, which was defined based upon available evidence-based guidelines (Agency for Health Care Policy and Research, 1993; American Psychiatric Association, 1998, 2000, 2002, 2004; Lehman & Steinwachs, 1998). Treatment was considered at least minimally adequate if the patient received either pharmacotherapy (at least two months of an appropriate medication for the focal disorder plus at least four visits to any type of medical doctor) or psychotherapy (at least eight visits with any health care or human services professional lasting an average of 30 minutes or longer). The decision to require at least four physician visits for pharmacotherapy was based upon the fact that at least four visits for medication evaluation, initiation, and monitoring are generally recommended during the acute and continuation phases of treatment in available guidelines (Agency for Health Care Policy and Research, 1993; American Psychiatric Association, 1998, 2000, 2002, 2004; Lehman & Steinwachs, 1998).

Appropriate medications for disorders included antidepressants for depressive disorders; mood stabilizers or antipsychotics for bipolar disorders; antidepressants or anxiolytics for anxiety disorders; antagonists or agonists (e.g., disulfiram, naltrexone, methodone) for alcohol and substance disorders; and any psychiatric drug for externalizing disorders (Schatzberg & Nemeroff, 2004). At least eight sessions were required for minimally adequate psychotherapy based upon the fact that clinical trials demonstrating effectiveness have generally included at least eight psychotherapy visits (Agency for Health Care Policy and Research, 1993; American Psychiatric Association, 1998, 2000, 2002, 2004; Lehman & Steinwachs, 1998). For alcohol and substance disorders, self-help visits of any duration were counted as psychotherapy visits. Treatment adequacy was defined separately for each 12-month disorder (i.e., a respondent with comorbid disorders could be classified as receiving minimally adequate treatment for one disorder but not for another). Respondents who began treatments shortly before the NCS-R interview may not have had time to fulfill requirements, even though they were in the early stages of adequate treatment. Furthermore, very brief treatments have been developed for certain disorders (Ballesteros, Duffy, Querejeta, Arino, & Gonzalez-Pinto, 2004; Ost, Ferebee, & Furmark, 1997). As a result, the authors created a broader definition of minimally adequate treatment for sensitivity analyses that consisted of receiving at least two visits to an appropriate treatment sector (one visit for presumptive evaluation/diagnosis and at least one visit for treatment) or being in ongoing treatment at interview.

Results

Trends in Prevalence

Estimated 12-month prevalence of any DSM-IV disorder did not differ significantly between the two surveys (29.4% in 1990–2, 30.5% in 2001–3, p = .52). There was no significant change in prevalence of serious (5.3% vs. 6.3%, p = .27), moderate (12.3% vs. 13.5%, p = .30), or mild (11.8% vs. 10.8%, p = .37) disorders and no statistically significant interactions between time and socio-demographics in predicting prevalence (for more details, see Kessler, Demler et al., 2005.)

TRENDS IN TREATMENT

Prevalence of 12-month treatment for emotional problems was 12.2% in 1990–2 and 20.1% in 2001–3, with a risk ratio (RR) of 1.7, p < .001 (Table 7.1). The association between severity and treatment was positive and significant (p < .001), although substantively modest in the pooled data, with a Pearson's Contingency Coefficient (C), an extension of the phi coefficient for ordinal data that are not dichotomous, of .14. The association between severity and treatment did not differ significantly over time. Only a minority of respondents with serious disorders received treatment (24.3% in 1990–2; 40.5% in 2001–3). Approximately half of patients who received treatment had none of the disorders considered here.

Trends in sector-specific treatment were similar to overall trends in two respects. First, severity was significantly related to treatment in each sector (p < .001). Second, these associations did not change over time (p = .399–.975). A significant difference in treatment trends was found, though, across sectors (p < .001). GM treatment increased from 3.9% to 10.0% (RR = 2.6, p < .001), PSY from 2.4% to 5.2% (RR = 2.2, p < .001), OMH from 5.3% to 8.4% (RR = 1.6, p < .001), and HS from 2.6% to 3.5% (RR = 1.3, p = .05). CAM decreased from 3.3% to 2.7% (RR = 0.8, p = .10). Furthermore, a distributional shift occurred in treatment because of these within-sector differences. GM changed from 31.5% to 49.6% (p < .001) of all treatment, PSY from 19.6% to 25.8% (p = .007), OMH from 43.5% to 41.9% (p = .59), HS from 21.5% to 17.2% (p = .11), and CAM from 26.8% to 13.2% (p < .001). These distributional changes did not vary by severity (p = .89–.99).

SOCIO-DEMOGRAPHIC CORRELATES OF TREATMENT

The authors examined pooled associations of socio-demographic variables with the treatment measures (for more details, see Kessler, Demler et al., 2005). Statistically significant predictors of any treatment included being older than 24, female, Non-Hispanic White, and non-married. Predictors of sector-specific treatment included age (related positively to GM and negatively to OMH), female (related positively to GM and negatively to CAM), marital status (the non-married more likely than the married to receive OMH), and education (related negatively to GM). However, these associations were all modest in magnitude (Pearson C = .04–.07). Interactions with time and severity were all non-significant, indicating that the increases in treatment over time occurred in all major segments of society defined by the socio-demographic variables studied.

LIFETIME PREVALENCE OF DSM-IV DISORDERS IN THE NCS-R

As prevalence estimates of comparably assessed disorders did not differ between the two surveys, the authors focus the remainder of the discussion of prevalence

Table 7.1 Twelve-Month Treatment of DSM-IV/CIDI Disorders by Severity and Sector among NCS (n=5388) and NCS-R (n=4319) Respondents Ages 18–54

	Any[1]		PSY[1]		OMH[1]		GM[1]		HS[1]		CAM[1]	
	%	(se)	%	(se)	%	(se)	%	(se)	%	(se)	%	(se)
I. NCS (1990-92)[2]												
Serious	24.3	(3.8)	7.3	(2.2)	11.4	(2.5)	8.2	(3.0)	4.5	(1.9)	8.4	(1.9)
Moderate	25.4	(2.4)	5.8	(1.2)	13.6	(1.6)	8.6	(1.4)	5.5	(1.1)	7.1	(1.2)
Mild	13.3	(2.4)	2.5	(1.2)	4.9	(1.3)	4.3	(1.4)	3.0	(1.2)	3.0	(0.8)
Any	20.3	(1.5)	4.8	(0.8)	9.7	(1.0)	6.8	(1.0)	4.3	(0.7)	5.7	(0.7)
None	8.8	(0.7)	1.4	(0.3)	3.5	(0.4)	2.6	(0.4)	1.9	(0.3)	2.3	(0.3)
Total	12.2	(0.6)	2.4	(0.3)	5.3	(0.3)	3.9	(0.4)	2.6	(0.3)	3.3	(0.3)
II. NCS-R (2001-03)[2]												
Serious	40.5	(4.7)	14.4	(3.3)	19.4	(3.5)	22.1	(3.5)	6.5	(1.6)	6.2	(1.5)
Moderate	37.2	(3.0)	13.0	(1.6)	15.8	(1.8)	19.5	(2.4)	5.5	(1.2)	4.6	(1.0)
Mild	23.0	(3.8)	5.1	(1.3)	9.0	(2.2)	11.8	(2.9)	3.9	(1.5)	2.9	(0.9)
Any	32.9	(2.0)	10.5	(1.0)	14.1	(1.3)	17.3	(1.3)	5.1	(0.8)	4.3	(0.6)
None	14.5	(0.9)	2.9	(0.4)	5.9	(0.6)	6.8	(0.6)	2.7	(0.4)	1.9	(0.3)
Total	20.1	(0.8)	5.2	(0.3)	8.4	(0.5)	10.0	(0.5)	3.5	(0.3)	2.7	(0.3)
III. NCS-R:NCS[3]	RR	(se)	RR	(se)	RR	(se)	RR	(se)	RR	(se)	RR	(se)
Serious	1.68	(0.35)	2.01	(0.84)	1.72	(0.49)	2.91	(1.33)	1.53	(0.70)	0.74	(0.25)
Moderate	1.47*	(0.19)	2.27*	(0.57)	1.17	(0.19)	2.29*	(0.46)	1.01	(0.29)	0.65	(0.17)

Mild	1.74*	(0.35)	2.17	(1.14)	1.85	(0.57)	2.82	(1.04)	1.34	(0.64)	0.97	(0.38)
Any	1.62*	(0.15)	2.21*	(0.40)	1.46*	(0.18)	2.58*	(0.41)	1.19	(0.25)	0.76	(0.14)
None	1.65*	(0.16)	2.05*	(0.50)	1.71*	(0.26)	2.57*	(0.46)	1.42	(0.32)	0.86	(0.14)
Total	1.65*	(0.10)	2.17*	(0.27)	1.59*	(0.15)	2.59*	(0.29)	1.32	(0.19)	0.81	(0.10)

IV. Statistical Significance[4]

	χ^2	(p)	χ^2	(p)	χ^2	(p)	χ^2	(p)	χ^2	(p)	χ^2	(p)
Severity (S)	194.6	(.000)	112.2	(.000)	118.1	(.000)	105.3	(.000)	23.0	(.000)	82.9	(.000)
Time (T)	56.8	(.000)	34.5	(.000)	22.7	(.000)	72.4	(.000)	3.3	(.069)	3.3	(.067)
T X S	0.5	(.928)	0.2	(.975)	3.0	(.399)	0.3	(.958)	0.9	(.825)	1.2	(.759)

Originally published in Kessler, R. C., Demler, O., Frank, R. G., Olfson, M., Pincus, H. A., Walters, E. E., Wang, P. S., Wells, K. B., Zaslavsky, A. M. (2005). Prevalence and treatment of mental disorders, 1990 to 2003. *New England Journal of Medicine* 352(24), 2515–2523. Copyright © 2005, Massachusetts Medical Society. All Rights reserved. Used with permission.

* Significant at the .05 level, two-sided test.

1 Any = Any treatment; PSY = Psychiatrist; OMH = Other mental health specialist; GM = General medical; HS = Human services; CAM = Complementary-alternative medicine

2 % = Proportion of respondents in the total sample who received either any treatment or treatment in the treatment sector indicated in the column heading. se = Design-based multiply imputed standard error of the % estimate.

3 RR = Risk Ratio, the proportional increase in prevalence in NCS-R compared to NCS. For example, a RR of 1.5 corresponds to the NCS-R prevalence being 50% higher than the NCS prevalence. Note that RR does not always equal the ratio of the % estimates in Parts I and II. This is because the Multiple Imputation method calculates % and RR as means of these estimates in pseudo-samples. The mean of a within-pseudo-sample ratio does not necessarily equal the ratio of the within-pseudo-sample means of the % estimates.

4 The significance tests for severity (S) evaluate the significance of differences in treatment proportions across the four categories of the severity variable pooled across the two surveys. Each severity χ^2 test has 3 degrees of freedom (serious, moderate, and mild vs. none). The significance tests for time (T) evaluate the significance of differences in treatment proportions in the two surveys controlling for differences in severity. Each time χ^2 test has 1 degree of freedom (1990-2 vs. 2001-3). The significance tests for interactions between time and severity (T X S) evaluate the significance of differential change across the two surveys depending on severity. Each T X S χ^2 test has 3 degrees of freedom.

on the more recent of the two surveys, the NCS-R, which used DSM-IV criteria rather than DSM-III-R criteria and assessed a wider range of disorders than the NCS.

The lifetime prevalence estimate of any disorder in the NCS-R was 46.4%, with 27.7% of respondents estimated to have two or more lifetime disorders and 17.3% three or more. The most prevalent class of disorders was estimated to be anxiety disorders (28.8%), followed by externalizing disorders (24.8%), mood disorders (20.8%), and substance use disorders (14.6%). The most prevalent individual lifetime disorders were estimated to be major depressive disorder (16.6%), alcohol abuse (13.2%), specific phobia (12.5%), and social phobia (12.1%).

DISTRIBUTIONS OF THE AGE-OF-ONSET OF MENTAL DISORDERS

Median ages-of-onset (AOO; i.e., the 50th percentile on the AOO distribution) were estimated to be earlier for anxiety disorders (age 11) and externalizing disorders (age 11) than for substance use disorders (age 20) or mood disorders (age 30). AOO was also found to be concentrated in a very narrow age range for most disorders, with the inter-quartile range (IQR; the number of years between the 25th and 75th percentiles of the AOO distributions) only eight years (ages 7–15) for externalizing disorders, nine years (ages 18–27) for substance use disorders, and 15 years (ages 6–21) for anxiety disorders. The AOO IQR was wider, though, for mood disorders (25 years, ages 18–43).

COHORT EFFECTS IN LIFETIME RISK OF MENTAL DISORDERS

Discrete-time survival analysis was used to predict lifetime risk of mental disorders in various age groups. Generally significant positive associations were found between recency of cohorts and risk of mental disorders. One possible explanation for these apparent cohort effects is that lifetime risk might actually be constant across cohorts but appeared to vary with cohort because onsets occur earlier in more recent than later cohorts (as might happen if there were secular changes in environmental triggers or to age-related differences in AOO recall accuracy). Another possible explanation is that mortality might have an increasing impact on sample selection bias as age increases. To study these possibilities, the cohort model was examined to see whether inter-cohort differences decrease significantly with increasing age. There was no evidence of decreasing cohort effects with increasing age for anxiety or mood disorders. For substance use disorders, though, there were much higher cohort effects in the teens and 20s than in either childhood or the 30s through 50s (Kessler, Berglund et al., 2005).

SOCIO-DEMOGRAPHIC PREDICTORS OF LIFETIME RISK OF MENTAL DISORDERS

Survival analyses that adjusted for cohort effects found women to have significantly higher risk of anxiety and mood disorders than men and found men to have significantly higher risk of externalizing and substance use disorders than women. Non-Hispanic Blacks and Hispanics were found to have significantly lower risk of anxiety, mood, and substance use disorders (the latter only among Non-Hispanic Blacks) than Non-Hispanic Whites. Education was found to be inversely related to risk of substance disorders. Three out of four disorder classes (not externalizing disorders) were associated with marital disruption (for more details, see Wang, Berglund et al., 2005).

To examine whether the increasing prevalence of disorders in recent cohorts is concentrated in certain subgroups, interactions between socio-demographic correlates and cohort were studied. At least one significant interaction was found for each socio-demographic predictor although patterns were generally not consistent in these interactions. Of note, gender differences in anxiety, mood, and externalizing disorders did not differ across cohort, but women were found to be more similar to men in substance disorders in recent than earlier cohorts. Significant associations of low education and not being married with substance use disorders were observed only in recent cohorts.

Delays in Initial Treatment Contact

Survival analysis was used to examine the proportion of cases in the NCS-R who made treatment contact in the year of first onset of the disorder and the median delay among people who eventually made treatment contact. Proportions of cases making treatment contact in the year of disorder onset ranged from highs of 37.4–41.6% for the mood disorders to lows of 1.0–3.4% for phobias and separation anxiety disorder. The median duration of delay also differed greatly across disorders, from lows of 6–8 years for mood disorders to highs of 20–23 years for specific phobia and separation anxiety disorder (for more details, see Wang, Berglund et al., 2005).

Predictors of Failure and Delay in Initial Treatment Contact

The predictors of failure to ever make treatment contact among NCS-R respondents with lifetime disorders were very similar to predictors of delay among respondents who eventually made treatment contact. Cohort was the strongest predictor, with both failure and delay highest in the earliest cohorts and lowest in recent cohorts. This finding documents a steady increase in treatment across time. AOO was also a significant predictor of delay in treatment contact, with the longest delays associated with the earliest AOO. Less consistency was found for socio-demographic predictors of failure and delay.

Prevalence and Severity of 12-Month Disorders

The most common 12-month disorders in the NCS-R were estimated to be specific phobia (8.7%), social phobia (6.8%), and major depressive disorder (6.7%) (Table 7.2). Among classes, anxiety disorders were estimated to be the most

Table 7.2 Twelve-Month Prevalence and Severity of DSM-IV/CIDI Disorders (n=9282)

| | Total | | Severity[a] | | | | | |
| | | | Serious | | Moderate | | Mild | |
	%	(se)	%	(se)	%	(se)	%	(se)
I. Anxiety Disorders								
Panic disorder	2.7	(0.2)	44.8	(3.2)	29.5	(2.7)	25.7	(2.5)
Agoraphobia without panic	0.8	(0.1)	40.6	(7.2)	30.7	(6.4)	28.7	(8.4)
Specific phobia	8.7	(0.4)	21.9	(2.0)	30.0	(2.0)	48.1	(2.1)
Social phobia	6.8	(0.3)	29.9	(2.0)	38.8	(2.5)	31.3	(2.4)
Generalized anxiety disorder	3.1	(0.2)	32.3	(2.9)	44.6	(4.0)	23.1	(2.9)
Post-traumatic stress disorder[b]	3.5	(0.3)	36.6	(3.5)	33.1	(2.2)	30.2	(3.4)
Obsessive-compulsive disorder[c]	1.0	(0.3)	50.6	(12.4)	34.8	(14.1)	14.6	(5.7)
Separation anxiety disorder[d]	0.9	(0.2)	43.3	(9.2)	24.8	(7.5)	31.9	(12.2)
Any anxiety disorder[c]	18.1	(0.7)	22.8	(1.5)	33.7	(1.4)	43.5	(2.1)
II. Mood Disorders								
Major depressive disorder	6.7	(0.3)	30.4	(1.7)	50.1	(2.1)	19.5	(2.1)
Dysthymia	1.5	(0.1)	49.7	(3.9)	32.1	(4.0)	18.2	(3.4)
Bipolar I-II disorders	2.6	(0.2)	82.9	(3.2)	17.1	(3.2)	0.0	(0.0)
Any mood disorder	9.5	(0.4)	45.0	(1.9)	40.0	(1.7)	15.0	(1.6)
III. Externalizing Disorders								
Oppositional-defiant disorder[d]	1.0	(0.2)	49.6	(8.0)	40.3	(8.7)	10.1	(4.8)
Conduct disorder[d]	1.0	(0.2)	40.5	(11.1)	31.6	(7.5)	28.0	(9.1)
Attention-deficit/hyperactivity disorder[d]	4.1	(0.3)	41.3	(4.3)	35.2	(3.5)	23.5	(4.5)
Intermittent explosive disorder	2.6	(0.2)	23.8	(3.3)	74.4	(3.5)	1.7	(0.9)
Any externalizing disorder[d, f]	8.9	(0.5)	32.9	(2.9)	52.4	(3.0)	14.7	(2.3)
IV. Substance use Disorders								
Alcohol abuse[b]	3.1	(0.3)	28.9	(2.6)	39.7	(3.7)	31.5	(3.3)

178

Alcohol dependence[b]	1.3	(0.2)	34.3	(4.5)	65.7	(4.5)	0.0	(0.0)
Drug abuse[b]	1.4	(0.1)	36.6	(5.0)	30.4	(5.8)	33.0	(6.8)
Drug dependence[b]	0.4	(0.1)	56.5	(8.2)	43.5	(8.2)	0.0	(0.0)
Any substance use disorder[b]	3.8	(0.3)	29.6	(2.8)	37.1	(3.5)	33.4	(3.2)
V. Any Disorder								
Any[c]	26.2	(0.8)	22.3	(1.3)	37.3	(1.3)	40.4	(1.6)
One disorder[e]	14.4	(0.6)	9.6	(1.3)	31.2	(1.9)	59.2	(2.3)
Two disorders[e]	5.8	(0.3)	25.5	(2.1)	46.4	(2.6)	28.2	(2.0)
Three or more disorders[e]	6.0	(0.3)	49.9	(2.3)	43.1	(2.1)	7.0	(1.3)

Originally published in Kessler, R. C., Chiu, W. T., Demler, O., Walters, E. E. (2005). Prevalence, severity, and comorbidity of twelve-month DSM-IV disorders in the National Comorbidity Survey Replication (NCS-R). *Archives of General Psychiatry* 62(6), 620. Copyright © (2005), American Medical Association. All Rights reserved. Used with permission.

[a] Percentages in the three severity columns are repeated as proportions of all cases and sum to 100% across each row.
[b] Assessed in the Part II sample (n = 5692)
[c] Assessed in a random one-third of the Part II sample (n = 1808)
[d] Assessed in the Part II sample among respondents aged 18–44 years (n = 3199)
[e] Estimated in the Part II sample. No adjustment is made for the fact that one or more disorders in the category were not assessed for all Part II respondents.
[f] The estimated prevalence of any externalizing disorder is larger than the sum of the individual disorders because the prevalence of intermittent explosive disorder, the only externalizing disorder that was assessed in the total sample, is reported here for the total sample rather than for the sub-sample of respondents among whom the other externalizing disorders were assessed (Part II respondents in the age range 18–44). The estimated prevalence of any externalizing disorder, in comparison, is estimated in the latter sub-sample. Intermittent explosive disorder has a considerably higher estimated prevalence in this sub-sample than in the total sample.

prevalent (18.1%), followed by mood disorders (9.5%), externalizing disorders (8.9%), and substance use disorders (3.8%). The 12-month prevalence of any disorder was 26.2%, with over half of cases (14.4% of the total sample) having only one disorder and smaller proportions having two (5.8%) or more (6.0%).

Of 12-month cases, 22.3% were classified serious, 37.3% moderate, and 40.4% mild. Having a serious disorder was strongly related to comorbidity, with 9.6% of those with one diagnosis, 25.5% with two, and 49.9% with three or more diagnoses classified as serious cases. Among disorder classes, mood disorders had the highest percentage of serious cases (45.0%) and anxiety disorders the lowest (22.8%). The anxiety disorder with the greatest proportion of serious cases was obsessive-compulsive disorder (50.6%), while bipolar disorder had the highest proportion of serious cases (82.9%) among mood disorders, oppositional-defiant disorder the highest (49.6%) among externalizing disorders, and drug dependence the highest (56.5%) among substance disorders.

BIVARIATE ANALYSES OF 12-MONTH COMORBIDITY

Table 7.3 shows tetrachoric correlations between hierarchy-free 12-month DSM-IV disorders in the NCS-R. Tetrachoric correlations are correlations between two presumed normally distributed latent liabilities based on observed associations between pairs of dichotomies that are assumed to be defined by making cut-points on these presumed liabilities. Nearly all of these correlations are positive (98%) and statistically significant (72%). Only four correlations are negative, all of which involve either OCD or separation anxiety disorder (SAD), both of which are uncommon disorders. The 12 highest correlations, each exceeding .60, involve well-known syndromes: bipolar disorder (major depressive episode with mania-hypomania), double-depression (major depressive episode with dysthymia), anxious-depression (major depressive episode with generalized anxiety disorder), comorbid mania-hypomania and attention-deficit/hyperactivity disorder, panic disorder with agoraphobia, comorbid social phobia with agoraphobia, and comorbid substance disorders (both alcohol abuse and dependence with drug abuse and dependence).

PROBABILITY OF 12-MONTH SERVICE USE

In the year prior to interview, 17.9% of NCS-R respondents used mental health services, including 41.1% of those with 12-month DSM-IV disorders and 10.1% of those without 12-month DSM-IV disorders (see Table 7.4). The proportion of cases in treatment ranged from a low of 29.6% for intermittent explosive disorder to a high of 67.5% for dysthymic disorder. Most of those treated received services in one of the Health Care sectors (15.3% of respondents, representing 85.5% of those in treatment). Among those treated in the Health Care sectors, most received services in the General Medical sector (9.3% of respondents, representing 52.0% of those in treatment).

NUMBER OF VISITS IN THE PRIOR YEAR

The median number of 12-month visits among those receiving any treatment was 2.9 and was significantly higher among those with disorders (4.5) than without (1.9; z = 5.8, p < .001) (for more details, see Wang, Lane et al., 2005). Respondents with no disorder made up most of the patients (74.6%), accounting for 33.2% of all visits. The median number of within-sector visits was lowest for the General Medical (1.6) and highest for CAM (9.2) sectors. Mean numbers of visits were consistently much higher than medians. For example, among patients receiving any treatment the median was 2.9 vs. a mean of 14.7. Patients with disorders had a significantly higher mean number of visits (16.9) than those without (11.6; z = 3.1, p = .001). Mean within-sector visits were lowest for General Medical (2.6), higher for Human Services (7.1), Psychiatrist (7.5), Non-Psychiatrist Specialty (16.1), and highest for CAM (29.8). The proportion of all visits made in specific sectors was highest for Non-Psychiatrist Specialty (39%) and CAM (32%), lower for Psychiatrist (13%), and lowest for General Medical (9%) and Human Services (9%).

The fact that the means were higher than the medians implies that a relatively small number of patients received a disproportionately high share of all visits. More detailed analyses showed that although nearly 60% of patients seen by psychiatrists made fewer than five visits in the year, they accounted for only one-sixth of all visits to psychiatrists (Wang, Lane et al., 2005). On the other hand, those making 50 or more visits to psychiatrists in the year, while representing only 1.6% of all patients seen by psychiatrists, accounted for 20.2% of all psychiatrist visits. The proportion of patients who account for 50% of all visits to the sector ranged between 6.4% for the Human Services sector to 23.6% for the General Medical sector.

MINIMALLY ADEQUATE TREATMENT IN THE PRIOR YEAR

Among treated patients with disorders in the NCS-R, only 32.7% were classified as receiving at least minimally adequate treatment in the prior year. The probability was lowest in the General Medical sector (12.7%) and highest in the Mental Health Specialty sectors (44.5% in the Psychiatrist sector and 46.5% in the Non-Psychiatrist Specialty sector). Using a broad definition of minimally adequate treatment (i.e., receiving at least two visits to an appropriate sector or being in ongoing treatment at the time of interview) in sensitivity analyses, the percent of patients receiving at least minimally adequate treatment increased to 47.8%. The probabilities were lowest in the General Medical sector (33.2%), higher in Human Services (46.9%) and Non-Psychiatrist Specialty (51.1%), and highest in the Psychiatrist (53.3%) sector.

SOCIO-DEMOGRAPHIC PREDICTORS OF 12-MONTH TREATMENT

Receiving any 12-month mental health treatment was unrelated to the socio-demographic variables included in our analysis after controlling for mental disorders. No significant socio-demographic correlates were found of treatment adequacy

Table 7.3 Tetrachoric Correlations among Hierarchy-Free 12-Month DSM-IV/CIDI Disorders and Factor Loadings from a Principal Axis Factor Analysis of the Correlation Matrix (n=3199)[a]

	PD	AG	SP	SoP	GAD	PTSD
I. Anxiety Disorders						
Panic disorder (PD)	1.0					
Agoraphobia (AG)	0.6*	1.0				
Specific phobia (SP)	0.5*	0.6*	1.0			
Social phobia (SoP)	0.5*	0.7*	0.5*	1.0		
Generalized anxiety disorder (GAD)	0.5*	0.4*	0.4*	0.5*	1.0	
Post-traumatic stress disorder (PTSD)	0.5*	0.5*	0.4*	0.4*	0.4*	1.0
Obsessive-compulsive disorder (OCD)[b]	0.4	0.4	0.2	0.2	0.3	0.6*
Separation anxiety disorder (SAD)	0.4*	0.3	0.3*	0.3*	0.4*	0.5*
II. Mood Disorders						
Major depressive episode (MDE)	0.5*	0.5*	0.4*	0.5*	0.6*	0.5*
Dysthymia (DYS)	0.5*	0.4*	0.4*	0.6*	0.6*	0.5*
Manic-hypomanic episode (MHE)	0.5*	0.5*	0.4*	0.5*	0.5*	0.4*
III. Externalizing Disorders						
Oppositional-defiant disorder (ODD)	0.4*	0.5*	0.4*	0.5*	0.3*	0.5*
Conduct disorder (CD)	0.3	0.2	0.2	0.3*	0.1	0.3
Attention-deficit/hyperactivity disorder (ADHD)	0.4*	0.4*	0.3*	0.5*	0.5*	0.4*
Intermittent explosive disorder (IED)	0.3*	0.4*	0.3*	0.3*	0.3*	0.2*
IV. Substance Disorders						
Alcohol abuse (AA)	0.3*	0.2	0.1	0.2*	0.2*	0.3*
Alcohol dependence (AD)	0.2	0.3	0.2*	0.3*	0.3*	0.3*
Drug abuse (DA)	0.2	0.1	0.1	0.2*	0.2*	0.1
Drug dependence (DD)	0.3	0.3	0.3	0.4*	0.4*	0.2
Prevalence	3.4	1.6	10.1	8.8	4.4	3.7
Percent comorbid	80	97	62	74	85	75
Factor 1[c]	0.7	0.8	0.6	0.7	0.6	0.6
Factor 2[c]	0.1	0.1	0.0	0.2	0.2	0.2

Originally published in Kessler, R. C., Chiu, W. T., Demler, O., Walters, E. E. (2005). Prevalence, severity, and comorbidity of 12-month DSM-IV disorders in the National Comorbidity Survey Replication (NCS-R). Archives of General Psychiatry 62(6), 621. Copyright © (2005), American Medical Association. All Rights reserved. Used with permission.

* Significant at the .05 level, two-sided test
[a] Part II respondents aged 18–44 years (n=3199)
[b] Assessed in a random one-third of the Part II sample among respondents aged 18–44 years (n = 1025)
[c] Varimax rotation. Similar results were obtained in a promax rotation.

OCD	SAD	MDE	DYS	MHE	ODD	CD	ADHD	IED	AA	AD	DA	DD
1.0												
-0.8	1.0											
0.4*	0.4*	1.0										
0.4	0.4*	0.9*	1.0									
0.4	0.4*	0.6*	0.6*	1.0								
0.5	0.5*	0.5*	0.5*	0.6*	1.0							
-0.8	-0.1	0.1	0.3	0.3*	0.5*	1.0						
0.3	0.4*	0.5*	0.5*	0.6*	0.6*	0.4*	1.0					
0.2	0.3	0.4*	0.4*	0.4*	0.4*	0.4*	0.4*	1.0				
0.3*	0.1	0.2*	0.3*	0.4*	0.3	0.4*	0.3*	0.4*	1.0			
0.2	0.1	0.4*	0.4*	0.4*	0.4	0.4	0.3	0.4*	1.0*	1.0		
0.3	0.1	0.2*	0.4*	0.4*	0.4	0.4	0.4*	0.3*	0.7*	0.6*	1.0	
0.4	-0.8*	0.4*	0.6*	0.4*	0.4	0.4	0.6*	0.4*	0.6*	0.7*	1.0*	1.0
1.3	0.9	10.3	2.4	3.8	1.1	1.0	4.1	6.6	5.0	2.2	2.4	0.7
65	71	76	99	87	93	70	78	70	77	100	79	100
–	–	0.8	0.7	0.7	0.6	0.3	0.6	0.4	0.1	0.2	0.1	0.3
–	–	0.2	0.3	0.3	0.3	0.5	0.3	0.4	0.9	0.9	0.9	0.9

Table 7.4 Prevalence of 12-Month Mental Health Service Use in Separate Service Sectors by 12-Month DSM-IV/CIDI Disorder

	Health Care					Non-Health Care				
	Mental health specialty			General Medical[e]	Any	Human Services[d]	CAM[c]	Any	Any service use	n[a]
	Psychiatrist	Non-psychiatrist[b]	Any							
	% (se)	% (se)	% (se)	% (se)	% (se)	% (se)	% (se)	% (se)	% (se)	
I. Anxiety Disorders										
Panic disorder	21.5 (2.5)	24.6 (2.8)	34.7 (2.6)	43.7 (3.3)	59.1 (3.3)	10.8 (1.9)	8.0 (2.0)	17.3 (2.3)	65.4 (3.3)	251
Agoraphobia without panic	—	—	—	—	45.8 (7.0)	—	—	—	52.6 (7.4)	79
Specific phobia	12.1 (1.6)	13.6 (1.4)	19.0 (1.8)	21.2 (1.5)	32.4 (2.0)	8.6 (0.9)	7.0 (0.8)	13.5 (1.0)	38.2 (1.9)	812
Social phobia	15.2 (1.5)	18.8 (1.5)	24.7 (1.5)	25.3 (1.7)	40.1 (1.9)	7.7 (1.1)	7.7 (1.0)	13.4 (1.1)	45.6 (1.9)	632
Generalized anxiety disorder	14.2 (2.4)	17.0 (2.5)	25.5 (2.9)	31.7 (2.6)	43.2 (3.0)	14.0 (3.5)	10.1 (1.8)	21.7 (3.5)	52.3 (2.9)	247
Post-traumatic stress disorder	22.6 (2.4)	26.1 (2.3)	34.4 (2.9)	31.3 (2.5)	49.9 (3.3)	10.7 (2.4)	12.6 (2.0)	19.7 (2.4)	57.4 (3.3)	203
Obsessive-compulsive disorder	—	—	—	—	—	—	—	—	—	—
Separation anxiety disorder	—	—	—	—	—	—	—	—	—	—
Any anxiety disorder	13.0 (1.0)	16.0 (1.0)	21.7 (1.2)	24.3 (1.0)	36.9 (1.4)	8.2 (0.9)	7.3 (0.6)	13.5 (0.7)	42.2 (1.3)	1036
II. Mood Disorders										
Major depressive disorder	20.6 (1.8)	23.2 (1.9)	32.9 (1.6)	32.5 (2.3)	51.7 (2.2)	10.7 (1.2)	9.0 (1.3)	16.8 (1.7)	56.8 (2.2)	623
Dysthymia	27.7 (3.7)	23.3 (3.2)	36.8 (4.1)	39.6 (5.1)	61.7 (4.5)	13.3 (3.2)	7.1 (2.3)	17.5 (3.9)	67.5 (4.1)	135

										N
Bipolar I-II disorders	22.5 (2.2)	27.1 (2.2)	33.8 (2.3)	33.1 (3.0)	48.8 (2.7)	11.7 (2.2)	12.2 (2.7)	21.6 (3.2)	55.5 (3.0)	244
Any mood disorder	21.0 (1.3)	24.1 (1.5)	32.9 (1.3)	32.8 (1.8)	50.9 (1.8)	11.0 (1.2)	9.8 (1.3)	18.1 (1.6)	56.4 (1.8)	884
III. Externalizing Disorders										
Intermittent explosive disorder	7.1 (1.7)	9.2 (1.7)	13.9 (2.3)	12.6 (2.4)	22.8 (2.6)	7.6 (2.3)	3.7 (1.2)	10.9 (2.6)	29.6 (2.9)	243
IV. Substance use Disorders										
Alcohol abuse	12.8 (1.7)	20.2 (2.7)	25.6 (2.3)	16.4 (2.1)	33.4 (2.5)	7.0 (1.8)	7.4 (1.9)	12.8 (2.2)	37.2 (2.6)	176
Alcohol dependence	19.6 (2.9)	28.0 (5.8)	35.1 (4.4)	19.3 (3.7)	43.6 (4.9)	8.2 (2.8)	14.5 (3.3)	19.6 (3.9)	48.4 (5.4)	76
Drug abuse	15.5 (3.7)	26.3 (4.8)	32.8 (4.9)	21.8 (4.1)	40.5 (4.9)	7.1 (3.9)	7.7 (2.7)	14.2 (5.5)	43.1 (4.8)	79
Drug dependence	30.4 (10.5)	29.4 (8.1)	42.9 (10.0)	23.9 (7.3)	49.8 (9.8)	0.0 (0.0)	6.0 (3.6)	6.0 (3.6)	51.5 (9.9)	24
Any substance disorder	13.2 (1.5)	21.0 (2.9)	26.2 (2.5)	18.1 (1.7)	34.5 (2.6)	7.8 (2.1)	7.2 (1.7)	13.7 (2.6)	38.1 (2.7)	219
V. Composite										
Any disorder	12.3 (0.7)	16.0 (0.9)	21.7 (0.9)	22.8 (0.9)	36.0 (1.1)	8.1 (0.8)	6.8 (0.6)	13.2 (0.7)	41.1 (1.0)	1443
No disorder	1.9 (0.2)	3.0 (0.3)	4.4 (0.4)	4.7 (0.3)	8.3 (0.5)	1.8 (0.2)	1.4 (0.2)	3.0 (0.3)	10.1 (0.6)	4249
Total sample	4.5 (0.3)	6.3 (0.4)	8.8 (0.5)	9.3 (0.4)	15.3 (0.6)	3.4 (0.3)	2.8 (0.2)	5.6 (0.4)	17.9 (0.7)	5692

Originally published in Wang, P. S., Lane, M., Kessler, R. C., Olfson, M., Pincus, H. A., Wells, K. B. (2005). Twelve-month use of mental health services in the U.S.: Results from the National Comorbidity Survey Replication (NCS-R). *Archives of General Psychiatry* 62(6), 632. Copyright © (2005), American Medical Association. All Rights reserved. Used with permission.

a Weighted number of respondents meeting criteria for each 12-month DSM-IV/ CIDI disorder

b Non-psychiatrist defined as psychologists or other non-psychiatrist mental health professional in any setting, social worker or counselor in a mental health specialty setting, use of a mental health hotline

c General Medical defined as primary care doctor, other general medical doctor, nurse, any other health professional not previously mentioned

d Human Services Professional defined as religious or spiritual advisor, social worker, or counselor in any setting other than a specialty mental health setting

e Complementary-Alternative Medicine defined as any other type of healer, participation in an Internet support group, or participation in a self-help group

185

among those receiving General Medical sector care. Significant predictors of adequate treatment in the Mental Health Specialty sector care included high education and living in a rural area.

TREATMENT AMONG PEOPLE WHO DID NOT HAVE DISORDERS

Somewhat more than half the NCS-R respondents who received treatment in the 12 months before interview despite not having a 12-month DSM-V/CIDI diagnosis had a lifetime diagnosis (Druss et al., 2007). The majority of those without a lifetime diagnosis had either a sub-threshold 12-month diagnosis, multiple days out of role in the year due to emotional problems despite not having a diagnosis, or a serious psychosocial stressor that led them to seek treatment. Among the small proportion of service users with neither a diagnosis nor another potential indication for service use, a disproportionately large percentage of visits were delivered in the CAM or HS sectors. These findings indicate that there is little inappropriate use of mental health services among people who have no need for treatment.

Discussion

STUDY LIMITATIONS

The results reported here should be interpreted with a number of limitations in mind. First, the NCS and NCS-R surveys excluded homeless and institutionalized people, people who do not speak English, and people who were too ill to be interviewed. However, as these exclusions apply only to a small proportion of the population, the results reported here can be extrapolated to the vast majority of the population, although it is important to recognize that the excluded population segments probably have a higher prevalence of mental disorders than the population included in the study. A related exclusion is that the interviews did not assess all DSM disorders. This means that some respondents in treatment classified as not having a disorder might actually have met criteria for a disorder not assessed.

Second, systematic survey non-response (i.e., people with mental disorders having a higher survey refusal rate than those without disorders) or systematic non-reporting (i.e., recall failure, conscious non-reporting, or error in the diagnostic evaluation) could lead to bias in the estimates of disorder prevalence or unmet need for treatment. Given what we know about the associations between true prevalence and these errors (Allgulander, 1989; Cannell, Marquis, & Laurent, 1977; Eaton, Anthony, Tepper, & Dryman, 1992; Kessler et al., 2004; Turner et al., 1998), it is likely that disorder prevalence was underestimated.

Third, the CIDI is a lay-administered interview that generates diagnoses imperfectly related to clinical diagnoses. However as reported elsewhere (Haro et al., 2006), a clinical reappraisal study using the Structured Clinical Interview for DSM-IV (SCID) (First, Spitzer, Gibbon, & Williams, 2002) found generally good individual-level concordance between the CIDI and SCID and conservative estimates of prevalence compared to the SCID. This finding that CIDI prevalence estimates are conservative adds to other evidence suggesting that the prevalence estimates reported here are conservative.

Noteworthy Trends

With these limitations in mind, the trend analyses reviewed here documented five noteworthy results. The first is that no substantial change occurred in the prevalence or severity of mental disorders in the United States in the decade between the NCS and NCS-R. Two explanations consistent with this result are that prevalence would have been higher were it not for increased treatment, and that increased treatment was ineffective in causing a decrease in disorders. Consistent with the first possibility, the economic recession of the early 2000s began shortly before and deepened throughout the NCS-R field period, while the 9/11 attacks occurred in the middle of the field period. Mental disorders might have increased in the absence of increased treatment. However, more evidence is consistent with the second explanation. Studies show that most treatment for mental disorders falls below minimum quality standards (Wang et al., 2000). In addition, this treatment is typically of short duration, which means it would influence episode duration more than 12-month prevalence. Finally, increased treatment was provided largely in the GM sector to patients without DSM-IV disorders. Controlled treatment trials find no evidence that pharmacotherapy significantly improves such mild cases, making it unlikely that it could prevent a significant secular increase in disorder prevalence.

The second noteworthy trend is that a substantial increase occurred between the two surveys in the proportion of the population treated for emotional problems. This was true even though the majority of people with disorders still received no treatment. The increased treatment could have been due to a number of things, including the following: aggressive direct-to-consumer marketing of new psychotropic medications (Rosenthal et al., 2002); development of new community programs to promote awareness, screening, and help-seeking for mental disorders (Jacobs, 1995); expansion of primary care, managed care, and behavioral "carve-out" systems of mental health services (Sturm & Klap, 1999); and new legislation and policies to reduce barriers to service use (Bender, 2002). Increased access presumably played an independent role (Frank, Huskamp, & Pincus, 2003). Insurance coverage expanded throughout the decade, while consumer cost-sharing declined.

The third noteworthy trend is that the proportional increase in treatment between the two surveys varied across sectors, leading to a compositional shift in treatment, the most notable aspect being a 150% increase in treatment in the GM sector. Despite hope that mental disorders would be treated more efficiently because of this shift, data show that many patients in GM treatment for emotional problems failed to complete the clinical assessment, delivery of treatment, and appropriate ongoing monitoring consistent with accepted standards of care (Wang et al., 2000). In addition, a high proportion of patients continued to receive treatments of uncertain benefit in the HS and CAM sectors despite the increase in treatment.

The fourth noteworthy trend is that the increase in treatment was unrelated to socio-demographic correlates. As a result, increased treatment did not reduce the socio-demographic disparities in treatment found in the baseline NCS (Kessler et al., 1999). Indeed, these inequalities increased in absolute terms. For example, although Non-Hispanic Blacks were only 50% as likely to receive PSY treatment as Non-Hispanic Whites with the same disorder severity in both surveys, the fact that PSY treatment increased by more than 100% means that this consistent difference resulted in the absolute Black-White treatment gap more than doubling.

The final noteworthy trend is that only a small positive association was found in the surveys between severity and treatment. Furthermore, severity did not inter-act with time in predicting treatment. This means that the proportional increase in treatment was the same for all levels of severity. The positive association between severity and treatment has previously been interpreted as evidence of rationality in allocation of treatment resources (Kessler et al., 1999). However, the fact that roughly half of patients do not meet criteria for any DSM disorder assessed in sur-veys has led to controversy regarding the relationship between severity and treat-ment need (Mechanic & McAlpine, 1999; Regier et al., 1998). Some commentators argue that treatment resources should be focused on serious cases (Narrow, Rae, Robins, & Regier, 2002). Others argue that it might be more cost-effective to focus on treating mild cases (Wakefield & Spitzer, 2002) or treating sub-threshold syn-dromes to prevent onset of future serious disorders (Kessler et al., 2003). No com-parative cost-effectiveness data exist to adjudicate between these contending views.

Turning to the more fine-grained prevalence estimates, these results are broadly consistent with those in other U.S. community surveys in showing that half of the general population is afflicted by mental disorders at some time in their life (Regier et al., 1998). This chapter's authors' finding, that anxiety and mood disor-ders are both common, is also consistent with these earlier studies. What may be more surprising, given the paucity of prior lifetime data, is the high prevalence of externalizing disorders, which are estimated in the NCS-R to be more common on a lifetime basis than either mood disorders or substance use disorders.

In addition to their high prevalence, the mental disorders examined here are notable for their ages of onset, which are concentrated in the first two decades of life. Consistent with previous epidemiological surveys (Christie et al., 1988; WHO International Consortium in Psychiatric Epidemiology, 2000), anxiety disorders were found to have the earliest AOO and mood disorders the latest. However in spite of any between-disorder variation, it is critical to note that mental disorders are uniquely burdensome in that they typically attack the young while almost all chronic physical disorders have conditional risks that increase with age, typically peaking in late middle or old age (Murray & Lopez, 1996).

The cohort effect in the NCS-R, with increasing prevalence of disorders in more recent cohorts, deserves further consideration. It varies in plausible ways (e.g., largest with substance disorders, which are known independently to have increased among cohorts that went through adolescence beginning in the 1970s), socio-demographic correlates are substantively plausible (e.g., increasing similarity of women and men in substance use disorders in recent cohorts), and there was no evidence for convergence among cohorts with increasing age. These data argue that the cohort effects are at least partly due to substantive rather than to methodological factors. Nonetheless, residual effects of methodological factors are likely based on the fact that longitudinal studies show mental disorders to be associated with early mortality (Bruce & Leaf, 1989) and the fact that resolved mental disorders reported in baseline interviews often are not reported in follow-up interviews (Badawi, Eaton, Myllyluoma, Weimer, & Gallo, 1999). To the extent that these biases are at work, the high prevalence found in the younger NCS-R cohorts might also apply to older cohorts.

Taken together, the findings of high lifetime prevalence and early AOO suggest that greater attention be paid to public health interventions that target the childhood and adolescent years. With appropriately balanced considerations of potential risks and benefits, focus is also needed on early interventions aimed at preventing the progression of primary disorders and the onset of comorbid disorders (see Chapter 8 in this volume on children & adolescents, and see Chapter 12 in this volume on co-occurring addictive and mental disorders).

The NCS-R 12-month prevalence results show episodes of DSM-IV disorders to be highly prevalent during the prior year, affecting over one-quarter of Americans. Although many cases are mild, the prevalence of moderate and serious cases is still substantial, affecting 14.0% of the population. The 5.7% with a serious 12-month disorder is remarkably close to the estimated prevalence of Serious Mental Illness (SMI) defined by SAMHSA in the original NCS (Kessler et al., 1996). Consistent with prior studies (Bijl et al., 2003; Demyttenaere et al., 2004), anxiety disorders are the most common class of disorders, but the proportion of serious cases is lower than for other classes; mood disorders are the next most common and have the highest proportion of serious cases. Externalizing disorders, which have been neglected in previous epidemiological studies, are present in over one-third of cases and also have a higher proportion of serious cases.

A striking finding from the NCS-R 12-month prevalence data is that more than 40% of cases in the prior year also have comorbid disorders. Patterns of bivariate comorbidity are broadly consistent with the ECA and original NCS in showing that the vast majority of disorders are positively correlated. Relative magnitudes of associations are also quite similar across the three surveys, with high rank-order correlations of odds ratios among comorbid pairs in the NCS-R versus published odds ratios (Kessler, 1995) in both the NCS (.79) and the ECA (.57). Major internal patterns of comorbidity are also quite consistent across surveys, such as the stronger odds ratios within the mood disorders than the anxiety disorders, very high odds ratios between anxiety and mood disorders, and odds ratios between anxiety and mood disorders generally being higher than between pairs of anxiety disorders. Severity is strongly related to comorbidity. The sociodemographic correlates of having 12-month disorders are broadly consistent with previous surveys in finding that mental disorders are associated with a general pattern of disadvantaged social status, including being female, unmarried, and having low socioeconomic status (Bland, Orn, & Newman, 1988; Canino et al., 1987; Demyttenaere et al., 2004; Hwu, Yeh, & Chang, 1989; Lee et al., 1990; Lépine et al., 1989; J. E. Wells, Bushnell, Hornblow, Joyce, & Oakley-Browne,

1989; WHO International Consortium in Psychiatric Epidemiology, 2000; Wittchen, Essau, von Zerssen, Krieg, & Zaudig, 1992).

The NCS-R lifetime data on use of mental health services reveal large and underappreciated needs for mental health treatment in the United States. A large number of lifetime cases never seek help. This is especially true for substance and externalizing disorders, where nearly half of all lifetime cases failed to ever make any treatment contact. The second source of unmet need is pervasive delay in initial treatment contact. The typical delay persists for years or even decades for some disorders. This has not been a focus of previous research, as mental health services research has traditionally focused on treatment of current episodes for established cases (Hu, Snowden, Jerrell, & Nguyen, 1991; Joseph & Boeckh, 1981; Leaf, Bruce, & Tischler, 1986; Leaf et al., 1988; Leaf et al., 1985; Padgett, Patrick, Burns, & Schlesinger, 1994; Temkin-Greener & Clark, 1988). These NCS-R findings suggest that the focus needs to be expanded to address the speed of initial help-seeking since, even for disorders where eventual treatment is typical, long delays are pervasive.

There was considerable variation between disorders in the probability of eventually making treatment contacts and in typical durations of delay. The higher initial treatment contact and shorter delays for mood disorders may be because they have been targeted by educational campaigns, primary care quality improvement programs, and treatment advances (Hirschfeld et al., 1997; Jacobs, 1995; Olfson et al., 2002; Pincus, Hough, Houtsinger, Rollman, & Frank, 2003; Schatzberg & Nemeroff, 2004). Panic disorder is often accompanied by prominent and dysphoric somatic symptoms which may explain why treatment contact for it is more common and rapid than for other anxiety disorders (Katerndahl & Realini, 1995; Katon, Von Korff, & Lin, 1992). Greater failure and delays for some anxiety disorders (e.g., phobias and SAD) could also be due to their earlier ages of onset, mild impairments, and even fear of providers or treatments (Leaf et al., 1988; Leaf et al., 1985; Solomon & Gordon, 1988).

Consistent with prior research (Christiana et al., 2000; Kessler, Olfson, & Berglund, 1998; Olfson, Kessler, Berglund, & Lin, 1998; Wang, Berglund, Olfson, & Kessler, 2004), we found that early-onset disorders are associated with longer delays and lower probabilities of help-seeking. Minors may need the help of parents or other adults, and recognition of disorders by these adults may be low unless symptoms are extreme (Janicke, Finney, & Riley, 2001; Morrissey-Kane & Prinz, 1999). Early onset may also lead to normalization of symptoms or coping strategies (e.g., social withdrawal) that interfere with help-seeking during adulthood. Child mental health services may also not be available. Socio-demographic correlates of failure and delay in making initial treatment contact (e.g., older age, male sex, being poorly educated, or racial-ethnic minority status) may reflect negative attitudes toward mental health treatments as well as financial and other barriers to care.

The shorter delays and higher proportions of cases making treatment contacts among more recent cohorts provide some grounds for optimism as well as clues for improving failure and delays in the future. This secular change could be due, at least in part, to recent programs to destigmatize and increase awareness of mental illness, screening and outreach initiatives, the introduction and direct-to-consumer promotion of new treatments, and expansion of some insurance programs (Bender, 2002; Bhugra, 1989; Hirschfeld et al., 1997; Jacobs, 1995; Kessler & Wang, 1999;

Leucht et al., 1999; Mechanic & McAlpine, 1999; Olfson et al., 2002; Regier et al., 1988; Ridgely & Goldman, 1989; Rosenthal et al., 2002; Ross, 1993; Schatzberg & Nemeroff, 2004; Spitzer, Kroenke, & Williams, 1999; Sturm & Klap, 1999; Weissman et al., 2000; Williams, 1998; Williams et al., 1999).

Additional large-scale public education programs (e.g., the NIMH Depression Awareness, Recognition, and Treatment [DART] program) and expanded use of National Screening Days continue to hold great promise for hastening detection and treatment (Jacobs, 1995; Morrissey-Kane & Prinz, 1999; Regier et al., 1988). School-based screening programs using brief self-report and/or informant scales may be needed to detect early-onset mental disorders (Aseltine & DeMartino, 2004; Connors, 1994). Demand management and other outreach strategies could also help reduce critical delays and failures in initial help-seeking once mental disorders are identified (Carleton et al., 1996; Velicer, Hughes, Fava, Prochaska, & DiClemente, 1995). Training non-health care professionals to recognize individuals with mental disorders and make timely referrals for health care should also be explored (Wang, Berglund, & Kessler, 2003; Weaver, 1995). Although preclinical (Post & Weiss, 1998), epidemiological studies (Forthofer, Kessler, Story, & Gotlib, 1996; Kessler, 1997; Kessler, Berglund et al., 1997; Kessler, Foster, Saunders, & Stang, 1995; Kessler & Price, 1993; Kessler, Walters, & Forthofer, 1998) and even trials (Meltzer et al., 2003) suggest there would be benefits to reducing these delays, definitively answering how much earlier treatment improves outcomes will need to wait until long-term trials of aggressive outreach and treatment of new cases are complete (Beidel, Turner, & Morris, 2000; Dierker et al., 2001; MTA Cooperative Group, 1999).

NCS-R findings on 12-month use of mental health services shed light on under-use of services, poor quality regimens, use of unproven modalities, and sub-optimal allocation of services. On one hand, the NCS-R reveals that mental health service use remains disturbingly low, with the majority of cases not receiving any care in the prior year. Among those receiving services, many go outside of health care sectors. For example, CAM treatments account for 32% of all mental health visits despite a paucity of data supporting their efficacy (Eisenberg et al., 1998; Eisenberg et al., 1993; Hypericum Depression Trial Study Group, 2002; Weaver, 1995). Even those using health care sectors fail to get sufficient visits for clinical assessments, delivery of treatments, and appropriate ongoing monitoring (National Committee for Quality Assurance, 1997; Olfson et al., 2002; Substance Abuse and Mental Health Services Administration, 1996). Because of these and other problems, only one-third of treatments meet minimal standards of adequacy based on evidence-based treatment guidelines (Agency for Health Care Policy and Research, 1993; American Psychiatric Association, 1998, 2000, 2002, 2004; Lehman & Steinwachs, 1998). A shift also appears to be occurring between sectors, with expanded use of the general medical sector for mental health services (by 17.9% of NCS-R respondents vs. 13.3% a decade earlier in the original NCS) (Kessler et al., 1999). However, this trend is of concern in light of the particularly low rate of treatment adequacy in the general medical sector.

On the other hand, a considerable number of mental health services are being consumed by respondents without apparent disorders. For example, respondents without disorders make up such a large majority of the population that they account for nearly one-third of all visits. As we showed in our analysis of these cases, some services are being used appropriately to treat disorders not assessed in the NCS-R, sub-threshold symptoms, and to provide secondary prevention of lifetime disorders. However, it remains concerning that such a high proportion of treatment resources are being potentially diverted to individuals with low severity when unmet needs among people with well-defined disorders are so great (Narrow et al., 2002). Another potential problem in the allocation of mental health care is suggested by the highly skewed distribution of visits, with a small proportion of patients using the majority of services. Developing and implementing a principled basis for optimally allocating treatment resources remains an enormous challenge.

The NCS-R results reveal that service use varies across disorders, with generally greater use for disorders marked by distress or impairment (e.g., panic disorder) and lower use for externalizing disorders (e.g., substance disorders and intermittent explosive disorder), which may be accompanied by diminished perceived needs for treatment. The socio-demographic predictors of 12-month service use confirm earlier studies in showing the greatest risks of under-treatment or ineffective treatment among vulnerable groups such as the elderly, racial-ethnic minorities, those with low education or incomes, the uninsured, and residents of rural areas (Fischer, Wei, Solberg, Rush, & Heinrich, 2003; Katz, Kessler, Lin, & Wells, 1998; Klap, Unroe, & Unutzer, 2003; Leaf et al., 1988; Leaf et al., 1985; McLean, Campbell, & Cornish, 2003; Rost, Fortney, Fischer, & Smith, 2002; Wang et al., 2002; Wells, Manning, Duan, Newhouse, & Ware, 1986).

Implications for Mental Health

These results suggest three directions for future research and policy analysis. First, as most people with a mental disorder receive no treatment, efforts are needed to increase access and demand for treatment. The persistence of low treatment among traditionally underserved groups calls for special initiatives (Smedley, Stith, & Nelson, 2003). The Surgeon General's report on under-treatment among racial-ethnic minorities (U.S. Department of Health and Human Services, 1999) and the NIMH initiative on under-treatment among men (National Institute of Mental Health, 2003) may provide useful models and should be evaluated. Programs to expand treatment resources in targeted locations could also be of value (Rost et al., 2002), as could initiatives such as legislation to encourage mental health service use among vulnerable elderly patients (Bender, 2002). Interventions to increase access and initiation of treatments could include renewed community awareness and screening programs, new means for financing mental health services, and expansion of treatment resources for underserved areas (Bender, 2002; Hirschfeld et al., 1997; Jacobs, 1995; Mechanic & McAlpine, 1999; Rost et al., 2002).

Second, our results show that interventions also are needed to improve the intensity and effectiveness of care that is given to patients with mental disorders. A related challenge is to understand why non–health care treatments such as CAM have such great appeal and whether legitimate aspects of this appeal (e.g., greater patient-centeredness) could be adopted in evidence-based treatments.

Proven disease management programs that enhance treatment adequacy and adherence (Katon et al., 2002; Katon et al., 1995; Schoenbaum et al., 2001;

Simon et al., 2001; K. B. Wells et al., 2000) as well as establishing performance standards hold promise for enhancing treatments and monitoring the impacts of interventions in the future (National Committee for Quality Assurance, 1997; Substance Abuse and Mental Health Services Administration, 1996). However, increasing uptake of such successful programs and treatment models will almost certainly require addressing existing barriers, such as competing clinical demands and distorted incentives for effectively treating mental disorders, as well as providing purchasers with metrics to help them understand what their return-on-investment (ROI) will be for improving mental health service use in the United States (Frank et al., 2003; Klinkman, 1997; Pincus et al., 2003; Wang, Simon, & Kessler, 2003; Williams, 1998; Williams et al., 1999).

Third, efforts are needed to evaluate the effectiveness of widely used treatments for which no effectiveness data exist and to increase use of evidence-based treatments. The expansion of disease management programs, treatment quality assurance programs, and "report cards" are important steps in this direction. Substantial barriers continue to exist, though, including competing clinical demands and distorted treatment incentives (Klinkman, 1997; Williams, 1998). Initiatives aimed at overcoming these barriers are under way (Pincus et al., 2003; Wang, Simon et al., 2003). Future trend surveys need to include data on treatment processes, like those in the NCS-R, to allow changes in treatment quality to be tracked.

Acknowledgments

Portions of this chapter have previously appeared in Kessler, R. C., Demler, O., Frank, R. G., Olfson, M., Pincus, H. A., Walters, E. E., Wang, P. S., Wells, K. B., Zaslavsky, A. M. Prevalence and treatment of mental disorders, 1990 to 2003. *New England Journal of Medicine*, 352(24), 2515–2523. © 2005 Massachusetts Medical Society; Kessler, R. C., Chiu, W. T., Demler, O., Walters, E. E. Prevalence, severity, and comorbidity of twelve-month DSM-IV disorders in the National Comorbidity Survey Replication (NCS-R). *Archives of General Psychiatry*, 62(6), 617–627; and Wang, P. S., Lane, M., Kessler, R. C., Olfson, M., Pincus, H. A., Wells, K. B. Twelve-month use of mental health services in the U.S.: Results from the National Comorbidity Survey Replication (NCS-R). *Archives of General Psychiatry*, 62(6), 629–640. Both © 2005 American Medical Association. Used with permission. And Kessler, R. C., Berglund, P. A., Chiu, W.-T., Demler, O. Glantz, M., Lane, M. C., Jin, R., Merikangas, K. R., Nock, M., Olfson, M., Pincus, H. A., Walters, E. E., Wang, P. S., Wells, K. B. (2008). The National Comorbidity Survey Replication (NCS-R): Cornerstone in improving mental health and mental health care in the United States. In R. C. Kessler & T. B. Üstün (Eds.), *The WHO World Mental Health Surveys: Global Perspectives on the Epidemiology of Mental Disorders* (pp. 165–209). New York: Cambridge University Press, 2008. Reprinted with permission.

Preparation of this chapter was supported, in part, by the National Institute of Mental Health grants U01-MH60220 and R01-MH070884. The views expressed in this article do not necessarily represent the views of the NIMH, NIH, HHS, or the United States Government.

References

Agency for Health Care Policy and Research. (1993). *Depression Guideline Panel: Vol 2, Treatment of Major Depression, Clinical Practice Guideline, No 5*. Rockville, MD: U.S. Department of Health and Human Services, Public Health Service, Agency for Health Care Policy and Research.

Allgulander, C. (1989). Psychoactive drug use in a general population sample, Sweden: Correlates with perceived health, psychiatric diagnoses, and mortality in an automated record-linkage study. *American Journal of Public Health, 79*, 1006–1010.

American Psychiatric Association. (1998). *Practice Guideline for Treatment of Patients with Panic Disorder*. Washington, DC: American Psychiatric Association Press.

American Psychiatric Association. (2000). *Practice Guideline for Treatment of Patients with Major Depressive Disorder* (2nd ed.). Washington, DC: American Psychiatric Association Press.

American Psychiatric Association. (2002). *Practice Guideline for Treatment of Patients with Bipolar Disorder* (2nd ed.). Washington, DC: American Psychiatric Association Press.

American Psychiatric Association. (2004). *Practice Guideline for Treatment of Patients with Schizophrenia* (2nd ed.). Washington, DC: American Psychiatric Association Press.

Aseltine, R. H., Jr., & DeMartino, R. (2004). An outcome evaluation of the SOS Suicide Prevention Program. *American Journal of Public Health, 94*, 446–451.

Badawi, M. A., Eaton, W. W., Myllyluoma, J., Weimer, L. G., & Gallo, J. (1999). Psychopathology and attrition in the Baltimore ECA 15-year follow-up 1981–1996. *Social Psychiatry and Psychiatric Epidemiology, 34*, 91–98.

Ballesteros, J., Duffy, J. C., Querejeta, I., Arino, J., & Gonzalez-Pinto, A. (2004). Efficacy of brief interventions for hazardous drinkers in primary care: Systematic review and meta-analyses. *Alcohol: Clinical and Experimental Research, 28*, 608–618.

Beidel, D. C., Turner, S. M., & Morris, T. L. (2000). Behavioral treatment of childhood social phobia. *Journal of Consulting and Clinical Psychology, 68*, 1072–1080.

Bender, E. (2002, August 16). Better access to geriatric mental health care goal of new house bill. *Psychiatric News*, p. 2.

Bhugra, D. (1989). Attitudes towards mental illness: A review of the literature. *Acta Psychiatrica Scandinavica, 80*, 1–12.

Bijl, R. V., de Graaf, R., Hiripi, E., Kessler, R. C., Kohn, R., Offord, D. R., et al. (2003). The prevalence of treated and untreated mental disorders in five countries. *Health Affairs (Millwood), 22*, 122–133.

Bland, R. C., Orn, H., & Newman, S. C. (1988). Lifetime prevalence of psychiatric disorders in Edmonton. *Acta Psychiatrica Scandinavica Supplement, 338*, 24–32.

Bruce, M. L., & Leaf, P. J. (1989). Psychiatric disorders and 15-month mortality in a community sample of older adults. *American Journal of Public Health, 79*, 727–730.

Canino, G. J., Bird, H. R., Shrout, P. E., Rubio-Stipec, M., Bravo, M., Martinez, R., et al. (1987). The prevalence of specific psychiatric disorders in Puerto Rico. *Archives of General Psychiatry, 44*, 727–735.

Cannell, C. F., Marquis, K. H., & Laurent, A. (1977). A summary of studies of interviewing methodology. *Vital Health and Statistics 2*, i–viii, 1–78.

Carleton, R. A., Bazzarre, T., Drake, J., Dunn, A., Fisher, E. B., Jr., Grundy, S. M., et al. (1996). Report of the Expert Panel on Awareness and Behavior Change to the Board of Directors, American Heart Association. *Circulation, 93*, 1768–1772.

Christiana, J. M., Gilman, S. E., Guardino, M., Kessler, R. C., Mickelson, K., Morselli, P. L., et al. (2000). Duration between onset and time of obtaining initial treatment among people with anxiety and mood disorders: An international survey of members of mental health patient advocate groups. *Psychological Medicine, 30*, 693–703.

Christie, K. A., Burke, J. D., Jr., Regier, D. A., Rae, D. S., Boyd, J. H., & Locke, B. Z. (1988). Epidemiologic evidence for early onset of mental disorders and higher risk of drug abuse in young adults. *American Journal of Psychiatry, 145*, 971–975.

Connors, C. K. (1994). The Connors Rating Scales: Use in clinical assessment, treatment planning and research. In M. Maruish (Ed.), *Use of Psychological Testing for Treatment Planning and Outcome Assessment*. Hillsdale, NJ: Lawrence Erlbaum Associates.

Demyttenaere, K., Bruffaerts, R., Posada-Villa, J., Gasquet, I., Kovess, V., Lépine, J. P., et al. (2004). Prevalence, severity and unmet need for treatment of mental disorders in the World Health Organization World Mental Health surveys. *Journal of the American Medical Association, 291*, 2581–2590.

Dierker, L. C., Albano, A. M., Clarke, G. N., Heimberg, R. G., Kendall, P. C., Merikangas, K. R., et al. (2001). Screening for anxiety and depression in early adolescence. *Journal of the American Academy of Child and Adolescent Psychiatry, 40*, 929–936.

Druss, B. G., Wang, P. S., Sampson, N. A., Olfson, M., Pincus, H. A., Wells, K. B., et al. (2007). Understanding mental health treatment in persons without mental diagnoses: Results from the National Comorbidity Survey Replication. *Archives of General Psychiatry, 64*, 1196–1203.

Eaton, W. W., Anthony, J. C., Tepper, S., & Dryman, A. (1992). Psychopathology and attrition in the Epidemiologic Catchment Area Study. *American Journal of Epidemiology, 135*, 1051–1059.

Eisenberg, D. M., Davis, R. B., Ettner, S. L., Appel, S., Wilkey, S. A., van Rompay, M., et al. (1998). Trends in alternative medicine use in the United States, 1990–1997: Results of a follow-up national survey. *Journal of the American Medical Association, 280*, 1569–1575.

Eisenberg, D. M., Kessler, R. C., Foster, C., Norlock, F. E., Calkins, D. R., & Delbanco, T. L. (1993). Unconventional medicine in the United States: Prevalence, costs, and patterns of use. *New England Journal of Medicine, 328*, 246–252.

Endicott, J., Spitzer, R. L., Fleiss, J. L., & Cohen, J. (1976). The gobal asessment sale: A procedure for measuring overall severity of psychiatric disorders. *Archives of General Psychiatry, 33*, 766–771.

First, M. B., Spitzer, R. L., Gibbon, M., & Williams, J. B. W. (2002). *Structured Clinical Interview for DSM-IV Axis I Disorders, Research Version, Non-patient Edition (SCID-I/NP)*. New York: Biometrics Research, New York State Psychiatric Institute.

Fischer, L. R., Wei, F., Solberg, L. I., Rush, W. A., & Heinrich, R. L. (2003). Treatment of elderly and other adult patients for depression in primary care. *Journal of the American Geriatric Society, 51*, 1554–1562.

Food and Drug Administration. (2004). Antidepressant use in children, adolescents, and adults [Electronic Version]. Available online at http://www.fda.gov/cder/drug/antidepressants/default.htm. Accessed May 7, 2007.

Forthofer, M. S., Kessler, R. C., Story, A. L., & Gotlib, I. H. (1996). The effects of psychiatric disorders on the probability and timing of first marriage. *Journal of Health and Social Behavior, 37*, 121–132.

Frank, R. G., Huskamp, H. A., & Pincus, H. A. (2003). Aligning incentives in the treatment of depression in primary care with evidence-based practice. *Psychiatric Services, 54*, 682–687.

Haro, J. M., Arbabzadeh-Bouchez, S., Brugha, T. S., de Girolamo, G., Guyer, M. E., Jin, R., et al. (2006). Concordance of the Composite International Diagnostic Interview Version 3.0 (CIDI 3.0) with standardized clinical assessments in the WHO World Mental Health surveys. *International Journal of Methods in Psychiatric Research, 15*, 167–180.

Hirschfeld, R. M. A., Keller, M. B., Panico, S., Arons, B. S., Barlow, D., Davidoff, F., et al. (1997). The national depressive and manic-depressive association consensus statement on the under-treatment of depression. *Journal of the American Medical Association, 277*, 333–340.

Holahan, J., & Cook, A. (2005). Changes in economic conditions and health insurance coverage, 2000–2004. *Health Affairs (Millwood)*, (Supplemental Web Exclusives), W5-498–508.

Hu, T. W., Snowden, L. R., Jerrell, J. M., & Nguyen, T. D. (1991). Ethnic populations in public mental health: Services choice and level of use. *American Journal of Public Health, 81*, 1429–1434.

Hwu, H. G., Yeh, E. K., & Chang, L. Y. (1989). Prevalence of psychiatric disorders in Taiwan defined by the Chinese Diagnostic Interview Schedule. *Acta Psychiatrica Scandinavica, 79*, 136–147.

Hypericum Depression Trial Study Group. (2002). Effect of hypericum perforatum (St. John's wort) in major depressive disorder: A randomized controlled trial. *Journal of the American Medical Association, 287*, 1807–1814.

Institute of Medicine. (2006). *Improving the Quality of Health Care for Mental and Substance-Use Conditions: Quality Chasm Series*. Washington, DC: National Academy of Sciences.

Jacobs, D. G. (1995). National depression screening day: Educating the public, reaching those in need of treatment and broadening professional understanding. *Harvard Review of Psychiatry, 3*, 156–159.

Janicke, D. M., Finney, J. W., & Riley, A. W. (2001). Children's health care use: A prospective investigation of factors related to care-seeking. *Medical Care, 39*, 990–1001.

Joseph, A. E., & Boeckh, J. L. (1981). Locational variation in mental health care utilization dependent upon diagnosis: A Canadian example. *Social Science and Medicine, 15*, 395–440.

Kaiser Commission on Medicaid and the Uninsured. (2006). The uninsured, a primer: Key facts about Americans without health insurance [Electronic Version]. Available online at www.kff. org. Accessed April 20, 2006.

Katerndahl, D. A., & Realini, J. P. (1995). Where do panic attack sufferers seek care? *Journal of Family Practice, 40*, 237–243.

Katon, W. J., Roy-Byrne, P., Russo, J., & Cowley, D. (2002). Cost-effectiveness and cost offset of a collaborative care intervention for primary care patients with panic disorder. *Archives of General Psychiatry, 59*, 1098–1104.

Katon, W. J., Von Korff, M., & Lin, E. (1992). Panic disorder: Relationship to high medical utilization. *American Journal of Medicine, 92*, 7S–11S.

Katon, W. J., Von Korff, M., Lin, E., Walker, E., Simon, G. E., Bush, T., et al. (1995). Collaborative management to achieve treatment guidelines: Impact on depression in primary care. *Journal of the American Medical Association, 273*, 1026–1031.

Katz, S. J., Kessler, R. C., Lin, E., & Wells, K. B. (1998). Medication management of depression in the United States and Ontario. *Journal of General Internal Medicine, 13*, 137–139.

Kessler, R. C. (1995). Epidemiology of psychiatric comorbidity. In M. T. Tsuang, M. Tohen, & G. E. P. Zahner (Eds.), *Textbook in Psychiatric Epidemiology* (pp. 179–197). New York: John Wiley & Sons.

Kessler, R. C. (1997). The prevalence of psychiatric comorbidity. In S. Wetzler & W. C. Sanderson (Eds.), *Treatment Strategies for Patients with Psychiatric Comorbidity*. New York: John Wiley & Sons.

Kessler, R. C., Berglund, P., Chiu, W. T., Demler, O., Heeringa, S., Hiripi, E., et al. (2004). The US National Comorbidity Survey Replication (NCS-R): Design and field procedures. *International Journal of Methods in Psychiatric Research, 13*, 69–92.

Kessler, R. C., Berglund, P., Demler, O., Jin, R., Merikangas, K. R., & Walters, E. E. (2005). Lifetime prevalence and age-of-onset distributions of DSM-IV disorders in the National Comorbidity Survey Replication. *Archives of General Psychiatry, 62*, 593–602.

Kessler, R. C., Berglund, P. A., Foster, C. L., Saunders, W. B., Stang, P. E., & Walters, E. E. (1997). Social consequences of psychiatric disorders, II: Teenage parenthood. *American Journal of Psychiatry, 154*, 1405–1411.

Kessler, R. C., Berglund, P. A., Zhao, S., Leaf, P. J., Kouzis, A. C., Bruce, M. L., et al. (1996). The 12-month prevalence and correlates of serious mental illness (SMI). In R. W. Manderscheid & M. A. Sonnenschein (Eds.), *Mental Health, United States, 1996* (pp. 59–70). Washington, DC: U.S. Government Printing Office.

Kessler, R. C., Chiu, W. T., Demler, O., Merikangas, K. R., & Walters, E. E. (2005). Prevalence, severity, and comorbidity of 12-month DSM-IV disorders in the National Comorbidity Survey Replication. *Archives of General Psychiatry, 62*, 617–627.

Kessler, R. C., Demler, O., Frank, R. G., Olfson, M., Pincus, H. A., Walters, E. E., et al. (2005). Prevalence and treatment of mental disorders, 1990 to 2003. *New England Journal of Medicine, 352*, 2515–2523.

Kessler, R. C., Foster, C. L., Saunders, W. B., & Stang, P. E. (1995). Social consequences of psychiatric disorders: I, Educational attainment. *American Journal of Psychiatry, 152*, 1026–1032.

Kessler, R. C., Frank, R. G., Edlund, M., Katz, S. J., Lin, E., & Leaf, P. (1997). Differences in the use of psychiatric outpatient services between the United States and Ontario. *New England Journal of Medicine, 336*, 551–557.

Kessler, R. C., Haro, J. M., Heeringa, S. G., Pennell, B. E., & Üstün, T. B. (2006). The World Health Organization World Mental Health Survey Initiative. *Epidemiologia e Psichiatria Sociale, 15*, 161–166.

Kessler, R. C., McGonagle, K. A., Zhao, S., Nelson, C. B., Hughes, M., Eshleman, S., et al. (1994). Lifetime and 12-month prevalence of DSM-III-R psychiatric disorders in the United States: Results from the National Comorbidity Survey. *Archives of General Psychiatry, 51*, 8–19.

Kessler, R. C., Merikangas, K. R., Berglund, P., Eaton, W. W., Koretz, D. S., & Walters, E. E. (2003). Mild disorders should not be eliminated from the DSM-V. *Archives of General Psychiatry, 60*, 1117–1122.

Kessler, R. C., Olfson, M., & Berglund, P. A. (1998). Patterns and predictors of treatment contact after first onset of psychiatric disorders. *American Journal of Psychiatry, 155*, 62–69.

Kessler, R. C., & Price, R. H. (1993). Primary prevention of secondary disorders: A proposal and agenda. *American Journal of Community Psychology, 21*, 607–633.

Kessler, R. C., & Üstün, T. B. (2004). The World Mental Health (WMH) Survey Initiative Version of the World Health Organization (WHO) Composite International Diagnostic Interview (CIDI). *International Journal of Methods in Psychiatric Research, 13*, 93–121.

Kessler, R. C., Walters, E. E., & Forthofer, M. S. (1998). The social consequences of psychiatric disorders: III, Probability of marital stability. *American Journal of Psychiatry, 155*, 1092–1096.

Kessler, R. C., & Wang, P. S. (1999). Screening measures for behavioral health assessment. In G. Hyner, K. Peterson, J. Travis, J. Dewey, J. Foerster, & E. Framer (Eds.), *In SPM Handbook of Health Assessment Tools* (pp. 33–40). Pittsburgh, PA: Society for Prospective Medicine.

Kessler, R. C., Wittchen, H.-U., Abelson, J. M., McGonagle, K. A., Schwarz, N., Kendler, K. S., et al. (1998). Methodological studies of the Composite International Diagnostic Interview (CIDI) in the US National Comorbidity Survey. *International Journal of Methods in Psychiatric Research, 7*, 33–55.

Kessler, R. C., Zhao, S., Katz, S. J., Kouzis, A. C., Frank, R. G., Edlund, M., et al. (1999). Past-year use of outpatient services for psychiatric problems in the National Comorbidity Survey. *American Journal of Psychiatry, 156*, 115–123.

Klap, R., Unroe, K. T., & Unutzer, J. (2003). Caring for mental illness in the United States: A focus on older adults. *American Journal of Geriatric Psychiatry, 11*, 517–524.

Klinkman, M. S. (1997). Competing demands in psychosocial care: A model for the identification and treatment of depressive disorders in primary care. *General Hospital Psychiatry, 19*, 98–111.

Leaf, P. J., Bruce, M. L., & Tischler, G. L. (1986). The differential effect of attitudes on the use of mental health services. *Social Psychiatry, 21*, 187–192.

Leaf, P. J., Bruce, M. L., Tischler, G. L., Freeman, D. H., Jr., Weissman, M. M., & Myers, J. K. (1988). Factors affecting the utilization of specialty and general medical mental health services. *Medical Care, 26*, 9–26.

Leaf, P. J., Livingston, M. M., Tischler, G. L., Weissman, M. M., Holzer, C. E., III, & Myers, J. K. (1985). Contact with health professionals for the treatment of psychiatric and emotional problems. *Medical Care, 23*, 1322–1337.

Lee, C. K., Kwak, Y. S., Yamamoto, J., Rhee, H., Kim, Y. S., Han, J. H., et al. (1990). Psychiatric epidemiology in Korea: Part I, Gender and age differences in Seoul. *Journal of Nervous and Mental Disease, 178*, 242–246.

Lehman, A. F., & Steinwachs, D. M. (1998). Translating research into practice: Schizophrenia patient outcomes research team (PORT) treatment recommendations. *Schizophrenia Bulletin, 24,* 1–10.

Leon, A. C., Olfson, M., Portera, L., Farber, L., & Sheehan, D. V. (1997). Assessing psychiatric impairment in primary care with the Sheehan Disability Scale. *International Journal Psychiatry in Medicine, 27,* 93–105.

Lépine, J. P., Lellouch, J., Lovell, A., Teherani, M., Ha, C., Verdier-Taillefer, M. G., et al. (1989). Anxiety and depressive disorders in a French population: Methodology and preliminary results. *Psychiatric Psychobiology, 4,* 267–274.

Leucht, S., Pitschel-Walz, G., Abraham, D., & Kissling, W. (1999). Efficacy and extrapyramidal side effects of the new antipsychotics olanzapine, quetiapine, risperidone, and sertindole compared to conventional antipsychotics and placebo: A meta-analysis of randomized controlled trials. *Schizophrenia Research, 35,* 51–68.

Mark, T. L., Coffey, R. M., McKusick, D. R., Harwood, H., King, E., Bouchery, E., et al. (2005). *National Estimates of Expenditures for Mental Health Services and Substance Abuse Treatment, 1991–2001.* SAMHSA Pub no. SMA 05-3999. Rockville, MD: Substance Abuse and Mental Health Services Administration.

McLean, C., Campbell, C., & Cornish, F. (2003). African-Caribbean interactions with mental health services in the UK: Experiences and expectations of exclusion as (re)productive of health inequalities. *Social Science and Medicine, 56,* 657–669.

Mechanic, D., & McAlpine, D. D. (1999). Mission unfulfilled: Potholes on the road to mental health parity. *Health Affairs (Millwood), 18,* 7–21.

Meltzer, H. Y., Alphs, L., Green, A. I., Altamura, A. C., Anand, R., Bertoldi, A., et al. (2003). Clozapine treatment for suicidality in schizophrenia: International Suicide Prevention Trial (InterSePT). *Archives of General Psychiatry, 60,* 82–91.

Morrissey-Kane, E., & Prinz, R. J. (1999). Engagement in child and adolescent treatment: The role of parental cognitions and attributions. *Clinical Child and Family Psychology Review, 2,* 183–198.

MTA Cooperative Group. (1999). A 14-month randomized clinical trial of treatment strategies for attention-deficit/hyperactivity disorder: Multimodal Treatment Study of Children with ADHD. *Archives of General Psychiatry, 56,* 1073–1086.

Murray, C. J. L., & Lopez, A. D. (Eds.). (1996). *The Global Burden of Disease: A Comprehensive Assessment of Mortality and Disability from Diseases, Injuries, and Risk Factors in 1990 and Projected to 2020.* Cambridge, MA: Harvard University Press.

Narrow, W. E., Rae, D. S., Robins, L. N., & Regier, D. A. (2002). Revised prevalence estimates of mental disorders in the United States: Using a clinical significance criterion to reconcile 2 surveys' estimates. *Archives of General Psychiatry, 59,* 115–123.

National Committee for Quality Assurance. (Ed.). (1997). *HEDIS 3.0: Narrative; What's In It and Why It Matters.* Washington, DC: National Committee for Quality Assurance.

National Institute of Mental Health. (2003). Real Men/Real Depression Program. Available online at http://menanddepression.nimh.nih.gov. Accessed July 9, 2004.

Olfson, M., Kessler, R. C., Berglund, P. A., & Lin, E. (1998). Psychiatric disorder onset and first treatment contact in the United States and Ontario. *American Journal of Psychiatry, 155,* 1415–1422.

Olfson, M., Marcus, S. C., Druss, B., Elinson, L., Tanielian, T., & Pincus, H. A. (2002). National trends in the outpatient treatment of depression. *Journal of the American Medical Association, 287,* 203–209.

Ost, L. G., Ferebee, I., & Furmark, T. (1997). One-session group therapy of spider phobia: Direct versus indirect treatments. *Behaviour Research and Therapy, 35,* 721–732.

Padgett, D. K., Patrick, C., Burns, B. J., & Schlesinger, H. J. (1994). Ethnicity and the use of out-patient mental health services in a national insured population. *American Journal of Public Health, 84,* 222–226.

Pincus, H. A., Hough, L., Houtsinger, J. K., Rollman, B. L., & Frank, R. G. (2003). Emerging models of depression care: Multi-level ('6 P') strategies. *International Journal of Methods in Psychiatric Research*, *12*, 54–63.

Post, R. M., & Weiss, S. R. (1998). Sensitization and kindling phenomena in mood, anxiety, and obsessive-compulsive disorders: The role of serotonergic mechanisms in illness progression. *Biological Psychiatry*, *44*, 193–206.

President's New Freedom Commission on Mental Health. (2003). Achieving the promise: Transforming mental health care in america. Available online at http://www.mentalhealth commission.gov/reports/finalreport/fullreport.htm

Regier, D. A., Hirschfeld, R. M., Goodwin, F. K., Burke, J. D., Jr., Lazar, J. B., & Judd, L. L. (1988). The NIMH Depression Awareness, Recognition, and Treatment Program: Structure, aims, and scientific basis. *American Journal of Psychiatry*, *145*, 1351–1357.

Regier, D. A., Kaelber, C. T., Rae, D. S., Farmer, M. E., Knauper, B., Kessler, R. C., et al. (1998). Limitations of diagnostic criteria and assessment instruments for mental disorders: Implications for research and policy. *Archives of General Psychiatry*, *55*, 109–115.

Ridgely, M. S., & Goldman, H. H. (1989). Mental health insurance. In D. A. Rochefort (Ed.), *Handbook on Mental Health Policy in the United States* (pp. 341–361). Westport, CT: Greenwood Press.

Robins, L. N., & Regier, D. A. (Eds.). (1991). *Psychiatric Disorders in America: The Epidemiologic Catchment Area Study*. New York: The Free Press.

Robins, L. N., Wing, J., Wittchen, H. U., Helzer, J. E., Babor, T. F., Burke, J., et al. (1988). The Composite International Diagnostic Interview: An epidemiologic instrument suitable for use in conjunction with different diagnostic systems and in different cultures. *Archives of General Psychiatry*, *45*, 1069–1077.

Rosenthal, M. B., Berndt, E. R., Donohue, J. M., Frank, R. G., & Epstein, A. M. (2002). Promotion of prescription drugs to consumers. *New England Journal of Medicine*, *346*, 498–505.

Ross, J. (1993). Social phobia: The consumer's perspective. *Journal of Clinical Psychiatry*, *54*(Suppl.), 5–9.

Rost, K., Fortney, J., Fischer, E., & Smith, J. (2002). Use, quality, and outcomes of care for mental health: The rural perspective. *Medical Care Research and Review*, *59*, 231–265.

Schatzberg, A. F., & Nemeroff, C. B. (2004). *Textbook of Psychopharmacology*. Washington, DC: American Psychiatric Publishing.

Schoenbaum, M., Unutzer, J., Sherbourne, C., Duan, N., Rubenstein, L. V., Miranda, J., et al. (2001). Cost-effectiveness of practice-initiated quality improvement for depression: Results of a randomized controlled trial. *Journal of the American Medical Association*, *286*, 1325–1330.

Simon, G. E., Katon, W. J., VonKorff, M., Unutzer, J., Lin, E. H., Walker, E. A., et al. (2001). Cost-effectiveness of a collaborative care program for primary care patients with persistent depression. *American Journal of Psychiatry*, *158*, 1638–1644.

Smedley, B. D., Stith, A. Y., & Nelson, A. R. (Eds.). (2003). *Unequal Treatment: Confronting Racial and Ethnic Disparities in Health Care*. Washington, DC: National Academy Press.

Solomon, P., & Gordon, B. (1988). Comparison of outpatient care of discharged state hospital and non-hospitalized psychiatric emergency room patients. *Psychiatric Quarterly*, *59*, 23–36.

Spitzer, R. L., Kroenke, K., & Williams, J. B. (1999). Validation and utility of a self-report version of PRIME-MD: The PHQ primary care study. Primary Care Evaluation of Mental Disorders, Patient Health Questionnaire. *Journal of the American Medical Association*, *282*, 1737–1744.

Sturm, R., & Klap, R. (1999). Use of psychiatrists, psychologists, and master's-level therapists in managed behavioral health care carve-out plans. *Psychiatric Services*, *50*, 504–508.

Substance Abuse and Mental Health Services Administration. (1996). *Consumer-Oriented Mental Health Report Card*. Rockville, MD: Center for Mental Health Services, SAMSHA.

Temkin-Greener, H., & Clark, K. T. (1988). Ethnicity, gender, and utilization of mental health services in a Medicaid population. *Social Science and Medicine*, *26*, 989–996.

Turner, C. F., Ku, L., Rogers, S. M., Lindberg, L. D., Pleck, J. H., & Sonenstein, F. L. (1998). Adolescent sexual behavior, drug use, and violence: Increased reporting with computer survey technology. *Science, 280*, 867–873.

U.S. Department of Health and Human Services. (1999). Mental health: Culture, race, and ethnicity, a supplement to mental health; A report of the surgeon general. Available online at http://www.surgeongeneral.gov/library/mentalhealth. Accessed July 9, 2004.

Velicer, W. F., Hughes, S. L., Fava, J. L., Prochaska, J. O., & DiClemente, C. C. (1995). An empirical typology of subjects within stage of change. *Addictive Behaviors, 20*, 299–320.

Wakefield, J. C., & Spitzer, R. L. (2002). Lowered estimates—but of what? *Archives of General Psychiatry, 59*, 129–130.

Wang, P. S., Berglund, P., & Kessler, R. C. (2000). Recent care of common mental disorders in the United States: Prevalence and conformance with evidence-based recommendations. *Journal of General Internal Medicine, 15*, 284–292.

Wang, P. S., Berglund, P. A., & Kessler, R. C. (2003). Patterns and correlates of contacting clergy for mental disorders in the United States. *Health Services Research, 38*, 647–673.

Wang, P. S., Berglund, P. A., Olfson, M., & Kessler, R. C. (2004). Delays in initial treatment contact after first onset of a mental disorder. *Health Services Research, 39*, 393–415.

Wang, P. S., Berglund, P., Olfson, M., Pincus, H. A., Wells, K. B., & Kessler, R. C. (2005). Failure and delay in initial treatment contact after first onset of mental disorders in the National Comorbidity Survey Replication. *Archives of General Psychiatry, 62*, 603–613.

Wang, P. S., Demler, O., & Kessler, R. C. (2002). Adequacy of treatment for serious mental illness in the United States. *American Journal of Public Health, 92*, 92–98.

Wang, P. S., Lane, M., Olfson, M., Pincus, H. A., Wells, K. B., & Kessler, R. C. (2005). Twelve-month use of mental health services in the United States: Results from the National Comorbidity Survey Replication. *Archives of General Psychiatry, 62*, 629–640.

Wang, P. S., Simon, G., & Kessler, R. C. (2003). The economic burden of depression and the cost-effectiveness of treatment. *International Journal of Methods in Psychiatric Research, 12*, 22–33.

Weaver, A. J. (1995). Has there been a failure to prepare and support parish-based clergy in their role as frontline community mental health workers: A review. *Journal of Pastoral Care, 49*, 129–147.

Weissman, E., Pettigrew, K., Sotsky, S., & Regier, D. A. (2000). The cost of access to mental health services in managed care. *Psychiatric Services, 51*, 664–666.

Wells, J. E., Bushnell, J. A., Hornblow, A. R., Joyce, P. R., & Oakley-Browne, M. A. (1989). Christchurch Psychiatric Epidemiology Study: Part I, Methodology and lifetime prevalence for specific psychiatric disorders. *Australian and New Zealand Journal of Psychiatry, 23*, 315–326.

Wells, K. B., Manning, W. G., Duan, N., Newhouse, J. P., & Ware, J. E., Jr. (1986). Sociodemographic factors and the use of outpatient mental health services. *Medical Care, 24*, 75–85.

Wells, K. B., Sherbourne, C., Schoenbaum, M., Duan, N., Meredith, L., Unutzer, J., et al. (2000). Impact of disseminating quality improvement programs for depression in managed primary care: A randomized controlled trial. *Journal of the American Medical Association, 283*, 212–220.

WHO International Consortium in Psychiatric Epidemiology. (2000). Cross-national comparisons of the prevalences and correlates of mental disorders. *Bulletin of the World Health Organization, 78*, 413–426.

Williams, J. W., Jr. (1998). Competing demands: Does care for depression fit in primary care? *Journal of General Internal Medicine, 13*, 137–139.

Williams, J. W., Jr., Rost, K., Dietrich, A. J., Ciotti, M. C., Zyzanski, S. J., & Cornell, J. (1999). Primary care physicians' approach to depressive disorders: Effects of physician specialty and practice structure. *Archives of Family Medicine, 8*, 58–67.

Wittchen, H.-U., Essau, C. A., von Zerssen, D., Krieg, C. J., & Zaudig, M. (1992). Lifetime and six-month prevalence of mental disorders in the Munich Follow-up Study. *European Archives of Psychiatry and Clinical Neuroscience, 241*, 247–225.

Chapter 8

CHILDREN AND ADOLESCENTS

Sharon Green-Hennessy, PhD

Children, after all, are not just adults-in-the-making. They are people whose current needs and rights and experiences must be taken seriously.

Kohn, 1993

FOR DECADES, a variety of voices within the children's mental health field have advocated modifying the approach to children and adolescents' mental health to reflect the understanding that "young people" are not "little adults" (Achenbach, 1978; Shirk, 1988; U.S. Department of Health and Human Services [USDHHS], 1999). Developmental psychopathology has answered this call by providing a much needed framework for conceptualizing childhood psychopathology (Cicchetti, 1984; Masten, 2006). Although this work is far from complete and at times controversial, it is no longer assumed that diagnostic criteria created for adults require but minor alterations to duration requirements to make them applicable to youth. In fact, the pendulum has swung so far that current controversies center on whether the field is giving too much latitude to developmental issues in conceptualizing disorders (Chang, 2007; Wozniak et al., 2005). Developmental psychopathology has transformed the understanding of the mental illness of youth, causing many to shed the view that they are but "little adults."

In contrast to widespread advances in the conceptualization of child and adolescent psychopathology, progress has been piecemeal when it comes to providing intervention services to those same youth (Huang et al., 2005; Tolan & Dodge, 2005). This reflects a variety of factors, not the least of which is the failure of the field to achieve consensus around a unifying organizational framework (Bickman, Noser, & Summerfelt, 1999; Glied & Cuellar, 2003; Holden & Blau, 2006; Tolan & Dodge, 2005; Weisz, Sandler, Durlak, & Anton, 2006; Westen, Novotny, & Thompson-Brenner, 2004). Although frameworks have been advanced, specifically the systems of care model and evidence-based treatment, no one model has as yet gained acceptance from a preponderance of the stakeholders who figure prominently in the child and adolescent mental health services landscape. However, the notion that the field and its providers must "choose" one model to the exclusion of the others is misleading (Weisz, Sandler et al., 2006). Systems of care, evidence-based practices, and developmental psychopathology target different components of child and adolescent mental health services: nothing precludes them from being integrated into a single broader approach. Moreover, such broad, encompassing mindsets are needed or else the conclusions reached, and the well-intentioned public policies they will spawn, will fail to achieve the desired end of improving mental health services for children and youth.

The aim of this chapter is to examine the pathway to successful mental health treatment in children and adolescents, freely drawing upon the tenets inherent in the paradigms mentioned above as applicable. The structure here is sequential, initially addressing issues of treatment entry and retention, with subsequent attention to the interventions' effectiveness.

The Scope of the Problem: Prevalence Rates and Service Use

Epidemiological data on child and adolescent psychopathology, though growing, still remain scarce in comparison to adult epidemiological data. The majority of studies assess older children and adolescents and lack uniformity in diagnostic measures, impairment criteria, time frames, and informants (Costello, Mustillo, Keeler, & Angold, 2004; Romano, Tremblay, Vitaro, Zoccolillo, & Pagini, 2001). This is the state of affairs despite recent findings from the adult epidemiological literature that nearly half of all lifetime mental disorders have an onset by mid-adolescence (Kessler et al., 2007; Kessler et al., 2005), a finding which begs the question of exactly how many disorders should populate the Diagnostic and Statistical Manual's category of *Disorders Usually First Diagnosed in Infancy, Childhood, or Adolescence.*

Despite these methodological difficulties, several broad findings can be discerned regarding prevalence rates. Globally, approximately one out of every five youth has a psychiatric disorder (Belfer, 2008; Canino et al., 2004; Costello, Angold, Burns, Stangl et al., 1996; Romano et al., 2001). When a significant functional impairment criteria is added, prevalence rates generally decrease by roughly half (Bird et al., 1988; Canino et al., 2004; Costello, Angold, Burns, Erkanli et al., 1996; Costello, Egger, & Angold, 2005; Romano et al., 2001). Psychopathology extends down to the youngest ages, with several studies recording significant mental health problems among preschoolers and toddlers (McDonnell & Glod, 2003; Skovgaard et al., 2007). The data also indicate a gender difference, with female adolescents more likely to experience internalizing problems, while male adolescents tend toward externalizing disorders (Rescorla et al., 2007).

While acknowledging that psychiatric diagnosis with impairment is not necessarily equal to the concept of "need," it can serve as a useful proxy (Ford, 2008). Although methodological problems also plague service use data (Reid, Tobon, & Shanley, 2008), estimates of the percentage of youth in need of mental health care who receive specialized mental health services hover around 20% for the United States, Canada, and Great Britain (Kataoka, Zhang, & Wells, 2002;

Staghezza-Jaramillo, Bird, Gould, & Canino, 1995; Waddell, Offord, Shepherd, Hua, & McEwan, 2002), with lower rates recorded in other countries (Eapen, Jakka, & Abou-Saleh, 2003; Sayal, 2006; Sourander et al., 2001) (see Chapter 6 in this volume for more information).

Youth with mental health needs access support from non-specialty mental health providers (i.e., school personnel, primary care providers, etc.) at a higher rate than they do specialty mental health providers (Ford, 2008). Moreover, most mental health services are accessed through the school as opposed to the mental health system (Bradshaw, Buckley, & Ialongo, 2008; Canino et al., 2004; Farmer, Burns, Phillips, Angold, & Costello, 2003). Analysis of youth data from the United States indicates inpatient services are used less frequently than outpatient treatment (Pottick et al., 2004), with a historical trend of decreasing inpatient lengths of stay (Case, Olfson, Marcus, & Siegel, 2007). Estimates for duration of outpatient mental health treatment vary, but studies generally indicate that outpatient treatment for youth is quite brief (Farmer et al., 2003). Most youth experience an average of six to seven outpatient visits (Martin & Leslie, 2003; Zuvekas, 2001), with the distribution being positively skewed, as illustrated by Harpaz-Rotem and colleagues' finding that 45% of new patients discontinue treatment within 30 days (Harpaz-Rotem, Leslie, & Rosenheck, 2004). Further, use of psychotropic medications has been increasing in the young (Martin & Leslie, 2003).

When examining data from the United States, striking differences between youth and adult mental health services are apparent. Youth are more likely to be referred to mental health care by community agencies (e.g., education, juvenile justice, social services) and less likely by themselves (Crider et al., 2006). Compared to adults, a lesser portion of children and adolescents' mental health care is delivered in 24-hour settings (i.e., inpatient, residential) (Crider et al., 2006), they have fewer outpatient visits than adults up to age 65 (Zuvekas, 2001), and they are more likely to be privately insured (Barry & Busch, 2007). Even accounting for their percentage in the total population, less money is spent on youth mental health and substance abuse treatment than for adults, with a greater percentage of that money going toward specialty mental health and substance abuse treatment organizations (Mark et al., 2008). This is consistent with international findings that show degree of coverage and mental health services provided for youth were less than those for adults (Levav, Jacobsson, Tsiantis, Kolaitis, & Ponizovsky, 2004; World Health Organization [WHO], 2005).

In summary, although a sizable percentage of youth are in need of mental health care, only one in five receives it. The pathway by which youth come to experience mental health treatment differs from that of adults, specifically in being more systemically based. Moreover, the resources that are available to youth, should they find their way to treatment, are both different in nature and lesser in amount than those for adults (see Chapter 7 in this volume for more information).

Service Models and Problem Recognition: Individual vs. System

The road to successful mental health treatment normally begins with problem recognition, for without such awareness there is no impetus to begin the journey

(Roberts, Alegria, Roberts, & Chen, 2005). It is the first of many steps that occurs before a child or adolescent is exposed to a moment of mental health treatment. To better understand this first step, as well as subsequent steps in help-seeking, the child and adolescent mental health services field reflexively turned toward adult models for guidance (Andersen, 1995; Andersen & Newman, 1973; Becker & Maiman, 1975; Prochaska & Di Clemente, 1982), with little initial acknowledgment that the process might differ according to developmental level (Logan & King, 2001). Traditionally, adult models have contained implicit assumptions that help-seeking is a rational, sequential process, whereby the individual, after assessing the situation cognitively, exercises his or her choice to enter into a health care system. While it is debatable if such notions truly capture adults' help-seeking patterns (Pescosolido, Gardner, & Lubell, 1998), they are not valid for describing the process in youth (Logan & King, 2001; Shanley, Reid, & Evans, 2008; Stiffman, Pescosolido, & Cabassa, 2004).

Recently, a number of specific child and adolescent models have been advanced that differ from adult models in several ways (Cauce et al., 2002; Eiraldi, Mazzuca, Clarke, & Power, 2006; Logan & King, 2001; Stiffman et al., 2004; Zwaanswijk, van der Ende, Verhaak, Bensing, & Verhulst, 2005). These youth-oriented models highlight the necessity of approaching treatment entry and access in a developmental and systems-focused way, taking into account the role of culture, the profound influence of parents in directing treatment, the multiple system providers involved, the impact of contextual variables, and the wide range of services that families tap. These variables are remarkably similar to those espoused as the underlying principles in the system of care framework (Stroul & Friedman, 1986).

To begin with, fundamentally, youth models are based upon the premise that help-seeking in children and adolescents is not an individually based process, but a systemic one (Logan & King, 2001). Youth rarely self-identify as needing mental health treatment (Crider et al., 2006; Raviv, Sills, Raviv, & Wilansky, 2000; Srebnik & Cauce, 1996); adults then are tasked with the responsibility of recognizing problems, especially in younger children (Eiraldi et al., 2006; Sayal, 2006). In fact, everyday clinical practice for children typically involves an adult identifying and describing a child's problem to a professional (Hawley & Weisz, 2003; Yeh & Weisz, 2001). Despite wishes of some to be more inclusive of children and adolescents in the process (Davies & Wright, 2008), clinicians are not unique in raising concerns about whether children and even adolescents have the self-reflective and perspective-taking skills to provide an accurate account of their emotional state and behaviors (Day, 2008).

Perhaps it is not surprising then that adults close to the child (i.e., parents, primary care physicians, teachers) shoulder the responsibility for recognizing mental health problems in youth. It is understandable that parents are charged with this task given that minors need their permission to engage in mental health services (Stiffman et al., 2004). However, difficulty in accurately perceiving and reporting a child or adolescent's emotional state and behavior is not a problem solely confined to the youth (Day, 2008; Logan & King, 2002; Teagle, 2002). Despite extensive daily contact with the child or adolescent, parents often fail to discern mental health problems in their offspring. Logan and King (2002) found that 79% of parents whose adolescents had been diagnosed with a depressive disorder via the Structured Clinical Interview for DSM-IV Axis I Disorders failed to endorse a single symptom of depression when queried about their adolescent (using the Diagnostic Interview Schedule for Children). Similarly Teagle (2002) found among youth with diagnosable mental illnesses that 61% of parents did not report any problems. Further support for the notion that parents are often unaware of their offspring's mental health problems is found among studies showing poor concordance between parental and youth self-report of emotional and behavioral problems (Rescorla et al., 2007; Yeh & Weisz, 2001; Zahner & Daskalakis, 1998).

However, this difficulty with problem recognition is not unique to parents. General practitioners, despite their professional training, only identify between 25% and 50% of their young patients with psychiatric diagnoses or psychosocial problems (Brown, Riley, & Wissow, 2007; Sayal & Taylor, 2004; Zwaanswijk, Verhaak, Bensing, van der Ende, & Verhulst, 2003). Teachers manifest similar problems, despite their advantage of daily contact with the child or adolescent and well-developed norms regarding typical behavior for a given age (Moor et al., 2007; Sayal, Hornsey, Warren, MacDiarmid, & Taylor, 2006). Such noteworthy difficulty in detecting mental health issues, even in response to educational interventions to improve recognition (Moor et al., 2007), suggests a need to focus on what is impeding adults' ability to see what is before them.

Although research has found caregiver problem recognition to be related to child variables such as age, symptom severity, and functional impairment (Bussing, Zima, Gary, & Garvan, 2003; Teagle, 2002), problem recognition also relates to a variety of contextual factors. These factors include perceived parental/family burden (Angold et al., 1998; Logan & King, 2002; Sayal, Taylor, & Beecham, 2003; Teagle, 2002; Zwaanswijk et al., 2003), parental psychopathology (Teagle, 2002; Youngstrom, Izard, & Ackerman, 1999; Zwaanswijk et al., 2003), parental ethnicity (Roberts et al., 2005; Wachtel, Rodrigue, Geffken, Graham-Pole, & Turner, 1994), family size (Zwaanswijk et al., 2003), presence of a relative who used mental health services (Zwaanswijk et al., 2005), and cultural norms (Cauce et al., 2002; Eiraldi et al., 2006; Heiervang, Goodman, & Goodman, 2008; Weisz, Weiss, Suwanlert, & Chaiyasit, 2006). Moreover, even when a problem is recognized, it must still be encoded as a mental health problem and its deviance recognized before it will generate the impulse to seek mental health services (Srebnik & Cauce, 1996; Zwaanswijk, van der Ende, Verhaak, Bensing, & Verhulst, 2007). There is some suggestion that parents, even when they can identify a problem in their children, have a tendency to attribute it to a benign, self-limiting developmental issue ("He'll grow out of it") (Day, 2008; Logan & King, 2001; Morrissey-Kane & Prinz, 1999; Pescosolido et al., 2008; Thompson & May, 2006).

Hence, many predictors of youth mental health problem recognition are not characteristics of the youth at all, but rather aspects of the perceiver or environment. This suggests that interventions to increase adults' ability to recognize youth mental health problems need to go beyond a psychoeducational model of teaching cardinal symptoms of various agreed upon disorders to focus on the removal of barriers that deter recognition. These barriers can include limited confidence in dealing with mental health issues (Koller & Bertel, 2006; Rothi, Leavey, & Best, 2008; Walter, Gouze, & Lim, 2006) and incomplete or inaccurate definitions of problem behavior, such as in the United States, where definitions of the special education categories of "learning disabilities" or "emotionally and behaviorally disturbed" exclude certain youth. In addition, another important issue is gateway providers' tendency to recognize fewer problems when they feel overburdened or perceive few resources available for any problems they do identify (Stiffman et al., 2001, 2004). The latter tendency in particular highlights the importance of not only limiting providers' caseloads but of stressing systemic interagency collaboration, thereby increasing the initial contact person's awareness of the full range and number of services available (Stiffman et al., 2001, 2004).

Referral and Accessing Treatment: Sequential vs. Unordered

In addition to their greater emphasis on systemic issues, youth focused models of help-seeking also acknowledge that child and adolescent access of mental health care is often not a particularly rational, sequential, or cognitively driven process. Upon recognition, parents generally first attempt to address problems themselves (Srebnik & Cauce, 1996). If this fails, they often turn to informal supports (e.g., family members, teachers, pastors). The threshold for accessing these supports appears to be lower than that for professional supports (Srebnik & Cauce, 1996; Stiffman et al., 2004; Zwaanswijk et al., 2007). In fact, Zwaanswijk and colleagues (2005) found among children identified as exhibiting problems and whose parents thought they needed help, only 20% went directly to specialty mental health treatment. Strong, dense informal support networks can meet the parents' need for assistance or, conversely, delay or deter the parent from pursuing needed specialty care (Srebnik & Cauce, 1996), although exceptions are noted (Wong, 2007). African American parents report more frequent contact and support from their informal networks than do Caucasian parents, perhaps lessening the impetus to seek formal mental health treatment (Bussing et al., 2003; Eiraldi et al., 2006).

Youth who move beyond this level and receive formal mental health services tend to be Caucasian, older, exhibit higher symptom severity, and have parents who believe the youth's problems arose from either physical causes or traumatic experiences (Logan & King, 2001; Morrissey-Kane & Prinz, 1999; Rickwood & Braithwaite, 1994; Srebnik & Cauce, 1996; Yeh et al., 2005). In general, research describes a "leaky pipeline," whereby only a limited number of youth progress through each subsequent stage toward specialty mental health treatment (Bussing et al., 2003; Sawyer et al., 2001; Shanley et al., 2008; Sourander et al., 2001; Thompson & May, 2006; Zwaanswijk et al., 2005).

However, not all studies confirm this somewhat meandering but still fundamentally sequential pathway whereby parental problem recognition yields initial self-management, succeeded by informal care, and culminating in formal mental health services. First, although parental problem recognition is normally the first step in treatment, this is not always the case. At times, other systems (e.g., schools, child welfare, juvenile justice) force treatment initiation when parents do not see the need (Pavuluri, Luk, & McGee, 1996; Shanley et al., 2008) and conversely, a small number of youth will pursue informal means of help that do not require parental awareness or consent (Logan & King, 2001).

Second, informal help does not always precede formal mental health services. Research has shown that families concurrently seek both professional and informal services (Cohen, Kasen, Brook, & Struening, 1991; Shanley et al., 2008). In fact, the pathway to care for children and adolescents is frequently disorganized and characterized by multiple entry points that are sometimes accessed simultaneously (Farmer et al., 2003; Shanley et al., 2008).

Lastly, the pathway is not necessarily forward progressing. When strong barriers are encountered, families may revert back to earlier stages (Logan & King, 2001; Zwaanswijk et al., 2007). These barriers can be direct access issues (e.g., finances, service availability) or they can be more intangible ones. For example, if a parent accesses informal supports (i.e., friends, community advisors, etc.) who do not perceive the youth's problem as concerning or deviant, the parent may be persuaded to that viewpoint (Srebnik & Cauce, 1996). Alternatively, faced with youth resistance to mental health services, the parent (or parents) may revise their estimate of the need for such services (Zwaanswijk et al., 2007). This would be consistent with the finding that parents' perception that their child or adolescent will resist treatment is significantly associated with unmet need (Flisher et al., 1997).

As with problem recognition, child factors, such as symptom severity (Ford, 2008; Rickwood & Braithwaite, 1994; Sayal, 2006; Sourander et al., 2001; Yeh et al., 2005; Zahner & Daskalakis, 1998; Zwaanswijk et al., 2003), presence of a co-morbid physical illness (Ford, Hamilton, Meltzer, & Goodman., 2008; Zahner & Daskalakis, 1998; Zwaanswijk et al. 2003), presence of maltreatment (Garland, Landsverk, Hough, & Ellis-Macleod, 1996), and out-of-home placement by child welfare (Hurlburt et al., 2008; Leslie et al., 2005) do influence help-seeking and service use for children and adolescents. The overlap and interaction of age, ethnicity, impairment, and type of symptoms (internalizing versus externalizing) makes it difficult to discern the unique effects of each (Ford et al., 2008; Zwaanswijk et al., 2003), despite some findings that minorities, older youth, and those with impairing internalizing disorders are less likely to seek and receive care (Alegria et al., 2004; Bradshaw et al., 2008; Brannan & Heflinger, 2005; Bussing et al., 2003; Cabiya et al., 2006; Kataoka et al., 2002; Pottick et al., 2004; Rickwood & Braithwaite, 1994; Thompson & May, 2006; Sourander et al., 2001; Wu et al., 1999; Yeh et al., 2005; Zimmerman, 2005).

As important as child variables are, environmental or family variables are more potent predictors of help-seeking and service use in children and adolescents (Flisher et al., 1997; Zwaanswijk et al., 2005). These variables include parental psychopathology (Cornelius, Pringle, Jernigan, Kirisci, & Clark, 2001; Flisher et al., 1997; Ford et al., 2008; Zimmerman, 2005), parental perception of burden (Angold et al., 1998; Brannan & Heflinger, 2005; Ford et al., 2008; Logan & King, 2002; Sayal et al., 2003; Zwaanswijk et al., 2003), parental marital status (Ford, 2008; Sayal, 2006; Sourander et al., 2001), and geographical location (Strum, Ringel, & Andreyeva, 2003). Evidence is more mixed with respect to socioeconomic status and insurance, likely reflecting differences in payment systems (Ford, 2008; Sayal, 2006; Zimmerman, 2005).

In summary, variables that predict help-seeking and service initiation appear to fall roughly into three categories: 1) access issues (i.e., geographical location); 2) caregiver difficulty managing the youth's problems, regardless of whether the problem is severe or the coping resources limited (i.e., symptom severity, parental burden, parental psychopathology, and single parenthood); and 3) other system contacts (i.e., child having comorbid physical illness, child having been maltreated, out-of-home placement). This last grouping in particular supports the importance of interagency coordination as well as attention to improving organizational culture toward accessing mental health treatment in related services agencies (Glisson & Green, 2006). In addition, the observed non-sequential pattern of care access suggests a need for a limited number of clear demarcation points in the mental health system, as well as single agency responsibility within a collaborative interagency framework to avoid duplication of services and coordinated care. These concepts would all be consistent with those espoused by the system of care paradigm.

Treatment Initiation and Retention:
Self-Determination vs. Paternalism

A third means in which child and adolescent help-seeking models differ from those of adults pertains to the degree to which treatment entry and retention is an autonomous choice. While clearly not all adult treatment is voluntary, the majority of adult mental health treatment lacks overt coercion (Pescosolido et al., 1998). This is not the situation with child and adolescent care (Paul, Foreman, & Kent, 2000). Although the United Nations' Convention on the Rights of the Child's statement that "parties shall assure to the child who is capable of forming his or her own views the right to express those views freely in all matters affecting the child, the views of the child being given due weight in accordance with the age and maturity of the child" (United Nations, 1989, Part I, ¶ 23), typically children and adolescents are not asked their views regarding mental health treatment or given a choice as to attendance (Aubrey & Dahl, 2006; Roose & John, 2003). This is the status quo despite studies showing youth desire and expect to have meaningful involvement in their own therapy (Davies & Wright, 2008; Paul, Berriman, & Evans, 2008; Roose & John, 2003) and studies linking youth treatment satisfaction with the youth having a choice as to the initiation of treatment (Garland, Aarons, Saltzman, & Kruse, 2000). Mental health's stance of largely ceding primacy to parental wishes and perspective (Day, 2008) is at odds with the educational system's gradual enlargement of the youth's role in special education treatment planning through greater student participation in individual educational program (IEP) meetings (Van Dycke, Martin, & Lovett, 2006) (see Chapter 17 in this volume on school mental health).

Although clinical wisdom is that failure to engage parents in therapy is often tantamount to failed therapy (Karver, Handelsman, Fields, & Bickman, 2006; Nock & Kazdin, 2001), routinely according parental concerns and goals supremacy over the child or adolescent's concerns may be equally problematic. Parental perspectives often are not concurrent with the youth's view of his or her difficulties (Logan & King, 2002; Rescorla et al., 2007; Teagle, 2002; Yeh & Weisz, 2001; Zahner & Daskalakis, 1998). Yeh and Weisz (2001) noted that only 37% of clinic-referred parent-child pairs could agree on one problem that was bringing them into treatment. Therapists tend to concur with parents' opinions regarding the presenting problem(s) more than they do with the youth's, irrespective of the offspring's age (Hawley & Weisz, 2003). Weisz and colleagues' work portrays a system whereby a younger client's perceptions and goals are not the main ones guiding treatment, even as that client ages and supposedly becomes more competent by adult standards.

Given the lack of concordance regarding *what* is being treated, it is not surprising that participants also disagree on *how* to structure treatment (Shanley et al., 2008). This is particularly concerning given that, even when controlling for other family and child risk factors, parental perception of treatment relevance is a particularly robust predictor of youth treatment retention and outcome (Garcia & Weisz, 2002; Kazdin, Holland, & Crowley, 1997; Kazdin & Wassell, 1999; Morrissey-Kane & Prinz, 1999; Nock & Kazdin, 2001). There has been speculation as to what might make parents believe the therapist is mistaken in his or her conceptualization and proposed treatment. In particular, it is thought that parents may be particularly likely to reject treatments that are at odds with their belief as to what is causing the child's difficulties (Morrissey-Kane & Prinz, 1999; Yeh et al., 2005) or treatments that awaken concerns of being blamed for their offspring's difficulties (Brown, 2008; Morrissey-Kane & Prinz, 1999; Shanley et al., 2008). Whatever the cause for why a parent feels a treatment course is erroneous, it is noteworthy that it is *parental* perception that has been shown to correlate with treatment retention. Interestingly, a study of older children and teens found that youth being in agreement with their therapist on treatment goals was not significantly related to retention, while agreement with their parents on treatment goals was (Brookman-Frazee, Haine, Gabayan, & Galand, 2008).

These data suggest that therapy for youth is often dictated by the beliefs and agenda of the non-identified client: their parents or caretakers. Parents exert a strong influence regarding whether the child or adolescent enters and stays in treatment, as well as what the treatment goals are and how they are pursued. This process is at odds with adult help-seeking models' portrayal of the client exercising choice about their treatment. This distinction between adult and youth psychotherapy is particularly interesting in light of recent efforts to draw parallels between the system of care philosophy and those of the recovery movement (Friesen, 2007; Oswald, 2006). While there is much in common, the two paradigms diverge over the concept of self-determination, with the systems of care movement strongly emphasizing family and parents' role in treatment, while the recovery movement theoretically would champion a position of increasing autonomy of the youth in treatment decisions (Friesen, 2007). Given that perceived treatment relevance is an important predictor variable for outcome with parents, one might imagine it would also be so for youth, with the lack of it likely harming youth's motivation, the therapeutic alliance, and ultimately therapy outcomes (Hawley & Weisz, 2003). Moreover, such a parent-focused system would also appear to undermine or be undermined by developmentally appropriate aspirations for greater autonomy as the youth progresses into adolescence. Although there are clearly challenges to greater inclusion of youth voices, work has already begun to improve the sparse literature on how to incorporate youth input in a developmentally informed manner (MacDonald et al., 2007; Worrall-Davies & Marino-Francis, 2008).

In contrast, while the system of care philosophy emphasizes that the service system should empower the often disenfranchised parents and families making them true partners in therapy, it has been slow to fully extend that role to the youth client (Gyamfi, Keens-Douglas, & Medin, 2007). This is exemplified in its motto that systems of care services are "youth guided" but "family driven" (Matarese, McGinnis, & Mora, 2005), with the latter term defined as "families have a primary decision-making role in the care of their own children as well as the policies and procedures governing care for all children" (Substance Abuse and Mental Health Services Administration [SAMHSA], "Working definition of family-driven care," ¶ 1).

Paradigms for Guiding Youth Mental Health Services

SYSTEMS OF CARE

As noted above, the systems of care paradigm is a multi-faceted one. Its core values are that mental health services should be comprehensive and community-based, offering a continuum of care that allows for individualized services and promotes youth being maintained in the least restrictive setting. Early intervention and inter-agency service coordination is prioritized, as is culturally competent care that is family driven and youth guided (Cook & Kilmer, 2004; Friesen, 2007; Huang et al., 2005). Systems of care philosophy became embodied by the Child and Adolescent Service System Program (CASSP) launched by the National Institute of Mental Health in 1984 and later was superseded in this role by the Substance Abuse and Mental Health Services Administration's (SAMHSA's) Comprehensive Community Mental Health Services for Children and Their Families Program (or Children's Mental Health Initiative, or CMHI) in 1992. CMHI had a budget of 102 million dollars for fiscal year 2008 and currently funds 85 grantees (SAMHSA, n.d; White House, n.d.).

Research evaluating the systems of care paradigm has found it to have positive results regarding accessing services. Systems of care sites have been associated with greater access and receipt of recommended care, wider continuum of care, and decreases in concrete barriers to access (Bickman et al., 1999; Tebes et al., 2005). CMHI programs have been shown to disproportionately enroll a greater number of poor minority youth despite a lack of mandate to do so (Miech et al., 2008). Systems of care can impact access to care, particularly among difficult to reach youth.

In contrast to its impact on systemic level variables such as access, systems of care interventions have not been shown to reliably impact youth clinical or functional outcomes when rigorous research designs are used (Cook & Kilmer, 2004; Bickman, Lambert, Andrade, & Penaloza, 2000; Bickman et al., 1999). This is despite a significantly higher cost for implementation, although some portion of the higher expenditures may reflect cost-shifting (Foster & Connor, 2005).

The systems of care approach has an impact, but one primarily manifested at the system level of service access and delivery (Hernandez & Hodges, 2003). As a paradigm, it has highlighted the need to focus on systemic forces impacting problem recognition and service use. In heralding the importance of providing a continuum of services embedded in the community to increase accessibility, it has paved the way for community-based interventions such as school-based mental health treatment (see Chapter 17 in this volume for more information on school mental health), which can provide unparalleled, if incomplete, access to youth in mental health need (Paternite, 2005). Nevertheless, the systems of care approach, despite being generously funded and extensively advanced through public policy, has not convincingly demonstrated it can impact clinical and functional variables. This indicates that the field must take additional steps to address the needs of youth with mental illness (Bickman, Noser et al., 1999; Bickman, Lambert et al., 2000). If the ultimate goal is to improve the lives of youth suffering from mental illness (Hohmann & Shear, 2002), then a systems of care approach, by itself, is inadequate.

EVIDENCE-BASED TREATMENT

Evidence-based treatments (EBTs) are interventions supported by empirical evidence. Meta-analyses indicate that youth receiving EBTs had better clinical and functional levels when compared to those receiving typical community-based care, with one recent meta-analysis showing that the average EBT youth had better outcomes than 62% of the youth who had not received EBTs (Weisz, Jensen-Doss, & Hawley, 2006). In addition, other reviews indicate the superiority of EBTs to controls in a variety of specific domains (Barrett, Farrell, Pina, Peris, & Piacentini, 2008; Curtis, Ronan, & Borduin, 2004; David-Ferdon & Kaslow, 2008; Eyberg, Nelson, & Boggs, 2008; Huey & Polo, 2008; Rogers & Vismara, 2008; Silverman, Ortiz et al., 2008; Silverman, Pina, & Viswesvaran, 2008; Waldron & Turner, 2008; Watanabe, Hunot, Omori, Churchill, & Furukawa, 2007; Weisz, McCarty, & Valeri, 2006). To improve dissemination of such treatments, lists of EBTs are available in journal articles (Barrett et al., 2008; David-Ferdon & Kaslow, 2008; Eyberg et al., 2008; Herschell, McNeil, & McNeil, 2004; Rogers & Vismara, 2008; Silverman, Pina et al., 2008; Silverman, Ortiz et al., 2008; Waldron & Turner, 2008) and via organizational websites, such as the American Psychological Association Division 53 website http://sccap.tamu.edu/EST/ or the NAMI's family guide http://www.nami.org/Content/Microsites186/NAMI_Maine/Home174/ FAMILY_Newsletter-_Winter_2006/ChoosingRightTreatment1.pdf.

A somewhat different approach has been taken with SAMHSA's National Registry of Evidence-Based Programs and Practices (NREPP) in its eschewal of categories. Instead, NREPP provides extensive descriptive information with associated ratings on various elements related to the internal and external validity of interventions (http://www.nrepp.samhsa.gov). Whatever its source, it is difficult to argue against employing treatments that have been vetted as being treatments that work. However, the issue is more complex upon further investigation.

An initial problem with EBT is the vetting process. There are a plethora of definitions as to what constitutes "supported by empirical evidence" (Hoagwood, Burns, Kiser, Ringeisen, & Schoenwald, 2001; Weisz, Sandler, Durlak, & Anton, 2005). Variations regarding that definition as well as differences in research methodology and analytic approaches can result in different conclusions (Weisz, McCarty et al., 2006). This is apparent in recent summaries of EBTs for youth depression, which vary in their conclusions as to whether EBTs for depression are superior to active control groups and indicate markedly different effect sizes ranging from 0.34 to 1.27 (Watanabe et al., 2007; Weisz, McCarty et al., 2006).

Related to this notion are problems with the quality of the evidence-based research (Kazdin, 2008; Westen et al., 2004). In a review of the child and adolescent treatment literature between 1963 and 2003, Weisz et al. noted that only a quarter of the studies used DSM or ICD criteria to define their sample, only 13% of the studies employed clinically referred or treatment-seeking youth, the most common control comparison employed was a waitlist or no treatment group, and in only 4% of the studies was treatment provided in a clinical service setting (Weisz, Doss, & Hawley, 2005).

Focusing on the representativeness of the sample, it has been argued that EBTs have been developed and tested on youth with less severe psychopathology and fewer comorbid disorders, and therefore do not reflect "real world" cases (Weisz, Jensen-Doss, & Hawley, 2006). In fact, there are data supporting the notion that compared to university clinic samples, community clinic youth show greater comorbidity and are more likely to come from lower income and single-parent homes (Southam-Gerow, Weisz, & Kendall, 2003). While there is some evidence that comorbidity may not play a significant role in treatment outcome (Doss & Weisz, 2006), given the pivotal role familial and contextual variables have in determining service use, differences in terms of income and family structure are far from inconsequential to outcome (Southam-Gerow, Chorpita, Miller, & Gleacher, 2008). Variability in these contextual factors may partly explain the tendency for community-based effectiveness studies to show diminished outcomes compared to university-based efficacy studies (Curtis et al., 2004; Weisz, Donenberg, Han, & Weiss, 1995). Minimally, this reflects the need for the field to better understand what works when and for whom (Weisz, Sandler et al., 2005).

Even if a definition of what merits the term "evidence-based" could be agreed upon, many diagnoses and problems do not have established evidence-based treatments (Hoagwood et al., 2007; Schiffman, Becker, & Daleiden, 2006; Weisz, Doss et al., 2005). In fact, in a recent meta-analysis purporting to assess evidence-based youth psychotherapy as compared to usual care, less than 10% of the studies reviewed involved internalizing disorders (Weisz, Jensen-Doss et al., 2006). This suggests that although EBTs have potential benefit, it is still very much an emerging field.

Finally, difficulties with dissemination have also plagued EBTs. EBTs are not widely used in everyday clinical practice (Sheehan, Walrath, & Holden, 2007). Clinicians have complained that the often manualized EBTs impede rapport and alliance, stifle the therapist's creativity, and limit the clinician to applying a "one size fits all" treatment plan (Palinkas et al., 2008; Weisz, Jensen-Doss et al., 2006). Moreover, practitioners have leveled charges that EBTs have been designed with little eye to employing them in everyday practice, where a myriad of organizational and practical factors may impact their feasibility (Aarons & Palinkas, 2007; Weisz, Sandler et al., 2005). Some clinicians report feeling coerced to employ certain EBTs, either directly or through financing mechanisms, a state of affairs hardly to make practitioners embrace EBTs (Rieckmann, Kovas, Fussell, & Stettler, 2008; Wagner, Munt, & Briner, 2006).

In an attempt to address these latter issues, the EBT field has recently engaged in several efforts to increase the "real world" appeal of their interventions. These include Weisz and colleagues' deployment-focused model (Weisz, Jensen, & McLeod, 2005); the MacArthur Foundation Child System and Treatment

Enhancement Projects (Child STEPs) (Schoenwald, Kelleher, Weisz, & the Research Network on Youth Mental Health, 2008); the Availability, Responsiveness, and Continuity (ARC) Model (Glisson & Schoenwald, 2005); and Identifying Common Elements of Evidence-Based Interventions Model (Chorpita, Daleiden, & Weisz, 2005; Garland, Hawley, Brookman-Frazee, & Hurlburt, 2008; Karver, Handelsman, Fields, & Bickman, 2005; Karver et al., 2006). This movement has led Kazdin to argue for a new term of *evidence-based practices* which, in contrast to EBT, is defined more broadly as "clinical practice that is informed by evidence about interventions, clinical expertise, and patient needs, values, and preferences and their integration in making decisions about individual care" (Kazdin, 2008, p. 147). These changes appear to reflect a shift away from a unidirectional "science to services" model and toward a transactional model where science and services are mutually informative, as well as an acknowledgment that unless barriers to employing and accessing EBTs are overcome they are of little use despite their efficacy.

Policy Issues

As the above discussion suggests, all models, regardless of their philosophical origins, must be attentive to influences that impact their use in everyday clinical practice. Among these influences are several key policy issues—such as financing, workforce development, and the delivery of culturally appropriate care—that possess the ability to affect youth mental health care irrespective of service delivery paradigm.

With respect to financing, very few states report consistent support and funding for the mental health needs of children and adolescents across the age-span (Cooper, Aratani, Knitzer, et al., 2008). Moreover, reimbursement of effective case management and other coordinating services among mental health professionals has been identified as a critical financing issue (American Academy of Child and Adolescent Psychiatry Task Force on Mental Health, 2009). Concerning workforce development, acute shortages of both child and adolescent psychiatrists, and school-based mental health professionals are projected over the next decade (see Chapter 5 in this volume on workforce development). In addition, the lack of mental health competencies among providers in other environments responsible to the identification and treatment of mental health problems in youth (e.g., child welfare, child care, education, juvenile justice), the mismatch between training and typical practice settings, and the need to re-invigorate clinical training programs to promote resilience and strength-based concepts and intervention approaches are all identified as significant workforce development challenges (Annapolis Coalition, 2007). Regarding the delivery of culturally appropriate care, only three states have reported taking purposeful steps toward promoting such policies through competency-based training, workforce development infrastructure support, ongoing assessment and strategic planning, and stakeholder involvement (Cooper, Aratani, Knitzer et al., 2008). Given the scope of the identified challenges, efforts to address these policy issues will be essential to advancing any successful model of child and adolescent mental health service delivery.

Developmental Psychopathology: Implications for Mental Health

There are several planks that compose the foundation of the developmental psychopathology paradigm. Specifically, developmental psychopathology maintains that knowledge of normal development informs our understanding of abnormal processes (and vice versa). The model is a fluid one, emphasizing that no one variable determines outcome, but rather that one's development is influenced by a complex interplay among forces within and outside the individual (Masten, 2006). As such, it is actually a highly inclusive and hopeful paradigm.

Developmental psychopathology has been a successful overarching paradigm for conceptualizing child and adolescent psychopathology. It has the potential to serve a similar function for child and adolescent mental health services. A developmental psychopathology perspective would maintain that a child's outcome or course could be affected by intervention at multiple levels. Hence, it can accommodate the systems of care framework, which impacts the system-level variables of service referral, entry, use, and retention. It can be stretched to include a variety of other system level interventions such as those designed to reduce stigma among youth with mental health problems (Martin, Pescosolido, Olafsdottir, & McLeod, 2007; Pescosolido, Perry, Martin, McLeod, & Jensen, 2007; Pitre, Stewart, Adams, Bedard, & Landry, 2007; Spagnolo, Murphy, & Librera, 2008), increase the number of qualified service providers and offered services (Kalet et al., 2007; Kim & American Academy of Child and Adolescent Psychiatry Task Force on Workforce Needs, 2003; Knapp, Ammen, Arstein-Kerslake, Poulsen, & Mastergeorge, 2007; WHO, 2005), and create stable financing on par with that of adults (e.g., State Children's Health Insurance Program [S-CHIP], mental health parity).

At the same time, the developmental psychopathology framework is equally accommodating to paradigms, like evidence-based treatments, that exert their greatest impact on individual outcome variables such as functionality and symptom reduction. From the developmental psychopathology perspective, these varied interventions each represent legitimate, albeit different, levels of influence on the individual. Hence, in providing a broad framework, developmental psychopathology would allow the field to avoid the misleading notion of needing to elevate one paradigm over another.

It is important to note what a developmental psychopathology paradigm brings to the youth services picture in addition to its inclusive stance. First, by always conceptualizing abnormal in reference to normal development, it implicitly enlarges the focus from symptom reduction (tertiary care) to the broader goal of facilitating positive development (primary prevention). Without such a reminder of the importance of primary prevention, the services field is apt to neglect it (Ripple & Zigler, 2003; Waddell, McEwan, Peters, Hua, & Garland, 2007).

Second, with its elevation of the developmental principle, developmental psychopathology continually emphasizes what is unique about mental illness in children and adolescents. As articulated above, this reflects a basic reality. Children's mental health services *are* different than those of adults. They are structured and funded differently. They are more systemic, unordered, and paternalistic. Equally important is the fact that, in some fundamental ways, they *need* to be different from adult services. Analyses suggest that the majority of treatment interventions still are best characterized as downward adaptations of interventions designed for adults, with relatively little integration of salient developmental issues (Weisz & Hawley, 2002). As of 2002, only 7% of countries worldwide had a clearly articulated child and adolescent mental health policy and less than a third of nations have an institution or government agency responsible for children's mental health programming (WHO, 2005). If we hope to improve the lot of youth with mental health issues, we need to realize their unique needs, remove the largely contextual barriers to problem identification and service use, and, fundamentally, treat them as children and adolescents, not as little adults.

References

Aarons, G. A., & Palinkas, L. A. (2007). Implementation of evidence-based practice in child welfare: Service provider perspectives. *Administration and Policy in Mental Health and Mental Health Services Research, 34*, 411–419.

Achenbach, T. M. (1978). Psychopathology of childhood: Research problems and issues. *Journal of Consulting and Clinical Psychology, 46*, 759–776.

Alegria, M., Canino, G., Lai, S., Ramirez, F. F., Chavez, L., Rusch, D., et al. (2004). Understanding caregivers' help-seeking for Latino children's mental health care use. *Medical Care, 42*, 447–455.

American Academy of Child and Adolescent Psychiatry Task Force on Mental Health. (2009). Improving mental health services in primary care: Reducing administrative and financial barriers to access and collaboration. *Pediatrics, 123*, 1248–1251.

Andersen, R. M. (1995). Revisiting the behavioral model and access to medical care: Does it matter? *Journal of Health and Social Behavior, 36*, 1–10.

Andersen, R., & Newman, J. (1973). Societal and individual determinants of medical care utilization in the United States. *Millbank Memorial Fund Quarterly, 51*, 95–124.

Angold, A., Messer, S. C., Stangl, D., Farmer, E. M. Z., Costello, E. J., & Burns, B. J. (1998). Perceived parental burden and service use for child and adolescents psychiatric disorders. *American Journal of Public Health, 88*, 75–80.

Annapolis Coalition (2007). *An Action Plan for Behavioral Health Workforce Development.* Available online at www.annapoliscoalition.org/pages/. Accessed April 20, 2009.

Aubrey, C., & Dahl, S. (2006). Children's voices: The views of vulnerable children on their service providers and the relevance of services they receive. *British Journal of Social Work, 36*, 21–39.

Barrett, P. M., Farrell, L., Pina, A. A., Peris, T. S., & Piacentini, J. (2008). Evidence-based psychosocial treatments for child and adolescents obsessive-compulsive disorder. *Journal of Clinical Child & Adolescent Psychology, 37*, 131–155.

Barry, C. L., & Busch, S. H. (2007). Do state parity laws reduce the financial burden on families of children with mental health care needs? *Health Research and Educational Trust, 42*, 1061–1084.

Becker, M. H., & Maiman, L. A. (1975). Sociobehavioral determinants of compliance with health and medical care recommendations. *Medical Care, 8*, 10–24.

Belfer, M. L. (2008). Child and adolescent mental disorders: The magnitude of the problem across the globe. *Journal of Child Psychology and Psychiatry, 49*, 226–236.

Bickman, L., Lambert, E. W., Andrade, A. R., & Penaloza, R. V. (2000). The Fort Bragg continuum of care for children and adolescents: Mental health outcomes over 5 years. *Journal of Consulting and Clinical Psychology, 68*, 710–716.

Bickman, L., Noser, K., & Summerfelt, W. T. (1999). Long-term effects of a system of care on children and adolescents. *Journal of Behavioral Health Services & Research, 26*, 185–202.

Bird, H. R., Canino, G., Rubio-Stipec, M., Gould, M. S., Ribera, J., Sesman, M., et al. (1988). Estimates of the prevalence of childhood maladjustment in a community survey in Puerto Rico. *Archives of General Psychiatry, 45*, 1120–1126.

Bradshaw, C. P., Buckley, J. A., & Ialongo, N. S. (2008). School-based service utilization among urban children with early onset educational and mental health problems: The squeaky wheel phenomenon. *School Psychology Quarterly, 23*, 169–186.

Brannan, A. M., & Heflinger, C. A. (2005). Child behavioral health service use and caregiver strain: Comparison of managed care and fee-for-service Medicaid systems. *Mental Health Services Research, 7*, 197–211.

Brookman-Frazee, L., Haine, R. A., Gabayan, E. N., & Garland, A. F. (2008). Predicting frequency of treatment visits in community-based youth psychotherapy. *Psychological Services, 5*, 126–138.

Brown, J. (2008). We don't need your help, but will you please fix our children. *Australian and New Zealand Journal of Family Therapy, 29*, 61–69.

Brown, J. D., Riley, A. W., & Wissow, L. S. (2007). Identification of youth psychosocial problems during pediatric primary care visits. *Administration and Policy in Mental Health and Mental Health Services Research, 34*, 269–281.

Bussing, R., Zima, B. T., Gary, F. A., & Garvan, C. W. (2003). Barriers to detection in help-seeking and service use for children with ADHD symptoms. *Journal of Behavioral Health Services & Research, 30*, 176–189.

Cabiya, J. J., Canino, G., Chavez, L., Ramirez, L. R., Alegria, M., Shrout, P., et al. (2006). Gender disparities in mental health service use of Puerto Rican children and adolescents. *Journal of Child Psychology and Psychiatry, 47*, 840–848.

Canino, G., Shrout, P. E., Rubio-Stipec, M., Bird, H. R., Bravo, M., Ramirez, R., et al. (2004). The DSM-IV rates of child and adolescents disorders in Puerto Rico. *Archives of General Psychiatry, 61*, 85–93.

Case, B. G., Olfson, M., Marcus, S. C., & Siegel, C. (2007). Trends in the inpatient mental health treatment of children and adolescents in US community hospitals between 1990 and 2000. *Archives of General Psychiatry, 64*, 89–96.

Cauce, A. M., Domenech-Rodriguez, M., Paradise, M., Cochran, B. N., Shea, J. M., Sebrnik, D., et al. (2002). Cultural and contextual influences in mental health help seeking: A focus on ethnic minority youth. *Journal of Consulting and Clinical Psychology, 70*, 44–55.

Chang, K. (2007). Adult bipolar disorder is continuous with pediatric bipolar disorder. *Canadian Journal of Psychiatry, 52*, 418–424.

Chorpita, B. F., Daleiden, E. L., & Weisz, J. R. (2005). Identifying and selecting the common elements of evidence based interventions: A distillation and matching model. *Mental Health Services and Research, 7*, 5–20.

Cicchetti, D. (1984). The emergence of developmental psychopathology. *Child Development, 55*, 1–7.

Cohen, P., Kasen, S., Brook, J. S., & Struening, E. L. (1991). Diagnostic predictors of treatment patterns in a cohort of adolescents. *Journal of the American Academy of Child and Adolescent Psychiatry, 30*, 989–993.

Cook, J. R., & Kilmer, R. P. (2004). Evaluating systems of care: Missing links in children's mental health research. *Journal of Community Psychology, 32*, 655–674.

Cooper, J. L., Aratani, Y., Knitzer, J., Douglas-Hall, A., Masi, R., Banghart, P., et al. (2008). *Unclaimed Children Revisited: The Status of Children's Mental Health Policy in the United States.* New York: National Center for Children in Poverty.

Cornelius, J. R., Pringle, J., Jernigan, J., Kirisci, L., & Clark, D. B. (2001). Correlates of mental health service utilization and unmet need among a sample of male adolescents. *Addictive Behaviors, 26*, 11–19.

Costello, E. J., Angold, A., Burns, B. J., Erkanli, A., Stangl, D. K., & Tweed, D. L. (1996). The Great Smoky Mountain study of youth: Functional impairment and serious emotional disturbance. *Archives of General Psychiatry, 53*, 1137–1143.

Costello, E. J., Angold, A., Burns, B. J., Stangl, D. K., Tweek, D. L., Erkanli, A., et al. (1996). The Great Smoky Mountain study of youth: Goals, designs, methods, and the prevalence of *DSM-III-R* disorders. *Archives of General Psychiatry, 53*, 1129–1136.

Costello, E. J., Egger, H., & Angold, A. (2005). 10-year research update review: The epidemiology of child and adolescent psychiatric disorders: I, Methods and public health burden. *Journal of the American Academy of Child and Adolescent Psychiatry, 44*, 972–986.

Costello, E. J., Mustillo, S., Keeler, G., & Angold, A. (2004). Prevalence of psychiatric disorders in childhood and adolescence. In B. L. Levin, J. Petrila, & K. Hennessy (Eds.), *Mental Health Services: A Public Health Perspective* (2nd ed., pp. 111–128). New York: Oxford University Press.

Crider, R. A., Milazzo-Sayre, L. J., Foley, D. J., Manderscheid, R. W., Blacklow, B. G., & Male, A. A. (2006). Sources of referral for persons admitted to specialty mental health organizations, United States, 1997. In R. W. Manderscheid & J. T. Berry (Eds.), *Mental Health, United States, 2004* (pp. 237–246). DHHS Publication No. (SMA) -06-4195. Rockville, MD: Substance Abuse and Mental Health Services Administration.

Curtis, N. M., Ronan, K. R., & Borduin, C. M. (2004). Multisystemic treatment: A meta-analysis of outcome studies. *Journal of Family Psychology, 18*, 411–419.

David-Ferdon, C., & Kaslow, N. J. (2008). Evidence-based psychosocial treatment for child and adolescent depression. *Journal of Clinical Child & Adolescent Psychology, 37*, 62–104.

Davies, J., & Wright, J. (2008). Children's voices: A review of the literature pertinent to looked-after children's views of mental health services. *Child and Adolescent Mental Health, 13*, 26–31.

Day, C. (2008). Children's and young people's involvement and participation in mental health care. *Child and Adolescent Mental Health, 13*, 2–8.

Doss, A. J., & Weisz, J. R. (2006). Syndrome co-occurrence and treatment outcomes in youth mental health clinics. *Journal of Consulting and Clinical Psychology, 74*, 416–425.

Eapen, V., Jakka, M. E., & Abou-Saleh, M. T. (2003). Children with psychiatric disorders: The Al Ain community psychiatric survey. *Canadian Journal of Psychiatry, 48*, 402–407.

Eiraldi, R. B., Mazzuca, L. B., Clarke, A. T., & Power, T. J. (2006). Service utilization among ethnic minority children with ADHD: A model of help-seeking behavior. *Administration & Policy in Mental Health & Mental Health Service Research, 33*, 607–622.

Eyberg, S. M., Nelson, M. M., & Boggs, S. R. (2008). Evidence-based psychosocial treatments for children and adolescents with disruptive behavior. *Journal of Clinical Child & Adolescent Psychology, 37*, 215–237.

Farmer, E. M. Z., Burns, B. J., Phillips, S. D., Angold, A., & Costello, E. J. (2003). Pathways into and through mental health services for children and adolescents. *Psychiatric Services, 54*, 60–66.

Flisher, A. J., Kramer, R. A., Grosser, R. C., Alegria, M., Bird, H. R., Bourdon, K. H., et al. (1997). Correlates of unmet need for mental health service by children and adolescents. *Psychological Medicine, 27*, 1145–1154.

Ford, T. (2008). Practitioner review: How can epidemiology help us plan and deliver effective child and adolescent mental health services? *Journal of Child Psychology and Psychiatry, 49*, 900–914.

Ford, T., Hamilton, H., Meltzer, H., & Goodman, R. (2008). Predictors of service use for mental health problems among British schoolchildren. *Child and Adolescent Mental Health, 13*, 32–40.

Foster, E. M., & Connor, T. (2005). Public costs of better mental health services for children and adolescents. *Psychiatric Services, 56*, 50–55.

Friesen, B. J. (2007). Recovery and resilience in children's mental health: Views from the field. *Psychiatric Rehabilitation Journal, 31*, 38–48.

Garcia, J. A., & Weisz, J. R. (2002). When youth mental health care stops: Therapeutic relationship problems and other reasons for ending youth outpatient care. *Journal of Consulting and Clinical Psychology, 70*, 439–443.

Garland, A. F., Aarons, G. A., Saltzman, M. D., & Kruse, M. I. (2000). Correlates of adolescents' satisfaction with mental health services. *Mental Health Services Research, 2*, 127–139.

Garland, A. F., Hawley, K. M., Brookman-Frazee, L., & Hurlburt, M. S. (2008). Identifying common elements of evidence-based psychosocial treatments for children's disruptive behavior problems. *Journal of the American Academy of Child and Adolescent Psychiatry, 47*, 505–514.

Garland, A. F., Landsverk, J. L., Hough, R. L., & Ellis-Macleod, E. (1996). Type of maltreatment as a predictor of mental health service use for children in foster care. *Child Abuse and Neglect, 20*, 675–688.

Glied, S., & Cuellar, A. E. (2003). Trends and issues in child and adolescent mental health. *Health Affairs, 22*, 39–50.

Glisson, C., & Green, P. (2006). The effects of organizational culture and climate on the access to mental health care in child welfare and juvenile justice systems. *Administration and Policy in Mental Health and Mental Health Services Research, 33*, 433–448.

Glisson, C., & Schoenwald, S. K. (2005). The ARC organizational and community intervention strategy for implementing evidence-based children's mental health treatment. *Mental Health Services Research, 7*, 243–259.

Gyamfi, P., Keens-Douglas, A., & Medin, E. (2007). Youth and youth coordinators' perspectives on youth involvement in systems of care. *Journal of Behavioral Health Services & Research, 34*, 382–394.

Harpaz-Rotem, I., Leslie, D., & Rosenheck, R. A. (2004). Treatment retention among children entering a new episode of mental health care. *Psychiatric Services, 55*, 1022–1028.

Hawley, K. M., & Weisz, J. R. (2003). Child, parent, and therapist (dis)agreement on target problems in outpatient therapy: The therapist's dilemma and its implications. *Journal of Consulting and Clinical Psychology, 71*, 62–70.

Heiervang, E., Goodman, A., & Goodman, R. (2008). The Nordic advantage in child mental health: Separating health differences from reporting style in a cross-cultural comparison of psychopathology. *Journal of Child Psychology and Psychiatry, 49*, 678–685.

Hernandez, M., & Hodges, S. (2003). Building upon the theory of change for systems of care. *Journal of Emotional and Behavioral Disorders, 11*, 19–26.

Herschell, A. D., McNeil, C. B., & McNeil, D. W. (2004). Clinical child psychology's progress in disseminating empirically supported treatments. *Clinical Psychology: Science and Practice, 11*, 267–288.

Hoagwood, K., Burns, B. J., Kiser, L., Ringeisen, H., & Schoenwald, S. K. (2001). Evidence-based practice in child and adolescent mental health. *Psychiatric Services, 52*, 1179–1189.

Hoagwood, K. E., Olin, S., Kerker, B. D., Kratochwill, T. R., Crowe, M., & Saka, N. (2007). Empirically based school interventions targeted at academic and mental health functioning. *Journal of Emotional and Behavioral Disorders, 15*, 66–92.

Hohmann, A. A., & Shear, M. K. (2002). Community-based intervention research: Coping with the "noise" of real life in study design. *American Journal of Psychiatry, 159*, 201–207.

Holden, W. E., & Blau, G. M. (2006). An expanded perspective on children's mental health. *American Psychologist, 61*, 642–644.

Huang, L., Stroul, B., Friedman, R., Mrazek, P., Friesen, B., Pires, S., et al. (2005). Transforming mental health care for children and their families. *American Psychologist, 60*, 615–627.

Huey, S. J., & Polo, A. J. (2008). Evidence-based psychosocial treatments for ethnic minority youth. *Journal of Clinical Child & Adolescent Psychology, 37*, 262–301.

Hurlburt, M. S., Leslie, L. K., Landsverk, J., Barth, R. P., Burns, B. J., Gibbons, R. D., et al. (2008). Contextual predictors of mental health service use among children open to child welfare. *Archives of General Psychiatry, 61*, 1217–1224.

Kalet, A. L., Juszczak, L., Pastore, D., Fierman, A. H., Soren, K., Cohall, A., et al. (2007). Medical training in school-based health centers: A collaboration among five medical schools. *Academic Medicine, 82*, 458–464.

Karver, M. S., Handelsman, J. B., Fields, S., & Bickman, L. (2005). A theoretical model of common process factors in youth and family therapy. *Mental Health Services and Research, 7*, 35–51.

Karver, M. S., Handelsman, J. B., Fields, S., & Bickman, L. (2006). Meta-analysis of therapeutic relationship variables in youth and family therapy: The evidence for different relationship variables in the child and adolescent treatment outcome literature. *Clinical Psychology Review, 26,* 50–65.

Kataoka, S. H., Zhang, L., & Wells, K. B. (2002). Unmet need for mental health care among U.S. children: Variation by ethnicity and insurance status. *American Journal of Psychiatry, 159,* 1548–1555.

Kazdin, A. E. (2008). Evidence-based treatment and practice: New opportunities to bridge clinical research and practice, enhance the knowledge base, and improve patient care. *American Psychologist, 63,* 146–159.

Kazdin, A. E., Holland, L., & Crowley, M. (1997). Family experience of barriers to treatment and premature termination from child therapy. *Journal of Consulting and Clinical Psychology, 65,* 453–463.

Kazdin, A. E., & Wassel, G. (1999). Barriers to treatment participation and therapeutic change among children referred for conduct disorder. *Journal of Clinical Child Psychology, 28,* 160–172.

Kessler, R. C., Amminger, G. P., Aguilar-Gaxiola, S., Alonso, J., Lee, S., & Ustun, T. B. (2007). Age of onset of mental disorders: A review of recent literature. *Current Opinion in Psychiatry, 20,* 359–364.

Kessler, R. C., Berglund, P., Demler, O., Jin, R., Merikangas, K. R., & Walters, E. E. (2005). Lifetime prevalence and age-of-onset distributions of *DSM-IV* disorders in the national comorbidity survey replication. *Archives of General Psychiatry, 62,* 593–602.

Kim, W. J., & American Academy of Child, Adolescent Psychiatry Task Force on Workforce Needs. (2003). Child and adolescent psychiatry workforce: A critical shortage and national challenge. *Academic Psychiatry, 27,* 277–282.

Knapp, P. K., Ammen, S., Arstein-Kerslake, C., Poulsen, M. K., & Mastergeorge, A. (2007). Feasibility of expanding services for very young children in the public mental health setting. *Journal of the American Academy of Child and Adolescent Psychiatry, 46,* 152–161.

Kohn, A. (1993). Choices for children: Why and how to let students decide. *Phi Delta Kappan, 75,* 8–19.

Koller, J. P., & Bertel, J. M. (2006). Responding to today's mental health needs of children, families and schools: Revisiting the preservice training and preparation of school-based personnel. *Education and Treatment of Children, 29,* 197–217.

Leslie, L. K., Hurlburt, M. S., James, S., Landsverk, J., Slymen, D. J., & Zhang, J. (2005). Relationship between entry into child welfare and mental health service use. *Psychiatric Services, 56,* 981–987.

Levav, I., Jacobsson, L., Tsiantis, J., Kolaitis, G., & Ponizovsky, A. (2004). Psychiatric services and training for children and adolescents in Europe: Results of a country survey. *European Child and Adolescent Psychiatry, 13,* 395–401.

Logan, D. E., & King, C. A. (2001). Parental facilitation of adolescent mental health service utilization: A conceptual and empirical review. *Clinical Psychology: Science and Practice, 8,* 319–333.

Logan, D. E., & King, C. A. (2002). Parental identification of depression and mental health service use among depressed adolescents. *Journal of the American Academy of Child and Adolescent Psychiatry, 41,* 296–304.

MacDonald, E., Lee, E., Geraghty, K., McCann, K., Mohay, H., & O'Brien, T. (2007). Towards a developmental framework of consumer and carer participation in child and adolescent mental health services. *Australiasian Psychiatry, 15,* 504–508.

Mark, T. L., Harwood, H. J., McKusick, D. C., King, E. C., Vandivort-Warren, R., & Buck, J. A. (2008). Mental health and substance abuse spending by age, 2003. *Journal of Behavioral Health Services & Research, 35,* 279–289.

Martin, A., & Leslie, D. (2003). Psychiatric inpatient, outpatient, and medication utilization and costs among privately insured youths, 1997–2000. *American Journal of Psychiatry, 160,* 757–764.

Martin, J. K., Pescosolido, B. A., Olafsdottir, S., & McLeod, J. D. (2007). The construction of fear: Americans preferences for social distance from children and adolescents with mental health problems. *Journal of Health and Social Behavior*, *48*, 50–67.

Masten, A. S. (2006). Developmental psychopathology: Pathways to the future. *International Journal of Behavioral Pediatrics*, *30*, 47–54.

Matarese, M., McGinnis, L., & Mora, M. (2005). *Youth involvement in systems of care: A guide to empowerment*. Available online at http://www.systemsofcare.samhsa.gov/headermenus/docsHM/youthguidedlink.pdf. Accessed August 22, 2008.

McDonnell, M. A., & Glod, C. (2003). Prevalence of psychopathology in preschool-age children. *Journal of Child and Adolescent Psychiatric Nursing*, *16*, 141–152.

Miech, R., Azur, M., Dusablon, T., Jowers, K., Goldstein, A. B., Stuart, E. A., et al., (2008). The potential to reduce mental health disparities through The Comprehensive Community Mental Health Services for Children and Their Families Program. *Journal of Behavioral Health Services & Research*, *35*, 253–264.

Moor, S., Maguire, A., McQueen, H., Wells, E. J., Elton, R., Wrate, R., et al. (2007). Improving the recognition of depression in adolescence: Can we teach the teachers? *Journal of Adolescence*, *30*, 81–95.

Morrissey-Kane, E., & Prinz, R. J. (1999). Engagement in child and adolescent treatment: The role of parental cognition and attributions. *Clinical Child and Family Psychology Review*, *2*, 183–198.

Nock, M. K., & Kazdin, A. E. (2001). Parent expectancies for child therapy: Assessment and relation to participation in treatment. *Journal of Child and Family Studies*, *10*, 155–180.

Oswald, D. P. (2006). Recovery and children's mental health services. *Journal of Child and Family Studies*, *15*, 525–527.

Palinkas, L. A., Schoenwald, S. K., Hoagwood, K., Landsverk, J., Chorpita, B. F., Weisz, J. R., et al. (2008). An ethnographic study of implementation of evidence-based treatment in child mental health: First steps. *Psychiatric Services*, *59*, 738–746.

Paternite, C. E. (2005). School-based mental health programs and services: Overview and introduction to the special issue. *Journal of Abnormal Child Psychology*, *33*, 657–663.

Paul, M., Berriman, J. A., & Evans, J. (2008). Would I attend child and adolescent mental health services (CAMHS)? Fourteen to sixteen year olds decide. *Child and Adolescent Mental Health*, *13*, 19–25.

Paul, M., Foreman, D. M., & Kent, L. (2000). Out-patient clinic attendance consent from children and young people: Ethical aspects and practical considerations. *Clinical Child Psychology and Psychiatry*, *5*, 203–211.

Pavuluri, M. N., Luk, S. L., & McGee, R. (1996). Help-seeking for behavior problems by parents of preschool children: A community study. *Journal of the American Academy of Child and Adolescent Psychiatry*, *35*, 215–222.

Pescosolido, B. A., Gardner, C. B., & Lubell, K. M. (1998). How people get into mental health services: Stories of choice, coercion, and "muddling through" from "first-timers." *Social Science Medicine*, *46*, 275–286.

Pescosolido, B. A., Jensen, P. S., Martin, J. K., Perry, B. L., Olafsdottir, S., & Fettes, D. (2008). Public knowledge and assessment of child mental health problems: Findings from the national stigma study-child. *Journal of the American Academy of Child and Adolescent Psychiatry*, *47*, 339–349.

Pescosolido, B. A., Perry, B. L., Martin, J. K., McLeod, J. D., & Jensen, P. S. (2007). Stigmatizing attitudes and beliefs about treatment and psychiatric medications for children with mental illness. *Psychiatric Services*, *58*, 613–618.

Pitre, N., Stewart, S., Adams, S., Bedard, T., & Landry, S. (2007). The use of puppets with elementary school children in reducing stigmatizing attitudes towards mental illness. *Journal of Mental Health*, *16*, 415–429.

Pottick, K. L., Warner, L. A., Issacs, M., Henderson, M. J., Milazzo-Sayre, L., & Manderscheid, R. W. (2004). Children and adolescents admitted to specialty mental health care programs in the United States, 1986 and 1997. In R. W. Manderscheid & M. J. Henderson (Eds.), *Mental Health, United States, 2002* (pp. 314–326). DHHS Publication No. (SMA) 3938. Rockville, MD: Substance Abuse and Mental Health Services Administration.

Prochaska, J. O., & Di Clemente, C. C. (1982). Transtheoretical therapy: Toward a more integrative model of change. *Psychotherapy: Theory, Research, and Practice, 19*, 276–288.

Raviv, A., Sills, R., Raviv, A., & Wilansky, P. (2000). Adolescents' help-seeking behaviour: The difference between self- and other-referral. *Journal of Adolescence, 23*, 721–740.

Rieckmann, T. R., Kovas, A. E., Fussell, H. E., & Stettler, N. M. (2008). Implementation of evidence-based practice for treatment of alcohol and drug disorders: The role of the state authority. *Journal of Behavioral Health Services & Research, 36*, 407–419.

Reid, G. J., Tobon, J. I., & Shanley, D. C. (2008). What is a mental health clinic? How to ask parents about help-seeking contacts within the mental health system. *Administration and Policy in Mental Health, 35*, 241–249.

Rescorla, L., Achenbach, T. M., Ivanova, M. Y., Dumenci, L., Almqvist, F., Bilenberg, N., et al. (2007). Epidemiological comparisons of problem and positive qualities reported by adolescents in 24 countries. *Journal of Consulting and Clinical Psychology, 75*, 351–358.

Rickwood, D. J., & Braithwaite, V. A. (1994). Social-psychological factors affecting help- seeking for emotional problems. *Social Science & Medicine, 39*, 563–572.

Ripple, C. H., & Zigler, E. (2003). Research, policy, and the federal role in prevention initiatives for children. *American Psychologist, 58*, 482–490.

Roberts, R. E., Alegria, M., Roberts, C. R., & Chen, I. G. (2005). Mental health problems of adolescents as reported by their caregivers. *Journal of Behavioral Health Services & Research, 32*, 1–13.

Rogers, S. J., & Vismara, L. A. (2008). Evidence-based comprehensive treatments for early autism. *Journal of Clinical Child & Adolescent Psychology, 37*, 8–38.

Romano, E., Tremblay, R. E., Vitaro, F., Zoccolillo, M., & Pagani, L. (2001). Prevalence of psychiatry diagnoses and the role of perceived impairment: Findings from an adolescent community sample. *Journal of Child Psychology and Psychiatry, 42*, 451–461.

Roose, G. A., & John, A. M. (2003). A focus group investigation into young children's understanding of mental health and their view on appropriate services for their age group. *Child: Care, Health, & Development, 29*, 545–550.

Rothi, D. M., Leavey, G., & Best, R. (2008). On the front-line: Teachers as active observers of pupils' mental health. *Teaching and Teacher Education, 24*, 1217–1231.

Sawyer, M. G., Arney, F. M., Baghurst, P. A., Clark, J. J., Graetz, B. W., Kosky, R. J., et al. (2001). The mental health of young people in Australia: Key findings from the child and adolescent component of the national survey of mental health and well-being. *Australia & New Zealand Journal of Psychiatry, 35*, 806–814.

Sayal, K. (2006). Annotation: Pathways to care for children with mental health problems. *Journal of Child Psychology and Psychiatry, 47*, 649–659.

Sayal, K., Hornsey, H., Warren, S., MacDiarmid, F., & Taylor, E. (2006). Identification of children at risk for attention deficit/hyperactivity disorder. *Social Psychiatry and Psychiatric Epidemiology, 41*, 860–813.

Sayal, K., & Taylor, E. (2004). Detection of child mental health disorders by general practitioners. *British Journal of General Practice, 54*, 348–352.

Sayal, K., Taylor, E., & Beecham, J. (2003). Parental perceptions of problems and mental health service use for hyperactivity. *Journal of the American Academy of Child and Adolescent Psychiatry, 42*, 1410–1414.

Schiffman, J., Becker, K. D., & Daleiden, E. L. (2006). Evidence-based services in a statewide public mental health system: Do the services fit the problems? *Journal of Clinical Child and Adolescent Psychology, 35*, 13–19.

Schoenwald, S. K., Kelleher, K., Weisz, J. R., & The Research Network on Youth Mental Health. (2008). Building bridges to evidence-based practice: The MacArthur Foundation Child System and Treatment Enhancement Projects (Child STEPs). *Administration and Policy in Mental Health, 35,* 66–72.

Shanley, D. C., Reid, G. J., & Evans, B. (2008). How parents seek help for children with mental health problems. *Administration and Policy in Mental Health, 35,* 135–146.

Sheehan, A. K., Walrath, C. M., & Holden, E. W. (2007). Evidence-based practice use, training, and implementation in the community-based service setting: A survey of children's mental health service providers. *Journal of Child Family Studies, 16,* 169–182.

Shirk, S. R. (1988). *Cognitive Development and Child Psychotherapy.* New York: Plenum.

Silverman, W. K., Ortiz, C. D., Viswesvaran, C., Burns, B. J., Kolko, D., Putnam, F. W., et al. (2008). Evidence-based psychosocial treatments for children and adolescents exposed to traumatic events. *Journal of Clinical Child & Adolescent Psychology, 37,* 156–183.

Silverman, W. K., Pina, A. A., & Viswesvaran, C. (2008). Evidence-based treatments for phobic and anxiety disorders in children and adolescents. *Journal of Clinical Child & Adolescent Psychology, 37,* 105–130.

Skovgaard, A. M., Houmann, T., Christiansen, E., Landorph, S., Jorgensen, T., Olsen, E. M., et al. (2007). The prevalence of mental health problems in children 1 1/2 years of age—the Copenhagen Child Cohort 2000. *Journal of Child Psychology and Psychiatry, 48,* 62–70.

Sourander, A., Helstela, L., Ristkari, T., Ikaheimo, K., Helenius, H., & Piha, J. (2001). Child and adolescent mental health service use in Finland. *Social Psychiatry and Psychiatric Epidemiology, 36,* 294–298.

Southam-Gerow, M. A., Chorpita, B. F., Miller, L. M., & Gleacher, A. A. (2008). Are children with anxiety disorders privately referred to a university clinic like those referred from the public mental health system? *Administration and Policy in Mental Health, 35,* 168–180.

Southam-Gerow, M. A., Weisz, J. R., & Kendall, P. C. (2003). Youth with anxiety disorders in research and service clinics: Examining client differences and similarities. *Journal of Clinical Child and Adolescent Psychology, 32,* 375–385.

Spagnolo, A. B., Murphy, A. A., & Librera, L. A. (2008). Reducing stigma by meeting and learning from people with mental illness. *Psychiatric Rehabilitation Journal, 31,* 186–193.

Srebnik, D., & Cauce, A. M. (1996). Help-seeking pathways for children and adolescents. *Journal of Emotional and Behavioral Disorders, 4,* 210–220.

Staghezza-Jaramillo, B., Bird, H. R., Gould, M. S., & Canino, G. (1995). Mental health service utilization among Puerto Rican children ages 4 through 16. *Journal of Child and Family Studies, 4,* 399–418.

Stiffman, A. R., Pescosolido, B., & Cabassa, L. J. (2004). Building a model to understand youth service access: The gateway provider model. *Mental Health Services Research, 6,* 189–198.

Stiffman, A. R., Striley, C., Horvath, V. E., Hadley-Ives, E., Polgar, M., Elze, D., et al. (2001). Organizational context and provider perceptions as determinants of mental health service use. *Journal of Behavioral Health Services & Research, 28,* 188–204.

Stroul, B. A., & Friedman, R. M. (1986). A system of care for children and youth with severe emotional disturbances. Washington, DC: Georgetown University Child Development Center, CASSP Technical Assistance Center.

Strum, R., Ringel, J. S., & Andreyeva, T. (2003). Geographical disparities in children's mental health care. *Pediatrics, 112,* 308–315.

Substance Abuse and Mental Health Services Administration (SAMHSA). (n.d.). *Origin of Family Driven Project.* Available online at http://www.systemsofcare.samhsa.gov/headermenus/family driven.aspx. Accessed August 22, 2008.

Substance Abuse and Mental Health Services Administration (n.d.). *About Child, Adolescent, and Family Branch.* Available online at http://mentalhealth.samhsa.gov/publications/allpubs/ KEN95-0016/default.asp#ccmhs. Accessed August 22, 2008.

Teagle, S. A. (2002). Parental problem recognition and child mental health service use. *Mental Health Services Research, 4,* 257–266.

Tebes, J. K., Bowler, S. M., Shah, S., Connell, C. M., Ross, E., Simmons, R., et al. (2005). Service access and service system development in a children's behavioral health system of care. *Evaluation and Program Planning, 28,* 151–160.

Thompson, R., & May, M. A. (2006). Caregivers' perception of child mental health needs and service utilization: An urban 8-year old sample. *Journal of Behavioral Health Services & Research, 33,* 474–482.

Tolan, P. H., & Dodge, K. A. (2005). Children's mental health as a primary care and concern: A system for comprehensive support and service. *American Psychologist, 60,* 601–614.

United Nations (1989, November 20). *Convention on the Rights of the Child.* Available online at http://www.un.org/documents/ga/res/44/a44r025.htm. Accessed August 12, 2008.

U.S. Department of Health and Human Services. (1999). *Mental Health: A Report of the Surgeon General.* Rockville, MD: U.S. Department of Health and Human Services, Substance Abuse and Mental Health Services Administration, Center of Mental Health Services, National Institutes of Health, National Institutes of Mental Health.

Van Dycke, J. L., Martin, J. E., & Lovett, D. L. (2006). Why is this cake on fire? Inviting students into the IEP process. *Teaching Exceptional Children, 38,* 42–47.

Wachtel, J., Rodrigue, J. R., Geffken, G. R., Graham-Pole, J., & Turner, C. (1994). Children awaiting invasive medical procedures: Do children and their mothers agree on child's level of anxiety? *Journal of Pediatric Psychology, 19,* 723–735.

Waddell, C., McEwan, K., Peters, R. D., Hua, J., & Garland, O. (2007). Preventing mental disorders in children: A public health priority. *Canadian Journal of Public Health, 98,* 174–178.

Waddell, C., Offord, D. R., Shepherd, C. A., Hua, J. M., & McEwan, K. (2002). Child psychiatric epidemiology and Canadian public policy-making: The state of the science and the art of the possible. *Canadian Journal of Psychiatry, 47,* 825–832.

Wagner, I., Munt, G., & Briner, P. (2006). Introducing evidence-based family assessment and therapy in child and youth mental health services. *Australian and New Zealand Journal of Family Therapy, 27,* 187–198.

Waldron, H. B., & Turner, C. W. (2008). Evidence-based psychosocial treatments for adolescent substance abuse. *Journal of Clinical Child & Adolescent Psychology, 37,* 238–261.

Walter, H. J., Gouze, K., & Lim, K. G. (2006). Teachers' beliefs about mental health needs in inner city elementary schools. *Journal of the American Academy of Child and Adolescent Psychiatry, 45,* 61–67.

Watanabe, N., Hunot, V., Omori, I. M., Churchill, R., & Furukawa, T. A. (2007). Psychotherapy for depression among children and adolescents: A systemic review. *Acta Psychiatry Scandanavia, 116,* 84–95.

Weisz, J. R., Donenberg, G. R., Han, S. S., & Weiss, B. (1995). Bridging the gap between laboratory and clinic in child and adolescent psychotherapy. *Journal of Consulting and Clinical Psychology, 63,* 688–701.

Weisz, J. R., Doss, A. J., & Hawley, K. M. (2005). Youth psychotherapy outcome research: A review and critique of the evidence base. *Annual Review of Psychology, 56,* 337–363.

Weisz, J. R., & Hawley, K. M. (2002). Developmental factors in the treatment of adolescents. *Journal of Consulting and Clinical Psychology, 70,* 21–43.

Weisz, J. R., Jensen-Doss, A., & Hawley, K. M. (2006). Evidence-based youth psychotherapies versus usual clinical care: A meta-analysis of direct comparisons. *American Psychologist, 61,* 671–689.

Weisz, J. R., Jenson, A., & McLeod, B. D. (2005). Development and dissemination of child and adolescent psychotherapies: Milestones, methods, and a new deployment-focused model. In E. D. Hibbs & P. S. Jensen (Eds.), *Psychosocial Treatments for Child and Adolescent Disorders: Empirically Based Strategies for Clinical Practice* (2nd ed., pp. 9–39). Washington, DC: American Psychological Association.

Weisz, J. R., McCarty, C. A., & Valeri, S. M. (2006). Effects of psychotherapy for depression in children and adolescents: A meta-analysis. *Psychological Bulletin, 132,* 132–149.

Weisz, J. R., Sandler, I. N., Durlak, J. A., & Anton, B. S. (2005). Promoting and protecting youth mental health through evidence-based prevention and treatment. *American Psychologist, 60,* 628–648.

Weisz, J. R., Sandler, I. N., Durlak, J. A., & Anton, B. S. (2006). A proposal to unite two different worlds of children's mental health. *American Psychologist, 61,* 644–645.

Weisz, J. R., Weiss, B., Suwanlert, S., & Chaiyasit, W. (2006). Culture and youth psychopathology: Testing the syndromal sensitivity model in Thai and American adolescents. *Journal of Consulting and Clinical Psychology, 74,* 1098–1107.

Westen, D., Novotny, C. M., & Thompson-Brenner, H. (2004). The empirical status of empirically supported psychotherapies: Assumptions, findings, and reporting in controlled clinical trials. *Psychological Bulletin, 130,* 631–663.

White House. (n.d.). *Expectmore.gov: Detailed Information on the Children's Mental Health Services Assessment.* Available online at http://www.whitehouse.gov/OMB/expectmore/detail/10000298.2002.html. Accessed August 22, 2008.

Wong, D. F. K. (2007). Crucial individuals in the help-seeking pathway of Chinese caregivers of relatives with early psychosis in Hong Kong. *Social Work, 52,* 127–135.

World Health Organization. (2005). *Child and Adolescent Atlas: Resources for Child and Adolescent Mental Health.* Geneva: World Health Organization.

Worrall-Davies, A., & Marino-Francis, F. (2008). Eliciting children's and young people's views of child and adolescent mental health services: A systemic review of best practices. *Child and Adolescent Mental Health, 13,* 9–15.

Wozniak, J., Biederman, J., Kwon, A., Mick, E., Faraone, S., Orlovsky, K., et al. (2005). How cardinal are the cardinal symptoms in pediatric bipolar? An examination of clinical correlates. *Biological Psychiatry, 58,* 583–588.

Wu, P., Hoven, C. W., Bird, H. R., Moore, R. E., Cohen, P., Alegria, M., et al. (1999). Depressive and disruptive disorders and mental health service utilization in children and adolescents. *Journal of the American Academy of Child and Adolescent Psychiatry, 38,* 1081–1090.

Yeh, M., McCabe, K., Hough, R. L., Lau, A., Fakhry, F., & Garland, A. (2005). Why bother with beliefs? Examining relationships between race/ethnicity, parental beliefs about causes of child problems, and mental health service use. *Journal of Consulting and Clinical Psychology, 73,* 800–807.

Yeh, M., & Weisz, J. R. (2001). Why are we here at the clinic? Parent-child (dis)agreement on referral problems at outpatient treatment entry. *Journal of Consulting and Clinical Psychology, 69,* 1018–1025.

Youngstrom, E., Izard, C., & Ackerman, B. (1999). Dysphoria-related bias in maternal ratings of children. *Journal of Consulting and Clinical Psychology, 67,* 905–916.

Zahner, G. E. P., & Daskalakis, C. (1998). Modeling sources of informant variance in parent and teacher ratings of child psychopathology. *International Journal of Methods in Psychiatric Research, 7,* 3–16.

Zimmerman, F. J. (2005). Social and economic determinants of disparities in professional help-seeking for child mental health problems: Evidence from a national sample. *Health Research and Educational Trust, 40,* 1514–1533.

Zuvekas, S. H. (2001). Trends in mental health service use and spending, 1987–1996. *Health Affairs, 20,* 214–224.

Zwaanswijk, M., van der Ende, J., Verhaak, P. F. M, Bensing, J. M., & Verhulst, F. C. (2005). Help-seeking for child psychopathology: Pathways for informal and professional services in the Netherlands. *Journal of the American Academy of Child and Adolescent Psychiatry, 44,* 1292–1300.

Zwaanswijk, M., van der Ende, J., Verhaak, P. F. M, Bensing, J. M., & Verhulst, F. C. (2007). The different stages and actors involved in the process leading to the use of adolescent mental health services. *Clinical Child Psychology and Psychiatry, 12,* 567–582.

Zwaanswijk, M., Verhaak, P. F. M., Bensing, J. M., van der Ende, J., & Verhulst, F. C. (2003). Help seeking for emotional and behavioural problems in children and adolescents: A review of recent literature. *European Child & Adolescent Psychiatry, 12,* 153–161.

Chapter 9

ADULTS

Alexander S. Young, MD, MSHS; and Noosha Niv, PhD

Introduction

During recent decades, there have been remarkable advances in mental health treatment. Vague classification schemes have been replaced by structured diagnoses (American Psychiatric Association, 2000a). Basic science research has irrefutably demonstrated that severe mental illnesses are brain-based conditions. Highly effective treatments have been developed for bipolar disorder, major depression, and schizophrenia (American Psychiatric Association, 2000b, 2002, 2004, 2007b). Medications can improve or eliminate psychotic and mood symptoms. Structured psychotherapies, such as interpersonal and cognitive-behavioral therapy, can reduce disabling depression and anxiety. Assertive Community Treatment, an intensive provision of a comprehensive array of services, allows people with treatment-resistant illnesses to live successfully in community settings. Rehabilitation interventions allow people with chronic psychotic disorders to obtain competitive, paid employment. The involvement of family members and caregivers in treatment reduces relapse rates. Finally, individuals with mental illness ("consumers") are themselves improving service delivery, working on clinical teams, and helping other consumers live successfully in the community.

Overall, outcomes are excellent when competent clinicians provide comprehensive, state-of-the-art treatments (President's New Freedom Commission on Mental Health, 2003). Unfortunately, effective treatments have only been disseminated to a small minority of people who would benefit from them (Institute of Medicine, 2006). In the United States, only one third of people with serious depression or anxiety disorders receive any effective treatment (Young, Klap, Sherbourne, & Wells, 2001). Treatment is no better in people with chronic illness. Despite a high level of persistent need, people with chronic depression or anxiety have only a one in four chance of being treated with medication, and a one in ten chance of receiving both psychotherapy and medication (Young, Klap, Shoai, & Wells, 2008). Even in severe disorders such as schizophrenia and bipolar disorder, only half of people have any contact with a professional during a given year (Wang, Demler, & Kessler, 2002), and treatment is often intermittent, inadequate, or inappropriate (Institute of Medicine, 2006; Young, Niv et al., 2008). Certain populations, such as African Americans, men, young adults, and the elderly are particularly unlikely to receive needed treatment (U.S. Surgeon General, 2001; Smedley, Stith, & Nelson, 2003).

As a result, actual outcomes for persons with mental illness are much worse than would be expected. In state-of-the-art treatment programs for schizophrenia, annual relapse rates are near zero, whereas half or more of patients relapse in a given year at typical community clinics (Kissling, 1994; Young, Niv et al., 2008). Without antipsychotic medication, 60–70% of patients with schizophrenia relapse within a year and 90% relapse within two years. Use of medication reduces the risk to less than 30% for individuals in the stable phase of illness (American Psychiatric Association, 2004). Cities have substantial populations of homeless persons with untreated mental illness, and many persons with mental illness are institutionalized in jails and prisons where they receive inadequate or no treatment (Criminal Justice Mental Health Consensus Project, 2002). In 2005, an estimated 56% of state prisoners, 45% of federal prisoners, and 64% of jail inmates had a mental health problem (U.S. Department of Justice, 2006). Of those who had mental health problems, only 34% of those in state prison, 24% of those in federal prison, and 17% of those in local jails received mental health treatment.

Although the United States spends more than $100 billion per year on mental health care, these are common disorders, and the economic burden that results from untreated or inadequately treated mental illness is much larger (Mark et al., 2007). Severe mental illnesses cost the United States at least $193 billion annually in lost earnings alone (Kessler et al., 2008). Mental illnesses are one of the leading causes of disability, and people with severe mental illness have a 2- to 3-fold increased risk of dying compared to the general population (Saha, Chant, & McGrath, 2007).

In summary, many people with disabling mental illness are not receiving effective treatments that would improve their health, well-being, and functioning. This is a problem with the *quality* of care. What accounts for this? A wide variety of ideological, social, economic, and political factors have hindered our ability to meet the needs of persons with mental illness. The authors introduce these factors by presenting three critical problems with U.S. mental health policy.

Critical Problems with U.S. Mental Health Policy

NO COMPREHENSIVE MENTAL HEALTH CARE SYSTEM

Current mental health delivery is a result of struggles between "conscience and convenience," strong negative attitudes and discrimination toward indigent groups, countless incremental policies, and marketplace pressures (Rothman, 1980;

U.S. Surgeon General, 1999; Frank & Glied, 2006; Mechanic, 2007). While comprehensive, community-based care has remained a stated national policy goal for over 40 years (U.S. President's Commission on Mental Health, 1978; President's New Freedom Commission on Mental Health, 2003), it has never been realized. Mental health services in the United States have not been organized into a coherent system. Rather, a patchwork of policies, laws, contracts, providers, and purchasers has evolved into highly complex sub-systems of care.

No Policy Regarding Health Care Financing

There is little or no policy regarding the appropriate overall level of spending or the allocation of this spending. As a result, health care in the United States is extremely inefficient. The United States spends more than 2.1 trillion dollars per year, or 16% of its gross national product on health care (Catlin, Cowan, Hartman, & Heffler, 2008). On a per-person basis, this is twice as much as any other industrialized nation. Despite this, health care quality and outcomes in the United States are among the worst of the industrialized nations (Davis, 2007; Docteur & Berenson, 2009). In 2008, the Commonwealth Fund reviewed national health, access, quality, equity, and efficiency. Compared with international and domestic benchmarks of 100, the United States averaged an overall score of 65 (Commonwealth Fund Commission on a High Performance Health System, 2008). The U.S. combination of high cost and low performance results from large sums being spent on expensive, high-technology treatments, many of which have little or no effect on patient outcomes, while millions of people have poor access to the most basic primary care. Poor access to basic primary care increases death rates in people with chronic medical illness and is a particular problem among the 46 million people in the United States with no insurance, and among people with mental illness (Lurie et al., 1986; Druss & von Esenwein, 2006; Morden, Mistler, Weeks, & Bartels, 2009; Roshanaei-Moghaddam & Katon, 2009).

The remarkably high level of U.S. health care expenditures has created strong pressure to cut costs wherever possible. Psychiatric disorders are an attractive target since they are among the top five costliest medical conditions to treat (Soni, 2009). In 2003, 6% of all U.S. health care expenditures were for the treatment of mental illness, and 1% were for the treatment of addictive disorders (Mark et al., 2007). The forces advocating for mental health spending are relatively weak. People with severe mental illness or addictive disorders are often unemployed, of relatively low socioeconomic status, strongly stigmatized, and can have difficulty advocating for themselves because of cognitive problems. Also, people with generous health care benefits through their employer pay little attention to their mental health benefits until they try to use them. Thus there is little incentive for purchasers or insurers to provide a good mental health benefit.

Over recent decades, awareness of and demand for mental health treatment has increased markedly. From 1996 to 2006, the number of people receiving mental health treatment nearly doubled from 19 million to 36 million (Soni, 2009). Prescriptions for psychotropic medication have become much more common and accepted (Harman, Edlund, & Fortney, 2009). Although brief counseling is also more common, access to intensive psychotherapy has been curtailed, and overall use of psychotherapy has remained unchanged at a low level. Funding for hospital treatment has been dramatically cut, funding for outpatient services has not increased to compensate for this, and many people have been "trans-institutionalized" to nursing homes, locked community facilities, jails, and prisons. There is intense pressure to limit mental health treatment, and the average per-patient treatment cost fell between 1996 and 2006. Treatment intensity remains quite low in people with serious, persistent illness (Young, Klap et al., 2008) (see Chapter 2 in this volume for additional information on financing and insurance).

LACK OF ATTENTION TO THE QUALITY OF MENTAL HEALTH SERVICES

For decades, there has been substantial work to evaluate and improve the quality of health care in America. Systems were developed in the 1970s and 1980s that accurately measured the quality of cardiac surgery (Fitch et al., 2001). These were implemented in New York state, where they led to improvement in hospitals' cardiac surgery programs and substantial reduced death rates (Chassin, 2002). In the Department of Veterans Affairs (VA), implementation of systematic quality improvement and computerized medical records in the 1990s transformed the VA into the national leader in health care quality (Jha, Perlin, Kizer, & Dudley, 2003; Asch et al., 2004). Starting in 2003, Medicare evaluated a two-year national demonstration of voluntary public reporting of health care quality and pay-for-performance by hospitals. Quality measures were developed and reported for the management of heart failure, acute myocardial infarction, and pneumonia. Hospitals were eligible for a payment bonus of 1% or 2% for high performance, or penalties of 1% or 2% for low performance. The quality of care improved significantly in both the public reporting hospitals and in the hospitals that combined public reporting with pay-for-performance (Lindenauer et al., 2007).

In mental health, there has been awareness regarding the magnitude of the quality problem, but much less done to address it. The President's New Freedom Commission (2003) and the Institute of Medicine (2006) concur that routine mental health care is usually not of high quality. The mental health workforce often lacks the competencies necessary to provide appropriate care (Hoge et al., 2005), and provider organizations routinely fail to make effective services available (National Association of State Mental Health Program Directors [NASMHPD] Research Institute, 2005; Young, Niv et al., 2008). Solutions to this problem have been elusive. A major barrier has been an inability to routinely measure the quality of care. In disorders such as diabetes, medical records contain all the information required to identify patients who are not receiving appropriate treatments or are doing poorly clinically. In mental health, medical records contain little reliable clinical information (Cradock, Young, & Sullivan, 2001; Young et al., 2007). As a result, most widely used quality measures are based only on billing or pharmacy data, and have a weak relationship with patient outcomes (Druss & Rosenheck, 1997; Young, 2003). For example, it is common to assess whether antidepressant medication is used in patients with a billing diagnosis of depression. However, the relationship of such a measure to patient outcomes is likely limited, since most patients with major depression are not diagnosed, the accuracy of billing diagnoses is questionable, and psychotherapy is often an equally effective treatment to medication. Medical records provide little information regarding whether or not evidence-based psychotherapies or rehabilitation interventions are provided (see Chapter 4 in this volume for more information on quality improvement).

The remainder of this chapter begins with a review of the major adult mental illnesses and their treatment, emphasizing severe disorders. It then provides an overview of homelessness, as well as key problems in the organization and delivery of mental health care. It concludes by discussing approaches to improving behavioral health services and policy.

The Major Mental Illnesses

As with health in general, mental health exists on a continuum. This extends from no problems, to normal sadness, grief and worrying, to moderate and severe mental illnesses that impair functioning and quality of life. The Diagnostic and Statistical Manual of Mental Disorders and the International Classification of Disease are similar and the most widely accepted schemes for defining mental illness (American Psychiatric Association, 2000a; American Medical Association, 2001). The most common mental illnesses are classified as anxiety disorders, mood disorders, schizophrenia, dementias, and addictive disorders, though there are a wide variety of other important disorders such as personality disorders and eating disorders. During a given year, about 20% of adults have a mental illness of serious or moderate severity (Kessler et al., 2005).

The most common adult mental illnesses are anxiety disorders, and these affect about 40 million or 18% of U.S. adults in a given year (Kessler et al., 2005). Persons with these disorders have disabling nervousness, worrying, or fearfulness. There are several types of anxiety disorders. Panic disorder consists of repeated episodes of intense fear that emerge without warning. Generalized anxiety disorder consists of ongoing, exaggerated worrying and tension about routine life activities. Obsessive-compulsive disorder consists of repetitive, intrusive thoughts, or compulsive behaviors that seem impossible to stop or control. Post-traumatic stress disorder occurs after experiencing a traumatic event and consists of re-experiencing the trauma, avoidance, and increased arousal that persist for more than a month. Phobias are overwhelming, disabling, and irrational fears of social or other specific situations or objects.

As with anxiety disorders, there are different types of mood disorders, including major depressive disorder, dysthymia, and bipolar disorder. Approximately 10% of the U.S. adult population has a mood disorder in a given year. Clinical depression is the most common disorder, affecting approximately 7% of the U.S. adult population. Persons with major depressive disorder feel sad or irritable most of the time, may cry often, have low energy, and feel worthless or that their life is meaningless. They can have changes in sleep and appetite, trouble concentrating, and are at increased risk for suicide. Dysthymia consists of depression that is less severe, but occurs on a daily basis for two years or more. Bipolar disorder is defined by the presence of one or more episodes of mania during which people can feel "high as a kite," have unreal, grandiose ideas, require little sleep, and engage in risky behaviors. Manic episodes often have severe negative consequences for the affected individual. Persons with bipolar disorder can have recurrent episodes of both mania and depression. Although manias are dramatic, major depression is the most common disorder of mood for most individuals with bipolar disorder and can be quite disabling.

Schizophrenia consists of chronic disorders of thought and occurs in about 1% of the population (Perala et al., 2007). People with schizophrenia have psychotic symptoms such as disorganization of thought and behavior, auditory or visual hallucinations, and paranoid and other delusional ideas. While symptoms of schizophrenia vary widely among individuals, they are often categorized as "positive," "negative," or "cognitive." Positive psychotic symptoms include hallucinations and delusions. Psychotic symptoms result in behavioral consequences, such as hospitalization, incarceration, or homelessness. Negative symptoms include blunting of affect, poverty of thought and speech, lack of motivation, and social withdrawal. Most individuals with schizophrenia have cognitive problems, including memory, attention, and social processing deficits. Cognitive deficits are the leading cause of social and vocational disability in schizophrenia. Schizoaffective disorder is similar to schizophrenia with the addition of a major mood syndrome.

Most mental illnesses are caused by a combination of genetic vulnerability and environmental stress (Ingram & Luxton, 2005). For instance, if one parent has schizophrenia, the odds of their child having the illness increases from 1% to about 13%. If both parents have schizophrenia, their children have a 46% chance of having the disorder (Gottesman & Moldin, 1999). Environmental stressors may interact with genetic vulnerability to cause illness. The nature of environmental stresses is poorly defined, but appears to include, for instance, interpersonal relationship problems for depression and perinatal injuries for schizophrenia.

Severe, persistent mental illness (SPMI) refers to any serious disorder that has a recurrent, profound effect on functioning and quality of life. While SPMI most commonly results from schizophrenia, bipolar disorder, and chronic depression, it can be caused by numerous other disorders. People with SPMI experience major difficulties in multiple areas, such as thought, mood, behavior, physical health, social interactions, or employment. A high proportion of people with SPMI cannot maintain continuous employment and so live in poverty. Persons with SPMI are at high risk for having co-occurring disorders, such as drug and alcohol misuse or cardiovascular disease. People with major depression, bipolar disorder, schizophrenia, and drug and alcohol disorders are at substantially elevated risk for suicide. For instance, up to 30% of people with schizophrenia attempt suicide, and between 4% and 10% succeed (Palmer, Pankratz, & Bostwick, 2005). People with SPMI also have an increased rate of death from homicide, general medical disorders, and accidents.

The prognosis with mental illness is highly variable. Major depression usually resolves within one year without treatment and within a few weeks or months with appropriate treatment. With prompt treatment, disability can be prevented (Wells et al., 2000). However, in 20% of individuals, a major depressive episode persists for more than two years. About 5% of the U.S. population has a long-term, continuous, or relapsing depressive or anxiety disorder (Young, Klap et al., 2008).

Schizophrenia and bipolar disorder have, by definition, a chronic course. When one examines people with schizophrenia two decades after onset of illness, between a third and a half have returned to the level of functioning they had before becoming ill (Harding & Zahniser, 1994). However, schizophrenia and bipolar disorder generally require medication treatment for many years, and the first decade of the illness tends to be the most severe.

Treatment of Serious Mental Illness

History

Because mental illness can affect many facets of a person's life, successful treatment requires attention to a range of biological, psychological, and social needs. During the latter half of the nineteenth and first half of the twentieth century, mental health services were primarily delivered in asylums, such as state mental hospitals and almshouses (Rothman, 1980). These were established as beneficent systems of care for various indigent groups, including immigrants, the poor, and persons with mental illnesses and other disabilities. At their peak in 1955, out of a total U.S. population of 165 million, 559,000 persons with mental illness were institutionalized in state mental hospitals (Lamb & Bachrach, 2001).

This asylum-oriented approach was reversed starting in the late 1950s by the "de-institutionalization" movement (Mechanic, 1986). The stated goal of this movement was to implement treatment alternatives in the community to replace round-the-clock care in mental hospitals. It was facilitated by the development of effective psychotropic medications and led by an alliance between civil libertarians and politicians eager to redirect revenues to purposes other than mental health care. Throughout the 1960s and 1970s, de-institutionalization released persons from "back wards" and chronic care hospitals. In 2004, out of a total U.S. population of 293 million, only about 167,000 were institutionalized at a state mental hospital (Manderscheid & Berry, 2006).

It proved much easier to release people from hospitals than to provide them with appropriate care in community settings. In 1963, the Mental Retardation Facilities and Community Mental Health Centers Construction Act set in motion national plans for a national community mental health center system that, by 1980, had only reached 40% of its goal (Lerman, 1982). Other efforts to improve community services included the Community Support Program guidelines of the 1970s and follow-up legislation in the 1980s and 1990s (Stroul, 1989). For instance, in 1986, the State Comprehensive Mental Health Services Plan Act encouraged the establishment of comprehensive state public mental health systems. It focused on people with chronic mental illness or at risk of homelessness and linked block grant funding to service system requirements, such as provision of a core set of services (Stockdill, 1990). In some locales, state-of-the-art services were implemented, and people with SPMI benefited from de-institutionalization. However, access to these services was not broadly provided, and the result has been widespread homelessness, frequent brief re-hospitalizations (the "revolving door" syndrome), and trans-institutionalization to squalid "board and care" homes, privately owned chronic care facilities, and jails and prisons (Criminal Justice Mental Health Consensus Project, 2002) (see Chapter 18 in this volume for more information on mental health treatment in criminal justice settings).

This problem was revisited in 2002 by the President's New Freedom Commission. The Commission declared that the U.S. mental health system was a "patchwork relic" that "presents barriers that all too often add to the burden of mental illnesses" (President's New Freedom Commission on Mental Health, 2003). It recommended fundamental transformation with goals that included improving public knowledge, consumer-driven care, early intervention, delivery of best practices, and use of technology to improve information. The U.S. Substance Abuse and Mental Health Services Administration (SAMHSA) was assigned with overseeing implementation, but provided with very little authority or resources. The VA has dedicated substantial resources toward implementing these recommendations in its national system. While some states have pursued transformation, overall there has been little federal leadership, and substantial reform has not occurred.

COMPREHENSIVE CARE

High quality care for mental illness begins with a health care system that has a wide variety of available treatment options and can deliver high quality treatments to each patient. The system must be prepared to attend to a range of needs, such as psychiatric treatment, rehabilitation, medical and dental care, and housing. Fortunately, there is now a very large body of science and clinical experience defining treatments that improve outcomes of mental illness (Schulberg, Katon, Simon, & Rush, 1999; American Psychiatric Association, 2000b; Lehman et al., 2004). A high quality health care system would offer at least these treatments to all individuals who could benefit from them and would provide education and outreach, since people with mental disorders often do not spontaneously seek treatment (Young et al., 2001). What has evolved, instead, are pockets of excellence—"model programs" that provide comprehensive care, but are not available to most affected individuals.

In people with SPMI, the problem is most severe. Individuals with disorders such as schizophrenia may not acknowledge they would benefit from treatment or may be unable to seek out treatment due to cognitive deficits or limited interpersonal effectiveness. In these circumstances, a specific intervention, "Assertive Community Treatment" or ACT, is effective (American Psychiatric Association, 2004). ACT starts with a team of treatment professionals that includes a psychiatrist. Clinicians have small caseloads. The team provides care in non-institutional settings and assertively reaches out to patients to ensure they have an opportunity to receive effective treatments. ACT was originally developed as a "hospital without walls," and it has proven to be highly effective in reducing homelessness, reducing hospitalizations, and improving outcomes among individuals who are homeless or at risk for re-hospitalization (Coldwell & Bender, 2007). It is more expensive than typical mental health treatment, but no more expensive than hospitalization or incarceration. Unfortunately, ACT has been disseminated to only a small fraction of people with SPMI who would benefit from it.

People with less severe mental illness can be successfully treated without ACT, but still require access to comprehensive care. The traditional locus for this care has been a solo clinician or community mental health center that makes extensive use of "case management." Traditional case management consists of linking patients by phone or referral to various services and coordinating service provision. Caseloads are quite large (100 or more patients per clinician), and the focus tends to be on care coordination and dealing with crises. For instance, people with SPMI often need disability payments, such as Supplemental Security Income (SSI) or Social Security Disability Income (SSDI); public health insurance, such as Medicaid or Medicare; and support for housing costs, such as "Section 8" vouchers. Case management is a nearly ubiquitous part of public mental health treatment organizations. Unfortunately, there is little reason to believe that typical case management improves patient outcomes (Holloway & Carson, 2001).

Appropriate care for people with SPMI can require interventions as diverse as vocational rehabilitation, antipsychotic medication, and supportive housing. It is not likely that any one clinician will have the skills to provide all needed treatments. Instead, the best approach is often team-based, with team members specializing in specific interventions while working together to deliver care (Young et al., 2000a). This has been operationalized as psychosocial rehabilitation programs or integrated service agencies (California Mental Health Association, 2000; President's New Freedom Commission on Mental Health, 2003). These programs use a holistic philosophy that extends beyond symptoms, emphasizing rehabilitation, illness self-management, peer support, patient empowerment, and "recovery" (Mueser et al., 2002). Recovery is a process of individual improvement based upon the belief that it is possible to regain purpose and meaning in life while having a serious disability (Anthony, 1993; SAMHSA Center for Mental Health Services, 2004b) (see Chapter 20 in this volume for more information on recovery). Psychosocial programs value natural supports and meaningful activities, as opposed to activities designed solely for people with mental illness. Programs include a variety of components, such as "clubhouses," consumer-run businesses, housing supports, money management assistance, outreach teams, skills training, peer support, and services for co-morbid substance abuse.

MEDICATION AND PSYCHOTHERAPY

Treatment begins with, and relies on, an accurate diagnosis. Anxiety disorders are treated with medication, psychotherapy, or both. In panic disorder, effective treatments include cognitive-behavioral psychotherapies, some antidepressant medications, and benzodiazepines (American Psychiatric Association, 2009). Effective treatments for generalized anxiety disorder include antidepressant medications, benzodiazepines, cognitive behavioral psychotherapies, and relaxation training (Canadian Psychiatric Association, 2006). Obsessive compulsive disorder improves with antidepressants that block serotonin re-uptake and with behavioral psychotherapy that focuses on stopping undesired behaviors using approaches such as exposure, desensitization, and response prevention (American Psychiatric Association, 2007a). Effective treatments for post-traumatic stress disorder include exposure psychotherapy and antidepressant medications (Bryant et al., 2008; Institute of Medicine, 2008b).

In major depression and dysthymia, effective treatments include antidepressant medications and cognitive-behavioral and interpersonal psychotherapies (American Psychiatric Association, 2000b; Barrett et al., 2001; Fochtmann & Gelenberg, 2005). Antidepressant medications were once poorly tolerated, potentially dangerous, and difficult to prescribe (Henry, 1992). This changed in the late 1980s with the release of fluoxetine (brand name Prozac) and the subsequent development of numerous other new medications that are typically safe and easy to use. There have also been major advances in our understanding of psychotherapy for depression. Unstructured counseling and psychodynamic psychotherapies may have some effectiveness, and research strongly supports the efficacy of certain structured psychotherapies. Cognitive behavioral therapy involves cognitive restructuring (working with patients to recognize and correct inaccurate thoughts associated with depressed feelings), behavioral activation (helping patients engage in enjoyable activities), and problem-solving skills. Interpersonal psychotherapy includes identification and management of stressful social situations.

The treatment of bipolar disorder begins with a mood stabilizer medication (American Psychiatric Association, 2002). Lithium was the first mood stabilizer to be discovered and remains quite effective. However, it has a high rate of unpleasant side-effects and is only safe and effective within a narrow dosage range. Other effective mood stabilizers, such as carbamazepine or valproate are easier to use. However, with any of these medications, many people continue to have episodes of depression or mania or suffer significant side-effects, such as weight gain or sedation. Antipsychotic medications are also effective in bipolar disorder, but carry potential side-effects of their own, including weight gain and tardive dyskinesia, a potentially irreversible movement disorder (Correll, Leucht, & Kane, 2004; Newcomer, 2007).

Depression during the course of bipolar disorder must be treated carefully, since treatments for depression can cause the patient to switch to mania. Effective treatments for bipolar depression include lithium, lamotrigine, cognitive behavioral therapy, social rhythm therapy, and interpersonal psychotherapy (American Psychiatric Association, 2002). With regard to preventing mania, no psychotherapies have been shown to be effective; however, there is support for educational interventions that improve illness self-management skills. Mania is treated with an appropriate level of care (often hospitalization), as well as mood stabilizer and antipsychotic medication.

The appropriate treatment of schizophrenia always includes an antipsychotic medication (American Psychiatric Association, 2004). The first antipsychotic medications, such as chlorpromazine (Thorazine), were identified and disseminated in the 1950s and 1960s. More than a dozen similar medications were developed over the next two decades. These were effective against positive psychotic symptoms, disorganization, and, to a lesser extent, negative symptoms. However, they had a high rate of very unpleasant side-effects, particularly motor side-effects such as muscle stiffness, severe restlessness, and tardive dyskinesia.

Fortunately, a number of "second generation" antipsychotic medications have been developed that cause fewer motor side-effects. The first of these was clozapine. Released in the United States in 1989, it was effective in the large proportion of patients who failed to respond fully to other antipsychotic medications, and it caused no motor side-effects. Clearly a breakthrough, it also caused a higher than usual rate of agranulocytosis, a temporary, though dangerous, disorder of the immune system. It has been reserved, therefore, for patients who have been unresponsive to at least two other medications.

Since the early 1990s, a number of other second generation medications have been made available (risperidone, olanzapine, quetiapine, ziprasidone, aripiprazole, paliperidone, and iloperidone). While these are no more effective than older "first generation" medications, they cause less motor restlessness and muscle stiffness and are easier to prescribe (Marder et al., 2002; Leucht et al., 2009). Second generation medications have captured almost all of the antipsychotic medication market. First generation antipsychotic medications cause tardive dyskinesia in about 4% of adults per year, while the second generation agents cause this side-effect at a much lower rate. Patients often prefer the second generation medications, but they do have important side-effects. The most common, serious side-effect is weight gain and resulting hyperlipidemia, diabetes, and hypertension (Marder et al., 2004; Newcomer, 2007). These problems substantially increase the risk of cardiovascular problems, such as stroke and heart attack, and reduce life expectancy. Olanzapine and clozapine have the greatest risk, with an average weight gain of 10 pounds during relatively brief research trials. A substantial proportion of patients continue to gain large amounts of weight with ongoing treatment. Ziprasidone and aripiprazole are associated with little or no weight gain. Risperidone, paliperidone, iloperidone, and quetiapine cause intermediate levels of weight gain.

Rehabilitation and Recovery

In people with SPMI, treatment often needs to move beyond medication and psychotherapy to include rehabilitation, services for concurrent disorders such as substance abuse, caregiver services, and peer support. A number of technologies improve outcomes in people with SPMI (Anthony, Cohen, Farkas, & Gagne, 2002). Just as medication treatment is based on diagnostic assessment, rehabilitation begins with an accurate functional assessment (Vaccaro, Pitts, & Wallace, 1992). Functional assessment includes evaluation of the patient's preferences regarding education, work, and leisure as well as their sources of motivation, resources, strengths, major problems, and deficits. Goals are identified and a rehabilitation plan developed. Illness self-management can be improved using psycho-educational and cognitive behavioral interventions that target medication compliance, relapse prevention, and coping with symptoms (Mueser et al., 2002).

Vocational functioning can be improved using Supported Employment (SE), an evidence-based approach that helps people find and keep competitive jobs. SE specialists provide assessment, job finding, and job supports. They provide both the patient and employer with continuing support (SAMHSA Center for Mental Health Services, 2004a). With SE, employment rates in people with SPMI increase from 10% to between 30% and 60% (American Psychiatric Association, 2004). Compared to traditional vocational rehabilitation, individuals receiving SE are more likely to be competitively employed and earn higher wages (Cook et al., 2005).

Outcomes in patients can also be substantially improved through the use of interventions that target family members and other caregivers (American Psychiatric Association, 2004; Glynn, Cohen, Dixon, & Niv, 2006; Cohen et al., 2008). Family psycho-education, a long-term form of family intervention, has a positive effect on outcomes for patients and their family members. Interventions vary, but generally include education regarding mental illness and its treatment, communication training, development of problem-solving skills, and assistance with crises. Interventions that educate and involve family members for at least nine months have consistently reduced relapse and facilitated recovery. Shorter-term family interventions increase knowledge and coping with the illness and decrease burden for family members, but have little to no impact on relapse rates or re-hospitalization. The National Alliance on Mental Illness, a leading national consumer organization, has disseminated structured "family to family" programs involving education and support.

Finally, there is increasing interest in peer support. Peer support is a structured process whereby people with SPMI provide assistance to each other (Davidson, Chinman, Sells, & Rowe, 2006a). It is based upon the belief that people with chronic disorders can help themselves and each other achieve better outcomes in their treatment and their lives. Though peer support groups are not widely available, they have been increasing in number. Schizophrenics Anonymous, Recovery Inc., and GROW are peer support organizations with groups operating around the world. In these organizations, persons with mental illness meet on a regular basis and discuss, for instance, stigma, employment, interpersonal issues, medication, symptoms, and how they are coping with their disorders. This process can provide new information and perspectives, while facilitating vicarious learning and enhancement of problem-solving skills (Chinman, Young, Hassell, & Davidson, 2006). Peer support may help individuals make best use of treatment while creating dense social networks and exposing them to role models who provide hope for recovery (Lucksted, McNulty, Brayboy, & Forbes, 2009).

Homelessness

Homelessness is a term that has been used to encompass a range of human conditions, from individuals who live on the streets every night to those who live in shelters, hotels, public facilities, vehicles, or with friends and family. In most cases, homelessness is a temporary circumstance. It has been estimated that 3.5 million people in the United States experience homelessness during a given year and 700,000 people are homeless on any given night (National Coalition for the Homeless, 2009a). When one focuses on the persistent "street homeless," about one-quarter have a serious mental illness, and two-thirds have an alcohol or drug use disorder (Koegel et al., 1999; SAMHSA Center for Mental Health Services, 2003).

A variety of factors contribute to homelessness (Sullivan, Burnam, Koegel, & Hollenberg, 2000; Bianco & Wells, 2001). Poverty is certainly the greatest contributor, and poor people must often choose between food, housing, health care, and child care. Other individual risk factors include having severe mental illness, a substance abuse disorder, a history of physical or sexual abuse, poor family relationships, and a childhood history of unstable housing. People who become homeless often have multiple risk factors. The lack of comprehensive services also contributes to homelessness.

Massive street homelessness, as we know it today, emerged in the 1980s, when employment and housing options began to diminish rapidly for people with low incomes (National Coalition for the Homeless, 2009b). Federal funding for affordable housing was cut by more than 75% (Lezak & Edgar, 1996). There was a loss of low-cost housing options, such as Single Room Occupancy hotels, that provide rooms by the week or month, and small, inexpensive rooms for rent. Shelters in major cities were eliminated. Housing that remained affordable was typically unsafe, in bad condition, or located far from mental health services and public transportation. Finally, starting in the 1980s, employment opportunities worsened for large segments of the workforce, and many people had their disability income terminated by the federal government. Those remaining on SSI and SSDI have had to cope with benefits that, over time, have fallen far below what would be required to obtain decent housing.

Inadequate access to affordable and appropriate housing has become an especially important problem for people with SPMI (O'Hara, 2007). For years, the disabled have not been part of mainstream housing policy debates, and no one agency has been responsible for the range of services necessary to meet a homeless person's needs (Bianco & Wells, 2001). Efforts to create services for the homeless often devolve into "not in my backyard" opposition. Within mental health, adequate housing has not consistently been considered part of treatment services (Newman, 2001). As a result, many clinical agencies lack evidence-based housing services, while housing agencies do not manage mental health and substance abuse services. At the same time, state vocational rehabilitation agencies have preferred to focus on people who do not have SPMI because they are easier to return to work.

Evidence-based care for the homeless with SPMI includes support for housing combined with mental health treatment (Martinez & Burt, 2006). The "housing first" approach starts by creating affordable housing options such as community residential facilities, supervised apartments, board and care homes, and SRO hotels. Treatment includes outreach to the homeless and assertive provision of mental health services (Rosenheck, Kasprow, W., Frisman, L., & Liu-Mares, 2003). This can be performed by ACT (Coldwell & Bender, 2007) or mobile treatment teams. In a New York City program, rapid housing placement was followed by assertive community-based treatment. In a population of homeless individuals with mental illness, 88% remained housed at five years, as opposed to 47% with traditional services (Tsemberis & Eisenberg, 2000). Unfortunately, high quality programs for the homeless are usually not available.

There have been many legislative, programmatic, and research activities with the goal of improving care for the homeless. In 1987, the first federal legislation, the McKinney-Vento Homeless Assistance Act, was passed. The McKinney-Vento Act established a variety of programs and services, such as emergency food and shelter programs, the PATH program (Projects for Assistance in Transition from

Homelessness), and community-based services for people who had a serious mental illness, co-occurring disorder, and were at risk for homelessness (Bianco & Wells, 2001). The homeless assistance grant programs created by the McKinney-Vento Act were reauthorized with the passing of the Homeless Emergency Assistance and Rapid Transition to Housing Act of 2008. Changes to existing programs include the expansion of homelessness prevention programs and new incentives for rapid re-housing, especially for homeless families. In 1988, The Fair Housing Amendments Act was passed to help decrease stigma and discrimination against persons with mental illness in the housing market.

The U.S. Department of Housing and Urban Development (HUD) supports a number of programs to promote a comprehensive housing and mental health community. To receive funds, communities must engage in a strategic planning and grant process called a Consolidated Plan. These are local housing and community development plans that consolidate applications for funds from various HUD programs. Also, HUD directly subsidizes rents for many people who are poor or disabled with the "Section 8" program. However, Section 8 is severely underfunded, and it can take years or be impossible for qualifying individuals to get a housing voucher.

Given the inadequate federal response to homelessness, state and local officials have employed a variety of prevention and treatment strategies. Eight-hundred sixty cities and counties have developed 10-year plans to end homelessness using a Housing First approach, and 49 states have established Interagency Councils on Homelessness. Examples of services for individuals with SPMI include providing substance abuse experts on ACT teams in Illinois; developing independent living skills training, support, and service linkages to people in scattered site apartments in Michigan; working with local Public Defenders in the release of jail inmates at risk for homelessness in Florida; enhancing crisis services in New York; developing an integrated community at Los Angeles Men's Place (LAMP); creating a non-profit housing development corporation in Rhode Island; and providing rent subsidies in Massachusetts. Creating these programs has required concerted efforts by key stakeholders to engage in strategic planning and maximize scarce resources from all levels of government (Marcos, Cohen, Nardacci, & Brittain, 1990; Lowery, 1992; Linkins, Brya, & Chandler, 2008).

There have been many successful "model" programs for homelessness. However, these have not generalized more broadly and have, therefore, only served a small fraction of homeless persons with SPMI. Model programs often have special, limited funding, either from a research grant, private foundation, or a governmental agency. They are typically designed to meet a defined need, such as demonstrating the effectiveness of a service model or convincing constituents that something is being done about a problem without actually allocating the necessary resources. Also, model programs are often not clearly defined or systematically evaluated. Program evaluations frequently lack adequate research methods and pay little attention to critical contextual factors (Newman, 2001). This has made it difficult to know how to proceed with program dissemination. Bridging the gap between research and practice in homelessness services is likely to require major policy changes and substantially more resources than is usually acknowledged.

Key Problems in Mental Health Care

POOR PUBLIC INFORMATION AND STIGMA

Many, if not most, people in the United States are poorly informed about mental illness, and stigma pervades all social, political, and economic domains associated with mental health care (Draine, Salzer, Culhane, & Hadley, 2002; Corrigan, 2004). For instance, press coverage often implies that too many people are taking antidepressants or getting counseling. In reality, while some people may be receiving unnecessary treatment, most people with mental illness get no treatment at all (McAlpine & Mechanic, 2000; Young et al., 2001). Similarly, there is a great deal of press when a person with untreated mental illness commits a violent crime. Although people with severe mental illness are at somewhat higher risk for violence than the general population, the vast majority of people with SPMI are not violent. Most risk for violence in people with SPMI is accounted for by other factors, primarily drug and alcohol abuse, or a history of physical abuse, recent divorce, unemployment, or victimization (Elbogen & Johnson, 2009).

Stigma has decreased over the past few decades. Clinicians have been increasingly likely to detect and diagnose depression and to prescribe antidepressant medications. Simultaneously, national rates of suicide have been decreasing substantially. However, both these trends reversed abruptly in late 2003, when the U.S. Food and Drug Administration warned that antidepressant medications can cause an increase in suicidal thinking in children (Libby, Orton, & Valuck, 2009). This increase occurs only during the first month of treatment, not one antidepressant-associated suicide has been identified, and there is no effect in people older than 25 years. The intention of the warning was to increase monitoring in children in order to detect this rare side-effect. However, the unintended result was a persistent, substantial decrease in the diagnosis and treatment of depression in adults, as well as an increase in rates of suicide in both children and adults.

Stigma and poor public information remain severe problems and continue to undercut appropriate demand for services. For instance, although mental illness is common among all socioeconomic groups, people do not believe they are at risk to develop mental illness. Therefore, they do not consider coverage for mental illness treatment when they choose their insurance, creating little demand for adequate coverage. Many people with private insurance do not even know that they have mental health coverage. A similar information problem exists with schizophrenia and bipolar disorder. People do not understand that they and their children have a substantial risk of developing SPMI, so they do not adequately support private insurance coverage or high quality public services for these disorders. Campaigns exist to "stamp out" stigma (www.nami.org), though there is clearly much more work to be done.

INADEQUATE ATTENTION TO TREATMENT QUALITY

To improve care, it is necessary to first understand the quality of current treatment services. Fortunately, it is possible to reliably and accurately measure the quality of health care, including mental health treatment (Hermann, 2005; Brook, 2009a). The Institute of Medicine has defined the quality of care as the extent to which health services "increase the likelihood of desired health outcomes and are consistent with current professional knowledge" (Institute of Medicine, 1999). Quality is measured in three domains: the structure, the process, and the outcomes of care (Donabedian, 1980). The *structure* of care includes organizational factors, such as insurance benefits, staffing, buildings, and hours of operation. For example, is there adequate financing and are there clinicians who are competent to provide needed services? The *process* of care consists of the services that patients actually receive. For instance, does someone with major depression receive psychotherapy or antidepressant medication? The *outcomes* of care are domains that are inherently important. For instance, does someone's depression improve, can they return to work, and how satisfied are they with the treatment received? Conceptually, the structure of care affects the process of care, which in turn affects the outcomes of care (Schuster, McGlynn, & Brook, 1998; Wells, 1999). Patient and environmental factors are also very important and directly affect both the process of care and outcomes. In fact, medical care has a weaker effect on patient outcomes than factors such as genetics, severity of illness, and available resources.

It seems appealing, at first, to study only the outcomes of care. For example, over time, do patients at a clinic get better, worse, or stay the same? Unfortunately, while outcomes are inherently important, poor outcomes have many causes. For instance, if patients at one clinic have worse quality of life than patients at a second clinic, this could be because the first clinic is particularly good at keeping severely ill patients in care (Young et al., 2000b). In addition, knowing outcomes provides little information about how to improve care. For example, patients at a clinic may have a high rate of psychotic symptoms. Is that because clinicians lack critical competencies, because patients do not receive appropriate medication treatment, or because needed medications are not on formulary? Since a major goal of quality measurement is to inform quality improvement, one must measure processes that strongly affect outcomes and that can be improved. This requires information regarding how often patients are accessing or dropping out of care, information on the clinical status of patients, and information on treatment delivery. Given a patient's clinical needs, are they receiving the appropriate treatments?

Quality problems can be grouped into three categories: under-use, over-use, and error (Chassin, 1996). Under-use occurs when an individual does not receive a treatment that would be beneficial. This is the most common problem in people with mental illness. Over-use occurs when people receive treatments that would be expected to provide little or no benefit. Unnecessary procedures should be avoided since they have little potential for benefit, leaving complications and side-effects as the predominant outcomes. Over-use is, for instance, a common problem with cardiac procedures and back surgery (Larequi-Lauber et al., 1997; Brook, 2009b). Error occurs when a mistake is made. For example, many patients with schizophrenia are receiving the wrong medication treatment and having unnecessary psychosis or side-effects (Young, Niv et al., 2008). It is important to note that while cost is often a consideration, it is not a domain of quality. However, it is possible to evaluate both the cost of a given treatment and the extent to which it improves patient outcomes. By examining a "cost-effectiveness" ratio or comparing the effectiveness of alternative treatments, policymakers can prioritize treatments when resources are limited (Gold, Siegel, Russell, & Weistein, 1996; Institute of Medicine, 2008a; Volpp & Das, 2009).

NEED FOR QUALITY IMPROVEMENT

In depressive and anxiety disorders, about two-thirds of people with a disorder receive no mental health treatment at all (Young et al., 2001). People are particularly unlikely to access mental health care if they have no insurance or insurance that is not managed (McAlpine & Mechanic, 2000; Wells et al., 2002). Only one-fifth of people with a disorder see a mental health specialist. However, 80% of people with a disorder have seen a health care professional within the past year. This is usually a visit in primary care, where rates of psychotherapy and medication treatment are low. For these reasons, efforts to improve care for depression should reach out to and identify people with a disorder, increasing the likelihood that they will receive treatment. Care models exist that do this in primary care. These care models are feasible and affordable to implement, and they substantially improve care and outcomes (Wells et al., 2000; Wells et al., 2004). Despite this, they have not been widely adopted. Even worse, organizations that adopted these care models during special projects have subsequently dropped them, despite evidence that they were improving care. While stigma contributes to this, a particular problem is that the costs of treating mental illness accrue to practices and insurance plans, while the benefits accrue to patients, families, and society. This leaves health care practices and insurance companies with little incentive to improve mental health care.

In bipolar disorder and schizophrenia, researchers have found different, though no less serious, quality problems. These disorders are usually managed by mental health specialists, often at busy, underfunded public mental health clinics. The most effective and efficient care is provided by a team of professionals that includes psychologists, social workers, nurses, psychiatrists, other mental health workers, and primary care practitioners. In an effort to minimize treatment costs, there has been an impressive loss of clinical professionals from these facilities over the past several decades. Whereas once doctoral staff had prominent roles at public mental health clinics, today the typical clinician is a masters-level social worker or a "mental health worker" with little clinical training (Hoge et al., 2005). New, effective treatments require highly trained staff who possess specific clinical competencies. "Competencies" are the values, knowledge, and skills that are required to deliver high quality care (Young et al., 2000a). National projects have developed sets of core competencies for the workforce caring for people with SPMI and have concluded that these are usually not present in current clinicians (Hoge et al., 2005).

To improve care broadly, it will be necessary to make quality measurement a routine part of mental health care. While this is not yet the case in mental health, there has been more progress in general medical care. Nationally, there are countless efforts evaluating the quality of medical care and providing information to guide health care purchasing, consumer choice, and quality improvement. This is clearly needed. Compared with other industrialized nations, the current U.S. health care system produces among the worst health outcomes at twice the cost.

Though this represents an unprecedented level of wasteful spending, vested inter-est groups, such as insurance companies, pharmaceutical manufacturers, hospitals, and physicians, are very powerful and have been an obstacle to quality improve-ment. For example, until the late 1990s, the Agency for HealthCare Policy and Research (AHCPR) funded numerous national projects to evaluate and improve the quality of care. In one project, experts concluded that most back surgery was unnecessary, a finding that was quite unpopular among surgeons. AHCPR was almost eliminated by the Congress, and it continued only with much reduced fund-ing and a narrower name, the Agency for Healthcare Research and Quality (AHRQ). No longer focused on policy, AHRQ now works to inform improvement in health care quality, costs, outcomes, and patient safety. AHRQ sponsors research, dis-seminates scientific findings, and develops an annual report on national trends in health care quality. For example, AHRQ has developed the National Guideline Clearinghouse, a comprehensive database of evidence-based clinical practice guide-lines, and the National Quality Measures Clearinghouse, a directory of evidence-based quality measures.

Efforts to improve the value of health care have been led primarily by purchas-ers, such as large corporations, Medicare, and the Department of Veterans Affairs. One central organization has been the National Council on Quality Assurance, an independent organization with substantial funding from insurance companies. It develops a report card, the Health Plan Employer Data and Information Set (HEDIS), which uses computerized data from health care organizations. HEDIS focuses on measures of quality that can be assessed using computerized data that already exist or that can be readily obtained. For instance, it is possible to use billing data to estimate vaccination rates. A limitation of this approach is that candidate measures should improve when health plans and providers improve their informa-tion systems. In mental health, better information often reveals that care is worse than expected. Failure to diagnose a disorder (such as depression) is not easily detected. Also, HEDIS reporting is voluntary. Not surprisingly, plans with poor performance are less likely to report their HEDIS results (McCormick et al., 2002).

In mental health, HEDIS started with one quality measure: the rate of outpa-tient follow-up after hospitalization for a mood disorder. The usefulness of this measure appears to be limited (Druss & Rosenheck, 1997). Subsequently, HEDIS has added measures, including antidepressant prescribing for patients diagnosed with a mood disorder. A limitation of this measure is that detection of depression is typically poor, and organizations that work to improve detection could actually look worse. In mood disorders, accurate quality measures may require systematic screening regarding which plan members have the disorder.

The VA has become a leader in quality measurement. Until the 1980s, the VA was regarded as a backwater of health care that delivered mediocre care at best. In the 1990s, the VA implemented routine, comprehensive assessment of quality. This was made feasible by moving to a fully electronic medical record. The pay and job performance ratings of VA medical center executives were linked to the perfor-mance of their health care systems. National report cards were developed with key indicators. With this focus on quality, the VA transformed into the national leader in health care quality (Jha et al., 2003; Asch et al., 2004). In mental health, however, performance improvement has been limited by the paucity of routine clinical information in the medical record (see Chapter 4 in this volume for additional information on quality).

There has also been a growing attentiveness to consumer's perspectives in the mental health system (Tomes, 2006; Happell, 2008). The recovery model emphasizes a service environment in which consumers have control over decisions about their care. The recovery model is based on the concepts of strengths, natural supports, and empowerment, positing that those who have greater control and choice in their treatment will be able to take increased control and initiative in their lives (Davidson et al., 2006b) (see Chapter 20 in this volume for more information on recovery).

As the concept of "consumer-centered care" has grown, there have been prominent efforts to measure consumer satisfaction with mental health treatment. In general medical care, experience of care and detailed consumer satisfaction have been widely assessed using instruments such as the Consumer Assessment of Health Plans Survey (see www.cahps.ahrq.gov). A companion survey for mental health is the Experience of Care and Health Outcomes (ECHO) survey (see http://www.cahps.ahrq.gov/cahpskit/ECHO/ECHOchooseQX1.asp). ECHO evaluates, from the patient's perspective, promptness of treatment, communication with clinicians, patient involvement in decision-making, information about self-help and treatment options, information regarding medication side effects, and policy administrative services (Eselius et al., 2008). In the public sector and patients with SPMI, a leading effort to evaluate satisfaction has been the Mental Health Statistical Improvement Program (MHSIP; www.mhsip.org). MHSIP includes a survey of satisfaction and subjective experience with care that has been used at mental health clinics across the nation (Jerrell, 2006).

There are challenges to the use of satisfaction surveys. The most important issue pertains to how people are selected to complete these surveys. Access is a major problem in private and public sector care, and one would like to survey all people in need of treatment, or, at the very least, the population of people with any clinician contact. However, to do this requires substantial effort. Especially in the public sector, most surveys focus on convenient groups of patients in regular care, patients who may not be representative of the population of interest (Young et al., 2000b). While satisfaction is inherently important, it is just one of several domains of quality. Correlations between satisfaction and the technical quality of care are modest (Edlund et al., 2003). Health care is complex, and few patients have the expertise to determine whether they are receiving appropriate care.

To obtain a comprehensive picture of organizational performance, "report cards" have been created that encompass a number of domains of health care quality. In research studies, these report cards have influenced consumer choice of health plans (Faber et al., 2009). However, their practical usefulness has been limited (Farley et al., 2002; Hibbard, Stockard, & Tusler, 2005). Individuals typically have few affordable health care choices. Even when there is more than one insurance plan available, there is often only one mental health plan. Also, quality information is complex, with many potential indicators. When individuals make purchasing decisions, such as buying a car, they may investigate the overall quality of the automobile by turning to their experience, friends, reviews, or Consumer

Reports. But they are not likely to study the quality of the transmission or water pump. For quality information to become useful, health care reform will need to create genuine choices for consumers and standardize methods for summarizing comprehensive quality assessment.

In the meantime, detailed report cards can be very useful for purchasers of health care, which are usually corporations and governments. Consequently, they are important for integrated health care systems whose care is being purchased. In the public sector, Medicare has begun experimenting with varying reimbursement by performance (Senate Finance Committee, 2009). To date, it has not been possible to affect enough reimbursement to make substantial changes in care. It is clear that this approach can work, if care is organized and the funder pays for a large proportion of a clinician's practice. Currently, financing is too fragmented to make this happen for most private-sector insurance. Organized systems of care, such as "Accountable Care Organizations," have been proposed for Medicare. Also, comprehensive electronic medical records can be used to align finance and quality, as well as disseminate quality improvement to the majority of U.S. clinicians who are found in solo or small group practices (Cys, 2009).

Improving the Quality of Care

FINANCING

Improving mental health care begins by ensuring that there is adequate financing to provide necessary services (Mechanic, 2001; President's New Freedom Commission on Mental Health, 2003). Effective new medication and rehabilitation technologies have been developed and demand has increased, but funding has not increased correspondingly. Mental health treatments are more cost-effective than many other health care services, including many widely used organ transplantation procedures or treatments for cancer. Yet funding is not available to provide comprehensive services to people diagnosed with mental illness, and the large population with a mental disorder but no treatment could overwhelm currently available resources.

Private insurance usually includes benefits for mental health and substance abuse treatment. However, these benefits are much more limited than other components of health care. Over the past decade, national mental health organizations worked to get "parity" legislation enacted to ensure that co-payments, deductibles, and insurance limits are the same as for general medical care. Many states passed parity legislation, and this improved coverage under insurance plans that previously had limited mental health benefits (Branstrom & Sturm, 2002). However, federal law exempts insurance plans of large corporations from state legislation. In the late 1990s, the federal government mandated parity in the health benefits program used by federal employees. A research evaluation of this large experiment found that parity reduced out-of-pocket costs for families and individuals affected by mental illness, with little or no increase in overall costs (Goldman et al., 2006). This experience provided support for a federal parity mandate. The Wellstone-Domenici Mental Health Parity and Addiction Equity Act was enacted in 2008 and took effect in 2010. This Act applies to corporations with 50 or more employees if they choose to provide mental health or substance abuse coverage. Under such benefits, all financial requirements (e.g. co-payments) and treatment limitations (e.g. number of visits) must be no more restrictive than medical or surgical benefits.

Parity legislation would not help the more than 47 million people in the United States who have no health insurance. It has been estimated that one-third of these individuals have a mental illness. Federal health care reform that provides insurance to this population would be expected to substantially increase access to mental health insurance.

Although funding is necessary to improve care, it is not sufficient. The evaluation of federal employee parity found that parity did not improve the quality of care (Busch et al., 2006). The prevailing insurance arrangement for mental health is managed behavioral health care, which improves access to low intensity care, such as medication treatment or counseling for acute depressive disorder (Merrick et al., 2009). However, it also limits access to high intensity treatments, such as supported employment, housing, education, or assertive community treatment. Requests for high intensity treatments are often shifted to the public sector, which lacks resources to provide them. Parity of benefit design, including that mandated by the Wellstone-Domenici Act, would not be expected to change these arrangements. Equity of coverage remains elusive (Burnam & Escarce, 1999).

IMPLEMENTING EFFECTIVE TREATMENTS

While current funding levels are too low to provide high quality care to the majority of people with need, important improvements in care are possible within existing budgets. Indeed, these improvements may be a prerequisite to increased funding, since purchasers are often reluctant to increase funding to systems that cannot demonstrate that they are efficiently using existing resources.

Because mental health systems have been plagued by fragmentation of funding, management, and policy, many had assumed that improving coordination would improve care (Kahn & Kamerman, 1992). However, multiple projects to improve system integration have been evaluated, and it has consistently been found that they do not improve the quality of care. The best example was the 1994 Robert Wood Johnson Foundation Program on Chronic Mental Illness. This program established centralized mental health authorities in nine communities across the United States. This consolidated funding and oversight, but did not improve patient care (Lehman et al., 1994).

To successfully improve care, mental health systems can draw on results from the growing field of implementation science (McLaughlin & Kaluzny, 1999; Schouten et al., 2008; Proctor et al., 2009). For example, contrary to popular belief, clinician education typically does not improve care (Davis, Thomson, Oxman, & Haynes, 1995). Little or no effectiveness has been found for continuing medical education, provision of guidelines, or feedback of data on patient status to clinicians. However, a number of multi-faceted approaches have improved service delivery and patient outcomes. The most effective strategies involve reorganizing care, establishing specialized clinics or planned visits, implementing new care models, or using non-physician staff to perform needed activities (Bodenheimer, Wagner, & Grumbach, 2002; Stone et al., 2002). Other effective interventions include patient reminders and changing patients' financial incentives.

There are multiple barriers to improving care for mental illness. In depressive and anxiety disorders, the majority of affected individuals receive no treatment but are seen in primary care settings (Young et al., 2001). As a result, collaborative care models have been developed that improve screening in primary care, create psychotherapy resources in primary care, and include care managers who ensure patient education and use of effective medications and psychotherapy. These care models improve treatment quality and quality of life, keep patients employed, and have positive economic benefits for patients, families, and society (Wells et al., 2004; Roy-Byrne et al., 2005).

In psychotic disorders, such as schizophrenia or bipolar disorder, most patients have treatment contacts at specialty mental health clinics, and evidence-based practices exist in multiple domains. Evidence-based practices include clozapine for persistent psychosis, adherence to mood stabilizers for bipolar disorder, medication changes and psycho-education for side-effects, supported employment for work, and family interventions. Most efforts to improve care will need to attend to the skills that clinicians must possess to provide effective care (Young et al., 2000a). More than three-quarters of clinicians in the United States caring for individuals with SPMI have a bachelor's degree or less education, with little training about severe mental illness or its treatment (Hoge et al., 2005). The situation is not much better in clinicians with masters or doctoral education, since training programs often include little attention to evidence-based practices for SPMI. Clinicians will need to be trained in evidence-based practices, both to ensure referrals and also to provide services (Young et al., 2005).

Clinician education will not be sufficient, however. Beyond education, challenges to improving care differ by domain (Brown et al., 2008). For example, supported employment requires collaboration between a mental health team and an employment specialist. However, the mental health and vocational rehabilitation systems are separated at the federal, state, and local levels. While most relevant funding goes toward rehabilitation, often these funds are allocated for pre-employment activities that do not improve outcomes in people with SPMI. A project to implement supported employment in six states and the District of Columbia was successful, due to a major focus on working with state policymakers to reorganize policies, procedures, and funding (Drake, Becker, Goldman, & Martinez, 2006).

Another approach to improving care is to engage in quality improvement. Traditional quality improvement, sometimes called "Continuous Quality Improvement" (CQI), consists of continually improving the underlying processes associated with providing services by monitoring and finding solutions within practice settings. When studied, CQI has generally not been effective in improving health care (Fischer, Solberg, & Zander, 2001). Some CQI efforts are driven by line clinicians or managers and make too little use of research evidence regarding organizational changes that are necessary to improve outcomes. Other CQI projects are driven by experts, but pay too little attention to the context of care, resulting in limited updates by clinicians and patients. Since both have often not worked, an alternative approach has been developed. "Evidence-Based Quality Improvement" includes partnerships between providers and experts to tailor research evidence to community settings. This has improved the quality of care, though changes have so far been modest (Rubenstein et al., 2006).

IMPROVING CLINICAL INFORMATION

Quality improvement requires accurate data regarding the clinical status of patients. To be feasible, broad quality improvement will likely require electronic medical records (EMRs) that contain this clinical information. The most striking examples of improving care have occurred in integrated health care systems that combined comprehensive EMRs with systematic quality improvement (Jha et al., 2003; Paulus, Davis, & Steele, 2008). These systems keep clinicians informed regarding their patients, and they can be used to monitor treatment quality and identify problems in care to be addressed. It is important to realize that information systems are tools, and as such they can be poorly or well designed and only achieve their potential if they are used to improve care. For example, the VA has succeeded in improving diabetes care. This became possible because the VA EMR contains all the information required to identify patients whose diabetes is poorly controlled or who are not getting appropriate treatments. The VA used this data to improve organizational performance.

In mental health, charts are usually paper-based, and documentation is highly inconsistent with little reliable clinical information (Cradock et al., 2001; Owen et al., 2004). Data on service utilization or billing are, on the other hand, often computerized. Utilization data were used, for example, by the VA to identify and remediate problems in access to and over-use of mental health services (Fontana & Rosenheck, 1997; Rosenheck & Cicchetti, 1998). However, identifying patients who are doing poorly has been nearly impossible. There have been efforts to have clinicians routinely document structured assessments. However, clinicians are generally not trained in assessment instruments, have little time or interest in performing them, and the data produced have not been accurate (Niv et al., 2007). The most promising approach to obtaining clinical data for quality improvement has been to have patients perform self-assessments of psychological status, functioning, and unmet needs, using validated instruments. These can be accurately delivered using forms or computerized kiosks (Chinman et al., 2003) and have been used to improve care (Priebe et al., 2007).

Implications for Mental Health

In the United States, the service system for adults with mental illness has both severe problems and also the potential to produce remarkably good outcomes. An impressive array of effective treatments exists for common disorders such as depression and severe disorders such as schizophrenia. When an individual with mental illness is cared for by competent clinicians and has access to a comprehensive set of psychosocial and medical treatments, outcomes are often excellent. Symptoms can be controlled, side-effects minimized, quality of life improved, and people can return to education and competitive employment. Whereas many people with mental illness once spent years in state hospitals or back rooms, disabled or with poor quality of life, they can now live satisfying, productive lives in the community.

Unfortunately, with the current system, positive outcomes remain the exception, rather than the rule. The most pressing mental health challenge in the United States today is to bring effective care to the *majority* of those in need. This will only be possible with changes in financing, purchasing that is tied to quality, and improvement in the delivery of care. The passage of mental health insurance parity was an important advance. While it will not improve care, it will protect many individuals and families from the risk of very high treatment costs due to mental illness. Health care reform efforts seek to increase the number of people with insurance. This would provide insurance to a large population of individuals with mental illness, thereby providing access to care that is currently lacking. However, even with these advances, people with serious mental illness will continue to lack financing for interventions that are critical for their recovery, such as assertive community treatment or supported employment. To ensure access to medically necessary services, it will be necessary to have insurance coverage that is equal to the coverage provided for other illnesses.

Improved services for mental illness would produce economic benefits for society, a more productive work force for employers, and reductions in homelessness and incarceration. They would strongly benefit ill individuals and their families, including some of the most vulnerable members of our society. However, at present, the costs of implementing services accrue to providers, while the economic benefits accrue to patients, families, and society. In this environment, services are only made available when they are mandated by the government or demanded by purchasers. Both of these are undercut by poor public information about mental illness and poor information about the quality of routine care. Most mental health care purchasing decisions are made by governments and corporations, both of which lack good information about the quality of care that is being provided. As a result, current purchasing decisions are made almost solely on the basis of cost. This has resulted in ongoing reductions in financing and too little improvement in access to needed treatments.

There is interest in improving the transparency of our health care system and improving measures of quality, including measures for mental health disorders. There are also major efforts to improve information, through implementation of both electronic medical records for providers and personal health records that are under the control of individuals. As information improves, consumers and purchasers will be able to tie payment for services to the quality of services received. To survive in an environment where value can be assessed, clinicians and provider organizations will need to form integrated systems that allow them to deploy electronic medical records and quality improvement systems. Although the science of implementation and quality improvement is in an early stage, there is experience from high performing systems, including Geisinger, Kaiser Permanente, and the VA, and opportunities now exist to substantially improve outcomes for individuals with mental illness.

Acknowledgments

This work was supported by the Department of Veterans Affairs and the UCLA-RAND NIMH Partnered Research Center for Quality Care (P30 MH082760). The authors thank Jennifer Magnabosco for contributions to earlier versions of this work. Opinions expressed are only the authors', and do not necessarily represent the views of any affiliated institutions.

References

American Medical Association. (2001). *International Classification of Diseases, 9th revision, Clinical Modification: Physician ICD-9-CM, 2002.* Chicago: AMA Press.

American Psychiatric Association. (2000a). *Diagnostic and Statistical Manual of Mental Disorders DSM-IV-TR.* Washington, DC: American Psychiatric Press.

American Psychiatric Association. (2000b). Practice guideline for the treatment of patients with major depressive disorder (revision). *American Journal of Psychiatry, 157*(Suppl. 4), 49.

American Psychiatric Association. (2002). Practice guideline for the treatment of patients with bipolar disorder (revision). *American Journal of Psychiatry, 159*(Suppl. 4), 1–50.

American Psychiatric Association. (2004). Practice guideline for the treatment of patients with schizophrenia, second edition. *American Journal of Psychiatry, 161*(Suppl. 2), 1–56.

American Psychiatric Association. (2007a). *Practice Guideline for the Treatment of Patients with Obsessive-Compulsive Disorder.* Available online at http://www.psych.org/psych_pract/treatg/pg/prac_guide.cfm. Accessed May 7, 2009.

American Psychiatric Association. (2007b). Treatment of patients with substance use disorders, second edition: American Psychiatric Association. *American Journal of Psychiatry, 164*(Suppl. 4), 5–123.

American Psychiatric Association. (2009). *Practice Guideline for the Treatment of Patients with Panic Disorder* (2nd ed.). Available online at http://www.psych.org/psych_pract/treatg/pg/prac_guide.cfm Accessed May 7, 2009.

Anthony, W. A. (1993). Recovery from mental illness: The guiding vision of the mental health service system in the 1990s. *Psychosocial Rehabilitation Journal, 16*(4), 11–23.

Anthony, W. A., Cohen, M., Farkas, M., & Gagne, C. (2002). *Psychiatric Rehabilitation.* Boston: Boston University Center for Psychiatric Rehabilitation.

Asch, S. M., McGlynn, E. A., Hogan, M. M., et al. (2004). Comparison of quality of care for patients in the Veterans Health Administration and patients in a national sample. *Annals of Internal Medicine, 141*(12), 938–945.

Barrett, J. E., Williams, J. W., Jr., Oxman, T. E., et al. (2001). Treatment of dysthymia and minor depression in primary care: a randomized trial in patients aged 18 to 59 years. *Journal of Family Practice, 50*(5), 405–412.

Bianco, C., & Wells, S. M. (2001). *Overcoming Barriers to Community Integration for People with Mental Illnesses.* Advocates for Human Potential. Available online at www.ahpnet.com/OvercomingBarriers.html. Accessed April 29, 2009.

Bodenheimer, T., Wagner, E. H., & Grumbach, K. (2002). Improving primary care for patients with chronic illness. *Journal of the American Medical Association, 288*(14), 1775–1779.

Branstrom, R. B., & Sturm, R. (2002). Economic grand rounds: An early case study of the effects of California's Mental Health Parity Legislation. *Psychiatric Services, 53*(10), 1215–1216.

Brook, R. H. (2009a). Assessing the appropriateness of care: Its time has come. *Journal of the American Medical Association, 302*(9), 997–998.

Brook, R. H. (2009b). The science of health care reform. *Journal of the American Medical Association*, *301*(23), 2486–2487.

Brown, A. H., Cohen, A. N., Chinman, M. J., et al. (2008). EQUIP: Implementing chronic care principles and applying formative evaluation methods to improve care for schizophrenia: QUERI Series. *Implementation Science*, *3*, 9.

Bryant, R. A., Mastrodomenico, J., Felmingham, K. L., et al. (2008). Treatment of acute stress disorder: A randomized controlled trial. *Archives of General Psychiatry*, *65*(6), 659–667.

Burnam, M. A., & Escarce, J. J. (1999). Equity in managed care for mental disorders. *Health Affairs*, *18*(5), 22–31.

Busch, A. B., Huskamp, H. A., Normand, S. L., et al. (2006). The impact of parity on major depression treatment quality in the Federal Employees' Health Benefits Program after parity implementation. *Medical Care*, *44*(6), 506–512.

California Mental Health Association. (2000). Gold Achievement Award: A comprehensive treatment program helps persons with severe mental illness integrate into the community; MHA Village, Long Beach, California. *Psychiatric Services*, *51*(11), 1436–1438.

Canadian Psychiatric Association. (2006). Clinical practice guidelines for the management of anxiety disorders: Generalized anxiety disorder. *Canadian Journal of Psychiatry*, *51*(2), 51S–55S.

Catlin, A., Cowan, C., Hartman, M., & Heffler, S. (2008). National health spending in 2006: A year of change for prescription drugs. *Health Affairs*, *27*(1), 14–29.

Chassin, M. R. (1996). Quality of health care: Part 3, Improving the quality of care. *New England Journal of Medicine*, *335*(14), 1060–1063.

Chassin, M. R. (2002). Achieving and sustaining improved quality: Lessons from New York State and cardiac surgery. *Health Affairs*, *21*(4), 40–51.

Chinman, M., Young, A. S., Hassell, J., & Davidson, L. (2006). Toward the implementation of mental health consumer provider services. *Journal of Behavioral Health Services and Research*, *33*(2), 176–195.

Chinman, M., Young, A. S., Rowe, M., et al. (2003). An instrument to assess competencies of providers treating severe mental illness. *Mental Health Services Research*, *5*(2), 97–108.

Cohen, A. N., Glynn, S. M., Murray-Swank, A. B., et al. (2008). The family forum: Directions for the implementation of family psychoeducation for severe mental illness. *Psychiatric Services*, *59*(1), 40–48.

Coldwell, C. M., & Bender, W. S. (2007). The effectiveness of assertive community treatment for homeless populations with severe mental illness: A meta-analysis. *American Journal of Psychiatry*, *164*(3), 393–399.

Commonwealth Fund Commission on a High Performance Health System. (2008). *Why Not the Best? Results from the National Scorecard on U.S. Health System Performance*. Available online at http://www.commonwealthfund.org/Content/Publications/Fund-Reports/2008/Jul/Why-Not-the-Best--Results-from-the-National-Scorecard-on-U-S--Health-System-Performance--2008.aspx. Accessed May 7, 2009.

Cook, J. A., Leff, H. S., Blyler, C. R., et al. (2005). Results of a multisite randomized trial of supported employment interventions for individuals with severe mental illness. *Archives of General Psychiatry*, *62*(5), 505–512.

Correll, C. U., Leucht, S., & Kane, J. M. (2004). Lower risk for tardive dyskinesia associated with second-generation antipsychotics: A systematic review of 1-year studies. *American Journal of Psychiatry*, *161*(3), 414–425.

Corrigan, P. (2004). How stigma interferes with mental health care. *American Psychologist*, *59*(7), 614–625.

Cradock, J., Young, A. S., & Sullivan, G. (2001). The accuracy of medical record documentation in schizophrenia. *Journal of Behavioral Health Services and Research*, *28*(4), 456–465.

Criminal Justice Mental Health Consensus Project. (2002). *Project Report*. Council of State Governments. Available online at http://consensusproject.org. Accessed May 7, 2009.

Cys, J. (2009). *Accountable Care Organizations: A New Idea for Managing Medicare*. Chicago: American Medical News. Available online at http://www.ama-assn.org/amednews/2009/08/31/gvsao831.htm. Accessed September 15, 2009.

Davidson, L., Chinman, M., Sells, D., & Rowe, M. (2006a). Peer support among adults with serious mental illness: A report from the field. *Schizophrenia Bulletin, 32*(3), 443–450.

Davidson, L., Tondora, J., Staeheli, M., et al. (2006b). Recovery guides: An emerging model of community-based care for adults with psychiatric disabilities. In A. Lightburn & P. Sessions (Eds.), *Handbook of Community-Based Clinical Practice* (pp. 476–513). New York: Oxford University Press.

Davis, D. A., Thomson, M. A., Oxman, A. D., & Haynes, R. B. (1995). Changing physician performance: A systematic review of the effect of continuing medical education strategies. *Journal of the American Medical Association, 274*(9), 700–705.

Davis, K. (2007). Uninsured in America: Problems and possible solutions. *British Medical Journal, 334*(7589), 346–348.

Docteur, E., & Berenson, R. A. (2009). *How Does the Quality of U.S. Health Care Compare Internationally?* Washington, DC: Urban Institute. Available online at http://www.urban.org/url.cfm?ID=411947. Accessed September 15, 2009.

Donabedian, A. (1980). *Explorations in Quality Assessment and Monitoring: Volume 1, The Definition of Quality and Approaches to Its Assessment*. Ann Arbor, MI: Health Administration Press.

Draine, J., Salzer, M. S., Culhane, D. P., & Hadley, T. R. (2002). Role of social disadvantage in crime, joblessness, and homelessness among persons with serious mental illness. *Psychiatric Services, 53*(5), 565–573.

Drake, R. E., Becker, D. R., Goldman, H. H., & Martinez, R. A. (2006). Best practices: The Johnson & Johnson-Dartmouth community mental health program; Disseminating evidence-based practice. *Psychiatric Services, 57*(3), 302–304.

Druss, B., & Rosenheck, R. (1997). Evaluation of the HEDIS measure of behavioral health care quality: Health Plan Employer Data and Information Set. *Psychiatric Services, 48*(1), 71–75.

Druss, B. G., & von Esenwein, S. A. (2006). Improving general medical care for persons with mental and addictive disorders: Systematic review. *General Hospital Psychiatry, 28*(2), 145–153.

Edlund, M. J., Young, A. S., Kung, F. Y., et al. (2003). Does satisfaction reflect the technical quality of mental health care? *Health Services Research, 38*(2), 631–645.

Elbogen, E. B., & Johnson, S. C. (2009). The intricate link between violence and mental disorder: Results from the National Epidemiologic Survey on Alcohol and Related Conditions. *Archives of General Psychiatry, 66*(2), 152–161.

Eselius, L. L., Cleary, P. D., Zaslavsky, A. M., et al. (2008). Case-mix adjustment of consumer reports about managed behavioral health care and health plans. *Health Services Research, 43*(6), 2014–2032.

Faber, M., Bosch, M., Wollersheim, H., et al. (2009). Public reporting in health care: How do consumers use quality-of-care information? A systematic review. *Medical Care, 47*(1), 1–8.

Farley, D. O., Elliott, M. N., Short, P. F., et al. (2002). Effect of CAHPS performance information on health plan choices by Iowa Medicaid beneficiaries. *Medical Care Research and Review, 59*(3), 319–336.

Fischer, L. R., Solberg, L. I., & Zander, K. M. (2001). The failure of a controlled trial to improve depression care: A qualitative study. *Joint Commission Journal on Quality Improvement, 27*(12), 639–650.

Fitch, K., Bernstein, S., Aguilar, M. D., et al. (2001). *The RAND/UCLA Appropriateness Method User's Manual*. Santa Monica, CA: RAND.

Fochtmann, L. J., & Gelenberg, A. J. (2005). *Guideline Watch: Practice Guideline for the Treatment of Patients with Major Depressive Disorder* (2nd ed.). Available online at http://www.psychiatryonline.com/content.aspx?aid=148217. Accessed September 8, 2009.

Fontana, A., & Rosenheck, R. (1997). Effectiveness and cost of the inpatient treatment of post-traumatic stress disorder: Comparison of three models of treatment. *American Journal of Psychiatry, 154*(6), 758–765.

Frank, R. G., & Glied, S. (2006). Changes in mental health financing since 1971: Implications for policymakers and patients. *Health Affairs, 25*(3), 601–613.

Glynn, S. M., Cohen, A. N., Dixon, L. B., & Niv, N. (2006). The potential impact of the recovery movement on family interventions for schizophrenia: Opportunities and obstacles. *Schizophrenia Bulletin, 32*(3), 451–463.

Gold, M. R., Siegel, J. E., Russell, L. B., & Weinstein, M. C. (Eds). (1996). *Cost-Effectiveness in Health and Medicine*. New York: Oxford University Press.

Goldman, H. H., Frank, R. G., Burnam, M. A., et al. (2006). Behavioral health insurance parity for federal employees. *New England Journal of Medicine, 354*(13), 1378–1386.

Gottesman, I. I., & Moldin, S. O. (1999). *Schizophrenia & Genetic Risks: A Guide to Genetic Counseling for Consumers, Their Families, and Mental Health Workers*. Available online at www.pbs.org/wgbh/amex/nash/filmmore/ps_genetic.pdf. Accessed May 7, 2009.

Happell, B. (2008). Determining the effectiveness of mental health services from a consumer perspective: Part 2, Barriers to recovery and principles for evaluation. *International Journal of Mental Health Nursing, 17*(2), 123–130.

Harding, C. M., & Zahniser, J. H. (1994). Empirical correction of seven myths about schizophrenia with implications for treatment. *Acta Psychiatrica Scandinavica, 90*(Suppl. 384), 140–146.

Harman, J. S., Edlund, M. J., & Fortney, J. C. (2009). Trends in antidepressant utilization from 2001 to 2004. *Psychiatric Services, 60*, 611–616.

Henry, J. A. (1992). Toxicity of antidepressants: Comparisons with fluoxetine. *International Clinical Psychopharmacology, 6*(Suppl. 6), 22–27.

Hermann, R. C. (2005). *Improving Mental Healthcare: A Guide to Measurement-Based Quality Improvement* Arlington, VA: American Psychiatric Publishing.

Hibbard, J. H., Stockard, J., & Tusler, M. (2005). Hospital performance reports: Impact on quality, market share, and reputation. *Health Affairs, 24*(4), 1150–1160.

Hoge, M. A., Paris, M., Jr., Adger, H., Jr., et al. (2005). Workforce competencies in behavioral health: An overview. *Administration and Policy in Mental Health, 32*(5–6), 593–631.

Holloway, F., & Carson, J. (2001). Case management: An update. *International Journal of Social Psychiatry, 47*(3), 21–31.

Ingram, R. E., & Luxton, D. D. (2005). Vulnerability-Stress Models. In J. Abela (Ed.), *Development of Psychopathology: Stress-Vulnerability Perspectives*. New York: Sage.

Institute of Medicine. (1999). *Measuring the Quality of Health Care*. Washington, DC: National Academies Press.

Institute of Medicine. (2006). *Improving the Quality of Health Care for Mental and Substance-Use Conditions: Quality Chasm Series*. Washington, DC: National Academies Press.

Institute of Medicine. (2008a). *Knowing What Works in Health Care: A Roadmap for the Nation*. Washington, DC: The National Academies Press.

Institute of Medicine. (2008b). *Treatment of Posttraumatic Stress Disorder: An Assessment of the Evidence*. Washington, DC: National Academies Press. Available online at http://www.nap.edu/catalog/11955.html. Accessed September 15, 2009.

Jerrell, J. M. (2006). Psychometrics of the MHSIP Adult Consumer Survey. *Journal of Behavioral Health Services and Research, 33*(4), 483–488.

Jha, A. K., Perlin, J. B., Kizer, K. W., & Dudley, R. A. (2003). Effect of the transformation of the Veterans Affairs Health Care System on the quality of care. *New England Journal of Medicine, 348*(22), 2218–2227.

Kahn, A. J., & Kamerman, S. B. (1992). *Integrating Services Integration: An Overview of Initiatives, Issues, and Possibilities*. New York: National Center for Children.

Kessler, R. C., Chiu, W. T., Demler, O., et al. (2005). Prevalence, severity, and comorbidity of 12-month DSM-IV disorders in the National Comorbidity Survey Replication. *Archives of General Psychiatry*, *62*(6), 617–627.

Kessler, R. C., Heeringa, S., Lakoma, M. D., et al. (2008). Individual and societal effects of mental disorders on earnings in the United States: Results from the national comorbidity survey replication. *American Journal of Psychiatry*, *165*(6), 703–711.

Kissling, W. (1994). Compliance, quality assurance and standards for relapse prevention in schizophrenia. *Acta Psychiatrica Scandinavica*, *382*(Suppl.), 16–24.

Koegel, P., Sullivan, G., Burnam, A., et al. (1999). Utilization of mental health and substance abuse services among homeless adults in Los Angeles. *Medical Care*, *37*(3), 306–317.

Lamb, H. R., & Bachrach, L. L. (2001). Some perspectives on deinstitutionalization. *Psychiatric Services*, *52*(8), 1039–1045.

Larequi-Lauber, T., Vader, J. P., Burnand, B., et al. (1997). Appropriateness of indications for surgery of lumbar disc hernia and spinal stenosis. *Spine*, *22*(2), 203–209.

Lehman, A. F., Kreyenbuhl, J., Buchanan, R. W., et al. (2004). The Schizophrenia Patient Outcomes Research Team (PORT): Updated treatment recommendations 2003. *Schizophrenia Bulletin*, *30*(2), 193–217.

Lehman, A. F., Postrado, L. T., Roth, D., et al. (1994). Continuity of care and client outcomes in the Robert Wood Johnson Foundation program on chronic mental illness. *Milbank Q*, *72*(1), 105–122.

Lerman, P. (1982). *Deinstitutionalization and the Welfare State*. Piscataway, NJ: Rutgers University Press.

Leucht, S., Corves, C., Arbter, D., et al. (2009). Second-generation versus first-generation antipsychotic drugs for schizophrenia: A meta-analysis. *Lancet*, *373*(9657), 31–41.

Lezak, A. D., & Edgar, E. (1996). *Preventing Homelessness among People with Serious Mental Illnesses: A Guide for States*. Policy Research Associates & National Resource Center on Homelessness and Mental Illness. Available online at http://www.nrchmi.samhsa.gov/Resource/View.aspx?id=37525. Accessed May 7, 2009.

Libby, A. M., Orton, H. D., & Valuck, R. J. (2009). Persisting decline in depression treatment after FDA warnings. *Archives of General Psychiatry*, *66*(6), 633–639.

Lindenauer, P. K., Remus, D., Roman, S., et al. (2007). Public reporting and pay for performance in hospital quality improvement. *New England Journal of Medicine*, *356*(5), 486–496.

Linkins, K. W., Brya, J. J., & Chandler, D. W. (2008). *Frequent Users of Health Services Initiative: Final Evaluation Report*. California Endowment and California HealthCare Foundation. Available online at http://documents.csh.org/documents/fui/FUHSIEvaluationReportFINAL.pdf

Lowery, M. (1992). LAMP in L.A.'s skid row: A model for community-based support services. *New Directions for Mental Health Services*, *56*, 89–98.

Lucksted, A., McNulty, K., Brayboy, L., & Forbes, C. (2009). Initial evaluation of the Peer-to-Peer program. *Psychiatric Services*, *60*(2), 250–253.

Lurie, N., Ward, N. B., Shapiro, M. F., et al. (1986). Termination of Medi-Cal benefits: A follow-up study one year later. *New England Journal of Medicine*, *314*(19), 1266–1268.

Manderscheid, R. W., & Berry, J. T. (Eds.). (2006). *Mental Health, United States, 2004*. Rockville, MD: Center for Mental Health Services, Substance Abuse and Mental Health Services Administration.

Marcos, L. R., Cohen, N. L., Nardacci, D., & Brittain, J. (1990). Psychiatry takes to the streets: The New York City initiative for the homeless mentally ill. *American Journal of Psychiatry*, *147*(11), 1557–1561.

Marder, S. R., Essock, S. M., Miller, A. L., et al. (2002). The Mount Sinai conference on the pharmacotherapy of schizophrenia. *Schizophrenia Bulletin*, *28*(1), 5–16.

Marder, S. R., Essock, S. M., Miller, A. L., et al. (2004). Physical health monitoring of patients with schizophrenia. *American Journal of Psychiatry*, *161*(8), 1334–1349.

Mark, T. L., Levit, K. R., Buck, J. A., et al. (2007). Mental health treatment expenditure trends, 1986–2003. *Psychiatric Services*, *58*(8), 1041–1048.

Martinez, T. E., & Burt, M. R. (2006). Impact of permanent supportive housing on the use of acute care health services by homeless adults. *Psychiatric Services*, *57*(7), 992–999.

McAlpine, D. D., & Mechanic, D. (2000). Utilization of specialty mental health care among persons with severe mental illness: The roles of demographics, need, insurance, and risk. *Health Services Research*, *35*(1, Pt. 2), 277–292.

McCormick, D., Himmelstein, D. U., Woolhandler, S., et al. (2002). Relationship between low quality-of-care scores and HMOs' subsequent public disclosure of quality-of-care scores. *Journal of the American Medical Association*, *288*(12), 1484–1490.

McLaughlin, C. P., & Kaluzny, A. D. (1999). *Continuous Quality Improvement in Health Care: Theory, Implementation, and Applications*. Boston: Jones & Bartlett Publishers.

Mechanic, D. (1986). The challenge of chronic mental illness: A retrospective and prospective view. *Hospital and Community Psychiatry*, *37*(9), 891–896.

Mechanic, D. (2001). Closing gaps in mental health care for persons with serious mental illness. *Health Services Research*, *36*(6, Pt. 1), 1009–1017.

Mechanic, D. (2007). Barriers to help-seeking, detection, and adequate treatment for anxiety and mood disorders: Implications for health care policy. *Journal of Clinical Psychiatry*, *68*(Suppl. 2), 20–26.

Merrick, E. L., Horgan, C. M., Garnick, D. W., et al. (2009). Accessing specialty behavioral health treatment in private health plans. *Journal of Behavioral Health Services and Research*, *36*(4), 420–435.

Morden, N. E., Mistler, L. A., Weeks, W. B., & Bartels, S. J. (2009). Health care for patients with serious mental illness: Family medicine's role. *Journal of the American Board of Family Medicine*, *22*(2), 187–195.

Mueser, K. T., Corrigan, P. W., Hilton, D. W., et al. (2002). Illness management and recovery: A review of the research. *Psychiatric Services*, *53*(10), 1272–1284.

National Association of State Mental Health Program Directors Research Institute. (2005). *Results of a Survey of State Directors of Adult and Child Mental Health Services on Implementation of Evidence-Based Practices*. Alexandria, VA: National Association of State Mental Health Program Directors. Available online at http://www.nri-inc.org/reports_pubs/2005/EBPLilly FullReport2005.pdf. Accessed May 7, 2009.

National Coalition for the Homeless. (2009a). *How Many People Experience Homelessness?* Available online at http://www.nationalhomeless.org/factsheets/How_Many.html. Accessed September 20, 2009.

National Coalition for the Homeless. (2009b). *Why Are People Homeless?* Available online at http:// www.nationalhomeless.org/factsheets/why.html. Accessed September 20, 2009.

Newcomer, J. W. (2007). Metabolic considerations in the use of antipsychotic medications: A review of recent evidence. *Journal of Clinical Psychiatry*, *68*(Suppl. 1), 20–27.

Newman, S. J. (2001). Housing attributes and serious mental illness: Implications for research and practice. *Psychiatric Services*, *52*(10), 1309–1317.

Niv, N., Cohen, A. N., Mintz, J., et al. (2007). The validity of using patient self-report to assess psychotic symptoms in schizophrenia. *Schizophrenia Research*, *90*(1–3), 245–250.

O'Hara, A. (2007). Housing for people with mental illness: Update of a report to the President's New Freedom Commission. *Psychiatric Services*, *58*(7), 907–913.

Owen, R. R., Thrush, C. R., & Cannon, D., et al. (2004). Use of electronic medical record data for quality improvement in schizophrenia treatment. *Journal of the American Medical Informatics Association*, *11*(5), 351–357.

Palmer, B. A., Pankratz, V. S., & Bostwick, J. M. (2005). The lifetime risk of suicide in schizophrenia: A reexamination. *Archives of General Psychiatry*, *62*(3), 247–253.

Paulus, R. A., Davis, K., & Steele, G. D. (2008). Continuous innovation in health care: Implications of the Geisinger experience. *Health Affairs, 27*(5), 1235–1245.

Perala, J., Suvisaari, J., Saarni, S. I., et al. (2007). Lifetime prevalence of psychotic and bipolar I disorders in a general population. *Archives of General Psychiatry, 64*(1), 19–28.

President's New Freedom Commission on Mental Health. (2003). *Achieving the Promise: Transforming Mental Health Care in America*. Available online at http://www.mentalhealth commission.gov/reports/reports.htm. Accessed May 7, 2009.

Priebe, S., McCabe, R., Bullenkamp, J., et al. (2007). Structured patient-clinician communication and 1-year outcome in community mental healthcare: Cluster randomised controlled trial. *British Journal of Psychiatry, 191*, 420–426.

Proctor, E. K., Landsverk, J., Aarons, G., et al. (2009). Implementation research in mental health services: An emerging science with conceptual, methodological, and training challenges. *Administration and Policy in Mental Health, 36*(1), 24–34.

Rosenheck, R., & Cicchetti, D. (1998). A mental health program report card: A multidimensional approach to performance monitoring in public sector programs. *Community Mental Health Journal, 34*(1), 85–106.

Rosenheck, R., Kasprow, W., Frisman, L., & Liu-Mares, W. (2003). Cost-effectiveness of supported housing for homeless persons with mental illness. *Archives of General Psychiatry, 60*(9), 940–951.

Roshanaei-Moghaddam, B., & Katon, W. (2009). Premature mortality from general medical illnesses among persons with bipolar disorder: A review. *Psychiatric Services, 60*(2), 147–156.

Rothman, D. (1980). *Conscience and Convenience: The Asylum and Its Alternatives in Progressive America*. Boston: Little, Brown & Company.

Roy-Byrne, P. P., Craske, M. G., Stein, M. B., et al. (2005). A randomized effectiveness trial of cognitive-behavioral therapy and medication for primary care panic disorder. *Archives of General Psychiatry, 62*(3), 290–298.

Rubenstein, L. V., Meredith, L. S., Parker, L. E., et al. (2006). Impacts of evidence-based quality improvement on depression in primary care: A randomized experiment. *Journal of General Internal Medicine, 21*(10), 1027–1035.

Saha, S., Chant, D., & McGrath, J. (2007). A systematic review of mortality in schizophrenia: Is the differential mortality gap worsening over time? *Archives of General Psychiatry, 64*(10), 1123–1131.

SAMHSA Center for Mental Health Services. (2003). *Homelessness: Provision of Mental Health and Substance Abuse Services*. Department of Health and Human Services (U.S.). Available online at http://mentalhealth.samhsa.gov/publications/allpubs/homelessness/. Accessed September 8, 2009.

SAMHSA Center for Mental Health Services. (2004a). *Evidence-Based Practice Implementation Resource Kits*. Department of Health and Human Services (U.S.). Available online at http://www.mentalhealth.samhsa.gov/cmhs/communitysupport/toolkits/. Accessed April 29, 2009.

SAMHSA Center for Mental Health Services. (2004b). *National Consensus Statement on Mental Health Recovery*. Available online at http://mentalhealth.samhsa.gov/publications/allpubs/sma05-4129. Accessed May 7, 2009.

Schouten, L. M., Hulscher, M. E., van Everdingen, J. J., et al. (2008). Evidence for the impact of quality improvement collaboratives: Systematic review. *British Medical Journal, 336*(7659), 1491–1494.

Schulberg, H. C., Katon, W. J., Simon, G. E., & Rush, A. J. (1999). Best clinical practice: Guidelines for managing major depression in primary medical care. *Journal of Clinical Psychiatry, 60* (Suppl. 7), 19–26.

Schuster, M. A., McGlynn, E. A., & Brook, R. H. (1998). How good is the quality of health care in the United States? *Milbank Q, 76*(4), 517–563, 509.

Senate Finance Committee. (2009). *Transforming the Health Care Delivery System: Proposals to Improve Patient Care and Reduce Health Care Costs.* Washington, DC: Author. Available online at http://finance.senate.gov/sitepages/leg/LEG%202009/042809%20Health%20Care%20D escription%20of%20Policy%20Option.pdf. Accessed May 8, 2009.

Smedley, B. D., Stith, A. Y., & Nelson, A. R. (2003). *Institute of Medicine: Unequal Treatment; Confronting Racial and Ethnic Disparities in Health Care* (pp. 29–79). Washington, DC: National Academies Press.

Soni, A. (2009). *The Five Most Costly Conditions, 1996 and 2006: Estimates for the U.S. Civilian Noninstitutionalized Population. Statistical Brief #248.* Agency for Healthcare Research and Quality. Available online at http://www.meps.ahrq.gov/mepsweb/data_files/publications/ st248/stat248.pdf. Accessed September 8, 2009.

Stockdill, C. N. (1990). On the federal scene. *Administration and Policy in Mental Health, 17*(3), 193–197.

Stone, E. G., Morton, S. C., & Hulscher, M. E., et al. (2002). Interventions that increase use of adult immunization and cancer screening services: A meta-analysis. *Annals of Internal Medicine, 136,* 641–651.

Stroul, B. A. (1989). Community support systems for persons with long-term mental illness: A conceptual framework. *Psychological Rehabilitation Journal, 12*(3), 9–39.

Sullivan, G., Burnam, A., Koegel, P., & Hollenberg, J. (2000). Quality of life of homeless persons with mental illness: Results from the course-of-homelessness study. *Psychiatric Services, 51*(9), 1135–1141.

Tomes, N. (2006). The patient as a policy factor: A historical case study of the consumer/survivor movement in mental health. *Health Affairs, 25*(3), 720–729.

Tsemberis, S., & Eisenberg, R. F. (2000). Pathways to housing: Supported housing for street-dwelling homeless individuals with psychiatric disabilities. *Psychiatric Services, 51*(4), 487–493.

U.S. Department of Justice. (2006). *Mental Health Problems of Prison and Jail Inmates.* Available online at http://www.ojp.usdoj.gov/bjs/pub/pdf/mhppji.pdf. Accessed September 8, 2009.

U.S. President's Commission on Mental Health. (1978). *Report to the President.* Rockville, MD: Author.

U.S. Surgeon General. (1999). *Mental Health: A Report of the Surgeon General.* Rockville, MD: U.S. Department of Health and Human Services, Substance Abuse and Mental Health Services Administration, and the National Institute of Mental Health. Available online at http://www. surgeongeneral.gov/library/mentalhealth/home.html. Accessed May 7, 2009.

U.S. Surgeon General. (2001). *Mental Health: Culture, Race, and Ethnicity; A Supplement to Mental Health: A Report of the Surgeon General.* SMA-01-3613. Rockville, MD: U.S. Department of Health and Human Services and Substance Abuse and Mental Health Services Administration. Available online at http://www.surgeongeneral.gov/library/mentalhealth/cre/. Accessed May 7, 2009.

Vaccaro, J. V., Pitts, D. B., & Wallace, C. J. (1992). Functional assessment. In R. P. Liberman (Ed.), *Handbook of Psychiatric Rehabilitation* (pp. 78–94). New York: Macmillan Publishing.

Volpp, K. G., & Das, A. (2009). Comparative effectiveness: Thinking beyond medication A versus medication B. *New England Journal of Medicine, 361*(4), 331–333.

Wang, P. S., Demler, O., & Kessler, R. C. (2002). Adequacy of treatment for serious mental illness in the United States. *American Journal of Public Health, 92*(1), 92–98.

Wells, K. B. (1999). The design of Partners in Care: Evaluating the cost-effectiveness of improving care for depression in primary care. *Social Psychiatry & Psychiatric Epidemiology, 34*(1), 20–29.

Wells, K. B., Sherbourne, C., Schoenbaum, M., et al. (2000). Impact of disseminating quality improvement programs for depression in managed primary care: A randomized controlled trial. *Journal of the American Medical Association, 283*(2), 212–220.

Wells, K., Sherbourne, C., Schoenbaum, M., et al. (2004). Five-year impact of quality improvement for depression: Results of a group-level randomized controlled trial. *Archives of General Psychiatry, 61*(4), 378–386.

Wells, K. B., Sherbourne, C. D., Sturm, R., et al. (2002). Alcohol, drug abuse, and mental health care for uninsured and insured adults. *Health Services Research, 37*(4), 1055–1066.

Young, A. S. (2003). Dosages and outcomes. *Psychiatric Services, 54*(11), 1547.

Young, A. S., Chaney, E., Shoai, R., et al. (2007). Information technology to support improved care for chronic illness. *Journal of General Internal Medicine, 22*(Suppl. 3), 425–430.

Young, A. S., Chinman, M., Forquer, S. L., et al. (2005). Use of a consumer-led intervention to improve provider competencies. *Psychiatric Services, 56*(8), 967–975.

Young, A. S., Forquer, S. L., Tran, A., et al. (2000a). Identifying clinical competencies that support rehabilitation and empowerment in individuals with severe mental illness. *Journal of Behavioral Health Services and Research, 27*(3), 321–333.

Young, A. S., Grusky, O., Jordan, D., & Belin, T. R. (2000b). Routine outcome monitoring in a public mental health system: The impact of patients who leave care. *Psychiatric Services, 51*(1), 85–91.

Young, A. S., Klap, R., Sherbourne, C. D., & Wells, K. B. (2001). The quality of care for depressive and anxiety disorders in the United States. *Archives of General Psychiatry, 58*(1), 55–61.

Young, A. S., Klap, R., Shoai, R., & Wells, K. B. (2008). Persistent depression and anxiety in the United States: Prevalence and quality of care. *Psychiatric Services, 59*(12), 1391–1398.

Young, A. S., Niv, N., Cohen, A. N., et al. (2008). The appropriateness of routine medication treatment for schizophrenia. *Schizophrenia Bulletin*. http://schizophreniabulletin.oxfordjournals.org/cgi/reprint/sbn138

Chapter 10

OLDER ADULTS

Stephen J. Bartels, MD, MS; Aricca D. Van Citters, MS; and
Tina Crenshaw, PhD, MSEd, MLS

Introduction

Over the next 20 years, the aging of the "baby boomer" cohort will result in a near
doubling in the number of older adults with major psychiatric illnesses, challenging
the nation's capacity to finance and provide mental health services for older adults
(Jeste et al., 1999). Unless substantial reforms are instituted, this demographic tsu-
nami will provide the context for a "perfect storm" due to a fragmented system of
care, a lack of trained providers, and inadequate financing of services. In this chapter, the authors provide an overview of these major issues pertaining to mental
health policy and aging, including 1) the prevalence and economic impact of geriatric mental disorders; 2) the mental health service delivery system for older adults;
3) the impact of federal regulatory and policy initiatives; 4) financing geriatric mental health services; and 5) future policy directions and challenges.

Prevalence and Economic Implications of
Geriatric Mental Disorders

Approximately 20% of adults aged 55 years and older have a mental disorder.
Among the most common mental health problems in older adults are anxiety,
depression, and dementia (Hybels & Blazer, 2003). By the year 2030, the number
of older adults with mental health disorders will equal or exceed the number with
mental illness in younger age groups (Jeste et al., 1999; U.S. Census Bureau, 2000).
However, mental disorders in older adults are frequently underdiagnosed, owing
to 1) misattribution of psychiatric symptoms due to cognitive disorders, physical

health disorders, or normal aging; 2) a lack of age-appropriate diagnostic criteria for certain psychiatric problems; and 3) under-reporting of symptoms by older people due to increased prevalence of cognitive disorders and stigma associated with psychiatric illness (Jeste et al., 1999).

Left untreated, late-life mental disorders are associated with compromised quality of life, impaired ability to live independently in the community, poor health outcomes, cognitive impairment, increased disability, and greater caregiver stress (Bartels, 2003). In addition, medical comorbidity is highly prevalent in older adults with psychiatric disorders and is associated with a high rate of premature mortality. According to a recent multi-state study, consumers of public mental health services die 25 to 30 years earlier than the general population, largely due to cardiovascular disease and other chronic medical conditions (Colton & Manderscheid, 2006) (see Chapter 12 in this volume for additional information on co-occurring disorders).

Psychiatric disorders in older adults are also associated with increased utilization and costs of health care services. For example, total health care costs for older primary care patients with depression are approximately 50% higher than for those without depression, an association that persists after controlling for comorbid physical health problems (Unützer et al., 1997). Fortunately, integrated treatment of geriatric depression can be provided within primary care settings using collaborative models of care that are cost effective. On average, collaborative care for depression can be delivered at a cost of less than $150 per older adult per year (Katon et al., 2005). Older adults who receive this type of treatment have greater rates of long-term recovery from depression and experience approximately $3,360 lower average total health care costs over a four-year period, compared to older adults who receive traditional care (Unützer et al., 2008). These long-term savings are more than adequate to cover the cost of this evidence-based treatment for geriatric depression.

The economic costs of caring for individuals with cognitive impairment disorders are also considerable and are projected to rapidly increase, as adults over age 85 are highly vulnerable to this disorder and also constitute the fastest growing segment of the population. Recent estimates suggest that 3.4 million adults aged 71 years and older have dementia (Plassman et al., 2007), representing nearly 14% of this age group. While total costs of caring for Alzheimer's disease vary widely across different studies (Bloom, de Pouvourville, & Straus, 2003), dementia in national samples of Medicare beneficiaries is associated with 3.3 times greater expenditures compared to beneficiaries without dementia, with the excess costs attributable to hospitalizations (Bynum et al., 2004).

Service utilization and the costs of caring for people with Alzheimer's disease and other forms of dementia are increased when behavioral and psychiatric symptoms are present. Older adults with dementia complicated by mixed agitation and depression, compared to other adults with dementia, have significantly higher rates of hospitalization, have a greater severity of medical problems, and receive higher numbers of psychiatric medications (Bartels, Horn et al., 2003). Approximately 30% of the total annual costs of care for people with Alzheimer's disease are associated with the management of behavioral symptoms (Beeri, Werner, Davidson, & Noy, 2002).

The costs of psychiatric disorders among older adults differ by age, service type, payer, diagnosis, and symptom severity. For example, Medicaid outpatient mental health expenditures for older adults are highest in the "young old" (aged 60 to 69 years) and decline with age, resulting in the lowest expenditures for adults aged 85 years and older. (Gilmer et al., 2006). In contrast, combined Medicaid and Medicare expenditures (including outpatient, inpatient, emergency room, pharmacy, and nursing home costs) increase with advancing age, with the highest per-person expenditures among the oldest old (age 85+) due to the high costs of acute and long-term care (Bartels, Clark, Peacock, Dums, & Pratt, 2003).

Regardless of payer, the greatest overall expenditures among older adults are associated with schizophrenia and bipolar disorder compared to expenditures associated with depression, anxiety, substance use disorders, or cognitive disorders (Gilmer et al., 2006). Among older adults with psychiatric illness, more impaired community living skills, negative symptoms, and greater cognitive impairment are associated with the highest service use (Bartels, Miles, Dums, & Pratt, 2003).

Mental Health Service Delivery Systems for Older Persons

Mental health service delivery systems for older adults are fragmented, underfinanced, lacking in trained and accessible providers, and disproportionately underserve older adults in need of care (Bartels, 2003; Borson, Bartels, Colenda, Gottlieb, & Meyers, 2001). Older adults who meet diagnostic criteria for a mental disorder are less likely than young or middle-aged adults to receive appropriate mental health care (Klap, Unroe, & Unützer, 2003). Cross-cutting features that complicate the financing, delivery, and organization of mental health services for older adults include underutilization of specialty mental health services and a diverse array of providers and settings ranging from institutional long-term care to acute home- and community-based services.

INSTITUTION-BASED CARE

Acute and long-term institution-based care account for the greatest mental health service expenditures for older adults (Administration on Aging [AoA], 2001). Acute inpatient hospitalizations account for almost half (48%) of all Medicare mental health expenditures (Health Care Financing Administration [HCFA], 2000), and older adults are disproportionately represented in long-term hospitalizations.

Older adults with psychiatric disorders are also overrepresented in nursing homes. From 65% to 91% of nursing home residents have a significant mental disorder (Burns, Taube, Fogel, Furino, & Gottlieb, 1990; Smyer, Shea, & Streit, 1994; Tariot, Podgorski, Blazin, & Leibovici, 1993). The most common mental health problems in nursing homes are associated with cognitive impairment disorders. Over 80% of cognitively impaired residents of nursing homes have neuropsychiatric symptoms, including delusions, hallucinations, depressed mood, anxiety, apathy, agitation, and physical aggression. Behavioral and psychiatric symptoms in dementia are associated with high costs, and distress to both staff and patients

(Zuidema, Koopmans, & Verhey, 2007). Depression is also common among nursing home residents, affecting approximately 30% of residents. Yet access to mental health services in nursing homes is limited, varies widely in quality, and largely consists of medication therapy (Linkins, Lucca, Housman, & Smith, 2006). The use of nursing homes as substitutes for long-term psychiatric institutions stimulated regulatory reforms in the late 1980s aimed at reducing inappropriate admissions through Preadmission Screening and Resident Review (PASRR). However, recent trends suggest that nursing homes are once again becoming the destination of last resort for middle-aged and older adults with serious mental illness (SMI). Limited community-based services for older adults with SMI, combined with growing numbers of unfilled beds in nursing homes nationwide, is once again resulting in an influx of older adults with SMI into institutional long-term care settings (Madhusoodanan & Brenner, 2007).

Home and Community-Based Mental Health Services

Less than half of community-residing older adults with a diagnosable mental disorder receive needed mental health care, and the majority of those who receive services obtain them from their primary care provider (Klap et al., 2003). Older people with mental disorders are less likely to receive care from mental health specialists than are other age groups; less than 7% of adults aged 65 years and older receive specialty outpatient mental health treatment, a rate that is lower than that of any other adult age group (Klap et al., 2003). A variety of reasons have been cited for the reluctance of older adults to receive specialty mental health services, including the perceived stigma associated with mental health care and a lack of access to specialty care. Other perceived barriers for older adults include a lack of transportation and the cost of services, as well as the belief that they could solve the problem on their own (Li, Proctor, & Morrow-Howell, 2005). In contrast, mental health treatment provided by primary care providers is perceived as more convenient (occurring within medical visits) and better coordinated (taking into account the interaction between medical and mental disorders) (USDHHS, 1999). However, providing mental health care in a busy routine medical practice is especially challenging when treating older adults who commonly have multiple medical problems requiring attention. In addition, most primary care providers have limited training in geriatric psychiatry (U.S. Department of Health and Human Services [USDHHS], 1999) or in geriatrics (Institute of Medicine, 2008) (see Chapter 16 in this volume for more information on integrating primary care and specialty mental health care).

Other alternatives to specialty mental health services that have been shown to be effective for older adults include community outreach teams. These service delivery models generally include interdisciplinary providers who are trained in the identification of mental disorders and the delivery of brief interventions. A series of randomized trials of geriatric mental health outreach teams providing services in senior housing and independent home-based settings confirms that these models are effective in treatment of depression in older adults (Van Citters & Bartels, 2004).

Various other community-based programs supplement formal mental health services and may provide a context for screening and delivery of mental health services. For example, adult day centers provide rehabilitative training and health maintenance programs for older functionally and cognitively impaired individuals (AoA, 2001). Community support services funded by the Older American's Act also provide support for senior centers, congregate meal sites, and other community services that potentially provide settings for screening and delivery of mental health services. In addition, support and peer counseling programs offer older adults a less formal approach to accessing support, information, and a broader social network.

Informal caregivers are often neglected in descriptions of the service delivery system for people with mental illness, yet they provide the majority of support services to older adults with mental disorders. Older adults with depressive symptoms receive from 4.3 to 6 hours of informal caregiving per week at an estimated yearly cost of $9 billion, compared to 2.9 hours received by non-depressed older adults (Langa, Valenstein, Fendrick, Kabeto, & Vijan, 2004). Family caregivers often provide essential assistance to adults with schizophrenia and other serious mental illnesses who live in the community.

Likewise, family caregivers provide support and care to older adults with dementia. Nearly 70% of people with Alzheimer's disease live at home, with family and friends providing almost three-quarters of their care (Alzheimer's Association, 2010). The current and future shortage of formal geriatric health care providers has led to calls for greater attention to providing training and support for this critical "shadow workforce."

Reforms Promoting Community Integration for Older Adults with Mental Disorders

The past three decades have witnessed a series of reforms in legislative policies and regulatory initiatives promoting a progressive shift away from a system of institutional care for older adults with mental disorders, toward greater integration in home and community-based settings. Following the development of a system of asylums embracing "moral treatment" of the mentally ill, there were more hospital beds dedicated to psychiatric institutional care by the middle of the twentieth century than all medical hospital beds combined. In 1963, this trend was reversed by the Community Mental Health Centers Act, aimed at decreasing unnecessary institutionalization of individuals with mental illness and promoting community-based care. Despite the early success of de-institutionalization in discharging younger patients, many older patients were not transferred to the community, but instead, were "trans-institutionalized" to nursing homes (Burns & Taube, 1990). This phenomenon, combined with inadequate community-based mental health services for psychiatric patients, resulted in burgeoning numbers of individuals with mental health needs in nursing homes.

The use of nursing homes as default "mental institutions" was addressed in the context of a variety of federal nursing home reforms under the Omnibus Budget Reconciliation Acts (OBRA) of 1987 and 1989. OBRA 1987 mandated the use of Preadmission Screening and Resident Review (PASRR) to identify and prevent potential admissions of people with serious mental illness who did not otherwise meet nursing home criteria. While PASRR slowed the rate of inappropriate nursing-home admissions and reduced the inappropriate use of restraints and over-use of psychotropic medications, its enactment had limited effectiveness in improving quality of care (USDHHS, 1999).

In an effort to improve access to mental health services in long-term care, OBRA 1987 and OBRA 1989 liberalized Medicare reimbursement for mental health services and expanded eligible providers by giving provider status to psychologists and social workers (Bartels & Colenda, 1998).

The failure of the PASRR process to prevent unnecessary and unwanted placement of individuals with mental disabilities in institutions precipitated an appeal to the U.S. Supreme Court in June of 1999. The subsequent "Olmstead Decision" defined federal policy regarding unnecessary or inappropriate institutional placement of individuals with disabilities. The *Olmstead v. L.C.* decision determined that maintaining individuals with disabilities in institutions who are capable of benefiting from living in the community is a violation of the Americans with Disabilities Act (ADA) (Williams, 2000). To comply with the Olmstead ruling, states were required to evaluate thousands of individuals residing in psychiatric institutions and nursing homes to determine whether they could be receiving care in a less restrictive community-based setting (National Council for Community Behavioral Healthcare [NCCBH], 2000) (for a more detailed discussion of the Olmstead decision and its aftermath, see Chapter 3 in this volume). Despite this ruling, a lack of community-based residential options for persons with serious mental illness remains a major impediment to achieving compliance with the Olmstead decision (Bartels & Van Citters, 2005).

In 2001, the New Freedom Initiative was established to improve integration of people with disabilities into the community. As a part of this initiative, the President's New Freedom Commission on Mental Health included a subcommittee with the directive to identify recommendations addressing the mental health needs of older adults. Three policy areas were identified by this subcommittee as essential to ensuring adequate and appropriate mental health care for older adults: access and continuity of services, quality of services, and workforce capacity. The commission noted that barriers to effective mental health care for older adults included discriminatory co-payments for mental health services, lack of Medicare insurance coverage for prescription drugs (at that time), inadequate reimbursements for providers, fragmentation of the health care delivery system, lack of correspondence between the system and the preferences of older adult consumers, and insufficient resources for training providers to meet the demand for services. The New Freedom Commission on Mental Health recommended broad reorganization of the system to promote integration of medical and mental health services, eradication of stigma associated with mental illness, more aggressive funding and reform of Medicare and Medicaid, and implementation of evidence-based practices (Bartels, 2003).

More recently, the unmet mental health needs of older adults were identified as a priority area in the 2005 White House Conference on Aging (WHCoA). Improving the detection and treatment of depression in older adults was listed among the top ten priorities in this national health policy event focusing on the needs of an aging population. Proposed strategies for improving mental health care included expanding Medicare mental health benefits, providing funding parity for mental health benefits, developing long-distance resources for delivering mental health services to older adults living in rural America, and providing financial incentives on both the federal and state levels to support advanced training and cultural competence in the geriatric mental health workforce (White House Conference on Aging, 2005).

Financing Geriatric Mental Health Services

The substantial growth in the number of older people with mental illness represents a major public health problem. This section describes the benefits and drawbacks of current financing of geriatric mental health care. Limitations in financing of mental health treatment can serve as a major barrier to providing adequate and effective care.

MEDICARE

Nearly all older Americans (95%) receive Medicare health insurance (Hoffman, Klees, & Curtis, 2007), and in 2000, more than half of the health care costs of older Americans were financed by Medicare (Assistant Secretary for Planning and Evaluation [ASPE], 2005). Medicare is the primary payer for mental health services for older adults, and includes four parts. Part A covers services associated with inpatient hospital care including charges for the hospital room, meals, and nursing services, as well as covering hospice care and acute home health care. Part B covers physician charges including hospital and outpatient visits, as well as laboratory tests, physical therapy or rehabilitation services, and ambulance services. Part C, introduced under the 1997 Balanced Budget Act, expanded Medicare to include Medicare Plus Choice managed care options. Advocacy over the past decade for mental health policy reform under Medicare has largely focused on two issues: the need for a prescription drug benefit and establishing parity for mental health coverage.

In 2003 the Medicare Prescription Drug, Improvement, and Modernization Act (MMA) was enacted under Medicare Part D, establishing a prescription drug benefit. Part D allows beneficiaries to choose among competing prescription drug plans with benefits that are administered by private insurers. The long-term impact of Medicare Part D on government and personal spending is not yet known. However, a report from the Congressional Budget Office (CBO) suggests that most Medicare beneficiaries have experienced reduced out-of-pocket expense for medications under Part D. The CBO estimates that the 2006 expenses for Part D participants were 37% less on average compared to expenses without the Part D benefit, with more dramatic savings (83% less) for those who received low-income subsidies (Rosenberg, 2007). However, many older adults appear to be confused by the multiple choices of plans under Part D, and may be unaware of available subsidies. According to a CBO estimate, 40% of Medicare beneficiaries who were eligible for a low-income subsidy in 2006 did not receive the subsidy (Rosenberg, 2007).

Despite cost savings for most beneficiaries, some provider organizations have expressed concerns about the effects of Part D on Medicare beneficiaries who have a mental illness. It is estimated that 25% of Medicare beneficiaries are treated with psychotropic medications, including many agents that are expensive and prescribed for long periods of time (Rosenberg, 2007). Implementation of Part D was met with complaints by providers that emergency supplies of psychiatric medications were not always available and formulary restrictions potentially prevented patients from receiving prescribed medications. According to the American Society of Consultant Pharmacists, some management strategies implemented by Part D insurers may encourage use of medications that are not appropriate for older adults through extensive use of prior authorization, use of step therapy requirements, and formulary restrictions. For example, some Part D plans encourage use of less costly medications within their formularies that are identified under the "Beers criteria" as medications to be avoided for older adults (American Society of Consultant Pharmacists, 2006).

Additional concerns voiced by providers include the unreimbursed costs associated with Part D administrative requirements (Wilk et al., 2008). For example, increased administrative burden for clinicians was associated with management strategies such as prior authorization, finding preferred drug lists that cover selected agents, and requirements to use step therapy strategies. With some plans, the administrative time approached an hour for every hour of direct patient care. In addition, psychiatrists reported making medication decisions based on whether appeals or exceptions would need to be pursued. In response to provider concerns, in February 2006, CMS proposed amendments to Part D, including a specialty tier for high-cost drugs (> $500 per month) with a 25% limit on cost-sharing. The proposed changes also included a requirement that residents of long-term care facilities must be given a 30-day emergency supply of a non-formulary drug during processing of an exception (Rosenberg, 2007).

Finally, effective reforms of Medicare Part D will require public disclosure and availability of detailed pharmacy data allowing comparison of different plans. Under the initial legislation, the Centers for Medicare and Medicaid Services (CMS) are only permitted to use drug claims data for payment purposes. This restriction does not allow entities such as congressional agencies, the Centers for Disease Control, the Food and Drug Administration, or independent health services researchers to evaluate the effectiveness, efficiency, and safety of the Part D program that services approximately 24 million people at an annual cost of about $50 billion. In March 2008, the Medicare Payment Advisory Commission (MedPAC) called on Congress to pass legislation to make Part D claims available "regularly and in a timely manner to congressional support agencies and selected executive branch agencies for purposes of program evaluation, public health, and safety" (Hargrave & Hoadley, 2008). The availability of these data is especially critical for ensuring positive outcomes for older adults with mental disorders who are particularly vulnerable to the potential adverse consequences of policies that may not appropriately accommodate psychiatric disorders and complex medical conditions.

The lack of parity between mental health and medical care coverage under Medicare has been a long standing priority for reform among consumer advocacy and provider organizations. In 1996, the first round of parity legislation was passed (Public Law 104-204, the "Mental Health Parity Act of 1996"), prohibiting insurers offering plans that serve over 50 employees from setting lower annual or lifetime dollar caps on mental health benefits than for other health benefits.

Despite objections raised by private payers, this legislation resulted in minimal impact on expenditures, utilization, and quality of mental health care (Druss, 2006; Hennessy & Goldman, 2001). In 2003, Senator Paul Wellstone proposed the "Mental Health Equitable Treatment Act" extending parity legislation to prohibit reduced benefits for mental health compared to other medical benefits through federally supported insurance. This reform highlighted the elimination of the required 50% co-payment for psychological services under Medicare, in contrast to the standard co-payment of 20% for medical care. This proposal was unsuccessful in achieving the necessary congressional support to become law.

In July 2008, the "Medicare Improvement for Patients and Providers Act of 2008" (Public Law No: 110-275) was enacted under the banner of the "Senator Paul Wellstone Parity Act" in honor of Senator Wellstone's longstanding advocacy for mental health reform. This legislation eliminates the lack of parity under Medicare between coverage for mental health treatments compared to medical or surgical visits by reducing the Medicare co-payment for outpatient mental health services to 20% over a period of six years (Association for the Advancement of Psychology, 2008). This legislation also contains provisions that will help ensure that beneficiaries will have access through Medicare Part D coverage to the medications they need, and it reverses scheduled cuts to the Medicare provider fee schedule, instead providing an increase of 1.1% for 2009.

MEDICAID

Medicaid is the largest insurance provider in the United States, exceeding Medicare (Henderson & Wilhide, 2005). Unlike Medicare, a federally funded health insurance plan, the federal contribution under Medicaid requires a 50% match by the states. Medicaid provides health care services to individuals who are poor, blind, or disabled, including individuals disabled by serious mental illness. Older adults and people with disabilities make up less than a third of Medicaid enrollees, yet account for almost three-quarters of Medicaid spending (Henderson & Wilhide, 2005). In 2006, approximately one-third of Medicaid expenditures were for long-term care, including care in nursing homes as well as home and community-based services (HCBS)(ASPE, 2007).

Medicaid is also responsible for a large portion of the costs for mental health services. Medicaid expenditures account for over one-fourth of all mental health expenditures, more than any other single payer (Mark & Buck, 2005). Older individuals eligible for both Medicare and Medicaid are referred to as "dually eligible." Because many dually eligible beneficiaries are both over age 65 years and have significant disabilities, older people with serious mental illness are overrepresented in this group. The dually eligible are a major contributor to the costs of Medicaid, accounting for an estimated 42% of Medicaid spending (Henderson & Wilhide, 2005).

Medicaid requires that states provide long-term care for individuals who are poor or disabled, but allows for waivers supporting home- and community-based alternatives to conventional nursing-home care. In addition, states may choose whether or not to cover such services as the Program for All-Inclusive Care for the

Elderly (PACE), or services for people age 65 years or older in mental institutions (Henderson & Wilhide, 2005).

Support Services for Older Adults Residing in the Community

Other critical services for older adults with mental health needs include a broad array of support and outreach services provided in the community under the Older Americans Act (OAA) of 1965. The OAA was developed to provide services to older adults at risk of losing their independence due to social and economic needs, as well as people with low incomes or minority status (Takamura, 1999). Through state agencies on aging and area agencies on aging, this act provides support for such services as transportation, screening and information, senior centers, adult day care, home care, home nutrition programs ("meals on wheels"), congregate meal programs, legal assistance, disease prevention, and health promotion.

The reauthorization of the OAA was identified as the single greatest priority of the 2005 White House Conference on Aging. The successful reauthorization in 2006 of the Older Americans Act Amendments of 2006, Pub. L. No. 109-365 (2006) included several new provisions not present in the original 1965 legislation. Under P.L. 109-365, state and area agencies on aging are required to provide programs and services specifically for older people who are at risk for institutional care and those with limited English proficiency. Also included in the reauthorization was a provision for developing systems of mental health screening and treatment for older people (O'Shaughnessy & Napili, 2006).

Future Challenges in Mental Health Policy and Aging

Policy and legislative initiatives enacted over the last three decades have defined the current financing and delivery system for older adults with mental illness. Several areas warrant future attention as major health policy challenges, including 1) the aging of the population with serious mental illness; 2) the evolving epidemic of Alzheimer's disease; 3) changes in long-term care, including home and community-based options; 4) the need for integrated mental and physical health care; 5) the workforce gap in geriatric providers; and 6) bridging the gap between research, practice, and policy.

Aging of the Population with Serious Mental Illness

Older adults with serious mental illness (SMI) present unique and complex challenges to the mental health service delivery system for older people. SMI (including schizophrenia, bipolar disorder, and treatment refractory depression) is associated with high rates of institution-based care. In the context of the closure and downsizing of state mental hospitals, many older adults with SMI now reside in nursing homes as the "new mental institution" in America. Two-thirds of older adults with SMI experience at least one hospitalization or nursing home admission annually and they are three times more likely to be admitted to a nursing home than older adults without SMI (Bartels, Forester, Miles, & Joyce, 2000). On average, Medicaid beneficiaries with schizophrenia, compared to Medicaid beneficiaries without a mental illness, enter nursing homes approximately thirteen years earlier and are four times more likely to be admitted to a nursing home between the ages of 50 and 65 (Andrews, Bartels, Xie, & Peacock, 2007).

In addition to greater use of long-term care in nursing homes, older adults with SMI have high rates of co-occurring physical health disorders associated with worse health status, more severe psychiatric symptoms, and increased mortality. They have a 25-to-30year decreased lifespan compared to persons without a mental illness, which lowers their age of death to approximately 53 years of age (Colton & Manderscheid, 2006). In addition, older adults with SMI are at substantial risk of receiving inadequate or inappropriate health care (Druss, Bradford, Rosenheck, Radford, & Krumholz, 2001). A number of organizations have taken a step toward reversing this direction by pledging to promote wellness and reduce early mortality of individuals with SMI within the next decade (Center for Mental Health Services, 2007).

To date, mental health service delivery has largely been focused on younger people with SMI. In recent years, however, our understanding of effective interventions for older adults with SMI has grown substantially. Redesign of the mental health service delivery system to accommodate the special needs of older adults with SMI should focus on factors that contribute most to the high rate of institutionalization for this group, including poor social skills and supports, high medical comorbidity, and inadequate independent living skills. New models of care, including age-appropriate psychosocial rehabilitation integrated with physical health care, will be needed to reduce the health disparity and address the needs of the increasing numbers of middle-aged and older individuals with SMI (Pratt, Van Citters, Mueser, & Bartels, 2008).

Evolving Epidemic of Alzheimer's Disease and Related Behavioral Disorders

Alzheimer's disease is a degenerative, neuropsychiatric illness that impairs cognitive and functional abilities, and most individuals with the disease also have significant secondary psychiatric symptoms, leading to decreased functioning, increased caregiver burden, and risk of institutionalization (Geldmacher, 2007). Historically, there has been a lack of consensus on the role of mental health services in the treatment of dementia (Bartels & Colenda, 1998). However, in 2002, the systematic exclusion of all individuals with an Alzheimer's disease diagnosis from eligibility for psychiatric services under Medicare was amended to allow coverage of mental health services, hospice care, or home health care (Hawryluk, 2002). Despite this legislation, psychiatric services under Medicare remain inconsistently reimbursed by Medicare intermediaries and private insurers. Reforms in policy and service delivery are needed to accommodate the increasing numbers of individuals with Alzheimer's disease complicated by psychiatric and behavioral symptoms. Addressing this challenge will require a coordinated health policy initiative that bridges health care, long-term care, mental health care, federal and state agencies, provider organizations, and, most importantly, consumer advocacy organizations such as the Alzheimer's Association and the National Alliance on Mental Illness (NAMI).

Changing Landscape of Long-Term Care: Home and Community-Based Options

Increasing demand by consumers for alternatives to nursing homes is evidenced by the proliferation of assisted living facilities, continuing care retirement communities, home health care options, and community-based aging network services. Some estimates suggest that between 30% and 56% of assisted living facility residents have a mental health problem (Becker, Stiles, & Schonfeld, 2002), while other research has found that two-thirds of assisted living residents have diagnosable dementia and over one-fourth have a non-cognitive psychiatric disorder (Rosenblatt et al., 2004). Studies also suggest high rates of mental illness among home health care populations (Bruce et al., 2002).

Many recent CMS reforms and state reforms in Medicaid are designed to promote home- and community-based long-term care alternatives. Between 1996 and 2006, Medicaid spending for Home and Community-Based Services (HCBS) increased from $11.2 billion to $38.5 billion (ASPE, 2007). The Deficit Reduction Act of 2005 (DRA) eliminated the requirement that individuals must be at risk of institutionalization before they can be given HCBS. The DRA also stipulated that states may provide special community-based services to individuals with chronic mental illness, including day treatment or partial hospitalization, psychosocial rehabilitation, and clinic services (Centers for Medicare and Medicaid Services [CMS], 2008).

A comparison of expenditures and health outcomes of people with dementia who receive long-term care in their homes through HCBS waivers compared to nursing home residents with dementia reveals that on average, overall expenditures are less for the waiver HCBS recipients (Sands et al., 2008). However, this same study also found that HCBS recipients are admitted to the hospital twice as frequently as nursing home residents. These findings suggest that better monitoring of waiver HCBS recipients with dementia and coordination with their primary care providers is needed.

As alternatives evolve to define the future long-term care system, policymakers will need to shift away from the bias toward acute and institution-based care. Future policy initiatives must also support provision of mental health services within home and community-based settings.

Implementation and Financing of Integrated Mental and Physical Health Care

Integration of physical and mental health care represents a departure from conventional models of mental health service delivery in which mental health services are "carved out" into separate organizations, with financing that is separate from general medical care. Integrated or collaborative physical and mental health treatment has been shown to have substantial benefits in primary care (Unützer, Schoenbaum, Druss, & Katon, 2006), home health care (Bruce, 2002), and long-term care (Bartels, Moak, & Dums, 2002). Older individuals with depression who receive integrated care have lower total health care costs (Unützer et al., 2008), and interdisciplinary care has been associated with improved survival, quality of life, and patient satisfaction (Institute of Medicine, 2008). For patients with substance abuse–related medical conditions, integrated care resulted in lower hospitalization rates, inpatient days, emergency room use, and medical costs (Parthasarathy, Mertens, Moore, & Weisner, 2003).

Unfortunately, "same day" separate billing for mental health and medical care remains uncovered under Medicare, presenting a major barrier to implementing integrated collaborative mental health care within primary care.

Recent reforms suggest that the long-standing segregation between mental and physical health care services is beginning to break down. For example, prior to January 1, 2008, only physicians were allowed to use Current Procedural Terminology (CPT) billing codes that would indicate time spent conferencing with providers from other disciplines for patient care planning. However, new CPT codes now allow psychologists or other non-physician providers to bill for such interdisciplinary team conferencing, potentially supporting reimbursement for care coordination in two-way dialogue between medical and mental health providers (American Psychological Association, 2008).

Despite these early signs of potential progress, further reforms are needed to support widespread adoption and reimbursement for the several evidence-based models of integrated collaborative care that have been proven to be effective in the treatment of geriatric depression and cognitive impairment disorders in primary care (Callahan et al., 2006; Unützer, Powers, Katon, & Langston, 2005) (see Chapter 16 in this volume for more information on integrating primary care and mental health care).

Addressing the Workforce Gap in Geriatric Providers

Demographic trends of increasing numbers of older adults needing treatment for mental illness or cognitive impairment project a dramatic shortfall in the number of trained providers who will be needed to provide services to an aging population (*Caring for Our Seniors*, 2008). Despite the clear need for increasing the workforce of health care providers with expertise in geriatrics, current training programs aimed at developing the next generation of providers will fail to meet this need. Despite efforts to expand capacity, over half of the geriatric psychiatry fellowship slots went unfilled in 2006 (Association of Directors of Geriatric Academic Programs, 2007). A recent Institute of Medicine (IOM) report underscores the problem of a diminishing geriatric care workforce (Institute of Medicine, 2008), and the American Association for Geriatric Psychiatry (AAGP) has recommended a follow-up study specifically examining the geriatric mental health care workforce. Among the most frequent concerns cited by training physicians reluctant to consider a career in geriatrics are the lower rates of reimbursement under Medicare in the context of significant personal debt due to student loans.

A number of legislative and policy initiatives have been introduced to provide incentives for health professionals to pursue geriatrics as a career choice. For example, the "Geriatricians Loan Forgiveness Act" (H.R. 2502), introduced in May 2007, would authorize repayment of $35,000 in educational loans for each year of geriatric medicine or geriatric psychiatry fellowship training. Another loan repayment bill, the "Caring for an Aging America Act of 2008" (S. 2708) includes loan forgiveness as well as other incentives to attract and retain geriatric care providers into the workforce. Other initiatives include calls for funding of the Geriatric Health Professions Programs and reforms in Medicare mental health coverage that reduce disincentives to providers specializing in geriatric mental health (*Caring for Our Seniors*, 2008) (see Chapter 5 in this volume for more information on workforce development).

BRIDGING THE GAP BETWEEN RESEARCH, PRACTICE, AND POLICY

The need to bridge the gap between what is known about effective mental health treatments and the services currently offered by health care providers is a federal priority (Institute of Medicine, 2006; National Institute of Mental Health [NIMH], 1998; USDHHS, 2003). While advances in geriatric psychiatry have defined a substantial set of evidence-based practices (EBPs) with known effectiveness in the prevention and treatment of mental disorders and substance abuse in older adults (Bartels & Drake, 2005; Blow, Bartels, Brockmann, & Van Citters, 2005), research has shown that it takes over a decade for findings on effective services to be routinely implemented by health care providers (Lenfant, 2003).

The recent national emphasis on the use of EBPs is designed to speed the process of introducing innovations into health care settings. However, several challenges must be overcome to implement EBPs for older adults with mental health or substance abuse problems. These include negative attitudes among health and social service providers, poor access to EBP guidelines that are specific to older adults, inadequate training resources, limited technical assistance, lack of expertise in assessing readiness and strategic planning, and insufficient management skills to create sustainable organizational change (Levkoff & Chen, 2006). Moreover, the implementation of EBPs for older adults is complicated by the different priorities, capacities, and levels of expertise among providers in primary care, long-term care, and specialty mental health or substance abuse settings.

Recent initiatives supported by the National Institute of Mental Health (NIMH), the Substance Abuse and Mental Health Services Administration (SAMHSA), and the Administration on Aging (AoA) are aimed at increasing the availability and use of EBPs. NIMH and SAMHSA have partnered to promote and support the use of evidence-based services in state mental health systems. This partnership involves increasing research to reduce the burden of mental illnesses and mental health disparities, expanding the National Registry of Evidence-based Programs and Practices (NREPP), developing toolkits that describe how to implement EBPs, and expanding the "Science-to-Services" agenda to further increase the use of EBPs (Substance Abuse and Mental Health Services Administration [SAMHSA], 2006).

SAMHSA also sponsors the Mental Health Transformation-State Incentive Grants (MHT-SIG) that support activities to improve the infrastructure of service delivery systems and help states plan for delivering effective mental health services. Aging services and the implementation of EBPs are priorities for some states that have received MHT-SIGs. Finally, the AoA has launched an initiative involving collaborations between federal agencies and private foundations to increase older people's access to effective programs that can reduce the risk of disease, disability, and injury.

State initiatives have also been introduced to encourage the adoption of EBPs (Marton, Daigle, & de la Gueronniere, 2005; National Association of State Mental Health Program Directors Research Institute [NRI], 2005). For example, Oregon passed legislation that requires 75% of state-supported substance abuse and mental health services to consist of EBPs by the year 2009. Other states have incorporated guidelines for the use of EBPs into their bidding and contracting processes, while others have used incentives to improve service provider behavior and promote EBPs. There has been limited attention, however, toward implementing services that are specifically designed for older adults.

Despite these signs of progress, additional strategies are needed to reduce the barriers to adopting EBPs for older adults. Potential areas of focus include increased emphasis on interventions that are designed to be used in real-world settings by real-world providers, development of financing options and incentives, improved educational opportunities for health and social service providers, and improved understanding of effective dissemination strategies.

Implications for Mental Health

This chapter summarizes a variety of key issues confronting the mental health service delivery system for older adults, including economic factors, regulatory and policy initiatives, financing, and future challenges. Many of the health policy recommendations that were articulated in the report of the President's New Freedom Commission on Mental Health (Bartels, 2003) remain even more relevant today, as the field must prioritize in the context of a challenging fiscal environment together with increasing numbers of people in need. Persistent challenges and promising directions include the dissemination and implementation of an array of evidence-based practices that have been proven to be effective in usual care settings with usual care providers.

There is also a clear need to continue to facilitate policy reform that advances the integration of mental and physical health care in both directions. This includes reforms in the financing and organization of services to routinely offer collaborative models of mental health care for older adults in primary care settings, as well as providing integrated physical health care in mental health settings to reverse the alarming health care disparity experienced by older persons with serious mental illness associated with a 25–30 year shorter life span.

Reform of payment and delivery of person-centered mental health services is also needed. These reforms include support for appropriate, timely, evidence-based treatment for older people with mental illness that incorporates the individual consumer's preferences, values, and informed choice.

Finally, the field is in danger of losing our capacity to advance progress in critical knowledge development aimed at discovering the causes and effective treatments of mental disorders in older adults. Despite major advances in research supported by the doubling of the NIH budget in the 1990s, this growth has been effectively wiped out by five consecutive years of NIH budgets that have been flat or below inflation. The overall success rate for NIH-sponsored research grants has decreased from 32% in 1999 to 24% in 2007, falling by one-quarter. This "research recession" has especially affected early career investigators. Of note, the average age for a first competitive independent R01 research grant has increased by four years (age 43 today) compared to age 39 in 1990.

Overall, these trends provide the foundation for the aforementioned "perfect storm" that threatens the very future of mental health care of older adults. A recent summit describing the endangered "pipeline" of geriatric mental health researchers identified a series of strategies to be adopted to reverse this trend (Bartels et al., in press). A variety of successful programs have been developed to mentor and advance early career researchers, yet these approaches need to be complemented by funding mechanisms to ease the financial pressures on early-career investigators. For example, increasing the availability of loan repayment programs and early career research awards is needed, combined with developing a substantial pool of trained and dedicated mentors in the field of geriatric mental health research. These approaches will be critical to reinvigorating the pipeline of researchers to inform future treatments and services for the rapidly growing population of older adults with mental health needs.

Acknowledgments

This work was supported by NIMH K24 MH66282 (PI: Bartels).

References

Administration on Aging. (2001). *Older Adults and Mental Health: Issues and Opportunities*. Rockville, MD: Author.

Alzheimer's Association. (2010). *Alzheimer's Disease Facts and Figures*. http://www.alz.org/alzheimers_disease_facts_figures.asp.

Association for the Advancement of Psychology. (2008). *AAP Legislative Issues*. Available online at http://www.aapnet.org/pdf/Practice_parity.pdf. Accessed on September 29, 2009.

American Psychological Association, Presidential Task Force on Integrated Care for an Aging Population. (2008). *Blueprint for Change: Achieving Integrated Health Care for an Aging Population*. Available online at www.apa.org/pi/aging/blueprint.html. Accessed June 25, 2009.

American Society of Consultant Pharmacists. (2006). *Letter to CMS from ASCP and Five Other Health Professional Organizations about Medicare Part D and Long-Term Care—Formulary Restrictions and Cost-Management Tools*. Available online at http://www.ascp.com/medicarerx/upload/LTCSignOnLetter.pdf. Accessed June 18, 2009.

Andrews, A. O., Bartels, S. J., Xie, H., & Peacock, W. (2007). *Early Nursing Home Admissions among Persons with Serious Mental Illness: New Hampshire Medicaid Beneficiaries 1995–2005*. Paper presented at the Annual Meeting of the American Association for Geriatric Psychiatry, New Orleans, Louisiana.

Assistant Secretary for Planning and Evaluation. (2005). *Long-Term Growth of Medical Expenditures: Public and Private*. Washington, DC: Office of the Assistant Secretary for Planning and Evaluation, Policy Information Center, U.S. Department of Health and Human Services.

Assistant Secretary for Planning and Evaluation. (2007). *Residential Care and Assisted Living Compendium: 2007*. Washington, DC: Office of the Assistant Secretary for Planning and Evaluation, Policy Information Center, U.S. Department of Health and Human Services.

Association of Directors of Geriatric Academic Programs. (2007). Fellows in geriatric medicine and geriatric psychiatry programs. *Training and Practice Update, 5*(2). http://129.137.5.214/GWPS/files/ADGAP%20Training%20and%20Practice%20Update%205_2.pdf

Bartels, S. J. (2003). Improving the system of care for older adults with mental illness in the United States: Findings and recommendations for the President's New Freedom Commission on Mental Health. *American Journal of Geriatric Psychiatry, 11*(5), 486–497.

Bartels, S. J., Clark, R. E., Peacock, W. J., Dums, A. R., & Pratt, S. I. (2003). Medicare and Medicaid costs for schizophrenia patients by age cohort compared with depression, dementia, and medically ill patients. *American Journal of Geriatric Psychiatry, 11*(6), 648–657.

Bartels, S. J., & Colenda, C. C. (1998). Mental health services for Alzheimer's disease: Current trends in reimbursement and public policy, and the future under managed care. *American Journal of Geriatric Psychiatry, 6*(2 Suppl. 1), S85–100.

Bartels, S. J., & Drake, R. E. (2005). Evidence-based geriatric psychiatry: An overview. *Psychiatric Clinics of North America, 28*(4), 763–784.

Bartels, S. J., Forester, B., Miles, K. M., & Joyce, T. (2000). Mental health service use by elderly patients with bipolar disorder and unipolar major depression. *American Journal of Geriatric Psychiatry, 8*(2), 160–166.

Bartels, S. D., Horn, S. D., Smout, R. J., Dums, A. R., Flaherty, E., Jones, J. K., et al. (2003). Agitation and depression in frail nursing home elderly with dementia: Treatment characteristics and service use. *American Journal of Geriatric Psychiatry, 11*(2), 231–238.

Bartels, S. J., Lebowitz, B. D., Reynolds, C. F., Bruce, M., Halpain, H., Faison, W. E., & Kriwin, P. D. (2010). A model for developing the pipeline of early career geriatric mental health researchers: Outcomes and implications for other fields. *Academic Medicine, 85*, 26–35.

Bartels, S. J., Miles, K. M., Dums, A. R., & Pratt, S. I. (2003). Factors associated with community mental health service use by older adults with severe mental illness. *Journal of Mental Health and Aging, 9*(2), 123–135.

Bartels, S. J., Moak, G. S., & Dums, A. R. (2002). Mental health services in nursing homes: Models of mental health services in nursing homes; A review of the literature. *Psychiatric Services, 53*(11), 1390–1396.

Bartels, S. J., & Van Citters, A. D. (2005). Community-based alternatives for older adults with serious mental illness: The Olmstead decision and deinstitutionalization of nursing homes. *Ethics, Law, and Aging Review, 11*, 3–22.

Becker, M., Stiles, P., & Schonfeld, L. (2002). Mental health service use and cost of care for older adults in assisted living facilities: Implications for public policy. *Journal of Behavioral Health Services & Research, 29*(1), 91–98.

Beeri, M. S., Werner, P., Davidson, M., & Noy, S. (2002). The cost of behavioral and psychological symptoms of dementia (BPSD) in community dwelling Alzheimer's disease patients. *International Journal of Geriatric Psychiatry, 17*(5), 403–408.

Bloom, B. S., de Pouvourville, N., & Straus, W. L. (2003). Cost of illness of Alzheimer's disease: How useful are current estimates? *Gerontologist, 43*(2), 158–164.

Blow, F. C., Bartels, S. J., Brockmann, L. M., & Van Citters, A. D. (2005). *Evidence-Based Practices for Preventing Substance Abuse and Mental Health Problems in Older Adults*. Available online at http://www.samhsa.gov/OlderAdultsTAC/EBPLiteratureReviewFINAL.pdf. Accessed June 25, 2009.

Borson, S., Bartels, S. J., Colenda, C. C., Gottlieb, G. L., & Meyers, B. (2001). Geriatric mental health services research: Strategic plan for an aging population; Report of the Health Services

Work Group of the American Association for Geriatric Psychiatry. *American Journal of Geriatric Psychiatry, 9*(3), 191–204.

Bruce, M. L. (2002). Mental health services in home healthcare: Opportunities and challenges. *Generations, 26*(1), 78–82.

Bruce, M. L., McAvay, G. J., Raue, P. J., Brown, E. L., Meyers, B. S., Keohane, D. J., et al. (2002). Major depression in elderly home health care patients. *American Journal of Psychiatry, 159*(8), 1367–1374.

Burns, B. J., & Taube, C. A. (1990). Mental health services in general medical care and nursing homes. In B. Fogel, A. Furino, & G. Gottlieb (Eds.), *Mental Health Policy for Older Americans: Protecting Minds at Risk* (pp. 63–84). Washington, DC: American Psychiatric Press.

Bynum, J. P., Rabins, P. V., Weller, W., Niefeld, M., Anderson, G. F., & Wu, A. W. (2004). The relationship between a dementia diagnosis, chronic illness, Medicare expenditures, and hospital use. *Journal of the American Geriatrics Society, 52*(2), 187–194.

Callahan, C., Boustani, M. A., Unverzagt, F. W., Austrom, M. G., Damush, T. M., Perkins, A. J., et al. (2006). Effectiveness of collaborative care for older adults with Alzheimer disease in primary care: A randomized controlled trial. *Journal of the American Medical Association, 295*(18), 2148.

Caring for an Aging America Act of 2008 (S. 2708), 110th Cong. (2). (2008).

Caring for Our Seniors: How Can We Support Those on the Frontlines? Senate Special Committee on Aging Committee Hearings, 110th Congress (2008).

Center for Mental Health Services. (2007, December 16). New web resource on wellness for people with mental illnesses. *CMHS Consumer Affairs E-News, 07–205.* Available online at http://mentalhealth.samhsa.gov/consumersurvivor/listserv/121607b.asp. Accessed July 28, 2009.

Centers for Medicare and Medicaid Services. (2008, March 31). Thousands more Medicaid enrollees could get home and community-based care under new rule. Press release. Available online at http://www.cms.hhs.gov/apps/media/press/release.asp?Counter=3018&intNumPerPage=10&checkDate=&checkKey=2&srchType=2&numDays=0&srchOpt=0&srchData=medicaid&keywordType=All&chkNewsType=1%2C+2%2C+3%2C+4%2C+5&intPage=&showAll=1&pYear=&year=0&desc=&cboOrder=date. Accessed June 13, 2009.

Colton, C. W., & Manderscheid, R. W. (2006). Congruencies in increased mortality rates, years of potential life lost, and causes of death among public mental health clients in eight states. *Preventing Chronic Disease: Public Health Research, Practice, and Policy, 3*(2), 1–14.

Druss, B. (2006). Mental health parity, access, and quality of care. *Medical Care, 44*(6), 497–498.

Druss, B. G., Bradford, W. D., Rosenheck, R. A., Radford, M. J., & Krumholz, H. M. (2001). Quality of medical care and excess mortality in older patients with mental disorders. *Archives of General Psychiatry, 58*(6), 565–572.

Geldmacher, D. S. (2007). Treatment guidelines for Alzheimer's disease: Redefining perceptions in primary care. *Primary Care Companion to The Journal of Clinical Psychiatry, 9*(2), 113–121.

Geriatricians Loan Forgiveness Act of 2007, H.R. 2502, 110th Cong. (2007).

Gilmer, T., Ojeda, V. D., Folsom, D., Fuentes, D., Criado, V., Garcia, P., et al. (2006). Costs of community-based public mental health services for older adults: Variations related to age and diagnosis. *International Journal of Geriatric Psychiatry, 21*(12), 1121–1126.

Hargrave, E. & Hoadley, J. (2008). *Facilitating access to Medicare Part D drug claims data.* Washington, DC: MedPAC. Available online at http://www.medpac.gov/documents/Mar08_PartD_CONTRACTOR_RS.pdf. Accessed June 25, 2009.

Hawryluk, M. (2002). Medicare ends routine Alzheimer's denials [Electronic version]. *American Medical News.* Available online at http://www.ama-assn.org/amednews/2002/04/22/gvsa0422.htm. Accessed June 25, 2009.

Health Care Financing Administration. (2000). *Medicare 2000: 35 Years of Improving Americans' Health and Security.* Washington, DC: Health Care Financing Administration, Department of Health and Human Services.

Henderson, T. M., & Wilhide, S. (2005). *Medicaid: Overview and Policy Issues.* Leawood, KS: American Academy of Family Physicians.

Hennessy, K. D., & Goldman, H. H. (2001). Full Parity: Steps toward Treatment Equity for Mental and Addictive Disorders. *Health Affairs, 20*(4), 58–68.

Hoffman, E. D., Jr., Klees, B. S., & Curtis, C. A. (2007). *Brief Summaries of Medicare and Medicaid Title XVIII and Title XIX of The Social Security Act.* Baltimore: Office of the Actuary, Centers for Medicare and Medicaid Services, Department of Health and Human Services.

Hybels, C. F., & Blazer, D. G. (2003). Epidemiology of late-life mental disorders. *Clinics in Geriatric Medicine, 19*(4), 663–696.

Institute of Medicine. (2006). *Improving the Quality of Health Care for Mental and Substance-Use Conditions: Quality Chasm Series.* Washington, DC: National Academies Press.

Institute of Medicine. (2008). *Retooling for an Aging America.* Washington, DC: The National Academies Press.

Jeste, D. V., Alexopoulos, G. S., Bartels, S. J., Cummings, J. L., Gallo, J. J., Gottlieb, G. L., et al. (1999). Consensus statement on the upcoming crisis in geriatric mental health: Research agenda for the next 2 decades. *Archives of General Psychiatry, 56*(9), 848–853.

Katon, W. J., Schoenbaum, M., Fan, M.-Y., Callahan, C. M., Williams, J., Jr., Hunkeler, E., et al. (2005). Cost-effectiveness of improving primary care treatment of late-life depression. *Archives of General Psychiatry, 62*(12), 1313–1320.

Klap, R., Unroe, K. T., & Unützer, J. (2003). Caring for mental illness in the United States: A focus on older adults. *American Journal of Geriatric Psychiatry, 11*(5), 517–524.

Langa, K. M., Valenstein, M. A., Fendrick, A. M., Kabeto, M. U., & Vijan, S. (2004). Extent and cost of informal caregiving for older Americans with symptoms of depression. *American Journal of Psychiatry, 161*(5), 857–863.

Lenfant, C. (2003). Shattuck lecture: Clinical research to clinical practice; Lost in translation? *New England Journal of Medicine, 349*(9), 868–874.

Levkoff, S., & Chen, H. (2006). Challenges to implementing evidence-based mental health practices. Personal communication.

Li, H., Proctor, E., & Morrow-Howell, N. (2005). Outpatient mental health service use by older adults after acute psychiatric hospitalization. *Journal of Behavioral Health Services and Research, 32*(1), 74–84.

Linkins, K. W., Lucca, A. M., Housman, M., & Smith, S. A. (2006). Use of PASRR programs to assess serious mental illness and service access in nursing homes. *Psychiatric Services, 57*(3), 325–332.

Madhusoodanan, S., & Brenner, R. (2007). Caring for the chronically mentally ill in nursing homes. *Annals of Long-Term Care, 15*(9), 29–32.

Mark, T. L., & Buck, J. A. (2005). Components of spending for Medicaid mental health services, 2001. *Psychiatric Services, 56*(6), 648.

Marton, A., Daigle, J., & de la Gueronniere, G. (2005). *Identifying State Purchasing Levers for Promoting the Use of Evidence-Based Practice in Substance Abuse Treatment.* Princeton, NJ: Center for Health Care Strategies, Inc.

National Association of State Mental Health Program Directors Research Institute. (2005). *Results of a Survey of State Directors of Adult and Child Mental Health Services on Implementation of Evidence-Based Practices.* Alexandria, VA: NASMHPD Author.

National Center for Health Statistics. (2004). *Nursing Home Residents: Mental Health. U.S. 1985–2004 (Source: National Nursing Home Survey):* National Center for Health Statistics, Trends in Health and Aging.

National Council for Community Behavioral Healthcare. (2000). *Olmstead: Department of Health and Human Services Urges Implementation of Olmstead.* Washington, DC: Author.

National Institute of Mental Health. (1998). *Bridging Science and Service.* No. 99-4353. Rockville, MD: Author.

O'Shaughnessy, C., & Napili, A. (2006). *The Older Americans Act: Programs, Funding, and 2006 Reauthorization (P.L. 109-365), CRS Report for Congress*. Washington, DC: Congressional Research Service.

Parthasarathy, S., Mertens, J., Moore, C., & Weisner, C. (2003). Utilization and cost impact of integrating substance abuse treatment and primary care. *Medical Care, 41*(3), 357–367.

Plassman, B. L., Langa, K. M., Fisher, G. G., Heeringa, S. G., Weir, D. R., Ofstedal, M. B., et al. (2007). Prevalence of dementia in the United States: The aging, demographics, and memory study. *Neuroepidemiology, 29*(1–2), 125–132.

Pratt, S. I., Van Citters, A. D., Mueser, K. T., & Bartels, S. J. (2008). Psychosocial rehabilitation in older adults with serious mental illness: A review of the research literature and recommendations for development of rehabilitative approaches. *American Journal of Psychiatric Rehabilitation, 11*(1), 7–40.

Rosenberg, J. M. (2007). Overview of Medicare Part D prescription drug benefit: Potential implications for patients with psychotic disorders. *American Journal of Health-System Pharmacists, 64*(Suppl. 1), S18–S23.

Rosenblatt, A., Samus, Q. M., Steele, C. D., Baker, A. S., Harper, M. G., Brandt, J., et al. (2004). The Maryland Assisted Living Study: Prevalence, recognition, and treatment of dementia and other psychiatric disorders in the assisted living population of central Maryland. *Journal of the American Geriatrics Society, 52*(10), 1618–1625.

Sands, L. P., Xu, H., Weiner, M., Rosenman, M. B., Craig, B. A., & Thomas, J., III. (2008). Comparison of resource utilization for Medicaid dementia patients using nursing homes versus home and community based waivers for long-term care. *Medical Care, 46*(4), 449–453.

Substance Abuse and Mental Health Services Administration. (2006, June 28). Transforming mental health care in America: The Federal Action Agenda; First Steps. Available online at http://www.samhsa.gov/Federalactionagenda/NFC_execsum.aspx. Accessed June 25, 2009.

Takamura, J. (1999). Getting ready for the 21st century: The aging of America and the Older Americans Act. *Health and Social Work, 24*(3), 232–238.

Unützer, J., Katon, W. J., Fan, M. Y., Schoenbaum, M. C., Lin, E. H., Della Penna, R. D., et al. (2008). Long-term cost effects of collaborative care for late-life depression. *American Journal of Managed Care, 14*(2), 95–100.

Unützer, J., Patrick, D. L., Simon, G., Grembowski, D., Walker, E., Rutter, C., et al. (1997). Depressive symptoms and the cost of health services in HMO patients aged 65 years and older: A 4 year prospective study. *Journal of the American Medical Association, 277*(20), 1618–1623.

Unützer, J., Powers, D., Katon, W., & Langston, C. (2005). From establishing an evidence-based practice to implementation in real world settings: IMPACT as a case study. *Psychiatric Clinics of North America, 28*(4), 1079–1092.

Unützer, J., Schoenbaum, M., Druss, B. G., & Katon, W. J. (2006). Transforming mental health care at the interface with general medicine: Report for the Presidents Commission. *Psychiatric Services, 57*(1), 37–47.

U.S. Census Bureau. (2000, January 13). *Projections of the Resident Population by Age, Sex, Race, and Hispanic Origin: 1999–2100*. Population Projections Program. Available online at http://www.census.gov/population/www/projections/natproj.html. Accessed June 25, 2009.

U.S. Department of Health and Human Services. (1999). *Mental Health: A Report of the Surgeon General*. Rockville, MD: Author.

U.S. Department of Health and Human Services. (2003). *New Freedom Commission on Mental Health: Achieving the Promise: Transforming Mental Health Care in America. Final Report*. No. DHHS pub no SMA-03-3832. Rockville, MD: Author.

Van Citters, A. D., & Bartels, S. J. (2004). A systematic review of the effectiveness of community-based mental health outreach services for older adults. *Psychiatric Services, 55*(11), 1237–1249.

White House Conference on Aging. (2005). *The Booming Dynamics of Aging: From Awareness to Action, Implementation Strategy Highlight Report*. Washington, D.C.: Author.

Wilk, J. E., West, J. C., Rae, D. S., Rubio-Stipec, M., Chen, J. J., & Regier, D. A. (2008). Medicare Part D prescription drug benefits and administrative burden in the care of dually eligible psychiatric patients. *Psychiatric Services, 59*, 34–39.

Williams, L. (2000). Long-term care after Olmstead v. L.C.: Will the potential of the ADA's integration mandate be achieved? *Journal of Contemporary Health Law and Policy, 17*(1), 205–239.

Zuidema, S., Koopmans, R., & Verhey, F. (2007). Prevalence and predictors of neuropsychiatric symptoms in cognitively impaired nursing home patients. *Journal of Geriatric Psychiatry & Neurology 20*(1), 41–49.

Chapter 11

THE TREATMENT SYSTEM FOR ALCOHOL AND DRUG DISORDERS

Dennis McCarty, PhD; and Traci Rieckmann, PhD

Introduction

Legacies of discrimination in access to health care, social control systems built upon incarceration, reliance on self-help, and emphasis on experiential training provide the context for contemporary alcohol and drug abuse treatment services. From 1935 to 1974, the primary treatment services for narcotic addiction were federally operated facilities that were more prison than rehabilitation in Lexington, Kentucky (Campbell, Olsen, & Walden, 2008), and Fort Worth, Texas. Alcoholics were regularly denied care in hospitals (Plaut, 1967) and confined in drunk tanks and county farms as recently as the 1960s and 1970s (President's Commission on Law Enforcement and Administration of Justice, Task Force on Drunkenness, 1967). Men and women in recovery advocated for changes in state and federal legislation and, through grassroots organization and community development, constructed and delivered treatment services for alcoholism and drug addiction. Today, treatments for alcohol and drug use disorders are an assortment of financing sources, a patchwork of small, independent and specialized services, and a loosely organized workforce that includes many individuals with personal experiences of addiction and recovery. As a result, substance abuse treatment services are, to a large degree, an idiosyncratic facet of health care systems in the United States.

This chapter provides an overview of the financing and organization of treatment services for alcohol and drug use disorders. Comparisons of expenditures for addiction treatment with treatment for mental health and general health reveal unique attributes of addiction treatment systems. An examination of specialty alcohol and drug treatment programs, a description of patient populations, and a review of the substance abuse treatment workforce provide more background for appreciating the distinctive nature of substance abuse services. The chapter concludes with a discussion of how the organization and financing of substance abuse treatment affect the potential for integration of care and adoption of evidence-based practices.

Expenditures for Treatment of Alcohol and Drug Use Disorders

A Center for Substance Abuse Treatment (CSAT) estimate suggests that total spending on treatment for alcohol and drug dependence and abuse was about $21 billion in 2003 (Mark et al., 2007; Mark et al., 2008) and projected to reach $35 billion in 2014 (Levit et al., 2008). This is more than a three fold increase compared to 1997's $11.4 billion in expenditures (Mark et al., 2000). The $21 billion represents about 17% of the nation's expenditures for the treatment of mental health and substance abuse and an almost trivial 1% of the nation's $1.6 trillion in total 2003 health care expenditures (Mark et al., 2007). Comparisons of the treatment providers and the payment sources for addiction treatments versus mental health and total health care services highlight unique features of substance abuse treatment systems.

Providers and Services

Specialty substance abuse treatment programs now account for about 41% of the total expenditures on treatment for drug and alcohol disorders (up from 33% in 1997) (Mark et al., 2007). An additional 24% of the treatment expenditures represent services from hospitals and physicians, and private practitioners account for 21% of total spending (Mark et al., 2007). Hospital expenditures primarily reflect inpatient services for detoxification and withdrawal management. Lengths of stay are brief (typically four days or less), and the cost per day for hospital beds is substantial. Multi-service mental health organizations account for only 6% of the total expenditures (Mark et al., 2007).

Finally, it is noteworthy that less than 1% of treatment expenditures in 2003 were for prescription medications. In contrast, pharmacotherapy accounted for 23% of mental health spending (Mark et al., 2007). Expenditures for medication assisted treatments are increasing. Sales of medications approved for treating alcohol abuse grew from $30 million in 2003 to $78 million in 2007; and sales of buprenorphine, approved for treating opiate dependence in 2002, increased from $5 million in 2003 to $327 million in 2007 (Mark, Kassed, Vandivort-Warren, Levit, & Kranzler, 2009). While recent sales gains are impressive, only a small portion of the potential patient population receive pharmacotherapy using approved medications.

In summary, expenditures for alcohol and drug abuse treatment services reflect a reliance on inpatient hospital services, the unique influence of specialty clinics, reluctance among independent practitioners to treat addictions, and a resistance to the use of medications. Thus, the idiosyncratic nature of the substance abuse treatment systems begins to emerge. An assessment of payers helps to more clearly describe the current systems of care.

PAYERS

Alcohol and drug abuse services receive a lower proportion of private insurance payments (10% of total 2003 expenditures) in comparison to payments for mental health services (22% from private insurance) (Mark et al., 2007). This disparity reflects historical reluctance among commercial health plans to provide coverage for alcohol and drug disorders and the persistent lack of parity in the benefits for substance abuse services. As a result, more than three-quarters of funds spent on services for substance abuse in 2003 were from public sources (78%): state and local funds (40%), Medicaid (18%), federal block grant and other federal funds (15%), and Medicare (5%) (Mark et al., 2007).

The resulting treatment systems are heavily dependent upon public revenues. The block grant and state revenues flow through state agencies that license and fund services for the treatment of alcohol and drug dependence. States have traditionally funded programs and facilities rather than practitioners. The resulting treatment infrastructures rely on community-based organizations rather than individual practitioners.

Multiple funding streams contribute to fragmentation of services delivery but are also evidence of creative strategies to support substance abuse treatment. Successful treatment centers often receive support from state, county, and local governments as well as federal block grants, Center for Substance Abuse Treatment capacity expansion grants, drug courts, corrections, parole, local foundations, many commercial health plans, Medicaid, Medicare, self-pay, and personal contributions. Data on the treatment programs add detail to the discussion of the addictions treatment system.

Treatment Centers, Workforce, and Patients

Institute of Medicine reviews of alcohol (Institute of Medicine, 1990a) and drug abuse (Institute of Medicine, 1990b) treatment provide excellent overviews of treatment modalities. Addiction treatment systems, however, continue to evolve and increasingly reflect a patient population using both alcohol and drugs (McCarty, Caspi, Panas, Krakow, & Mulligan, 2000; Substance Abuse and Mental Health Services Administration [SAMHSA], 2007). As a result, most addiction treatment facilities treat both alcohol and drug dependence. An overview of treatment centers, the workforce, and the patients they serve further illustrates key features of the nation's systems for addressing addiction.

ALCOHOL AND DRUG ABUSE TREATMENT CENTERS

The most comprehensive descriptive data on addiction treatment programs come from a census of known alcohol and drug abuse programs conducted annually by the Substance Abuse and Mental Health Services Administration (SAMHSA): The National Survey of Substance Abuse Treatment Services (N-SSATS). Annual N-SSATS updates are posted on the SAMHSA Web site (www.samhsa.gov).

The 2007 census identified a total of 13,648 specialty substance abuse treatment facilities (SAMHSA, 2008b). Most (61%) of the responding treatment facilities identified themselves as only providing services for alcohol and drug abuse (i.e., no medical or mental health services other than addictions treatment (SAMHSA, 2008b). About one in three (36%) facilities reported that they also provided mental health services, and 1.4% of facilities were located in general health care settings. Typically, substance abuse treatment programs were organized as private non-profit corporations (58%); 29% were private for-profit entities, and 13% operated as units of local, state, federal, or tribal government (SAMHSA, 2008b).

Facilities that provide addiction treatments delivered a range of services but focused on assessments for substance abuse (98%) and related counseling services: individual counseling (99%); group counseling (96%); and family therapy (72%) (SAMHSA, 2008b). More than half of the programs also reported providing urine screening for drug use (83%), after-care counseling (81%), case management (76%), and HIV education (56%). Treatment facilities were less likely to offer medical and support services: medications (47%); HIV testing (29%); employment counseling (34%); and child care (8%).

The programs that provide alcohol and drug treatment services tended to have small caseloads. The median daily caseload was 42 patients and 79% of the facilities served fewer than 120 patients a day (SAMHSA, 2008b).

The available information suggests that the programs serving individuals seeking treatment for alcohol and drug use disorders are an eclectic group of non-profit, for-profit, and governmental entities. The largest proportion, however, are the traditional freestanding non-profit corporations that specialize in treating substance abuse. The programs tend to have small caseloads, and services are primarily individual and group therapy, problem assessment, and urine screens for drugs of abuse. For the most part, even though patients have multiple needs, few programs provide ancillary and support services for housing, education, and legal problems. The limited data available on the staff in alcohol and drug abuse programs reinforces impressions about the unique nature of the treatment services and facilities.

WORKFORCE

Because the patients treated in alcohol and drug abuse treatment often have co-occurring legal, employment, mental health, family relationship, and housing problems, counselors need a wide range of knowledge and skills to address multiple patient needs. Training a workforce with the capabilities to respond to all of the treatment needs places heavy expectations on education programs to develop counselors with multi-faceted skills and to provide continuing education opportunities. Although descriptions of the substance abuse treatment workforce are limited, they are, nonetheless, informative.

Analyses of the individuals providing drug and alcohol counseling during the late 1970s and early 1980s suggest that much of the workforce practiced without graduate training. Between one in five (Camp & Kurtz, 1982) and one in three counselors (Birch & Davis, 1984) claimed a masters or doctoral degree. Rates of graduate training may have been even lower in programs that were classified as drug treatment (Aiken, LoSciuto, & Ausetts, 1985; LoSciuto, Aiken, & Ausetts, 1979). Many of those working without a college degree or a bachelor's degree identified themselves as "in recovery."

Contemporary assessments of the workforce continue to report that women account for a majority of the workforce and that about 50% of the counselors have graduate degrees (Gallon, Gabriel, & Knudsen, 2003; Harwood, 2002; Johnson, Knudsen, & Roman, 2002; Mulvey, Hubbard, & Hayashi, 2003). The National Drug Abuse Treatment Clinical Trials Network completed an extensive analysis of the workforce. Two of three (67%) individuals working in drug and alcohol treatment facilities within the Clinical Trials Network were women, and 36% reported having a master's or doctoral degree (McCarty et al., 2007a). Comparisons of counselors with managers/supervisors, medical staff, and support staff suggested that supervisors were more supportive of evidence-based behavioral therapies and medical staff were more supportive of pharmacotherapy (McCarty et al., 2007a) (see Chapter 5 in this volume for additional information on workforce issues in mental health).

ALCOHOL AND DRUG DEPENDENT INDIVIDUALS

The National Survey on Drug Use and Health (NSDUH) tracks the prevalence and incidence of illicit drug, alcohol, and tobacco use in the United States and estimates the need for treatment and the demand for treatment services. Annual updates are posted on the SAMHSA Web site (www.samhsa.gov). The 2007 Survey reported that 20 million individuals (8% of the population 12 years of age and older) used illicit drugs in the 30 days prior to the survey; 127 million (51% of the population) drank alcohol in the past month; and 17 million (7%) met criteria for heavy drinking (SAMHSA, 2008a). The survey also suggested that 22 million individuals (9% of the U.S. population 12 years and older) were in need of treatment for abuse or dependence on alcohol and drugs (SAMHSA, 2008a). Nearly 19 million met criteria for abuse or dependence on alcohol, and 7 million met criteria for drug abuse or dependence: 3.9 million for marijuana, 1.7 million for prescription opiates; and 1.6 million for cocaine (SAMHSA, 2008a).

Most alcohol and drug dependent and abusing individuals were not in treatment. The 22 million in need of treatment contrasts with the 4.0 million who reported receiving treatment in 2007. Respondents suggested that 1.7 million entered care in specialty substance abuse treatment programs and 2.2 million participated in self-help groups (SAMHSA, 2008a). Other estimates suggest that about 44% of the most severely dependent illicit drug users received treatment in the past year (Woodward et al., 1997). A "treatment gap," therefore, exceeds 50% for the individuals with greatest treatment priority and is much higher among alcohol dependent individuals and individuals with less severe drug problems.

Implications for Mental Health and Substance Abuse

The nation's addiction treatment systems stand relatively isolated from systems of care for health and mental health. There are, consequently, perennial policy issues: 1) a persistent gap in access to care and skepticism about the effectiveness of treatment; 2) limited coverage for alcohol and drug abuse treatment within health insurance; 3) poor integration with health care and criminal justice systems; and 4) challenges related to the adoption of evidence-based practices.

ACCESS TO CARE AND SKEPTICISM ABOUT THE VALUE OF CARE

The gap between the need for care and access to care is a product of patient factors (stigma of addiction and denial about the need for care), financing issues (limited funding and health care coverage for addiction treatments), poor linkages between service systems, and weak screening and referral mechanisms. Individuals dependent upon alcohol and other drugs often fail to recognize that they need treatment or may be ambivalent about entering care.

Treatment systems struggle with strategies to engage adults and adolescents who need care. Motivational interviewing techniques enhance patient motivation and controlled studies consistently find improvements in entry to and retention in care (Carroll et al., 2006; Miller & Rollnick, 2002; Miller & Wilbourne, 2002). However, facilitation of access and enhanced retention also require improved systems for patient placement (American Society of Addiction Medicine, 2001), assessment of patients (McLellan et al., 1992), and change in the delivery of services to enhance quality of care (Capoccia et al., 2007; Institute of Medicine, 1997, 1998, 2006; McCarty et al., 2007b; McCarty, Capoccia, Gustafson, & Cotter, 2008; McLellan & McKay, 1998; McLellan et al., 2003). In short, treatment providers and policymakers have numerous opportunities to improve treatment access and retention through restructuring of addiction treatment services. Programs participating in the Network for the Improvement of Addiction Treatment, for example, reduced days to treatment entry by 37% and improved retention in care from the first outpatient visit to the second visit by 17% (Hoffman, Ford, Choi, Gustafson, & McCarty, 2008; McCarty et al., 2007b).

Investigations consistently find that treatment for alcohol and drug dependence is associated with reductions in use and improvements in functioning (Institute of Medicine, 1990b, 1990a, 1998; Simpson, 1997). For example, comparisons of drug use at intake and 12 months after leaving treatment using data from the Treatment Outcome Prospective Study (TOPS) (intake interviews were completed in 1979 and 1980) and the Drug Abuse Treatment Outcomes Studies (DATOS) (intake interviews conducted in 1991, 1992, and 1993) suggested that about 50% of weekly and daily heroin and cocaine users reported "any use" at follow-up (Hubbard, Flynn, Craddock, & Fletcher, 2001). The likelihood of use, however, was lower in the DATOS cohort (heroin and cocaine = 47% reporting any use) than among patients who participated in the earlier TOPS investigation (heroin = 59%; cocaine = 65%) and suggests improvements in the effectiveness of treatment services (Hubbard et al., 2001).

Nonetheless, public and private policymakers continue to question the efficacy of alcohol and drug abuse treatment services. A comparison of treatment outcomes for addiction, asthma, diabetes, and heart disease provides an interesting perspective on efficacy; the analysis found similar rates of treatment compliance

(40 to 60%) and readmission to care (about 50%) for each disease (McLellan, Lewis, O'Brien, & Kleber, 2000). The essay argues that alcohol and drug dependence should be viewed as a chronic illness that requires continued treatment attention and advocates for substantive change in the ways in which care is delivered in order to provide long-term, low intensity services to help patients function and maintain without intensive acute care (McLellan et al., 2000).

FINANCING AND INSURANCE PARITY

Historically, health insurance plans have been reluctant to cover treatment for alcohol and drug dependence (Scott, Greenberg, & Pizarro, 1992). Concern with adverse selection inhibits liberal benefits: plans offering better coverage for alcoholism and drug abuse treatment services may attract members who need that service and could require expensive services (Frank, McGuire, Bae, & Rupp, 1997). To facilitate access to treatment, 41 states mandate coverage for treatment of alcohol and/or drug abuse, but the coverage tends to be limited to $500 of outpatient services (Scott et al., 1992). When available, inpatient benefits are heavily managed, making it difficult to use the nominal benefit.

The persistent disparity in coverage for alcohol and drug dependence prompted state and federal legislation to require parity: mental health and substance abuse treatment benefits with limits on duration of outpatient and inpatient care similar to the coverage available for most medical services. State parity legislation, however, usually excluded treatment for alcohol and drug use disorders. Only Oregon and Vermont provided full parity for addiction treatments. The federal government administratively required parity in coverage for services for mental illness and alcohol and drug use disorders in health plans for federal employees. An evaluation of the federal parity initiative reported that increases in the cost of health coverage were due to cyclical rises in the cost of health care and that parity requirements for mental health and substance abuse treatment did not have a significant impact on costs (Goldman et al., 2006).

Until 2008, federal parity legislation applied only to treatment for serious mental illness. The Wellstone-Domenici Mental Health Parity Act of 2008 represented a major change in federal policy. Group health plans that cover more than 50 employees are required to provide comparable coverage for mental health, substance abuse, and medical/surgical benefits if they cover mental health and substance abuse treatment services. The parity legislation became effective in January of 2010. With regulatory provisions of this legislation currently in development, it is premature to assess the impact of the legislation on access, utilization, and costs of care (see Chapter 2 in this volume for additional discussion of insurance, financing, and managed care).

INTEGRATION WITH HEALTH CARE

Most individuals with alcohol and drug problems are found in primary care settings rather than specialty clinics and criminal justice systems (Weisner, 2001).

Continued reluctance to identify and treat alcohol and drug dependent individuals, however, inhibits the integration of substance abuse treatment services with primary care. More integrated services, nonetheless, continue to promise economic and health care benefits.

A recent investigation conducted within a health maintenance organization assigned patients either to a primary care clinician located in the addiction treatment service unit or treatment as usual with a primary care clinician not located within the addiction treatment unit. Patients with substance abuse–related medical conditions were more likely to be abstinent six months post treatment when primary care was integrated with addiction treatment (69% versus 55% abstinence) (Weisner, Mertens, Parthasarathy, Moore, & Lu, 2001). Despite a slightly higher cost, the integrated care was more cost-effective (better outcomes with a modest increase in cost) (Weisner et al., 2001). Better integration of addiction services and primary care continues to be an aspiration.

Screening for alcohol disorders (using a brief standardized assessment) and simple 10- to 15-minute interventions in primary care medical settings have been shown to reduce self-reported alcohol use (Babor et al., 2007; Whitlock, Polen, Green, Orleans, & Klein, 2004). Interventions may be especially helpful for hazardous drinkers, those with moderate substance use disorders, medically ill patients who are abusing substances, minimally motivated patients, and those receiving substance abuse counseling services elsewhere (Samet, Friedmann, & Saitz, 2001). There is less research on screening for drug use disorders, and the U.S. Preventive Services Task Force concludes that current evidence is insufficient to recommend routine screening for drug misuse (Polen, Whitlock, Wisdom, Nygren, & Bougatsos, 2008). Nevertheless, significant evidence exists regarding the potential for screening and brief interventions with alcohol use/abuse. Investigations with other drug use are under way. In response, Medicaid, Medicare, and the American Medical Association have approved health care procedure codes and reimbursement rates to encourage widespread implementation of alcohol and drug screening in medical care settings (see Chapter 16 in this volume for additional discussion of the integration of primary care services with specialty mental health services).

An additional potential benefit from closer integration between substance abuse treatment and primary care is better access to medications. Despite recent advances in the development of pharmacotherapies for alcohol and drug dependence (Institute of Medicine, 2004), adoption of these medications has been slow (Horgan, Reif, Hodgkin, Garnick, & Merrick, 2008; Knudsen, Ducharme, & Roman, 2007; Mark et al., 2009; Rieckmann, Daley, Fuller, Thomas, & McCarty, 2007). A lack of access to primary care clinicians who can write prescriptions inhibits adoption in many freestanding alcohol and drug abuse treatment centers. Policymakers and practitioners continue to be challenged to find effective strategies for integrating treatment for alcohol and drug problems with primary care and mental health services. Participants in the Robert Wood Johnson Foundation's Advancing Recovery program (www.advancingrecovery.org) are making systems changes to promote access to addiction medications: linkages with physicians and mechanisms to pay for pharmacotherapies (see Chapter 21 in this volume for additional information on economic issues in psychotropic medication use).

COORDINATION WITH CRIMINAL JUSTICE SYSTEMS

Individuals struggling with alcohol and other drug abuse and dependence also appear frequently in the criminal justice system. The National Institute on Drug Abuse (NIDA) is supporting the Criminal Justice Drug Abuse Treatment Studies (CJ-DATS) to conduct systematic investigations that develop and test integrated treatment strategies for drug-involved criminal offenders (Friedmann, Taxman, & Henderson, 2007; Taxman, Yound, Wiersema, Rhodes, & Mitchell, 2007; Taxman, Perdoni, & Harrison, 2007). The nine research centers and coordinating center are conducting trials to develop better assessment tools, assess treatment progress, link criminal justice and treatment services, address adolescent offenders, and reduce risks for infectious diseases.

Drug courts have become a major part of the criminal justice response to drug crime. The courts remove drug offenders from crowded dockets and create a special venue for monitoring offenders and prescribing sanctions designed to promote the use of treatment services and recovery from drug dependence. The authority of the court persuades offenders to choose recovery over continuation of a criminal career. The first drug court began in 1989. Operating drug courts numbered 2,147 at the end of 2007 (Office of National Drug Control Policy, 2008). Federal funds fueled this tremendous growth. Reviews of the management of drug courts, however, report poor data collection and weak evaluation activities (U.S. General Accounting Office, 2002). While evaluation studies often conclude that drug courts have positive impacts upon offenders, evaluations often lack appropriate comparison groups, and it is difficult to attribute the apparent improvements to drug court involvement (Belenko, 2002; Cooper, 2003; Turner et al., 2002). Systematic research, however, has begun to identify the key components of the drug court intervention (Marlowe, Festinger, Dugosh, & Lee, 2005) (see Chapter 18 in this volume for additional information on specialty services in criminal justice systems).

EVIDENCE-BASED PRACTICE

Research is developing more comprehensive descriptions of the effects of chronic alcohol and drug use on neurobiology and identifying more effective behavioral and pharmacological interventions. Program directors and policymakers strive to encourage application of these findings in contemporary treatment services, but community drug and alcohol programs seem to be particularly resistant to the adoption of evidence-based practices (Garner, 2009; Institute of Medicine, 1998; Miller, Zweben, & Johnson, 2005).

Initiatives like the National Institute on Drug Abuse's National Drug Abuse Clinical Trials Network help research become more relevant to practitioners and encourage clinicians to read research findings. Studies conducted within the Clinical Trials Network document the effectiveness of buprenorphine (Amass et al., 2004; Ling et al., 2005; Woody et al., 2008), the value of low-cost incentives to encourage retention in outpatient (Petry et al., 2005), less drug use during methadone maintenance (Peirce et al., 2006), and the effectiveness of motivational interviewing (Carroll et al., 2006). The Addiction Technology Transfer Centers, moreover, collaborate with the Clinical Trials Network to produce user-friendly training materials so that dissemination can occur shortly after publication in peer-reviewed journals (Albright, 2006; Freese, 2006; Gallon, 2006). The manuals are available as a five compact disk set (without cost) from the National ATTC office (http://www.attcnetwork.org/explore/priorityareas/science/blendinginitiative/science_of_tx.asp). Despite progress on science and dissemination of research findings, the field continues to struggle with the challenge of enhancing workforce skills and the application of evidence-based practices.

Federal, state, and local initiatives foster increased adoption of evidence-based practices for treatment of alcohol and drug disorders. The National Registry of Evidence-Based Programs and Practices (NREPP) is the Substance Abuse and Mental Health Services Administration online resource for independently reviewed and rated evidence-based interventions for the prevention and treatment of mental health and substance use disorders (http://www.nrepp.samhsa.gov/).

Importantly, a National Quality Forum consensus panel identified five categories of evidence-based practices: 1) screening and brief intervention; 2) psychosocial interventions; 3) medications; 4) wrap-around services; and 5) after-care and recovery management. The consensus panel also identified four specific strategies designed to facilitate adoption of EBPs in substance abuse treatment, including 1) financial incentives and mechanisms; 2) use of regulations and accreditation; 3) education and training; and 4) infrastructure development (National Quality Forum, 2007). These strategies provide broad categories, leaving room for individual flexibility and state-specific efforts aimed at increasing implementation.

Translation of substance abuse research into clinical practice presents a complex set of workforce and organizational challenges for treatment agencies, research, and policy communities. As available evidence continues to confirm that empirically derived treatment strategies improve outcomes for those struggling with alcohol and drug abuse (McLellan & McKay, 1998; Miller & Wilbourne, 2002; Miller et al., 2005), the significant lag between development of such strategies and widespread adoption becomes increasingly problematic (Garner, 2009; Institute of Medicine, 1998; Marinelli-Casey, Domier, & Rawson, 2002).

Interventions that are empirically validated, however, may be irrelevant, too complicated, too expensive, and/or too narrowly focused (McGovern & Carroll, 2003). Intensive examination of factors that enhance technology transfer is critical for accelerating implementation of new practices in substance abuse treatment. Both counselor and organizational factors are important in the diffusion and translation of technology to practice (Ducharme, Knudsen, Roman, & Johnson, 2007; Simpson, 2002; Simpson & Flynn, 2007; Thomas, Wallack, Lee, McCarty, & Swift, 2003; Thomas & McCarty, 2004). Little is known, however, about the specific qualities or ingredients that facilitate implementation.

State agencies that license and fund prevention and treatment services can also affect the use of evidence-based practices in substance abuse treatment (Rieckmann, Kovas, Fussell, & Stettler, 2009). State authorities communicate their commitment to the use of evidence-based practices through language in contracts, licensing regulations, quality improvement and strategic plans, and design and language included in calls for proposals.

Contemporary alcohol and drug abuse treatment services have persisted despite limited resources and public ambivalence about the value of addictions treatment. To survive in the next decade, attention will focus on the development of quality improvement strategies to document effectiveness and promote greater account-ability. Therapists will enhance their skills, and the field will become more inte-grated into health care, mental health, and criminal justice systems. Systematic evolution will promote a continuing role for specialty alcohol and drug abuse treat-ment programming.

References

Aiken, L. S., LoSciuto, L., & Ausetts, M. (1985). Who is serving drug abuse clients? In R. S. Ashery (Ed.), *Progress in the Development of Cost-Effective Treatment for Drug Abusers*. Rockville, MD: National Institute on Drug Abuse.

Albright, L. (2006). *Promoting Awareness of Motivational Incentives*. Kansas City, MO: Addiction Technology Transfer Centers National Office.

Amass, L., Ling, W., Freese, T. E., Reiber, C., Annon, J. J., Cohen, A. J., et al. (2004). Bringing buprenorphine-naloxone detoxification to community treatment programs: The NIDA Clinical Trial Network field experience. *American Journal on Addictions, 13*, S42–S66.

American Society of Addiction Medicine. (2001). *Patient Placement Criteria for the Treatment of Substance Related Disorders, Second Edition Revised (ASAM PPC-2R)* (2nd rev. ed.). Chevy Chase, MD: American Society of Addiction Medicine.

Babor, T. F., McRee, B. G., Kassebaum, P. A., Grimaldi, P. L., Ahmed, K., & Bray, J. (2007). Screening, brief intervention, and referral to treatment (SBIRT): Toward a public health approach to the management of substance abuse. *Substance Abuse, 28*, 7–30.

Belenko, S. (2002). The challenges of conducting research in drug treatment court settings. *Substance Use & Misuse, 37*, 1635–1664.

Birch & Davis Associates. (1984). *Development of Model Professional Standards for Counselor Credentialing*. Rockville, MD: National Institute on Alcohol Abuse and Alcoholism.

Camp, J. M., & Kurtz, N. R. (1982). Redirecting manpower for alcoholism treatment. In *Prevention, Intervention, and Treatment: Concerns and Models* (pp. 371–397). DHHS Publication No. ADM-1192 ed. Rockville, MD: National Institute on Alcohol Abuse and Alcoholism.

Campbell, N. D., Olsen, J. P., & Walden, L. (2008). *The Narcotic Farm: The Rise and Fall of America's First Prison for Drug Addicts*. New York: Harry N. Abrams.

Capoccia, V. A., Cotter, F., Gustafson, D. H., Cassidy, E., Ford, J., Madden, L., et al. (2007). Making "stone soup": How process improvement is changing the addiction treatment field. *Joint Commission Journal on Quality and Patient Safety, 33*, 95–103.

Carroll, K. M., Ball, S. A., Nich, C., Martino, S., Frankforter, T. L., Farentinos, C., et al. (2006). Motivational interviewing to improve treatment engagement and outcome in individuals seeking treatment for substance abuse: A multisite effectiveness study. *Drug and Alcohol Dependence, 81*, 301–312.

Cooper, C. S. (2003). Drug courts: Current issues and future perspectives. *Substance Use & Misuse, 38*, 1671–1711.

Ducharme, L. J., Knudsen, H. K., Roman, P. M., & Johnson, J. A (2007). Innovation adoption in substance abuse treatment: Exposure, trialability, and the Clinical Trials Network. *Journal of Substance Abuse Treatment, 32*, 321–329.

Frank, R. G., McGuire, T. G., Bae, J. P., & Rupp, A. (1997). Solutions for adverse selection in behavioral health care. *Health Care Financing Review, 18*, 109–122.

Freese, T. E. (2006). *Short-Term Opioid Withdrawal Using Buprenorphine: Findings and Strategies from a NIDA Clinical Trials Network Study.* Kansas City, MO: Addiction Technology Transfer Center National Office.

Friedmann, P. D., Taxman, F. S., & Henderson, C. E. (2007). Evidence-based treatment practices for drug-involved adults in the criminal justice system. *Journal of Substance Abuse Treatment, 32*, 267–277.

Gallon, S. L. (2006). *Motivational Interviewing Assessment: Supervisory Tools for Enhancing Proficiency (MIA: STEP).* Kansas City, MO: Addiction Technology Transfer Center National Office.

Gallon, S. L., Gabriel, R. M., & Knudsen, J. (2003). The toughest job you'll ever love: A Pacific Northwest Treatment Workforce Survey. *Journal of Substance Abuse Treatment, 24*, 183–196.

Garner, B. (2009). Research on the diffusion of evidence-based treatments within substance abuse treatment: A systematic review. *Journal of Substance Abuse Treatment, 36*, 376–399.

Goldman, H. H., Frank, R. G., Burnam, M. A., Huskamp, H. A., Ridgely, M. S., Normand, S.-L. T., et al. (2006). Behavioral health insurance parity for federal employees. *New England Journal of Medicine, 354*, 1378–1386.

Harwood, H. J. (2002, November). Survey on behavioral health workplace. *Frontlines: Linking Alcohol Services Research & Practice, 3*.

Hoffman, K., Ford, J. H., Choi, D., Gustafson, D., & McCarty, D. (2008). Replication and sustainability of improved access and retention within the Network for the Improvement of Addiction Treatment. *Drug and Alcohol Dependence, 98*, 63–69.

Horgan, C. M., Reif, S., Hodgkin, D., Garnick, D. W., & Merrick, E. L. (2008). Availability of addiction medications in private health plans. *Journal of Substance Abuse Treatment, 34*, 147–156.

Hubbard, R. L., Flynn, P. M., Craddock, S. G., & Fletcher, B. W. (2001). Relapse after drug abuse treatment. In F. M. Tims, C. G. Leukefeld, & J. J. Platt (Eds.), *Relapse and Recovery in Addictions* (pp. 109–121). New Haven, CT: Yale University Press.

Institute of Medicine (1990a). *Broadening the Base of Treatment for Alcohol Problems.* Washington, DC: National Academy Press.

Institute of Medicine (1990b). *Treating Drug Problems.* Washington, DC: National Academy Press.

Institute of Medicine (1997). *Managing Managed Care: Quality Improvement in Behavioral Health.* Washington, DC: National Academy Press.

Institute of Medicine (1998). *Bridging the Gap between Practice and Research: Forging Partnerships with Community-Based Drug and Alcohol Treatment.* Washington, DC: National Academy Press.

Institute of Medicine (2004). *New Treatments for Addiction* Washington, DC: The National Acadmies Press.

Institute of Medicine (2006). *Improving the Quality of Health Care for Mental and Substance-Use Disorders: Quality Chasm Series.* Washington, DC: National Academy Press.

Johnson, J. A., Knudsen, H. K., & Roman, P. M. (2002). Counselor turnover in private facilities. *Frontlines: Linking Alcohol Services Research & Practice, November, 5, 8.*

Knudsen, H. K., Ducharme, L. J., & Roman, P. M. (2007). The adoption of medications in substance abuse treatment: Associations with organizational characteristics and technology clusters. *Drug and Alcohol Dependence, 87*, 164–174.

Levit, K. R., Kassed, C. A., Coffey, R. M., Mark, T. L., McKusick, D. R., King, E. C., et al. (2008). *Projections of National Expenditures for Mental Health Services and Substance Abuse Treatment 2004–2014.* SAMHSA Publication No. SMA 08-4326 ed. Rockville, MD: Substance Abuse and Mental Health Services Administration.

Ling, W., Amass, L., Shoptow, M., Annon, J. J., Hillhouse, M., Babcock, D., et al. (2005). A multicenter randomized trial of buprenorphine-naloxone versus clonidine for opioid detoxification: Findings from the National Institute on Drug Abuse's Clinical Trial Network. *Addiction, 100*, 1090–1100.

LoSciuto, L. A., Aiken, L. S., & Ausetts, M. A. (1979). *Professional and Paraprofessional Drug Abuse Counselors: Three Reports*. Rep. No. NIDA Services Research Monograph Series, DHHS Publication No. ADM 81-858. Rockville, MD: National Institute on Drug Abuse.

Marinelli-Casey, P., Domier, C., & Rawson, R. (2002). The gap between research and practice in substance abuse treatment. *Psychiatric Services, 53*, 984–987.

Mark, T. L., Coffey, R. M., King, E., Harwood, H., McKusick, D., Genuardi, J., et al. (2000). Spending on mental health and substance abuse treatment, 1987–1997. *Health Affairs, 19*, 108–120.

Mark, T. L., Harwood, H. J., McKusick, D., King, E., Vandivort-Warren, R., & Buck, J. A. (2008). Mental health and substance abuse spending by age, 2003. *Journal of Behavioral Health Services & Research, 35*(3), 279–289.

Mark, T. L., Kassed, C. A., Vandivort-Warren, R., Levit, K. R., & Kranzler, H. R. (2009). Alcohol and opioid dependence medications: Prescription trends, overall and by physician specialty. *Drug and Alcohol Dependence, 99*, 345–349.

Mark, T. L., Levit, K. R., Coffey, R. M., McKusick, D., Harwood, H. J., King, E., et al. (2007). *National Expenditures for Mental Health Services and Substance Abuse Treatment: 1993–2003*. SAMHSA Publication No. SMA 07-4227 ed. Rockville, MD: Substance Abuse and Mental Health Services Administration.

Marlowe, D. B., Festinger, D. S., Dugosh, K. L., & Lee, P. A. (2005). Are judicial status hearings a "key component" of drug court? Six and twelve months outcomes. *Drug and Alcohol Dependence, 79*, 145–155.

McCarty, D., Capoccia, V. A., Gustafson, D., & Cotter, F. (2009). Improving care for the treatment of alcohol and drug disorders. *Journal of Behavioral Health Services & Research, 36*(1), 52–60.

McCarty, D., Caspi, Y., Panas, L., Krakow, M., & Mulligan, D. H. (2000). Detoxification centers: Who's in the revolving door? *Journal of Behavioral Health Services & Research, 27*, 245–256.

McCarty, D., Fuller, B., Arfken, C. L., Miller, M., Nunes, E. V., Edmundson, E., et al. (2007a). Direct care workers in the National Drug Abuse Treatment Clinical Trials Network: Characteristics, opinions, and beliefs. *Psychiatric Services, 58*, 181–190.

McCarty, D., Gustafson, D. H., Wisdom, J. P., Ford, J., Choi, D., Molfenter, T., et al. (2007b). The Network for the Improvement of Addiction Treatment (NIATx): Enhancing access and retention. *Drug and Alcohol Dependence, 88*, 138–145.

McGovern, M., & Carroll, K. (2003). Evidence-based practices for substance use disorders. *Psychiatric Clinics of North America, 26*, 991–1010.

McLellan, A. T., Carise, D., & Kleber, H. D. (2003). Can the national addiction treatment infra-structure support the public's demand for quality care? *Journal of Substance Abuse Treatment, 25*, 117–121.

McLellan, A. T., Kushner, H., Metzger, D., Peters, R., Smith, I., Grisson, G. et al., (1992). The fifth edition of the Addiction Severity Index. *Journal of Substance Abuse Treatment, 9*, 199–213.

McLellan, A. T., Lewis, D. C., O'Brien, C. P., & Kleber, H. D. (2000). Drug dependence a chronic medical illness: Implications for treatment, insurance and outcomes evaluation. *Journal of the American Medical Association, 284*, 1689–1695.

McLellan, A. T., & McKay, J. R. (1998). The treatment of addiction: What can research offer practice? In Institute of Medicine (Ed.), *Bridging the Gap between Practice and Research: Forging Partnerships with Community-Based Drug and Alcohol Treatment* (pp. 147–185). Washington, DC: National Academy Press.

Miller, W. R., & Rollnick, S. (2002). *Motivational Interviewing: Preparing People for Change* (2nd ed.). New York: Guilford Press.

Miller, W. R., & Wilbourne, P. L. (2002). Mesa Grande: A methadological analysis of clinical trials of treatments for alcohol use disorders. *Addiction, 97*, 265–277.

Miller, W. R., Zweben, J., & Johnson, W. R. (2005). Evidence-based treatment: Why, what, where, when and how? *Journal of Substance Abuse Treatment, 29*, 267–276.

Mulvey, K. P., Hubbard, S., & Hayashi, S. (2003). A national study of the substance abuse treatment workforce. *Journal of Substance Abuse Treatment, 24,* 51–57.

National Quality Forum. (2007). *National Voluntary Consensus Standards for the Treatment of Substance Use Conditions: Evidence-Based Treatment Practices.* Washington, DC: National Quality Forum.

Office of National Drug Control Policy. (2008). *Drug Courts: Providing Treatment Instead of Jail for Non-Violent Offenders.* Washington, DC, Office of National Drug Control Policy.

Peirce, J. M., Petry, N. M., Stitzer, M. C., Blaine, J., Kellogg, S., Satterfield, F., et al. (2006). Effects of lower-cost incentives on stimulant abstinence in methadone maintenance treatment: A National Drug Abuse Treatment Clinical Trials Network Study. *Archives of General Psychiatry, 63,* 201–208.

Petry, N. M., Peirce, J. M., Stitzer, M. L., Blaine, J., Roll, J. D., Cohen, A., et al. (2005). Prize-based incentives increase retention in outpatient psychosocial treatment programs: Results of the National Drug Abuse Treatment Clinical Trials Network Study. *Archives of General Psychiatry, 62,* 1148–1156.

Plaut, T. F. X. (1967). *Alcohol Problems: A Report to the Nation by the Cooperative Commission on the Study of Alcoholism.* New York: Oxford University Press.

Polen, M. R., Whitlock, E. P., Wisdom, J. P., Nygren, P., & Bougatsos, C. (2008). *Screening in Primary Care Settings for Illicit Drug Use: Staged Systematic Review for the U.S. Preventive Services Task Force. Evidence Synthesis No. 48, Part 1.* Rockville, MD: Agency for Healthcare Research and Quality.

President's Commission on Law Enforcement and Administration of Justice, Task Force on Drunkenness. (1967). *Task Force Report: Drunkenness.* Washington, DC: U.S. Government Printing Office.

Rieckmann, T., Daley, M., Fuller, B., Thomas, C. P., & McCarty, D. (2007). Counselor and client attitudes toward the use of medications for the treatment of opioid dependence. *Journal of Substance Abuse Treatment, 32,* 207–215.

Rieckmann, T. R., Kovas, A. E., Fussell, H. E., & Stettler, N. M. (2009). Implementation of evidence-based practices for treatment of alcohol and drug disorders: The role of the state authority. *Journal of Behavioral Health Services & Research, 36*(4), 407–419.

Samet, J. M., Friedmann, P. D., & Saitz, R. (2001). Benefits of linking primary medical care and substance abuse services. *Archives of Internal Medicine, 161,* 85–91.

Scott, J. E., Greenberg, D., & Pizarro, J. (1992). A survey of state insurance mandates covering alcohol and other drug treatment. *Journal of Mental Health Administration, 19,* 96–118.

Simpson, D. D. (1997). Effectiveness of drug-abuse treatment: A review of research from field settings. In J. A. Egertson, D. M. Fox, & A. I. Leshner (Eds.), *Treating Drug Abusers Effectively* (pp. 41–73). Malden, MA: Blackwell Publishers.

Simpson, D. D. (2002). A conceptual framework for transferring research to practice. *Journal of Substance Abuse Treatment, 22,* 171–182.

Simpson, D. D., & Flynn, P. M. (2007). Moving innovations into treatment: A stage-based approach to program change. *Journal of Substance Abuse Treatment, 33,* 111–120.

Substance Abuse and Mental Health Services Administration. (2007). *National Survey of Substance Abuse Treatment Services (N-SSATS): 2006; Data on Substance Abuse Treatment Facilities.* Vols. DASIS Series: S-39, DHHS Publication No. (SMA) 07-4296. Rockville, MD: Substance Abuse and Mental Health Services Administration.

Substance Abuse and Mental Health Services Administration. (2008a). *Results from the 2007 National Survey on Drug Use and Health: National Findings.* DHHS Publication No SMA 08-4343 ed. Rockville, MD: Substance Abuse and Mental Health Services Administration.

Substance Abuse and Mental Health Services Administration, Office of Applied Studies. (2008b). *Results from the 2007 National Survey on Drug Use and Health: Detailed Tables.* Rockville, MD: Substance Abuse and Mental Health Services Administration.

Taxman, F. S., Perdoni, M. L., & Harrison, L. D. (2007). Drug treatment services for adult offenders: The state of the state. *Journal of Substance Abuse Treatment, 32*, 239–254.

Taxman, F. S., Yound, D. W., Wiersema, B., Rhodes, A., & Mitchell, S. (2007). The National Criminal Justice Treatment Practices survey: Multilevel survey methods and procedures. *Journal of Substance Abuse Treatment, 32*, 225–238.

Thomas, C. P., & McCarty, D. (2004). Adoption of drug abuse treatment technology in specialty and primary care settings. In H. J. Harwood (Ed.), *Immunotherapies and Depot Medications for the Treatment and Prevention of Drug Dependence.* Washington, DC: National Academy Press.

Thomas, C. P., Wallack, S., Lee, S. S., McCarty, D., & Swift, R. (2003). Research to practice: Factors affecting the adoption of naltrexone in alcoholism treatment. *Journal of Substance Abuse Treatment, 24*, 1–11.

Turner, S., Longshore, D., Wenzel, S., Deschenes, E., Greenwood, P., Fain, T., et al. (2002). A decade of drug treatment court research. *Substance Use & Misuse, 37*, 1489–1527.

U.S. General Accounting Office. (2002). *Drug Courts: Better DOJ Data Collection and Evaluation Efforts Needed to Measure Impact of Drug Courts.* Rep. No. GAO-02-434. Washington, DC: U.S. General Accounting Office.

Weisner, C. (2001). The provision of services for alcohol problems: A community perspective for understanding access. *Journal of Behavioral Health Services & Research, 28*, 130–142.

Weisner, C., Mertens, J., Parthasarathy, S., Moore, C., & Lu, Y. (2001). Integrating primary medical care with addiction treatment: A randomized controlled trial. *Journal of the American Medical Association, 286*, 1715–1723.

Whitlock, E. P., Polen, M. R., Green, C. A., Orleans, T., & Klein, J. (2004). Behavioral counseling interventions in primary care to reduce alcohol misuse by non-pregnant adults: A summary of the evidence for the U.S. Preventive Services Task Force. *Annals of Internal Medicine, 140*, 557–568.

Woodward, A., Epstein, J., Gfroerer, J., Melnick, D., Thoreson, R., & Willson, D. (1997). The drug abuse treatment gap: Recent estimates. *Health Care Financing Review, 18*, 5–17.

Woody, G. E., Poole, S. A., Subramaniam, G., Dugosh, K., Bogenschutz, M., Abbott, P., et al. (2008). Extended vs short-term buprenorphine-naloxone for treatment of opioid-addicted youth: A randomized trial. *Journal of the American Medical Association, 300*, 2003–2011.

Chapter 12

THE PUBLIC HEALTH IMPLICATIONS OF CO-OCCURRING ADDICTIVE AND MENTAL DISORDERS

Fred C. Osher, MD; and Jill G. Hensley, MA

Introduction

Despite increasing evidence that outcomes for persons with co-occurring addictive and mental disorders improve when care is provided in a comprehensive and inte-grated fashion (Drake, O'Neal, & Wallach, 2008; Drake, Mueser, & Brunette, 2007; Brunette, Mueser, & Drake, 2004; Drake et al., 2001; Drake, Mercer-McFadden, & Mueser, 1998), access to effective service remains elusive to most individuals with these conditions (Substance Abuse and Mental Health Services Administration [SAMHSA], 2007; Wang et al., 2005; Grant et al., 2004a; U.S. Department of Health and Human Services [DHHS], 1999). It is estimated that up to 10 million people in the United States meet criteria for co-occurring disorders in any given year (Center for Substance Abuse Treatment [CSAT], 2007; Center for Mental Health Services [CMHS], 1997). Without adequate treatment, one can predict a continuation of poor adjustment and sub-optimal quality of life among persons with co-occurring disorders (Institute of Medicine [IOM], 2006; Osher & Kofoed, 1989).

Clinicians, health care administrators, families, and consumers articulate a sense of frustration that not enough is being done to address the needs of persons with co-occurring disorders. These groups witness the "revolving door" nature of the service delivery system as these individuals cycle in and out of costly and inap-propriate treatment settings, such as emergency rooms and jails, and are consis-tently over-represented in surveys of homeless populations. This chapter will highlight the negative outcomes associated with co-occurring disorders, the need for screening and assessment, the heterogeneity of the population with co-occurring disorders, evidence-based practices and treatment principles associated with positive outcomes, barriers to service delivery, implications for behavioral health, and the efforts of this system of care to address the needs of persons with co-occurring mental and addictive disorders.

Negative Outcomes

Substance abuse among persons with mental illnesses has been associated with negative outcomes, including 1) *increased vulnerability to relapse and rehospitalization* (Mueser, Drake, Turner, & McGovern, 2006; Hammerbacher & Lyvers, 2006; Brady et al., 1990; Caton, Wyatt, Felix, Grunberg, & Dominguez, 1993; Seibel et al., 1993; Haywood, Kravitz, Grossman, Davis, & Lewis, 1995; Lyons & McGovern, 1989; Negrete, Knapp, Douglas, & Smith, 1986; Carpenter, Mulligan, Bader, & Meinzer, 1985); 2) *more psychotic symptoms* (Cannon et al., 2008; Addington & Addington, 2007; Carey, Carey, & Meisler, 1991; Drake, Osher, & Wallach, 1989; Osher et al., 1994); 3) *risk of pregnancy loss* (Gold, Dalton, Schwenk, & Hayward, 2007); 4) *greater depression and suicidality* (Ries, Yuodelis-Flores, Comtois, Roy-Byrne, & Russo, 2008; Joe, Baser, Breeden, Neighbors, & Jackson, 2006; Bartels, Drake, & McHugo, 1992); 5) *violence* (Pulay et al., 2008; Friedmann, Melnick, Jiang, & Hamilton, 2008; Clingempeel, Britt, & Henggeler, 2008; Cuffel, Shumway, & Chouljian, 1994; Yesavage & Zarcone, 1983); 6) *incarceration* (Peters, Bartoi, & Sherman, 2008; Osher, 2007; CSAT, 2005a; Hartwell, 2004; Abram & Teplin, 1991; Bureau of Justice Statistics, 1999); 7) *gambling* (Petry, Stinson, & Grant, 2005; CSAT, 2005b), 8) *inability to manage finances and daily needs* (Drake & Wallach, 1989); 9) *housing instability and homelessness* (North, Eyrich, Pollio, & Spitznagel, 2004; Burt & Aron, 2000; Caton, Shrout, Eagle, Opler, Felix, & Dominguez, 1994; Osher et al., 1994); 10) *noncompliance with medications and other treatments* (Manwani et al., 2007; Magura, Laudet, Mahmood, Rosenblum, & Knight, 2002; Alterman, Erdlen, LaPorte, & Erdlen, 1982; Drake et al., 1989; Miller & Tanenbaum, 1989; Drake, Mueser, Clark, & Wallach, 1996; Owen, Fischer, & Booth, 1996); 11) *anti-depressant-induced mania* (Manwani et al., 2006); 12) *increased vulnerability to HIV infection* (Meade, Graff, Griffin, & Weiss, 2008; Forney, Lombardo, & Toro, 2007; Reback, Kamien, & Amass, 2007; Krakow, Galanter, & Dermatis, 1997; Cournos & McKinnon, 1997; Kessler et al., 1996; Cournos et al., 1991) *and hepatitis* (Rosenberg et al., 2001); 13) *lower satisfaction with familial relationships* (Dixon, McNary, & Lehman, 1995); 14) *increased family burden* (Drapalski, Leith, & Dixon, 2009; Clark, 1994); and 15) *higher service utilization and costs* (Druss et al., 2006; Katon, 2003; Curran et al., 2003; Dickey & Azeni, 1996; Bartels et al., 1993).

Associations between substance use disorders among persons with mental illnesses and negative outcomes are not consistent across studies and establishing causality is complicated by several factors. Comparing persons with severe mental illness who abuse substances with those who do not assumes that the two groups are otherwise equivalent, and they clearly are not. For example, substance-abusing persons are more likely to be young and male (SAMHSA, 2007). They may also be different from patients who never abuse substances prior to the onset of symptoms. For example, between group differences have been described in the age of onset of the mental disorder (Kessler et al., 2005; Breakey, Goodell, Lorenz, & McHugh, 1974), in premorbid functioning (Arndt, Tyrrell, Flaum, & Andreasen, 1992), in premorbid sexual adjustment (Dixon, Haas, Weiden, Sweeney, & Frances, 1991), and in family history of substance use disorders (Noordsy, Drake, Biesanz, & McHugo, 1994).

Finally, the association of medication and treatment noncompliance, homelessness, and other social problems with psychiatric patients who abuse substances may account for their poor adjustment (Magura et al., 2002; Drake & Wallach, 1989; Osher et al., 1994). Despite the difficulty in establishing causality, the negative outcomes associated with the presence of co-occurring disorders in traditional treatment settings suggest non-traditional treatment approaches are required.

The Relationship between Substance Use and Psychiatric Disorders and the Role of Assessment

It is important to recognize the complex interaction of substance use and psychiatric disorders. The Substance Abuse and Mental Health Services Administration's (SAMHSA) Co-Occurring Center for Excellence (COCE) defines co-occurring disorders as an assessment of findings "when at least one disorder of each type can be established independent of the other and is not simply a cluster of symptoms resulting from [a single] disorder" (CSAT, 2006a). Sorting out the interaction is a sophisticated assessment task that may lead to classification, as outlined by Lehman, Myers, & Corty (1989), in which six possible relationships were identified: 1) acute and chronic substance abuse may produce psychiatric symptoms; 2) substance withdrawal can cause psychiatric symptoms; 3) substance use can mask psychiatric symptoms; 4) psychiatric disorders can mimic symptoms associated with substance use; 5) acute and chronic substance abuse can exacerbate psychiatric disorders; and 6) the two types of disorders can exist simultaneously and independently with a negative synergy. These authors suggest modifying the sixth category to read "acute and chronic psychiatric disorders can exacerbate the recovery process from addictive disorders."

In this classification scheme, the first two relationships do not qualify as co-occurring disorders and will principally require addiction interventions. The third and fourth relationships are not co-occurring disorders either and require mental health treatment. It is only the last two categories that qualify as co-occurring disorders, and they require integrated treatment strategies. Determining the nature of the relationship between substance use and abnormalities in mood, thinking, and behavior is a complex, yet critical, task. It is predicated on the assumption that clinicians in either mental health or addiction services actively search for the relationship. This must become a routine process in any behavioral health treatment setting.

Epidemiologic data provide compelling reasons for the importance of screening and assessment. *First, substance use disorders and psychiatric disorders occur at high rates.* Results from the National Epidemiologic Survey on Alcohol and Related Conditions (NESARC) revealed that associations between most substance use disorders and independent mood and anxiety disorders were positive and significant

(P<.05) (Grant et al., 2004a). Grant et al. (2004b) also found that the co-occurrence of personality disorders with alcohol and drug use disorders was positive and significant. The Epidemiological Catchment Area (ECA) study (Regier et al., 1990) assessed psychiatric and substance use disorders in over 20,000 persons living in the community and in various institutional settings and found that persons with a psychiatric disorder, especially those with a severe mental illness, were at increased risk for developing a substance use disorder over their lifetime. For example, persons with schizophrenia were more than four times as likely to have a substance use disorder during their lifetime than persons in the general population, and those with bipolar disorder were more than five times as likely to have had such a diagnosis (Regier et al., 1990). A new research report from the North American Prodrome Longitudinal Study also found that the presence of a substance use disorder roughly doubled the likelihood that youth at high risk for psychosis went from a symptomatic state to a diagnosable psychotic disorder during the 30-month study period (Cannon et al., 2008). (For additional information on the epidemiology of mental disorders, see Chapters 6 and 7 in this volume.)

Second, persons with co-occurring disorders frequently seek help. The 1992 National Longitudinal Alcohol Epidemiologic Survey (Grant, 1997) in which dually diagnosed persons were five times more likely to seek services then singly diagnosed respondents, as well as similar findings in the National Comorbidity Survey (Kessler et al., 1996), support this bias. Kessler and associates (1996) reported that 19% of alcohol dependent and 26% of drug dependent individuals without a co-occurring mental disorder received treatment in a 12-month period, but in the presence of a co-occurring disorder, the rates increase to 41% and 63% respectively. In a study which analyzed the 2002 National Survey on Drug Use & Health (NSDUH) data, Mojtabai & Singh (2007) reported a strong likelihood of wanting mental health treatment among persons who had also received substance abuse treatment. Among participants with drug use disorders who were recipients of substance abuse treatment, 56.2% also received mental health treatment or reported a need for mental health treatment that had gone unmet (Mojtabai & Singh, 2007). Large numbers of individuals with co-occurring disorders are likely to enter some type of treatment and require accurate screening and assessment.

Lastly, the most dramatic public health consideration is the vast numbers of persons with co-occurring disorders who receive no care at all. Grant et al. (2004a) found that only between approximately 6% and 13% of study respondents, with an alcohol or drug disorder during the past year, sought treatment and, of those who sought treatment, between 40% and 60% had at least one co-occurring mood disorder (Grant et al., 2004a). Similarly, approximately 26% of respondents with at least one mood disorder during the past year sought treatment and of those, 15% to 22% had a comorbid substance use disorder (Grant et al., 2004a).

NSDUH reported that of the 5.6 million adults with co-occurring serious psychological distress and a substance use disorder, 49.2% received no treatment, 39.6% received treatment for mental health problems only, 2.8% received treatment for substance use problems only, and 8.4% received treatment for both mental health and substance use problems (SAMHSA, 2007). In light of the negative factors associated with co-occurring disorders, improving access to care, and particularly integrated care, is of paramount importance.

Screening and Assessment of Co-Occurring Disorders

If you do not look for co-occurring disorders, you are not likely to find them. The concept of "universal screening" conveys the utility of screening for co-occurring conditions in all health service venues. SAMHSA has published several guidelines for screening and assessing co-occurring disorders in order to ensure that there is "no wrong door" for clients to enter in order to have their full array of needs determined and addressed. COCE's *Overview Paper 2: Screening, Assessment, and Treatment Planning for Persons with Co-Occurring Disorders* (CSAT, 2006b) provides an overview of the purposes and principles of integrated assessment, briefly reviews a 12-step assessment process (detailed more fully in SAMHSA's *Treatment Improvement Protocol 42 for Persons with Co-Occurring Disorders* [CSAT, 2005b]), and provides an introductory discussion on how to link integrated screening and assessment protocols to integrated treatment planning overall. SAMHSA's *Treatment Improvement Protocol 42* also provides an appendix with instruments that may be used in the assessment of co-occurring disorders (CSAT, 2005b). COCE's *Technical Assistance Report to the Co-Occurring State Incentive Grants on Assessment* also includes a table on several assessment instruments for consideration based upon a number of characteristics.

In general, screening and assessment for co-occurring disorders should enable a provider to determine the presence or absence of a co-occurring disorder and to further determine the client's readiness for change, the client's strengths and problem areas that may affect the treatment and recovery process, and finally, the willingness of the client to engage in an appropriate treatment plan.

Heterogeneity of the Population with Co-Occurring Disorders

Treatment planning and policy development require an accurate description of the problem to be addressed. Despite considerable progress in assessment tools and strategies, the identification and characterization of persons with co-occurring disorders remains a difficult task (DiClemente, Nidecker, & Bellack, 2008; Lehman, 1996). While the assessment process is complex and can be protracted, the identification of those individuals with co-occurring disorders is simply an early step in designing an appropriate response to their needs. It is critical that the heterogeneity of the population be acknowledged. Any substance of abuse can be combined with any mental disorder to meet criteria under this umbrella term. These two dimensions can be crossed with any set of demographic variables (age, gender, and/or culture) to create additional subgroups with special needs. If the frequent presence of other medical comorbidities is added, the classification of co-occurring disorders gains additional complexity. These interacting variables underline the adage that "if you've seen one person with co-occurring disorders, you've seen one person with co-occurring disorders."

For clinical and organizational purposes, the separation of persons with co-occurring disorders into subgroups based solely upon diagnosis or demographics will not lead to effective matching to treatment. Arguably the most important dimension to consider is the degree of dysfunction the two disorders produce in an individual. One useful model, the quadrant model, was developed in New York and endorsed by both the National Association of State Mental Health Program Directors and the National Association of State Alcohol and Drug Abuse Directors (NASMHPD & NASADAD, 1999).

The quadrant model provides a framework by which to organize the heterogeneous population of persons with co-occurring disorders who historically have differentially utilized systems of care based upon the severity of illness (McGovern, Clark, & Samnaliev, 2007). Further, it establishes a conceptual tool by which a focus on improving service delivery guides integration of services and allocation of resources (Keyser, Watkins, Vilamovska, & Pincus, 2008). Rather than focus on diagnoses, the model uses two dimensions: 1) the severity of the mental illness; and 2) the severity of the addiction to define four subgroups of persons with co-occurring disorders in a two-by-two matrix, assigning one side to high versus low severity of mental illness and the other to high versus low substance use severity. The model then assigns responsibility to 1) primary care providers with consultation from behavioral health specialists (for persons with low severity on each dimension), 2) and 3) one of the specialty sector systems (for persons with either severe mental illnesses or severe alcohol or drug abuse) with collaboration from the other specialty sector, or 4) to a set of providers delivering integrated care to the most disabled consumers, those with high severity in both dimensions.

The advantages of this model are that it encompasses the heterogeneity of the dual diagnosis population, it assigns responsibility to every system for providing some degree of care to persons with co-occurring disorders, and it is flexible enough to be adapted to most service settings. Significant overlap between systems is inherent in the model, and it more realistically corresponds to the multiple pathways used by this population to access care.

Evidence-Based Practices

Evidence-based practice (EBP) is not a novel concept. The term originated in the 1980s in Canada at the McMaster Medical School as an analogy to *evidence-based medicine* (McCabe, 2004). *Evidence*, in this case, has been defined with respect to scientific rigor and explicitly available facts regarding whether an intervention has been effective in producing desired behavioral change or a specific health outcome (Briss et al., 2000; Rychetnik, Hawe, Waters, Barratt, & Frommer, 2004). This concept of *evidence*, combined with protocols from medical research traditions, produced a public health decision-making process for the selection of interventions based upon the perceived capacity for effectiveness (Baker, Brennan-Ramirez, Claus, & Land, 2008). The contemporary use of EBPs in behavioral health settings is well established. Comprehensive literature reviews in this area (Deegear & Lawson, 2003; Nathan, 1998) have addressed various topics, including the benefits and drawbacks of EBPs and guidelines for implementation.

Given the high prevalence rates and the high morbidity and mortality associated with having co-occurring disorders, the identification of effective interventions for persons with co-occurring disorders has gained both immediacy and a growing database. Whereas a range of interventions have been identified and a call for integrated services initiated (Drake et al., 2007), the evidence base for these modified programs is still very recent and scant. Nonetheless, integrated services have emerged as evidence-based practice. Integrated treatment addresses two important issues: 1) improving access to care for both mental health and substance abuse services in one setting; and 2) improving the quality of care by combining the two interventions (Mueser, Noordsy, Drake, & Fox, 2003). Primarily, this integration occurs at both the program level and the interface of the provider and consumer. Ideally, integrated care also occurs at systems levels with efforts to standardize assessment tools, treatment protocols, and licensure standards, implement integrated evidence-based practices, and comprehensively train and prepare multidisciplinary treatment teams.

For the past 20 years, extensive efforts have been made to develop integrated models of care that bring together mental health and substance abuse treatment. The reported studies have focused primarily on individuals with serious mental illnesses and co-occurring substance use disorders. Recent evidence from more than a dozen studies shows that comprehensive integrated efforts help persons with dual disorders reduce substance use and attain remission (Drake et al., 2008; CMHS, 2003; Drake et al., 1998). Integrated approaches are also associated with a reduction in hospital utilization, psychiatric symptomatology, and other problematic negative outcomes.

Comprehensiveness is a critical component in successful interventions. Those programs that simply add a group or short-term treatment intervention to existing treatment protocols suffer high dropout rates and have little overall impact upon either rates of substance abuse or psychiatric disability. Comprehensive approaches are defined by the inclusion of a staged approach to care with motivational interventions, assertive outreach, intensive case management, individual counseling, long-term interventions, and family interventions. Positive outcomes include high rates of engaging and retaining patients in care, reduced hospital utilization, reduced substance use, and increased abstinence. This research base has allowed the development of treatment principles associated with positive outcomes. In addition, several evidence-based practices for co-occurring disorders have been documented, including Assertive Community Treatment (ACT) and Modified Therapeutic Communities (MTC) (CSAT, 2005b). SAMHSA also operates the National Registry of Evidence-Based Programs and Practices (NREPP) that can be searched for various terms of interest, including program models with evidence for addressing co-occurring disorders (http://www.nrepp.samhsa.gov/).

Principles of Care for Systems and Services

While historically mental health and substance abuse approaches to care are different, principles of care within the two fields converge on respect for the individual, reaching out to engage those who cannot yet trust, and the importance of community, family, and peers to recovery. SAMHSA's COCE has used the existing evidence base to identify principles for developing effective systems of care in its *Overview Paper #3: Overarching Principles to Address the Needs of Persons with Co-Occurring Disorders* (CSAT, 2006c). These principles serve to bridge the gap between the service orientations and characterize an effective system of care for persons with co-occurring disorders. They can be used for both planning and evaluation purposes. The first 6 principles guide systems of care of individuals with co-occurring disorders (COD), and principles 7–12 guide provider activity for individuals with COD:

1. *"Co-occurring disorders are to be expected in all behavioral health settings and system planning must address the need to serve people with COD in all policies, regulations, funding mechanisms, and programming"* (CSAT, 2006c, p. 2). Principle 1 is based upon epidemiological data and clinical studies that have reported high prevalence of COD in the general population and in the populations seeking treatment. Based upon these data, all systems of care must anticipate the need to address COD and appropriately fund systems to adequately identify and respond to the full set of needs among individuals with COD. To be effective, all programs within the system of care must achieve basic competencies in screening, assessing, and addressing co-occurring disorders.

2. *"An integrated system of mental health and addiction services that emphasizes continuity and quality is in the best interest of consumers, providers, programs, funders, and systems"* (CSAT, 2006c, p.2). Principle 2 implies the need for systems of care to develop a common vision of the full range of needs of their clients in order to develop programs and policies, identify staffing needs, and allocate resources to support services for these needs.

3. *"The integrated system of care must be accessible from multiple points of entry (i.e., "no wrong door") and be perceived as caring and accepting by the consumer"* (CSAT, 2006c, p. 2). Principle 3 requires that systems assume the responsibility for ensuring that individuals with COD entering their programs are able to access and receive care for their full set of needs. Any individual seeking help for a range of problems should not be turned away because the treatment system only addresses a subset of those issues. Individuals should be engaged in the treatment planning process, and systems must be prepared to respond to their range of concerns.

4. *"The system of care for COD should not be limited to a single "correct" model or approach"* (CSAT, 2006c, p. 3). Principle 4 emphasizes the reality that there is no single formula for providing integrated screening, assessment, and treatment for individuals with COD. Treatment plans must be customized based upon individual needs and preferences.

5. *"The system of care must reflect the importance of the partnership between science and service, and support both the application of evidence- and consensus-based practices for persons with COD and evaluation of the efforts of existing programs and services"* (CSAT, 2006c, p. 3). Principle 5 reminds systems of the advantages of utilizing evidence- and consensus-based practices in maximizing benefits to consumers across the mental health and substance abuse treatment fields. System designs for services should support the application of existing science and encourage participation in ongoing research and evaluation efforts to continue to expand and strengthen the science base for effective service provision.

6. *"Behavioral health systems must collaborate with professionals in primary care, human services, housing, criminal justice, and related fields in order to meet the complex needs of persons with COD"* (CSAT, 2006c, p. 3). Principle 6 is a reminder that individuals with COD are likely to have additional medical, social, and legal problems.

This complex range of needs requires collaborations across public health, housing, and justice systems in order to support a sustained recovery process for individuals with COD. Possible strategies include shared case management models, creation of local service coalitions, State use of special waivers, and interagency task forces.

7. *"Co-occurring disorders must be expected when evaluating any person, and clinical services should incorporate this assumption into all screening, assessment, and treatment planning"* (CSAT, 2006c, p. 3). Principle 7 shifts the emphasis from the systems level to the provider level with the need to acknowledge the high prevalence of individuals with COD and the workforce training that is needed to adequately screen, coordinate assessments, and develop treatment plans that recognize the full set of a client's needs.

8. *"Within the treatment context, both co-occurring disorders are considered primary"* (CSAT, 2006c, p. 4). Principle 8 acknowledges the interactive nature of COD and the need to continually assess individuals and adjust treatment plans to meet the ongoing variable needs and symptoms of each disorder, and the complex nature of their interaction.

9. *"Empathy, respect, and belief in the individual's capacity for recovery are fundamental provider attitudes"* (CSAT, 2006c, p. 4). Principle 9 focuses on the quality of the treatment relationship as the most important predictor of success and emphasizes the need for providers to adopt a recovery perspective in order to provide a positive and stable treatment relationship through the course of treatment, regardless of the ups and downs that will inevitably occur.

10. *"Treatment should be individualized to accommodate the specific needs, personal goals, and cultural perspectives of unique individuals in different stages of change"* (CSAT, 2006c, p. 4). As with Principle 4 for systems, Principle 10 focuses on the need to acknowledge, at the program level, the importance of individualized treatment plans in meeting the needs, goals, and perspectives of each individual client with COD.

11. *"The special needs of children and adolescents must be explicitly recognized and addressed in all phases of assessment, treatment planning, and service delivery"* (CSAT, 2006c, p. 4). Principle 11 calls attention to the need to acknowledge the unique differences of children and adolescents from adults in their treatment needs. This developmental perspective should guide all aspects of care at the provider level.

12. *"The contribution of the community to the course of recovery for consumers with COD and the contribution of consumers with COD to the community must be explicitly recognized in program policy, treatment planning, and consumer advocacy"* (CSAT, 2006c, p. 5). Principle 12 focuses on the need to accept and respond to the needs of individuals with COD as fellow citizens and community members. In implementing Principle 12, communities are called upon to continue to combat stigma and discrimination that may prevent individuals from seeking treatment. Similarly, individuals with COD are called on to work with providers to share their experiences and perspectives in developing effective programs (CSAT, 2006c).

While there is general acceptance of these principles, why are very few systems in the process of delivering services consistent with these ideas? The following paragraph will address this issue.

Barriers to Services Delivery

For persons with co-occurring disorders, barriers to accessing comprehensive care, embracing the principles outlined above, are formidable. This is primarily due to the fragmentation of existing service systems for people with numerous and complex clinical, social, and legal problems. The linkage of mental health and addiction service systems has wavered over time (IOM, 2006) and despite an understanding of the utility of coordination, these systems are currently predominantly separate. This non-integration of mental and addictive services exists at both administrative and clinical levels. Current efforts are under way to address the obstacles inherent in services that are fragmented and lacking in coordination. The Institute of Medicine recently provided a series of recommendations to improve the quality of health care for individuals with mental and substance use conditions, including recommendations that address obstacles to patient-centered care (IOM, 2006).

Barriers to Administrative Integration: A Federal Case Study

A review of the evolution of federal programs for mental health and addiction services illustrates the development of non-integrated systems and the resultant negative impact for approaches to co-occurring disorders at all levels of service delivery. The Mental Health Act of 1946 created the National Institute of Mental Health that assumed responsibility for mental health, alcohol, and drug issues. In the 1960s, in addition to its mental health focus, the National Institute of Mental Health (NIMH) actively advocated for more community based clinics for alcohol treatment. When Congress enacted the Narcotic Addict Rehabilitation Act in 1966, NIMH was authorized to make grants to establish community based drug treatment programs and supported numerous therapeutic communities and methadone maintenance programs. NIMH findings contributed to a growing awareness of the inadequate capacity for treating the disease of alcoholism and the enormous social costs of a burgeoning drug epidemic in the late 1960s. Passage of decriminalization laws in the late 1960s redirected punitive responses to the possession and use of drugs to treatment within the public health sector.

In 1970, Congress passed the Comprehensive Alcoholism Prevention, Treatment and Rehabilitation Act (PL 91-616) to support increased and improved services for people with alcoholism. The Act also created a federal agency, the National Institute on Alcohol Abuse and Alcoholism (NIAAA), to administer, among other programs, a formula grant that allocated money to the states based upon population and need.

In 1972, the Drug Office and Treatment Act (PL 92-255) authorized the establishment of the National Institute on Drug Abuse (NIDA) and created an analogous formula grant program for this agency to administer. An unintended effect of these positive developments for the alcohol and drug fields was to formalize services and operations separate from, and in competition with, the mental health establishment (i.e., NIMH). NIDA and NIAAA joined labor unions and state insurance commissions to promote insurance coverage for the treatment of alcohol and drug dependence. This successful effort, coupled with the new formula grant monies, resulted in a dramatic expansion of both private and public substance abuse employee assistance and chemical dependency programs in the 1970s.

Opening the floodgates to addictive disorder treatment dramatically increased the demand for care. Unfortunately, resources did not increase with this demand. Federal dollars for mental health and substance abuse treatment during the Ford, Carter, and Reagan administrations, adjusted for inflation, did not grow, and state and local governments experienced declining federal support (Baumohl & Jaffe, 1995). In response to widespread resource limitations, a narrowing of target populations and benefit limitations became management strategies of states to achieve cost containment. Considerable effort was placed upon defining eligibility for services with the goal being the identification of the "purest" target population, thereby keeping available resources for narrowly defined purposes.

In the context of this burgeoning demand for substance abuse and mental health treatment, with diminished resources and targeting of clearly defined populations, the exclusion of individuals with co-occurring disorders became commonplace. Parallel pressure was felt at the service level. Staff time became limited, and addressing the complex needs of individuals with co-occurring disorders was viewed as too labor intensive. It was during the early 1980s that the needs of individuals with co-occurring disorders began appearing in the mental health and addiction literature (Drake & Wallach, 1989; Pepper, Kirshner, & Ryglewicz, 1981).

In the most recent of a series of federal agency reorganizations, SAMHSA was created in 1992. It is comprised of the Center for Substance Abuse Prevention, the Center for Substance Abuse Treatment (CSAT), and the Center for Mental Health Services (CMHS). The enabling legislation also separated the alcohol and drug portion of the block grant (administered by CSAT) from the mental health portion (administered by CMHS). This case study illustrates how federal policy can promote policies and practice, implemented by either state, local, or private alcohol, drug, or mental health agencies, that impede the likelihood of persons with co-occurring disorders from receiving effective care.

It should be noted that as the problems associated with co-occurring disorders became more widely appreciated, initiatives to promote more effective responses at the federal level have emerged. In 2002, SAMHSA published its landmark "Report to Congress on the Prevention and Treatment of Co-Occurring Substance Abuse Disorders and Mental Disorders" that was mandated under the Children's Health Act of 2000. The Report included a Five-Year Blueprint for Action that set forth a number of initiatives by SAMHSA designed to ensure national accountability, capacity, and effectiveness in addressing co-occurring disorders. In 2003, SAMHSA began to implement many of the plans identified in the Blueprint. Among the funding initiatives that resulted were the development of co-occurring measures to enhance statewide accountability on serving individuals with co-occurring disorders; development of grant programs for states to enhance clinical capacity and infrastructure systems to better address co-occurring disorders (co-occurring state incentive grants [COSIGs]), and for states to develop Action Plans (co-occurring Policy Academy grants); development of a Science-to-Services Workgroup between SAMHSA and the National Institutes of Health (NIH); development of a new technical assistance center (the Co-Occurring Center for Excellence) and technical assistance materials (including *Treatment Improvement Protocol 42, the Integrated Dual*

Disorders Treatment Toolkit, and *Strategies for Developing Treatment Programs for People with Co-Occurring Substance Abuse and Mental Disorders*); further development of SAMHSA's *National Registry of Effective Programs and Practices* to include evidence-based programs for the prevention and treatment of co-occurring disorders; and development of a Taskforce with NASMHPD and NASADAD to examine state efforts to address co-occurring disorders.

Despite recent efforts to address co-occurring disorders at the federal level, separate administrative structures and funding sources continue to reinforce the separation of mental health and addiction systems.

Barriers to Clinical Integration: Lack of Cross-Training

With increased national attention on treating addictive disorders in the late 1960s and early 1970s, coupled with the expansion of treatment facilities, the need for human resource development became paramount. Responsibility for addictions services was in flux. Not until new theoretical models posited biologic underpinnings to addictions did the traditional health system begrudgingly reconsider its role in providing addiction treatment.

Jellinek's seminal work, *The Disease Concept of Alcoholism* (1960), is credited with providing a renewed rationale for medical personnel to treat alcoholism. Short-term inpatient stays with long-term AA/NA outpatient fellowship became the modal treatment across the country during the 1960s. Thus, even though addiction treatment returned to medical settings, it remained separate from mental health services. Through grants and contracts, NIAAA and NIDA sponsored "manpower training" with the goal of producing a large pool of practitioners around the country to positively affect current treatment efforts (Deitch & Carleton, 1992). Training in mental health was not typically a part of these efforts.

Recognizing that large numbers of people with addictive disorders were entering mental health treatment settings, academic psychiatric training centers found themselves under increasing pressure to insert addiction training into the curriculum, and specialty physician organizations (e.g., the American Society of Addiction Medicine) were founded. In 1989, the Accreditation Council for Graduate Medical Education required that all psychiatric residents receive training in addiction psychiatry. While these developments were welcome, they did not focus on the needs of individuals with co-occurring disorders, and integrated approaches were not emphasized.

While the alcohol and drug field moved to professionalize its human resources, distrust of the "medicalization" of addictions surfaced. To many, the use of mind-altering medications was antithetical to a drug-free lifestyle and often seen as a misguided shortcut to requisite abstinence. Battle lines were drawn as to whether psychiatric symptoms were simply the result of alcohol and drug abuse or this abuse was only a self-medication strategy for underlying mental disorder. Such conflicts were played out in the treatment planning for dually diagnosed individuals in a way that precluded coordinated approaches. Clinicians with expertise in addictions and consumers recovering from co-occurring disorders, who would improve the quality of care, are routinely excluded from jobs in the mental health system (Drake et al., 2001).

These different treatment philosophies and lack of cross-training result in inaccurate assessments, under-recognition of co-occurring disorders, and failure to implement appropriate interventions. Ongoing stereotyped attitudes derived from a common lack of information and understanding between the fields continue to create barriers to care.

However, efforts to address these obstacles in the workforce have begun, especially as evidenced above in SAMHSA's implementation of recommendations in the Report to Congress. In addition, SAMHSA convened a diverse group of experts to develop a national strategic plan on workforce development for the behavioral health field. This group, the Annapolis Coalition, formed seven strategic goals as a result of their planning, which focus on three main areas: 1) broadening the concept of "workforce" to include persons in recovery, children, youth, families, and communities; 2) strengthening the workforce related to enhancing recruitment and retention strategies, training and education, and leadership development; and 3) creating enhanced structural supports for the workforce (i.e., mechanisms for the provision of technical assistance, stronger human resource departments, improved information technology systems, and a national research and evaluation agenda) (SAMHSA, 2006).

Ensuring Access to Treatment for Persons with Co-Occurring Disorders

While it is possible to identify principles of care, it is more difficult to identify who, within the existing service systems, should be responsible for implementing these principles and engaging the person with co-occurring disorders in treatment. Persons with co-occurring disorders may seek help from mental health, substance abuse, or primary health care providers. The systems that support these providers have historically operated independent of one another with separate philosophies, administrative oversight, and financial support (IOM, 2006; Ridgely, Goldman, & Willenbring, 1990). Both public and private sector initiatives over the last twenty years have reinforced the separation of these systems (Osher & Drake, 1996), while persons with co-occurring disorders continue to flood clinical settings.

The debate surrounding appropriate models of care and the locus of responsibility for providing care is often acrimonious as administrators and policymakers struggle to stretch scarce resources over the spectrum of care required for effective treatment of "singly" diagnosed populations. Failure to resolve these barriers to care ensures that access to effective integrated care interventions is unavailable. In order to move the debate forward, there must be a shared language and vision for how to provide care to dually diagnosed individuals. Using a framework as outlined in the New York Model can serve as the basis for state and local strategies to ensure that the needs of persons with co-occurring disorders are addressed. The appropriate domain for service delivery and the eligibility criteria for various service settings will vary depending upon existing resources and programmatic structure.

Various mechanisms can be used to ensure accountability and manage client flow at the systems level. These include interagency agreements, joint program development, cross-training of providers, and the specific identification of individuals with co-occurring disorders as a priority population within all strategic planning initiatives (Ridgely & Dixon, 1995). At the community and program level, the comprehensive, continuous, integrated system of care (CCIS) model (Minkoff, 1999) outlines a process for implementing integrated services. This begins with the development of an integrated philosophy among all relevant stakeholders, from consumers to administrators. After agreement on an integrated mission and some principles of care, an assessment of current organizational capacity is performed, and service gaps are identified. Participants then prioritize modest steps toward creating a continuum of assessment and treatment services using evidence-based practices. Ongoing psychiatric and addiction training is provided to all staff. All of these strategies require strong and committed leadership.

Implications for Addictive and Mental Disorders

Important strides have been made in the identification and implementation of effective service for persons with co-occurring disorders. Nonetheless, further implementation research is needed to determine the effectiveness of the services currently being implemented (Sacks, Chandler, & Gonzales, 2008). In addition, access to these effective interventions is not widespread, and persons with co-occurring disorders continue to bounce between systems of care without sufficient progress on their recovery goals. As a public health concern, advocating for improved access and quality for persons with co-occurring disorders is of paramount importance. Translating the bright lights of effective treatment into a normative experience is possible. It will take concerted leadership and efficient use of existing and new resources. Not providing these services is ultimately more costly both in terms of dollars and quality of life.

Principles of care within mental health and addiction fields converge on respect for the individual, belief in the human capacity to change, and the importance of community, family, and peers to the recovery process. Consumers do not have the opportunity to separate their addiction from their mental illnesses, and there is a critical need to address the policies and practices that fail to reflect this reality.

Acknowledgments

The authors of this chapter are grateful to Ms. Donna L. Burton, Doctoral Student in the Department of Community & Family Health at the University of South Florida College of Public Health, for her generous contributions to this chapter.

References

Abram, K. M., & Teplin, L. A. (1991). Co-occurring disorders among mentally ill jail detainees. *American Psychologist, 46*, 1036–1045.

Addington, J., & Addington, D. (2007). Patterns, predictors, and impact of substance use in early psychosis: A longitudinal study. *Acta Psychiatrica Scandinavica, 115*(4), 304–309.

Alterman, A. I., Erdlen, D. L., LaPorte, D. J., & Erdlen, F. R. (1982). Effects of illicit drug use in an inpatient psychiatric population. *Addictive Behaviors, 7*, 231–242.

Arndt, S., Tyrrell, G., Flaum, M., & Andreasen, N. C. (1992). Comorbidity of substance abuse and schizophrenia: The role of pre-morbid adjustment. *Psychological Medicine, 22*, 379–388.

Baker, E. A., Brennan-Ramirez, L. K., Claus, J. M., & Land, G. (2008) Translating and disseminating research- and practice-based criteria to support evidence-based intervention planning. *Journal of Public Health Management & Practice, 14*(2), 124–130.

Bartels, S. J., Drake, R. E., & McHugo, G. J. (1992). Alcohol abuse, depression, and suicidal behavior in schizophrenia. *American Journal of Psychiatry, 149*, 394–395.

Bartels, S. J., Teague, G. B., Drake, R. E., Clark, R. E., Bush, P., & Noordsy, D. L. (1993). Substance abuse in schizophrenia: Service utilization and costs. *Journal of Nervous and Mental Disease, 181*, 227–232.

Baumohl, J., & Jaffe, J. R. (1995). The history of alcohol and drug treatment in America. In J. Jaffe (Ed.), *Encyclopedia of Drug and Alcohol* (vol. 3, pp. 1057–1077). New York: Mac Milan.

Brady, K., Anton, R., Ballenger, J. C., Lydiard, R. B., Adinoff, B., & Selander, J. (1990). Cocaine abuse among schizophrenic patients. *American Journal of Psychiatry, 147*, 1164–1167.

Breakey, W. R., Goodell, H., Lorenz, P. C., & McHugh, P. R. (1974). Hallucinogenic drugs as precipitants of schizophrenia. *Psychological Medicine, 4*, 255–261.

Briss, P. A., Zaza, S., Pappaioanou, M., et al. (2000). Developing an evidence-based guide to community preventive services: Methods. *American Journal of Preventive Medicine, 18*(Suppl. 1), 35–43.

Brunette, M. F., Mueser, K. T., & Drake, R. E. (2004). A review of research on residential programs for people with severe mental illness and co-occurring substance use disorders. *Drug and Alcohol Review, 23*, 471–481.

Bureau of Justice Statistics. (1999). *United States Department of Justice, Corrections Facts at a Glance.* Available online at http://www.ojp.usdoj.gov/bjs/glance/corr2.htm. Accessed October 29, 2009.

Burt, M., & Aron, L. (2000). *America's Homeless: II, Populations and Services.* Washington, DC: Urban Institute.

Cannon, T. D., Cadenhead, K., Cornblatt, B., Woods, S. W., Addington, J., Walker, E., et al. (2008). Prediction of psychosis in youth at high clinical risk: A multisite longitudinal study in North America. *Archives of General Psychiatry, 65*(1), 28–37.

Carey, M. P., Carey, K. B., & Meisler, A. W. (1991). Psychiatric symptoms in mentally ill chemical abusers. *Journal of Nervous and Mental Disease, 179*, 136–138.

Carpenter, M. D., Mulligan, J. C., Bader, I. A., & Meinzer, A. E. (1985). Multiple admissions to an urban psychiatric center: A comparative study. *Hospital and Community Psychiatry, 36*, 1305–1308.

Caton, C. L. M., Shrout, P. E., Eagle, P. F., Opler, L. A., Felix, A., & Dominguez, B. (1994). Risk factors for homelessness among schizophrenic men: A case-control study. *American Journal of Public Health, 84*, 265–270.

Caton, C. L. M., Wyatt, R. J., Felix, A., Grunberg, J., & Dominguez, B. (1993). Follow-up of chronically homeless mentally ill men. *American Journal of Psychiatry, 150*, 1639–1642.

Center for Mental Health Services (CMHS). (1997). *Addressing the Needs of Homeless Persons with Co-Occurring Mental Illness and Substance Use Disorders.* Rockville, MD: Substance Abuse and Mental Health Services Administration, U.S. Department of Health and Human Services.

Center for Mental Health Services. (2003). *Co-occurring Disorders: Integrated Dual Disorders Treatment, Implementation Resource Kit.* Rockville, MD: Substance Abuse and Mental Health Services Administration.

Center for Substance Abuse Treatment (CSAT). (2005a). *Substance Abuse Treatment for Adults in the Criminal Justice System.* Treatment Improvement Protocol (TIP) Series No. 44, DHHS Publication No. [SMA] 05-4056. Rockville, MD: Substance Abuse and Mental Health Services Administration.

Center for Substance Abuse Treatment. (2005b). *Substance Abuse Treatment for Persons with Co-Occurring Disorders.* Treatment Improvement Protocol (TIP) Series No. 42, DHHS

Publication No. [SMA] 05-3992. Rockville, MD: Substance Abuse and Mental Health Services Administration.

Center for Substance Abuse Treatment. (2006a). *Definitions and Terms Relating to Co-Occurring Disorders: COCE Overview Paper 1*. DHHS Publication No. (SMA) 06-4163. Rockville, MD: Substance Abuse and Mental Health Services Administration and Center for Mental Health Services.

Center for Substance Abuse Treatment. (2006b). *Screening, Assessment, and Treatment Planning for Persons with Co-Occurring Disorders: COCE Overview Paper 2*. DHHS Publication No. (SMA) 06-4164. Rockville, MD: Substance Abuse and Mental Health Services Administration and Center for Mental Health Services.

Center for Substance Abuse Treatment. (2006c). *Overarching Principles to Address the Needs of Persons with Co-Occurring Disorders: COCE Overview Paper 3*. DHHS Publication No. (SMA) 06-4165. Rockville, MD: Substance Abuse and Mental Health Services Administration and Center for Mental Health Services.

Center for Substance Abuse Treatment. (2007). *The Epidemiology of Co-Occurring Substance Use and Mental Disorders: COCE Overview Paper 8*. DHHS Publication No. (SMA) 07-4308. Rockville, MD: Substance Abuse and Mental Health Services Administration and Center for Mental Health Services.

Clark, R. E. (1994). Family costs associated with severe mental illness and substance use: A comparison of families with and without dual disorders. *Hospital and Community Psychiatry, 45*, 808–813.

Clingempeel, W. G., Britt, S. C., & Henggeler, S. W. (2008). Beyond treatment effects: Comorbid psychopathologies and long-term outcomes among substance-abusing delinquents. *American Journal of Orthopsychiatry, 78*(1), 29–36.

Cournos, F., Empfield, M., Horwath, E., McKinnon, K., Meyer, I., Schrage, H., et al. (1991). HIV seroprevalence among patients admitted to two psychiatric hospitals. *American Journal of Psychiatry, 148*, 1225–1230.

Cournos, F., & McKinnon, K. (1997). HIV seroprevalence among people with severe mental illness in the United States: A critical review. *Clinical Psychology Review, 17*, 259–269.

Cuffel, B. J., Shumway, M., & Chouljian, T. L. (1994). A longitudinal study of substance use and community violence in schizophrenia. *Journal of Nervous and Mental Disease, 182*, 342–348.

Curran, G. M., Sullivan, G., Williams, K., Han, X., Collins, K., Keys, J., et al. (2003). Emergency department use of persons with comorbid psychiatric and substance abuse disorders. *Annals of Emergency Medicine, 41*, 650–667.

Deegear, J., & Lawson, D. M. (2003). The utility of empirically supported treatments. *Professional Psychology: Research and Practice, 34*, 271–277.

Deitch, D. A., & Carleton, S. A. Education and training of clinical personnel. In J. H. Lowinson, P. Ruiz, & R. B. Millman (Eds.), *Substance Abuse: A Comprehensive Textbook* (pp. 970–982). Baltimore: Williams and Wilkins.

Dickey, B., & Azeni, H. (1996). Persons with dual diagnosis of substance abuse and major mental illness: Their excess costs of psychiatric care. *American Journal of Public Health, 86*, 973–977.

DiClemente, C. C., Nidecker, M., & Bellack, A. S. (2008). Motivation and the stages of change among individuals with severe mental illness and substance abuse disorders. *Journal of Substance Abuse Treatment, 34*, 25–35.

Dixon, L., Haas, G., Weiden, P. J., Sweeney, J., & Frances, A. J. (1991). Drug abuse in schizophrenic patients: Clinical correlates and reasons for use. *American Journal of Psychiatry, 148*, 224–230.

Dixon, L., McNary, S., & Lehman, A. (1995). Substance abuse and family relationships of persons with severe mental illness. *American Journal of Psychiatry, 152*, 456–458.

Drake, R. E., Essock, S., Shaner, A., Carey, K. B., Minkoff, K., Kola, L., et al. (2001). Implementing dual diagnosis services for clients with severe mental illness. *Psychiatric Services, 4*(52), 469–476.

Drake, R. E., Mercer-McFadden, C., & Mueser, K. T. (1998). A review of integrated mental health and substance abuse treatment for patients with dual disorders. *Schizophrenia Bulletin, 24,* 589–608.

Drake, R. E., Mueser, K. T., & Brunette, M. F. (2007). Management of persons with co-occurring severe mental illness and substance use disorder: Program implications. *World Psychiatry, 6,* 131–136.

Drake, R. E., Mueser, K. T., Clark, R. E., & Wallach, M. A. (1996). The course, treatment and outcome of substance disorder in persons with severe mental illness. In L. Davidson, C. Harding, & L. Spaniol (Eds.), *Recovery from Severe Mental Illnesses: Research Evidence and Implications for Practice* (vol. 1, pp. 100–114). Boston: Center for Psychiatric Rehabilitation.

Drake, R. E., O'Neal, E. L., & Wallach, M. A. (2008). Systematic review of psychosocial research on psychosocial interventions for people with co-occurring severe mental and substance use disorders. *Journal of Substance Abuse Treatment, 24,* 123–128.

Drake, R. E., Osher, F. C., & Wallach, M. A. (1989). Alcohol use and abuse in schizophrenia: A prospective community study. *Journal of Nervous and Mental Disease, 177,* 408–414.

Drake, R. E., & Wallach, M. A. (1989). Substance abuse among the chronic mentally ill. *Hospital and Community Psychiatry, 40,* 1041–1046.

Drapalski, A. L., Leith, J., & Dixon, L. (2009). Involving families in the care of persons with schizophrenia and other serious mental illnesses: History, evidence, and recommendations. *Clinical Schizophrenia & Related Disorders, 3*(1), 39–49.

Druss, B. G., Bornemann, T., Fry-Johnson, Y. W., McCombs, H. G., Politzer, R. M., & Rust, G. (2006). Trends in mental health and substance abuse services at the nation's community health centers: 1998–2003. *American Journal of Public Health, 96,* 1779–2003.

Forney, J. C., Lombardo, S., & Toro, P. A. (2007). Diagnostic and other correlates of HIV risk behaviors in a probability sample of homeless adults. *Psychiatric Services, 58*(1), 92–99.

Friedmann, P. D., Melnick, G., Jiang, L., & Hamilton, Z. (2008). Violent and disruptive behavior among drug-involved prisoners: Relationship with psychiatric symptoms. *Behavioral Sciences & the Law, 26*(4), 389–401.

Gold, K., Dalton, V. K., Schwenk, T. L., & Hayward, R. A. (2007). What causes pregnancy loss? Preexisting mental illness as an independent risk factor. *General Hospital Psychiatry, 29,* 207–213.

Grant, B. F. (1997) The influence of co-morbid major depression and substance use disorders on alcohol and drug treatment: Results from a national survey. In L. S. Onken, J. D. Blaine, S. Genser, & A.M. Horton, Jr. (Eds.), *Treatment of Drug Dependent Individuals with Comorbid Mental Disorders.* Research monograph 172. Rockville, MD: National Institute of Drug Abuse.

Grant, B. F., Stinson, F. S., Dawson, D. A., Chou, P., Dufour, M. C., Compton, W., et al. (2004a). Prevalence and co-occurrence of substance use disorders and independent mood and anxiety disorders. *Archives of General Psychiatry, 61,* 807–816.

Grant, B. F., Stinson, F. S., Dawson, D. A., Chou, P., Ruan, W. J., & Pickering, R. P. (2004b). Co-occurrence of 12-month alcohol and drug use disorders and personality disorders in the United States. *Archives of General Psychiatry, 61,* 361–368.

Hammerbacher, M., & Lyvers, M. (2006). Factors associated with relapse among clients in Australian substance disorder treatment facilities. *Journal of Substance Use, 11*(6), 387–394.

Hartwell, S. (2004). Triple stigma: Persons with mental illness and substance abuse problems in the criminal justice system. *Criminal Justice Policy Review, 15*(1), 84–99.

Haywood, T. W., Kravitz, H. M., Grossman, J. L., Davis, J. M., & Lewis, D. A. (1995). Predicting the "revolving door" phenomenon among patients with schizophrenic, schizoaffective, and affective disorders. *American Journal of Psychiatry, 152,* 856–861.

Institute of Medicine, Committee on Crossing the Quality Chasm, Adaptation to Mental Health and Addictive Disorders. (2006). *Improving the Quality of Health Care for Mental and Substance-Use Conditions.* Washington, DC: National Academy Press.

Jellinek, E. M. (1960).*The Disease Concept of Alcoholism*. New Brunswick: Hillhouse.

Joe, S., Baser, R. E., Breeden, G., Neighbors, H. W., & Jackson, J. S. (2006). Prevalence of and risk factors for lifetime suicide attempts among blacks in the United States. *Journal of the American Medical Association, 296*(17), 2112–2123.

Katon, W. (2003). Clinical and health services relationships between major depression, depressive symptoms, and general medical illness. *Biological Psychiatry, 54*, 216–226.

Kessler, R. C., Berglund, P. A., Demler, O., Jin, R., Merikangas, K. R., & Walters, E. E. (2005). Lifetime prevalence and age-of-onset distributions of DSM-IV disorders in the national comorbidity survey replication. *Archives of General Psychiatry, 62*, 593–602.

Kessler, R. C., Nelson C. B., McGonagle, K. A., Edlund, M. J., Frank, R. G., & Leaf, P. J. (1996). The epidemiology of co-occurring addictive and mental disorders: Implications for prevention and service utilization. *American Journal of Orthopsychiatry, 66*(1), 17–31.

Keyser, D. J., Watkins, K. E., Vilamovska, A., & Pincus, H. A. (2008). Improving service delivery for individuals with co-occurring disorders: New perspectives on the quadrant model. *Psychiatric Services, 59*(11), 1251–1253.

Krakow, D. S., Galanter, M., & Dermatis, H. (1997). HIV risk factors in dually diagnosed patients. *American Journal of Addictions, 7*, 74–80.

Lehman, A. F. (1996). Heterogeneity of person and place: Assessing co-occurring addictive and mental disorders. *American Journal of Orthopsychiatry, 66*(1), 32–41.

Lehman, A. F., Myers, C. P., & Corty, E. (1989). Assessment and classification of patients with psychiatric and substance abuse syndromes. *Hospital and Community Psychiatry, 40*, 1019–1030.

Lyons, J. S., & McGovern, M. P. (1989). Use of mental health services by dually diagnosed patients. *Hospital and Community Psychiatry, 40*, 1067–1068.

Magura, S., Laudet, A. B., Mahmood, D., Rosenblum, A., & Knight, E. (2002). Adherence to medication regimens and participation in dual-focus self-help groups. *Psychiatric Services, 53*, 310–316.

Manwani, S. G., Pardo, T. B., Albanese, M. J., Zablotsky, B., Goodwin, F. K., & Ghaemi, S. N. (2006). Substance use disorder and other predictors of antidepressant-induced mania: A retrospective chart review. *Journal of Clinical Psychiatry, 67*(9), 1341–1345.

Manwani, S. G., Szilagyi, K. A., Zablotsky, B., Hennen, J., Griffin, M. L., & Weiss, R. D. (2007). Adherence to pharmacotherapy in bipolar disorder patients with and without co-occurring substance use disorders. *Journal of Clinical Psychiatry, 68*(8), 1172–1176.

McCabe, L. O. (2004). Crossing the quality chasm in behavioral health care: The role of evidence-based practice. *Professional Psychology: Research and Practice 35*(6), 571–579.

McGovern, M. P., Clark, R. E., & Samnaliev, M. (2007). Co-occurring psychiatric and substance use disorders: A multi-state feasibility study of the quadrant model. *Psychiatric Services, 58*, 949–957.

Meade, C. S., Graff, F. S., Griffin, M. L., & Weiss, R. D. (2008). HIV risk behavior among patients with co-occurring bipolar and substance use disorders: Associations with mania and drug abuse. *Drug and Alcohol Dependence, 92*(1–3), 296–300.

Miller, F. T., & Tanenbaum, J. H. (1989). Drug abuse in schizophrenia. *Hospital and Community Psychiatry, 40*, 847–849.

Minkoff, K. (1999). *Model for the Desired Array of Services and Clinical Competencies for a Comprehensive, Continuous, Integrated System of Care*. Worcester: University of Massachusetts, Department of Psychiatry, Center for Mental Health Services Research.

Mojtabai, R., & Singh, P. (2007) Implications of co-occurring alcohol abuse for role impairment, health problems, treatment seeking, and early course of alcohol dependence. *American Journal on Addictions, 16*, 300–309.

Mueser, K. T., Drake, R. E., Turner, W., & McGovern, M. (2006). *Integrated Treatment for Dual Disorders*. New York: Guilford Press.

Mueser, K. T., Noordsy, D. L., Drake, R. E., & Fox, M. (2003). *Integrated Treatment for Dual Disorders: A Guide to Effective Practice*. New York: Guilford Press.

Nathan, P. E. (1998). Not yet ideal. *American Psychologist, 53,* 290–299.

NASMHPD and NASADAD (1999). *National Dialogue on Co-occurring Mental Health and Substance Use Disorders*. Washington, DC: National Association of State Alcohol and Drug Abuse Directors.

Negrete, J. C., Knapp, W. P., Douglas, D. E., & Smith, W. B. (1986). Cannabis affects the severity of schizophrenic symptoms: Results of a clinical survey. *Psychological Medicine, 16,* 515–520.

Noordsy, D. L., Drake, R. E., Biesanz, J. C., & McHugo, G. J. (1994). Family history of alcoholism in schizophrenia. *Journal of Nervous and Mental Disease, 182,* 651–655.

North, C. S., Eyrich, K. M., Pollio, D. E., & Spitznagel, E. L. (2004). Are rates of psychiatric disorders in the homeless population changing? *American Journal of Public Health, 94,* 103–108.

Osher, F. C. (2007). Integrated mental health/substance abuse responses to justice involved persons with co-occurring disorders. *Journal of Dual Diagnosis, 4*(1), 3–33.

Osher, F. C., & Drake, R. E. (1996). Reversing a history of unmet needs: Approaches to care for persons with co-occurring addictive and mental disorders. *American Journal of Orthopsychiatry, 66,* 4–12.

Osher, F. C., Drake, R. E., Noordsy, D. L., Teague, G. B., Hurlbut, S. C., Biesanz, J. C., & Beaudett, M. S. (1994). Correlates and outcomes of alcohol use disorder among rural outpatients with schizophrenia. *Journal of Clinical Psychiatry, 55,* 109–113.

Osher, F. C., & Kofoed, L. L. (1989). Treatment of patients with psychiatric and psychoactive substance abuse disorders. *Hospital and Community Psychiatry, 40,* 1025–1030.

Owen, R. R., Fischer, E. P., & Booth, B. M. (1996). Medication noncompliance and substance abuse among patients with schizophrenia. *Psychiatric Services, 47,* 853–858.

Pepper, B., Kirshner, M. C., & Ryglewicz, H. (1981). The young adult chronic patient: Overview of a population. *Hospital and Community Psychiatry, 32,* 463–467.

Peters, R. H., Bartoi, M. G., & Sherman, P. B. (2008). *Screening and Assessment of Co-Occurring Disorders in the Justice System*. Delmar, NY: CMHS National GAINS Center.

Petry, N. M., Stinson, F. S., & Grant, B. F. (2005). Comorbidity of DSM-IV pathological gambling and other psychiatric disorders: Results from the national epidemiologic survey on alcohol and related conditions. *Journal of Clinical Psychiatry, 66,* 564–574.

Pulay, A. J., Dawson, D. A., Hasin, D. S., Goldstein, R. B., Ruan, W. J., Pickering, R. P., et al. (2008). Violent behavior and DSM-IV psychiatric disorders: Results from the national epidemiologic survey on alcohol and related conditions. *Journal of Clinical Psychiatry, 69*(1), 12–22.

Reback, C. J., Kamien, J. B., & Amass, L. (2007). Characteristics and HIV risk behaviors of homeless, substance-using men who have sex with men. *Addictive Behaviors, 32*(3), 647–654.

Regier, D. A., Farmer, M. E., Rae, D. S., Locke, B. Z., Keith, S. J., Judd, L. L., & Goodwin, F. K. (1990). Comorbidity of mental disorders with alcohol and other drug abuse. *Journal of the American Medical Association, 264,* 2511–2518.

Ridgely, M. S., & Dixon, L. (1995). Financing and policy issues in dual diagnosis. In A. Lehman & L. Dixon (Eds.), *Double Trouble: Chronic Mental Illness and Substance Abuse*. New York: Harwood Academic Publishers.

Ridgely, M. S., Goldman, H. H., & Willenbring, M. (1990). Barriers to the care of persons with dual diagnoses: Organizational and financing issues. *Schizophrenia Bulletin, 16,* 123–132.

Ries, R. K., Yuodelis-Flores, C., Comtois, K. A., Roy-Byrne, P. P., & Russo, J. E. (2008). Substance-induced suicidal admissions to an acute psychiatric service: Characteristics and outcomes. *Journal of Substance Abuse Treatment, 34,* 72–79.

Rosenberg, S. D., Goodman L. A., Osher, F. C., Swartz, M., Essock, S. M., Butterfield, M. I., et al. (2001). Prevalence of HIV, Hepatitis B, and Hepatitis C in people with severe mental illness. *American Journal of Public Health, 91*(1), 31–37.

Rychetnik, L., Hawe, P., Waters, E., Barratt, A., & Frommer, M. (2004). A glossary for evidence-based public health. *Journal of Epidemiology and Community Health*, *58*(7), 538–545.

Sacks, S., Chandler, R., & Gonzales, J. (2008). Responding to the challenge of co-occurring disorders: Suggestions for future research. *Journal of Substance Abuse Treatment*, *34*, 139–146.

Seibel, J. P., Satel, S. L., Anthony, D., Southwick, S. M., Krystal, J. H., & Charney, D. S. (1993). Effects of cocaine on hospital course in schizophrenia. *Journal of Nervous and Mental Disease*, *181*, 31–37.

Substance Abuse and Mental Health Services Administration (SAMHSA). (2006). *A Thousand Voices: The National Action Plan on Behavioral Health Workforce Development*. Rockville, MD: Office of the Administrator.

Substance Abuse and Mental Health Services Administration. (2007). *Results from the 2006 National Survey on Drug Use and Health: National Findings*. Rockville, MD: Office of Applied Studies.

U.S. Department of Health and Human Services. (1999). *Mental Health: A Report of the Surgeon General*. Washington, DC: Office of the Surgeon General.

Wang, P. S., Berglund, P. A., Kessler, R. C., Olfson, M., Pincus, H. A., & Wells, K. B. (2005). Failure and delay in initial treatment contact after first onset of mental disorders in the National Comorbidity Survey Replication. *Archives of General Psychiatry*, *62*, 603–613.

Yesavage, J. A., & Zarcone, V. (1983). History of drug abuse and dangerous behavior in inpatient schizophrenics. *Journal of Clinical Psychiatry*, *44*, 259–261.

Section B

TREATMENT SETTINGS

Chapter 13

STATE MENTAL HEALTH AGENCIES

Theodore C. Lutterman, BA; Michael Hogan, PhD;
Bernadette E. Phelan, PhD; and Noel A. Mazade, PhD

THIS CHAPTER presents the evolution of state mental health agencies (SMHAs) from historically operating large state psychiatric hospitals to today's role in coordinating, funding, and planning community-based systems for adults with serious mental illness (SMI) and children with severe emotional disturbance (SED). In recent years, SMHAs have also promoted recovery-focused services and evidence-based practices, as well as coordinated general medical care, housing, and other programs for children, adults, and elders. However, as governmental roles and health care evolve, new challenges to the role of the SMHA have emerged. These include the responsibilities of coordinating complex community systems of care where the SMHA is becoming less of a direct operator and funder of mental health services and more of a governmental entity managing collaboration with local and federal agencies in a fiscal environment characterized by the worst state budget crises since the Great Depression.

This chapter reviews the evolution of the SMHAs' mission, how SMHAs are organized within state government, their clientele, what services SMHAs provide, and how these services are funded and organized. Finally, the chapter identifies a number of policy issues that SMHAs are currently addressing as well as future challenges.

Introduction and Overview

SMHAs are the state government agencies responsible for assuring the provision of high quality mental health services especially for adults with severe mental illness and children with severe emotional disturbances. Decades ago, SMHAs managed systems where all services were provided in large state-operated psychiatric hospitals. Today, the SMHA role has evolved to "provide a guaranteed supply of specialized care, political focus for advocates, and state police powers for social control" (Frank & Glied, 2006, p. 6). Today, every state has a designated SMHA that is responsible for funding and/or providing community mental health services as well as developing annual mental health plans that are submitted to the federal government as a condition of receiving federal Community Mental Health Block Grant funds from the federal Substance Abuse and Mental Health Services Administration (SAMHSA).

In addition to funding and/or operating community-based services, every state also operates psychiatric inpatient services, usually located within state-operated psychiatric hospital(s). SMHAs also serve a public safety function. The majority of persons served in state-operated psychiatric hospitals are either involuntarily committed to the hospital, having been judged to be a danger to themselves or others (involuntary civil status) or due to their involvement in the criminal justice system (involuntary forensic status). As state psychiatric hospitals have been drastically downsized over the last 50 years, the number of "voluntary" and involuntary civil status clients has reduced considerably. In 24% of reporting states, over half of all state psychiatric beds are occupied by forensic status clients (National Association of State Mental Health Program Directors Research Institute [NRI], 2008).

The role of SMHAs has shifted from management of a separate system of care to a leadership role within state government focused on coordinating care across multiple state agencies involving many state and federal funding streams. As consumers are mainstreamed from state psychiatric services into the broader community, the need to assure access to adequate housing, vocational and educational supports, and physical health services has become a major SMHA concern. While SMHAs directly provide some of these housing, vocational, and other support and case management services, SMHAs are increasingly responsible for coordinating with other agencies to ensure that mental health consumers have appropriate and timely access to these services and supports from other systems.

The dire need for coordination was highlighted in the report of the President's New Freedom Commission on Mental Health (2003), which concluded that the mental health system is fragmented and "in shambles." A set of transformation goals to develop a recovery-oriented, seamless system of services and supports that meet consumers' needs for high quality integrated care was recommended. The SMHAs embraced the Commission's goals and are now devoting significant efforts to transform state systems to meet the Commission's laudable goals. Through affiliation with the National Association of State Mental Health Program Directors (NASMHPD), the states have collectively passed position statements endorsing the Commission's goals. Individual states have engaged in a number of major reorganization initiatives targeted to one or more of the Commission's goals, including participation in a series of SAMHSA-funded Transformation Systems Improvement Grants (TSIGs) in nine states; development of state transformation workgroups and governor's commissions; and participation in SAMHSA's Transformation Transfer Initiative (TTI). A recent report by the independent NASMHPD Research Institute, Inc. (NRI) found that every SMHA was working to address a majority of the six Freedom Commission goals (Lutterman, Mayberg, & Emmett, 2006).

Today, SMHAs provide services to over 6 million individuals at an annual cost of over $31 billion. Over 95% of the consumers served by SMHA systems are currently served in community-based programs. While state psychiatric inpatient hospitals serve a relatively small percent (3%) of the persons served by SMHAs, the expenditures for these intensive inpatient services account for 29% of SMHA-controlled spending ($8 billion). Although all SMHAs plan and organize comprehensive community-based mental health systems, every state organizes and structures its SMHA system differently.

SMHAs

EVOLUTION OF SMHAs

> In the 1950s and 1960s mental health policy making was the domain of governors and their state mental health program directors. Organized psychiatry wielded great influence and was deeply involved in consequential debates about the future of mental health care in the United States. Today, by contrast, state Medicaid directors, the Social Security Commissioner, the administrator of the Centers for Medicare and Medicaid Services (CMS), and human resource directors in U.S. corporations are the voices of the greatest influence on the direction of mental health policy. These policy makers have little direct connection with the specialty mental health sector (Frank & Glied, 2006, p. 91).

As Frank and Glied (2006) observe, SMHAs were once the primary locus of mental health policy in America. Although the evolution of mental health services has witnessed new policymakers, funders, and delivery systems, every state government maintains an SMHA and vests within that agency responsibility for serving the needs of a population with mental illness dispersed across communities and including individuals primarily served in other systems (e.g. schools, foster care, mainstream supportive housing, and criminal justice).

State governments began providing mental health services before the United States became emancipated from Britain. In 1773, the Virginia Colonial government opened the first state facility constructed solely for the care and treatment of persons with mental illness (Virginia Department of Mental Health, Mental Retardation, and Substance Abuse Services, n.d.). This facility later became Virginia's Eastern State Hospital and marked the beginning of state governments assuming a central role in providing mental health care to their citizens.

During the early part of the 19th century, more states opened state psychiatric hospitals. For example, New York State opened its first state psychiatric hospital in 1806 (Stinger, 2008) and Connecticut in 1823 (Grob, 2008). However, many persons with mental illnesses who were not hospitalized ended up housed in jails, prisons, and poor-houses.

During the 1840s, Dorothea Dix led a national effort to establish humane care and treatment for persons with mental illnesses. Ms. Dix's efforts focused on state governments, and her advocacy led many state legislatures to build and expand state psychiatric hospitals (U.S. Department of Health and Human Services [USDHHS], 1980). By 1870, the U.S. Census Bureau counted 42 state psychiatric hospitals with 14,605 resident patients. The number of state psychiatric hospitals and the number of persons served in them grew steadily until, by the middle of the twentieth century, there were 332 state psychiatric hospitals with over 512,000 residents (Atay, Crider, & Foley, 2007).

The reasons for the expansion of asylums and institutionalized populations, as well as the reasons for their continued shrinkage in the last half of the twentieth century, are many and complex. Early optimism about the capacity of patients to recover and return home after a period of "moral treatment" involving structure and participation in the work of running the institution proved only partially correct. While many were successfully treated in state psychiatric hospitals, many others languished in the absence of effective treatments and the presence of primarily custodial care that emerged following the Industrial Revolution.

Up until the 1950s, state governments were responsible for providing and paying for most public mental health services, but these services were almost entirely inpatient services provided in state psychiatric hospitals. A few states offered outpatient clinic services, but statewide systems of community services barely existed since the SMHAs of that era were organized around supporting the state psychiatric hospitals. Given their primary role of operating state psychiatric hospitals, the SMHA directors were usually psychiatrists, and most of them acted as the state hospital superintendent (according to NASMHPD records, only one state SMHA Director was not a physician during the 1950s).

During World War II, over 1.75 million men were rejected for military service due to mental or emotional issues (USHHS, 1980). In addition, experience during the war with crisis care demonstrated improved effectiveness for brief interventions and early return to the community (one's military unit) (Lamb, 1998). These experiences led to increased awareness of the prevalence of mental illness in the civilian population and greater understanding of the role that psychiatrists could assume in the community.

Following the war, the mental health needs of returning military personnel led to a growing concern about what types of services were available. Simultaneously, a series of exposés (such as Albert Deutsch's *The Shame of the States*, 1948) demonstrated that many state psychiatric hospitals had become seriously overcrowded and therapeutic treatment was not being provided. In 1954, Congress passed the National Mental Health Act, which authorized the National Institute of Mental Health (NIMH) to provide leadership in research and improve the provision of services to persons with mental illnesses. Under NIMH's oversight, and building upon the World War II experience, the strategy of community-based mental health services emerged as a viable alternative to large state psychiatric hospitals. According to Frank and Glied (2006), the goal of moving consumers to the community was facilitated by the development of the first psychopharmacologic treatments for schizophrenia (Chlorpromazine and Haloperidol), which allowed mental health systems to explore alternatives to inpatient psychiatric services by maintaining patients in the community with supportive medications.

Perhaps the greatest contributing factor to the "decline" of hospitals as institutions was facilitated by a series of Supreme Court decisions. In *Souder v. Brennan*

(1973) the Court found that the use of unpaid patient labor in the hospitals was unconstitutional. The decision contributed to dramatically escalating operating costs in state psychiatric hospitals, since states could no longer rely on unpaid patients to reduce their labor costs. The Court's decision in *O'Connor v. Donaldson* (1975) found that the denial of personal liberty inherent in involuntary institutionalization was so substantial as to require a higher standard (now expressed in the familiar "dangerous to self or others by reason of mental illness") (see Chapter 3 in this volume for additional reading in the areas of law, services delivery, and policy).

THE RISE OF COMMUNITY-BASED MENTAL HEALTH CARE

Community care began to emerge as a priority, and states began to pass legislation to initiate community-based alternatives to state psychiatric hospitals. For example, in 1954, New York passed the first state legislation that established local community mental health boards (Hogan, 2008a). In 1963, Congress passed, and President John F. Kennedy signed, the Community Mental Health Centers Construction Act, Public Law No. 88-164, to construct and fund the operation of new local community mental health centers (CMHCs) throughout the nation. Based upon a public health population-based approach of 3,000 catchment areas nationwide, each CMHC was to serve 125,000 to 250,000 persons and provide a comprehensive array of six mandated mental health services that were predicted to reduce the need for state psychiatric hospitals. Required services included inpatient services, outpatient services, day treatment, consultation/education, and emergency services.

Despite a laudable public-health oriented strategy, eventual flaws and limits in the CMHC program blunted its impact. The Medicaid and Medicare programs, created just a few years later, would have a much more significant impact upon community mental health care. Medicaid initially provided no specialty benefit for mental health care, and thus it, did not assist states with the cost of their psychiatric hospitals. However, Medicaid would pay for brief inpatient care in general hospitals, thereby stimulating the development of psychiatric units in general hospitals that eventually became the preferred option for hospitalization. Since Medicaid added coverage of nursing home care, many elderly state hospital patients were transferred to these facilities. In 2005, only 4% of residents in state psychiatric hospitals were persons over age 64, down from 25% of the hospitals' population in 1985 (Hepburn & Sederer, 2009). Thus, Medicaid's payment for alternatives at the "front door" and "back door" of the state psychiatric hospitals contributed greatly to the downsizing of these facilities and started a long trend under which Medicaid would greatly impact mental health policy. During the 1960s and 1970s, SMHAs were heavily involved in both institutional reform sparked by class action lawsuits over conditions in state psychiatric hospitals such as *Wyatt v. Stickney* (1974) (first filed in 1970) and *Dixon v. Barry* (1997) (filed in 1974), and in developing community based mental health services.

Although the CMHC Act expanded community-based care by paying for the building and operation of hundreds of CMHCs, the funding mechanism of the CMHC Act was predicated on NIMH funds being provided directly to local CMHCs, thereby bypassing the SMHAs. Funds were also provided on a "start-up" cycle of seven years. By the time that the seven-year federal funding phased out, every CMHC needed to find "paying customers." Under the CMHC Act, CMHCs were not required to support, coordinate, or integrate with SMHAs, which were simultaneously developing their own community mental health systems. The lack of coordination between the federally funded CMHCs and the SMHAs (that still devoted the majority of their fiscal resources to state psychiatric hospitals) continued through the 1960s and 1970s. This lack of integration led President Jimmy Carter to establish a Mental Health Commission to plan for a new national initiative, the Mental Health Systems Act, which was passed in 1980, but immediately ended with President Reagan's first budget, which converted the CMHC program funding to support a block grant.

During the CMHC program era, transfers of elderly patients from state psychiatric hospitals to nursing homes continued. During the 1960s and 1970s, the number of patients in state psychiatric hospitals was reduced by one-half, supported under the new Medicaid program, which paid for nursing facility care, but not for state psychiatric hospitals. Despite this transfer, only a few state psychiatric hospitals were closed, leaving the majority of SMHA funds dedicated to maintaining the state psychiatric hospitals. In Fiscal Year 1981 (FY1981), over 69% of SMHA funds were spent in state psychiatric hospitals (NRI, 2008).

In 1982, under President Reagan, the Community Mental Health Block Grant (CMHBG) converted the CMHC direct funding into a block grant administered by the SMHAs. With the CMHBG funds flowing under control of SMHAs, a new tool was available to develop community mental health systems. The CMHBG required that SMHAs develop plans to expand community care and to minimize the use of state psychiatric hospitals. NIMH also supported the development of community mental health systems by initiating the "Community Support System" (CSP) for adults and "Child and Adolescent Service System Program" (CASSP) for children. NIMH provided grants to the SMHAs to plan for CSP and CASSP systems. Both focused on the provision of services to help consumers live in the community. Both CSP and CASSP model services moved beyond a focus of clinic-based mental health services to providing case management and other mental health services to consumers wherever they lived and worked.

Concurrently in the 1980s, states began to utilize Medicaid to pay for community-based mental health services. Initially, states used the Medicaid Clinic Option, which limited reimbursement to services provided in outpatient office settings. However, during the later part of the 1980s and throughout the 1990s, states began to modify their State Medicaid Plan to use the Rehabilitation Services Option and Targeted Case Management Option, which allowed reimbursement for treatment rehabilitation and case management services delivered in consumers' homes, the workplace, and in the streets. During the 1990s, Medicaid became the major source of new funds to SMHA systems (NRI, 2008).

Despite increased revenues, the burgeoning role of Medicaid as a dominant payer for community-based services has not been all positive to the SMHA systems. Since Medicaid is based upon a federal-state formula financial match, with the federal government contributing at least 50% of the funds in each state, shifting services to Medicaid allows states to greatly expand available fiscal resources beyond only state tax base-funded services. However, as a management strategy,

Medicaid introduced a complex array of rules, eligibility requirements, and a medical model orientation that required a consumer's eligibility determination for receiving Medicaid-reimbursed services be predicated on "medical necessity." The shift to use Medicaid to pay for mental health services brought with it another state government agency, the State Medicaid Agency, into the already complex community mental health system of services. In effect, these Medicaid-imposed regulatory stipulations and functions resulted in a functional shared authority between the State Medicaid Agency and the SMHA in the delivery of mental health services. As a result, in states where Medicaid holds responsibility for administering the community mental health portion of the Medicaid benefit, and /or where Medicaid established third-party managed care organizations to manage Medicaid reimbursed care, the role of the SMHA became both altered and diminished (Hogan, 2008b).

As the focus of SMHAs shifted from operating large state institutions to building comprehensive community based systems, the leadership in SMHAs shifted from physicians to other mental health professions. Governors began to hire SMHA Commissioners who had expertise either in community based mental health systems or who possessed either management or legal skills. By 2008, only four SMHA directors were psychiatrists, and many more have professional degrees in fields related to providing community-based services and/or managing community based systems (e.g., PhDs, MSWs, and MBAs). Today there are more SMHA Directors with law degrees and MBAs than there are psychiatrists. Currently, the SMHA must function within the larger fabric of state government, thereby subordinating the SMHA to controlling only a portion of all state government funds for public mental health services. The complexity of the SMHA role in assuring mental health services has continued to develop with "second order" changes, such as the incorporation of evidence-based practices and working "laterally" with other major state agencies (including Medicaid, housing, education, children's agencies, criminal justice, and corrections).

In the era following the 2003 President's Commission Report, two challenges for SMHAs have emerged: 1) directing hospital and community services not entirely under the SMHA's control; and 2) "managing laterally" by working through and cooperatively with other agencies, such as schools, foster care, juvenile justice, corrections, and primary health care, to improve the circumstances of people with a mental illness who are the primary responsibility of these other agencies.

Therefore, the overarching question revolves less around the role of the SMHA, but more on the level of coherence, integrity, and leadership needed within state government to best support policy changes and assure the well-being of people with mental illnesses in an environment of shared responsibility between the SMHAs and other state, local, and private entities.

Who Is Served by SMHAs Today?

In 2007, just over 6 million persons (2% of the U.S. population) received mental health services from the SMHAs' system of care (USDHHS, 2008). The vast majority (95%) of these individuals received services from community-based providers funded by the SMHA. Only 3% of consumers were served in state-operated psychiatric hospitals. An additional 7% received inpatient psychiatric services from other SMHA-funded providers including general hospitals and private psychiatric hospitals. Percentages total to more than 100% because individuals can be served in both hospital and community settings during the year.

States vary considerably on the percentage of their state population that receives mental health services from SMHA-funded service providers. The total number of persons reported as receiving mental health services from the SMHA system ranged from 9,756 in Delaware (1.4% of their population) to a high of 658,314 in California (1.8% of the population). While the average SMHA provided mental health services to 2% of its population, the median was 2.1% and ranged from 4.0% in New Jersey to 0.4% in Massachusetts (where the state's Medicaid managed care carve-out for psychiatric services is not considered part of the SMHA system). States in the northeastern region of the United States had the highest average utilization rates (2.6%), while states in the southwestern region of the United States had the lowest rates (1.6%).

CHARACTERISTICS OF PERSONS SERVED BY SMHA SYSTEMS

Persons served by SMHA mental health systems are often minorities, unemployed, eligible for Medicaid, and have a serious mental illness or serious emotional disturbance. Every year, each SMHA must report to the federal government's Center for Mental Health Services (CMHS) through the Uniform Reporting System (URS), a set of common data on the characteristics of persons served by the SMHA (Lutterman & Gonzalez, 2006). The annual URS reports, due to CMHS by December 1 of each year, include a set of standard tables depicting the age, gender, race, employment status, living situation, and other aspects of care provided to these consumers.

While the President's New Freedom Commission found that "the mental health system has not kept pace with the diverse needs of racial and ethnic minorities, often under-serving or inappropriately serving them" (New Freedom Commission, 2003, p. 49), the state mental health system is one arena where minorities are receiving a disproportionate share of the mental health services compared to the minorities' percentage distribution in the state population. Overall, SMHAs served more Whites (62%) than persons of any other race. However, minorities had higher utilization rates than Whites: African Americans (32 per 1,000 population), Native Hawaiians/Pacific Islanders (25.9 per 1,000 population), and American Indian/Alaskan Natives (25.1 per 1,000) compared to Whites (15.8 per 1,000 population). Moreover, children under age 21 represented 32.1% of all persons served by SMHA systems. Adolescents aged 13 to 17 had the highest utilization rate of any age group (37.7 per 1000 population), followed by adults (22.0). Older adults had much lower utilization rates in SMHA systems than any other age group.

With regard to employment, the majority of consumers served by SMHAs are either unemployed or "not in the labor force" (a category that includes persons who are disabled, retired, or otherwise not actively seeking employment). In 2007, only 21% of consumers were reported as competitively employed (as a percentage of those with any known employment status). Almost half of all SMHA consumers

Table 13.1 Characteristics of Persons Served by SMHAs: 2007

	Number Served by SMHAs	%	Utilization Rate Per 1,000 Population	States & Territories Reporting	Percent Living In Private Residence	Percent Competitively Employed
Age						
0 to 12	883,202	14.4%	16.9	58	(1)	
13 to 17	807,963	13.2%	37.7	58	84.4%	
18 to 20	273,626	4.5%	21.8	58	(2)	18%
21 to 64	3,866,031	63.2%	22.0	58	79.2%	22%
65 to 74	169,368	2.8%	9.0	58	(3)	(4)
75 and over	111,912	1.8%	6.1	57	69.9%	6%
Not Available	9,539	0.2%		31	71.3%	13%
TOTAL	6,121,641	100%	20.1	58	80.1%	21%
Gender						
Female	3,134,214	51.2%	20.3	58	83.5%	21%
Male	2,947,828	48.2%	19.7	58	76.5%	22%
Not Available	39,599	0.6%		38	84.0%	18%
TOTAL	6,121,641	100%	20.1	58	80.1%	21%
Race/Ethnicity						
American Indian/ Alaskan Native	72,878	1.2%	25.1	53	77.0%	
Asian	80,296	1.3%	6.1	56	81.4%	
Black/African American	1,228,744	20.1%	32.0	56	75.2%	
Native Hawaiian/ Pacific Islander	12,662	0.2%	25.9	50	79.4%	
White	3,794,159	62.0%	15.8	57	81.8%	
Hispanic*	215,485	3.5%	13.7	11	83.2%	
Multi-Racial	95,116	1.6%	22.4	46	78.2%	
Not Available	622,301	10.2%		34	79.9%	
TOTAL	6,121,641	100%	20.1	58	80.1%	
Hispanic Origin						
Hispanic or Latino	519,995	9.7%	17.0	48	83.1%	
Not Hispanic or Latino	4,116,658	77.1%	18.7	51	80.4%	
Hispanic Status Unknown	702,945	13.2%		53	74.3%	
TOTAL	5,339,598	100%	20.3	53	80.1%	

*Hispanic status was collected as a race category in 11 states.
Number "Not Available" differs by Age, Gender, and Race due to state variation in collecting data.
(1) Living Situation for Children are reported for a combined age 0 to 17 category
(2) Living Situation for Adults are reported for a combined age 18 to 64 category
(3) Living Situation for Older Adults are reported for a combined age 65 and over category
(4) Employment Status for Older Adults are reported for a combined age 65 and over category
Source: DHHS, CMHS Uniform Reporting System, 2007 data.

were reported with the status "not in the labor force," and 32% were unemployed. Note that the 21% employment rate is viewed as an optimistic level of employment since it likely includes many consumers who are employed only part-time and who do not work sufficient hours to either receive health benefits or to live without other federal and state supports.

With regard to the living situation of children and adolescents, the majority lived in private residences (84%), with the remaining living in a variety of settings including foster homes (6%), residential care (2%), children's residential treatment (1.1%), institutional settings (1.4%), and jail/correctional facilities (2%). A very small percentage (0.4%) of children and adolescents served by the SMHAs were either homeless or living in a shelter.

For adults, the majority lived in private residences (79%) while the remainder of adult consumers reported living in a variety of settings, including residential care (5%), institutional settings (4%), jail/corrections facilities (2%), and foster homes (0.8%). Nearly 4% of adult mental health consumers were homeless or living in shelters. Overall, more male consumers (4%) were homeless or living in a shelter than female consumers (2%). Of the racial groups, more African American consumers (5%) were homeless or living in a shelter. Hispanic/ Latino and Asian consumers had the lowest percentage of homeless consumers (2% each) (U.S. Department of Health and Human Services, 2008).

Medicaid Status of SMHA Consumers

Persons become eligible for Medicaid due to disabilities (including psychiatric disabilities) and/or low income. According to SAMHSA, Medicaid has grown to become the largest single payment source for mental health services in the country (Mark et al., 2007). The NRI's annual *SMHA-Controlled Revenues and Expenditures* study has documented that Medicaid is the fastest-growing revenue source for the SMHA system, with nearly one-half of SMHA revenues derived from Medicaid (NRI, 2007).

The 2007 CMHS URS data show that over half of all SMHA consumers (57%) utilized Medicaid to pay for some of their mental health services, with a substantial percent (43%) having no Medicaid coverage. Fifty-nine percent (59%) of all female consumers were covered by Medicaid, while 56% of male consumers had Medicaid as a payment source (U.S. Department of Health and Human Services, 2008).

Organization and Structure of SMHA Systems

How states organize their SMHAs, where they are organizationally located within the state government, and the specific mix of services and disabilities for which they are responsible vary widely from state to state. In every state, the SMHA either provides community mental health services directly or, more commonly, funds community mental health providers. Every SMHA is also responsible for administering the federal Community Mental Health Block Grant (CMHBG) and developing annual plans for their community mental health system. In addition, every state operates psychiatric inpatient facilities, but how these psychiatric beds relate to the SMHA also varies. Finally, every state has involuntary commitment statutes that vest in the SMHA the responsibility of insuring the public's safety in terms of allowing the commitment of individuals deemed dangerous to themselves or others. All states have statutes that allow the involuntary commitment of persons to state inpatient facilities, but an increasing number of states (37 in 2007) also have outpatient commitment statutes that allow persons to be required to participate in mental health treatment as a condition of living in their communities (NRI, 2008).

SMHAs are most frequently organized within state governments as a division or office located within a larger umbrella agency. In 2007, 29 SMHAs were located within state Departments of Human Services, seven were within the Health Department, and two were in some other state department (often departments that combine Health and Human Services). In 13 states, the SMHAs are independent departments of mental health.

In 10 states, the SMHA's director is a member of the Governor's Cabinet. In seven states, the SMHA's director is directly accountable to the governor, and in 38 states the SMHA director is accountable to another administrator such as the Cabinet Secretary of an umbrella agency. In five states, the SMHA director is accountable to other leadership such as a mental health board/commission.

Furthermore, many SMHAs are responsible for other disability services in addition to mental health. The two most common additional responsibilities of SMHAs are for substance abuse services and for intellectual disabilities and developmental disabilities (ID/DD). Over the last twenty years, many SMHAs have had responsibilities for providing ID/DD services moved out of the SMHA, while even more states have moved substance abuse services into the SMHA. In 26 states, the SMHA is also responsible for the provision of substance abuse (SA) treatment services (including alcohol and other drug abuse), while these two agencies (SMHA and SA) are located within the same state umbrella agency in 17 states. In seven states, interagency agreements exist between the SMHA and SA agencies to coordinate care. In 12 states, the SMHA is also responsible for the provision of

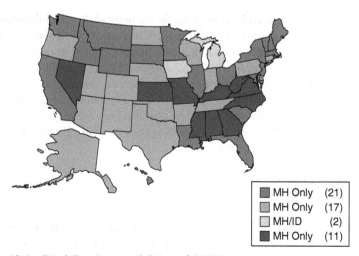

Figure 13.1 Disability Responsibilities of SMHAs: 2007. (*Source:* NRI State Mental Health Agency Profiles System.)

ID/DD services, while in 27 states the ID/DD agency is located within the same umbrella agency as the SMHA. In 11 states, all three disability services are co-located within the SMHA. The states with all three disabilities organized within a single state agency are most frequently located in the South.

Within the last two years, nine SMHAs have been organizationally relocated within state/district government (Colorado, District of Columbia, Florida, Kansas, New Jersey, New Mexico, Rhode Island, Texas, and Washington). In five states (Colorado, Nevada, Vermont, Florida, and Kentucky), the reorganization involved shifting additional disability services either into or out of the SMHA. For example, in Nevada, substance abuse services were moved into the SMHA, and in Florida the Agency for Persons with Disabilities was created and services for persons with ID/DD were moved from the SMHA. Twenty years ago, the substance abuse agency was co-located with mental health in 19 states. During the 1980s and early 1990s, the trend was to split mental health and substance abuse into separate agencies. However, in the later 1990s and this decade, this trend has reversed, and more states have reorganized to place these agencies into the same agency, while creating a separate agency responsible for ID/DD services.

SMHA Mental Health Agency Service Responsibilities

SMHAs vary widely on the extent of mental health services coverage for which they are responsible. Some SMHAs are responsible for mental health services across the lifespan: children, adults, and older adults. In some states, responsibilities for specific types of mental health services, such as forensics, brain injuries, or Alzheimer's disease, are carved out to a different state agency and are not part of the SMHA's responsibility.

Children/Adolescent Mental Health Services

In most states (30), the SMHA is responsible for both adult and child/adolescent mental health services; however, in three states (Connecticut, Delaware, and Rhode Island), the responsibility for providing mental health services to children/adolescents is vested to a separate state agency, usually a Department of Children and Families, that is primarily responsible for children's services including child welfare, juvenile justice, and other children's related social and health services. In 16 other states, the responsibility for children/adolescent's mental health services is shared between the SMHA and another state agency (see Chapter 8 in this volume on children and adolescent mental health).

State Psychiatric Hospitals

There are state-owned and -operated psychiatric inpatient beds in every state, which are used for persons who are in need of the most intensive level of mental health services. In most states (44), the operation of state psychiatric hospitals is the SMHA's responsibility. In six states (Colorado, New Hampshire, New Mexico,

Rhode Island, South Dakota, and Wyoming), a separate state government agency has this responsibility. In these states, the SMHA works with the state psychiatric hospitals and the other state agency to coordinate care between the state psychiatric hospital(s) and the SMHA's community mental health system. These states describe having special initiatives to help coordinate the transition of consumers from psychiatric hospitals into community mental health services (see Chapter 15 in this volume on specialty mental hospitals).

Forensic Mental Health Services

Forensic mental health services are services provided to persons who are found in need of mental health services by a court through the criminal justice system. Forensic services range from evaluations of competency to stand trial, to providing mental health services to persons found by courts to be incompetent to stand trial, not guilty by reason of insanity, and/or guilty but having a mental illness. In most states (33), the provision of forensic mental health services is the responsibility of the SMHA. In 10 states, this responsibility is shared with another agency, and in two states the responsibility for forensic mental health services is located in the State Department of Corrections (see Chapter 18 in this volume on mental health treatment in criminal justice settings).

Alzheimer's Disease and Organic Brain Syndromes (OBS)

In 35 states, the SMHA is responsible for providing services to persons with Alzheimer's disease and/or other organic brain syndromes. In ten states, responsibility for providing services to persons with Alzheimer's and OBS are shared with another state government agency (often the State Health Department), and in two states the SMHA has no responsibility for such services. However, even in states where the SMHA does not have responsibility for providing Alzheimer's and OBS services, data from state psychiatric hospitals often show that patients with these diagnoses are being served in the state psychiatric hospitals, often because they may have co-occurring mental health diagnoses or because there are no alternative placements for these individuals (see Chapter 10 in this volume on mental health policy and aging).

Traumatic Brain Injury (TBI) Services

In seven states, the SMHA is responsible for providing services to individuals with traumatic brain injuries. In 11 states, the responsibility for providing such services is shared between the SMHA and another state government agency, and in 25 states, the SMHA has no responsibility for these services.

Eligibility for SMHA Mental Health Services

SMHAs' eligibility criteria that consumers must meet to qualify for receiving mental health services from SMHA-operated or -funded providers vary across states.

Adult Mental Health Eligibility

In 19 states, mental health services paid for by state general or special funds are limited to serve adults with a serious mental illness (SMI), while in 21 states, eligibility criteria are used to provide services either to adults with serious mental illnesses or adults with any mental illness. For services funded by non-state sources such as Medicaid, 13 states restrict eligibility to only adults with SMI, while 25 states have service eligibility criteria for adults with SMI and adults with any mental illness.

States use a combination of specific diagnoses, functional status, and other criteria to establish SMI eligibility for adults receiving SMHA-funded or -operated mental health services. In 44 states, specific diagnoses are part of the eligibility criteria. In 40 states, an adult's functional status is part of the eligibility criteria, and in 11 states, some other additional criteria are used to establish eligibility (duration of illness, history of prior hospitalization, income, and risk) (see Chapter 9 in this volume for further information on adult mental health).

Child and Adolescent Eligibility

In 17 states, mental health services using state general or special funds are limited to children with Serious Emotional Disturbances (SED), while in 22 states, there are eligibility criteria for children with SED and children with any emotional disturbances. For services funded with non-state sources such as Medicaid, 12 states restrict eligibility to only children with SED, while 26 states have service eligibility criteria for both children with SED and children with any emotional disturbances.

States use a combination of specific diagnoses, functional status, and other criteria to establish eligibility for children's mental health services. In 39 states, specific diagnoses are part of the eligibility criteria. In 37 states, a child's functional status is part of the eligibility criteria, and in 8 states, some other additional criteria are used to establish eligibility (duration of illness in four states, history of prior hospitalization, income, and risk).

Mental Health Organizations Operated and/or Funded by SMHAs

In 2007, SMHAs funded and/or operated 11,681 mental health organizations (see Table 13.2). SMHAs collaborate with different types of mental health providers ranging from state psychiatric hospitals staffed by state employees to a variety of county- or city-based providers and a mixture of for-profit and not-for-profit community organizations. Most of the organizations that comprise the SMHA system are not operated by the SMHA, but are funded by the SMHA. These provider organizations usually receive funds from a variety of other funding sources including Medicaid, Medicare, city/county funds, private health insurance, and donations. In some states, the SMHA operates community mental health organizations that are state-owned (with state employees delivering the mental health services). Sixteen states reported that they operated a total of 338 community mental health organizations during 2007.

Table 13.2 Number of Mental Health Organizations Operated or Funded by SMHA (2007)

	State Psychiatric Hospitals	Community MH Providers	Private Psychiatric Hospitals	General Hospitals with Separate Psych Units	Nursing Homes & Other ICF-MI & SNF Providers	Total Mental Health Providers
State Operated	210	338		4	17	569
State Funded	15	10,641	98	273	85	11,112
Total	225	10,979	98	277	102	11,681

Source: NRI State Profiles: 2007.

In addition to funding and operating mental health organizations, in 21 states, the SMHA is responsible for licensing or certifying private mental health providers. In 18 of these states, the SMHA receives reports on the services provided by these private mental health providers.

In recent years, a number of states have explored privatizing some of their state-owned and -operated mental health programs. Two states (Florida and Kansas) reported that within the last year they have privatized one of their state-operated psychiatric hospitals. In Florida, the Treasure Coast Forensic Treatment Facility was entirely privatized, and in Kansas, the Rainbow Mental Health Facility children's program was privatized. Three states (Kansas, North Carolina, and South Dakota) reported they have privatized one or more of their state-operated community mental health programs.

Organization of SMHA's Community Mental Health Systems

In 2007, 96% (5.6 million persons with 49 states, the District of Columbia, and four U.S. Territories reporting) of mental health consumers served by SMHA systems received community mental health services. Some individuals who received community mental health services also received care in state psychiatric hospitals (3%) or other psychiatric inpatient settings (7%) during the year.

In 2005, SMHAs expended over 70% of their funds ($20.7 billion) for mental health services provided in communities. SMHAs used three primary methods to pay for or deliver community-based mental health services, with a number of states using combinations of these methods:

1. SMHAs directly contracted with local (usually not-for-profit) community-based mental health providers. This method was used in 36 states and is the primary method of funding community services in 27 states;
2. SMHAs funded local governments (city, county, or multi-county) mental health authorities, which in turn operated and contracted for community mental

health services. This method was used in 20 states and is the primary method used in 17 states; and,

3. SMHAs provided direct care using state employees in state-operated community mental health centers. This method was used in 12 states and is the primary method used in 7 states.

In several states, combinations of these mechanisms are used, with the SMHA operating a few mental health clinics and funding counties or private-not-for profit mental health providers for most community mental health services. Large-population states tend to use local governments to organize the delivery of community mental health services (56% of the U.S. population lives in 17 states that primarily use county/city governments to organize and deliver community mental health services), while smaller states often directly operate the community system with their own employees.

In addition to SMHAs funding community mental health systems through these three methods, in many states Medicaid funds are being delivered by a managed care contract that may follow the SMHA's method of working with local governments or private not-for-profits. However, in other states a Medicaid managed care waiver may be funding an additional network of community mental health providers. The use of managed care for mental health services in states is discussed in more detail below.

In the 17 states that report using county or city governments to provide mental health services, most (14) reported that counties or cities are used across the entire state, and 3 states (Arkansas, Georgia, and Kansas) reported that funds are used in parts of the state. In 16 states, some counties have merged together to form multi-county mental health authorities. Most large population states use county and city governments to coordinate the delivery of community mental health services as a way of ensuring a match of mental health services to local needs.

In 13 states, local governments contribute their own tax dollars to pay for community mental health services. In eight of these states, the local government

Table 13.3 Primary Methods Used by SMHAs to Fund Community Mental Health Services: 2007

Primary Mechanism used by SMHAs to Fund Community Mental Health	Number of States	Average State Population (using Method)	Percent of U.S. Population
SMHA Directly Contracts with Local Providers	27 SMHAs	4,133,742	37%
SMHA Funds Local Government (County/ City) MH Authorities	17 SMHAs	9,802,368	56%
SMHA Operates Community Providers with State Employees	7 SMHAs	3,021,025	7%

Source: NRI State Profiles: 2007.

contributions are required by the SMHA as a match for state funds. Ten states report that local counties/cities collect dedicated taxes for mental health services.

Community-Based Mental Health Services

In 82% of the SMHAs (37 of 45 states), the SMHA requires state-funded mental health service providers to offer a mandated set of mental health services. As shown on Table 13.4, case management and emergency services were the most commonly provided community-based services, which were offered by every reporting state for adult consumers.

For children and adolescents, case management, school-based services, outpatient services, and emergency services were the most frequently provided services. Specialized services such as in-home family services and family preservation/family psychoeducational services were also common.

For persons who enter the SMHA system through the criminal justice system (forensics), the most commonly offered services were services to courts, case

Table 13.4 Community-Based Serviced Targeted toward Specific Population Groups

Community-Based Services	Children/ Adolescent	Adults	Elderly	MI Forensic	MI Homeless
Case Management	41	44	34	27	36
Emergency	39	44	36	24	33
Dual DX: MI/SA	32	42	23	19	26
PsychoSocial Rehab	19	42	22	15	23
Outpatient	40	41	35	25	32
Housing	9	40	22	17	35
Acute Care Inpatient	32	38	26	20	20
Supportive Employment	6	38	9	12	18
Consumer Run Services	7	38	12	0	15
PACT/ACT	7	38	17	15	21
Employment/Voc Rehab	12	36	11	14	21
Residential	30	34	19	15	20
MI Deaf & Hearing Impaired Services	24	32	20	10	10
Intensive Case Management	28	31	22	18	25
Dual DX: MI/DD	25	27	15	12	10
Services to Courts	23	27	14	29	17
Extended Care Inpatient	20	24	20	18	14
Partial Day	23	24	15	8	12
Social Clubs	3	19	9	5	10
Family Preservation/Family PsychoEd	35	17	8	3	3
In-Home Family Services	40	13	10	2	2
School Based Services	42	4	2	0	1
Other Services	6	4	0	0	0

Source: NRI State Profiles: 2007.

management, and outpatient services. For persons who are homeless and have a mental illness, many states target specific services to meet their needs and engage them into services. The most common services were case management, housing, and emergency services.

CONSUMER OPERATED SERVICES

As Table 13.4 indicates, many SMHAs are using consumer-operated mental health services as part of their continuum of state-supported mental health services. SMHAs support these consumer-operated services in a variety of ways: providing direct funding (42 states), technical assistance (37 states), conference sponsorships (37 states), and providing office space (15) for consumer programs.

Twenty-nine SMHAs reported they provided a total of $62,003,065 for consumer-operated services. The median state spending for such services was $360,514, ranging from a high of $23,000,000 in Michigan to a low of $5,000 in South Dakota. SMHAs reported funding a total of 327 consumer-operated programs within 32 states, with a median of five consumer-operated programs per state, and a range from a high of 50 programs in Michigan to a low of one program in six states.

As Table 13.5 shows, SMHAs fund a variety of consumer-operated program activities. The most commonly funded activities are Peer/Mutual Support, Advocacy, Leadership Training, Drop-in Centers, and Promoting Positive Public Attitudes.

In some states, Medicaid funds are used to reimburse Peer Specialists who provide services to other mental health consumers. Georgia was one of the first

Table 13.5 Types of Consumer-Operated Services Funded by the SMHA

Services	Number of States
Peer/Mutual Support	46
Advocacy	40
Leadership skills training	35
Drop in centers	32
Promoting Positive public attitudes	32
Wellness/prevention services	28
Technical Assistance	23
Policy Development	22
Social Services (e.g., independent living skills, training, job development)	17
Vocational Rehabilitation/ employment	16
Client-staffed businesses	13
Research Activities	10
Non-Residential Crisis Interventions	8
Transitional/ Supported Housing	8
Case Management	7
Residential Crisis facility	4
Other	7

Source: NRI State Profiles: 2007.

states to train and certify mental health consumers as peer specialists, and the model has been viewed as successful in many states. There were 21 states that reported they reimburse adult consumer peer specialists through Medicaid. Two additional states (District of Columbia and Michigan) now also reimburse adolescent consumer peer specialists through Medicaid.

MANAGED CARE PRACTICES

In order to control the growth of mental health care costs, a number of states have elected to use a variety of managed care practices to deliver services paid for by Medicaid and state funds. The managed care practices of the SMHA include contracting with managed care organizations (MCOs), administrative service organizations (ASOs), and health maintenance organizations (HMOs).

- MCO: A managed care organization is an organization that contracts to manage a defined set of health benefits. For mental health, a set of behavioral health managed care organizations (usually either private for-profit or not-for-profit companies) are contracted to cover the mental health needs of a (carved out) group of consumers. MCOs are usually funded using capitation rates (per-member-per-month) and seek to control utilization to manage mental health costs.
- ASO: An administrative service organization is a contractual arrangement under which an independent organization (often an insurance company or MCO) handles the administration of claims, benefits, and other functions for a Medicaid Agency or SMHA. While an ASO manages risk, it usually does not assume any medical risk of its own.
- HMO: Health maintenance organizations: The Centers for Medicare and Medicaid Services (CMS) defines a health maintenance organization for Medicare as "a type of Medicare managed care plan where a group of doctors, hospitals, and other health care providers agree to give health care to Medicare beneficiaries for a set amount of money from Medicare every month" (U.S. Department of Health and Human Services, 2009, ¶2).

As noted in Table 13.6 below, most states (33) use a managed care practice to provide mental health services (27 states also used managed care to provide substance abuse services). Overall, in 2007, SMHAs provided managed behavioral health services to 2.2 million individuals, or 10% of the 22.3 million individuals covered by managed behavioral health plans.

Of the 33 states that are using managed care for mental health services, 18 have a Medicaid 1915(b) Waiver, ten states have a Medicaid Research and Demonstration (1115) Waiver, and five states have a Medicaid Home and Community-Based Waiver. Medicaid 1915(b) Waivers allow states to provide a continuum of services to disabled and elderly populations, such as nontraditional home and community-based services. Medicaid 1115 Waivers allow states to undertake new experimental and demonstration projects to test their efficacy. These projects often provide innovative services or services that are not otherwise covered. Medicaid Home

Table 13.6 Services Provided via Managed Care Plans

Services Provided Under Managed Care Plans	Number of States
Assessment and diagnosis	32
Outpatient therapy	30
Emergency/Crisis	28
Treatment planning	28
Acute hospitalization	27
Day treatment/partial hospitalization	25
Psychosocial rehabilitation	23
Intensive in-home services	23
Prescription drugs for mental health	20
Services in residential treatment centers	19
Wrap-around services (e.g. intensive case management, supported employment, respite services, etc)	16
Crisis residential services	15
Peer support	14
Long-term hospitalization	11
Consumer-run services	7

Source: NRI State Profiles: 2007.

and Community-Based Waivers allow states to offer traditional medical services and non-medical services. These services are sometimes provided by unpaid family members.

Most states (28) carve mental health benefits out of the basic benefit plan to specialty behavioral health care networks or managed behavioral health organizations. Some states (11) carve in mental health benefits with general health benefits provided by primary health care providers or HMOs.

EVIDENCE-BASED PRACTICES (EBPs)

> State-of-the-art treatments, carefully refined through years of research, are not being translated into community settings. . . . A gap persists in the broad introduction and application of these advances in service delivery to local communities, and many people with mental illness are being denied the most up-to-date and advanced forms of treatment (USDHHS, 1999, p. 455).

For a number of years, SMHAs have focused on improving the quality of the mental health services they provide to reflect the latest scientific research on effective services. However, for many years, the difficulty of moving the most effective treatments from clinical research studies into common practice has been recognized as a major issue in both general medicine and in public mental health services. To help public mental health systems address the difficulties of implementing EBPs, the SAMHSA's Center for Mental Health Services supported the development of six toolkits to help states, providers, clinicians, consumers, and families implement and use EBP services for adults with serious mental illnesses. Since the original six toolkits were published by CMHS, work on additional toolkits for supported housing, consumer-operated services, and a variety of child, adolescent, and older adult EBPs have been supported by CMHS.

SMHAs have responded to federal leadership on EBPs by focusing their attention on increasing the number and level of EBPs being provided. In 2007, every reporting state was implementing at least one of the CMHS toolkit EBPs, and most states were implementing multiple EBPs. Among EBPs designed for adults with serious mental illnesses, the most frequently implemented EBPs were Assertive Community Treatment (being implemented in 45 states), Integrated Mental Health and Substance Abuse Services (45 states), and Supported Employment (42 states).

As Table 13.7 shows, not all of these EBPs are being implemented statewide, but many of them are being implemented in regions within a state. For example, Assertive Community Treatment (ACT) teams may be offered only in the large urban areas of a state instead of statewide. In addition to the EBPs being implemented in parts of a state, there are several EBPs that are being piloted by SMHAs in selected settings. There are a number of EBPs that are not yet implemented by SMHAs, but for which SMHAs have announced plans to implement. For example, family psychoeducation programs were in the planning stage in 10 states during 2007.

As Table 13.8 reveals, among EBPs designed for children with mental illnesses, therapeutic foster care (35 states), multi-systemic therapy (31 states), and school-based interventions (30 states) constitute the most frequently implemented EBPs. Therapeutic foster care is the EBP with the most frequent statewide implementation (17 states), while school-based interventions and MST are most often not available statewide, but instead are offered in regions of a state.

Table 13.7 Implementation Status of Adult EBPs

Adult EBP	Implementing Statewide	Implementing Parts of State	Piloting	Planning to Implement	Total Implementing (Statewide or Part)
Assertive Community Treatment (ACT)	11	34	0	1	45
Integrated MH/SA	14	29	2	4	45
Supported Employment	20	24	1	1	45
Supported Housing	22	20	0	3	42
Consumer Operated Services	12	23	2	4	37
Illness Self-Management	7	22	2	6	31
Family Psycho-Education	6	20	0	9	26
Medication Algorithms (schizophrenia)	6	14	5	4	25
Medication Algorithms (bipolar)	4	8	1	5	13
Other Adult EBPs	3	13	1	2	17

Source: NRI State Profiles: 2007.

Table 13.8 Implementation of Children's EBPs: 2007

Children's EBPs	Implementing Statewide	Implementing Parts of State	Piloting	Planning to Implement	Total Implementing (Statewide or Part)
Therapeutic Foster Care	17	18	0	3	35
School-Based Interventions	5	24	1	1	30
MST (Conduct Disorders)	1	22	8	1	31
Functional Family Therapy	3	19	3	3	25
Other Child EBPs	4	8	0	5	12

Source: NRI State Profiles, 2007.

FINANCING SMHA SERVICES

In state FY2005, the 50 states and the District of Columbia collectively expended over $29.4 billion to provide mental health services. States averaged mental health expenditures of $100 per every resident in their state, and SMHA expenditures for mental health averaged almost 2% of total state government expenditures. As may be explained by the vast differences in how SMHAs are organized and structured, the array of mental health services they offer, and their priority treatment populations, there is considerable variation in the level of expenditures among the states. State mental health expenditures ranged from less than $60 per state resident, to over $200 per resident in several states. In FY2005 SMHAs reported that they provided mental health services to almost 6 million persons (USDHHS, 2008). The average expenditure per mental health service recipient was $4,738 and the median was $4,074 per client served (see Chapter 2 in this volume for more information on financing mental health and substance abuse services).

SHIFT FROM STATE PSYCHIATRIC HOSPITAL-BASED TO COMMUNITY-BASED MENTAL HEALTH

As described in Figure 13.2, over the last quarter-century, SMHAs have shifted their treatment paradigm to focus on providing comprehensive mental health services in the community. As a result, community mental health expenditures have grown much faster than state psychiatric hospital expenditures. In FY2005, community–mental health expenditures accounted for 70% of total SMHA-controlled expenditures, and state psychiatric hospital-inpatient expenditures accounted for 27%. This is a major shift from FY1981, when community–mental health expenditures accounted for 33% of SMHA expenditures and state psychiatric hospitals accounted for 63% of expenditures.

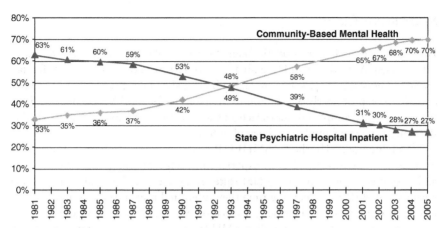

Figure 13.2 State Mental Health Agency Controlled Expenditures for State Psychiatric Hospital Inpatient and Community-Based Services as a Percentage of Total Expenditures FY1981 to FY2005. (*Source:* NRI FY2005 SMHA-Controlled Revenues and Expenditures Study.)

Overall, in FY2005, 63% (or approximately $18.8 billion) of SMHA funding came from state government sources. In addition, 31% (or approximately $9 billion) came from federal government sources (mostly Medicaid funds); 1% (or approximately $300 million) came from local government funds; and 5% (or approximately $1.3 billion) came from third-party funds and charitable contributions. Total Medicaid funds (state match and federal share) received by SMHA-funded programs represented $12.5 billion (42%) of SMHA resources.

Most of the new funds available for SMHA funded services have come from Medicaid. From FY2001 to FY2005, 62% of new SMHA funds were from Medicaid, while the other 30% came from state general revenues. Over the longer time period from FY1981 to FY2005, half (50%) of all new SMHA funds came from Medicaid, while state general funds represented the other 40%.

Moreover, most of the new Medicaid revenues for mental health have funded community mental health services. From FY1981 to FY2005, Medicaid funds for community mental health grew an average of 25% per year, which paid for $10 billion of the total SMHA-controlled community–mental health spending for the period.

Policy Issues Facing SMHAs

SMHAs are addressing a number of policy initiatives that will likely drive activities for the next several years. These policy initiatives include:

- Coping with the state fiscal crises;
- Health/mental health integration;
- Role of mental health in health care reform;
- Returning veterans from active duty;
- Promoting the use of EBPs; and
- Medicaid and other state government collaborations.

STATE FISCAL CRISIS

During the second half of 2008, the budget situation of many states began to drastically worsen. According to a December 2008 report from the National Conference
on State Legislatures, 41 states are facing budget shortfalls in 2009. States closed a
cumulative gap of nearly $40 billion in preparation for the FY2009 budget. Since
that budget was completed, states face an additional gap of $30 billion. One-half of
the states project a cumulative shortfall of $63.7 billion for 2010.

A study compiled by the NASMHPD Research Institute (Roberts & Lutterman,
2008) found that most SMHAs are experiencing budget cuts in the current (FY2009)
and next fiscal years. Forty-two (42) states responded to this study. Many states
have indicated that between the time they submitted their responses and the time
this study went to press, their budget situation has significantly deteriorated.

Thirty-two of the 42 responding SMHAs reported that their states are experiencing budget shortfalls in both the current fiscal year (FY2009) and next fiscal year
(FY2010). Thirteen of the 42 states are already expecting budget shortfalls in
FY2011. Of those 32 states receiving budget cuts, FY2009 reductions are averaging
4.9% with a median cut of 4.0%. Cuts range from a low of 0% (no cuts) to a high of
17.5%.

Of the 32 states expecting budget cuts in FY2010, the anticipated cuts average
8.2% with a median of 7.5%. Anticipated cuts range from a low of 1% to a high of
25%. Of the 13 SMHAs anticipating cuts in FY2011, anticipated cuts average 9.4%
with a median of 10%. The cuts range from a low of 3% to a high of 25%.

SMHAs were asked what strategies they are using to make required budget
cuts. As Figure 13.3 indicates, the most common approaches include freezing staff
hires; reducing administrative expenses; reducing services; reducing staff; reducing
the number of people served; and closing state psychiatric hospitals and wards.

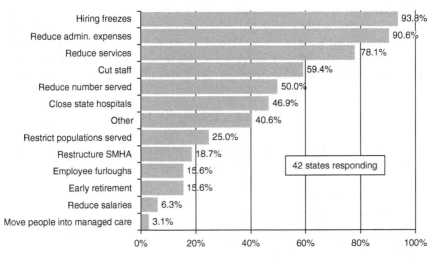

Figure 13.3   Responses to Cuts in Overall SMHA Budget.

Integration of Health/Mental Health

SMHAs have recently begun a major new focus on addressing the physical health needs of persons with mental illness, with a variety of efforts to look at the premature mortality of mental health consumers, excess rates of diabetes and obesity, and excessive smoking, all of which are major health concerns of mental health consumers. The NRI and NASMHPD Medical Directors developed a series of special reports that documented that consumers served by SMHA systems have up to 25 years of premature life lost (Lutterman et al., 2003; Colton & Manderscheid, 2006; Mauer, 2006). These findings of premature mortality among mental health consumers have led SMHAs to launch studies to determine the causes of premature mortality and to develop a set of recommendations for new physical health screening initiatives for new patients entering mental health systems, for increased collaborations with Community Health Centers and primary care physicians, and for smoking cessation initiatives (Mauer, 2008) (see Chapter 16 in this volume for further information on integration of primary care and specialty mental health services).

Mental Health within Health Care Reform

SMHAs, along with other mental health advocates, strongly supported the passage, in October 2008, of the landmark federal mental health Parity Law as part of the new economic stimulus package. The passage of mental health parity promises to improve access to mental health services for persons with health insurance. However, most persons who receive SMHA mental health services do not have private health insurance coverage.

President Obama's campaign promise for passage of national health care reform that includes mental health as a fundamental part of health care raises an opportunity to provide coverage for the majority of persons who are served by SMHAs: persons without health insurance or persons whose only coverage is Medicaid. Over the next few years, SMHAs are expected to be actively involved in ensuring that the needs of persons with serious mental illnesses and serious emotional disturbances become visible components of the national health care reform.

Mental Health Needs of Returning Veterans

Most SMHAs reported working with their state National Guard Units and Reserves, as well as with the U.S. Department of Veterans Affairs and Department of Defense to ensure that the mental health needs of veterans and their families are being met. With over 1.67 million veterans having served in Iraq and Afghanistan, the number of persons returning with PTSD, depression, anxiety, and brain injuries will require coordination among many providers and training for SMHA systems in evidence-based practices to meet these needs.

EVIDENCE-BASED PRACTICES

As discussed above, all SMHAs are working to increase the number of EBPs that are provided. However, there are a number of barriers to expanding the availability of EBPs, including new restrictions in Medicaid, lack of adequate training for practitioners, and the need to adapt EBP models to treat minorities and those in rural areas. In addition, new services that may become EBPs that address recovery and health-physical health services are being tested, but will need to be rolled out by SMHAs.

MEDICAID AND OTHER STATE GOVERNMENT COLLABORATIONS

As this chapter has emphasized, SMHAs are now only one part of the state government system that provides mental health services. The state Medicaid Agency, through its use of Medicaid options and managed care waivers, has had a major impact on the SMHA's system of care. Even other state agencies whose primary mission is not directly related to health service delivery, such as the state Corrections agencies, are now providing mental health services to prisoners and parolees. A number of SMHAs are now working to coordinate sharing health care information with Corrections or using SMHA staff to provide mental health treatment in prisons and jails.

The current budget shortages facing all states will make the cooperation and coordination among state government agencies that are providing mental health services and supports even more important as each agency's budget is reduced. States will have to make sure that all funds are used most efficiently.

Implications for Mental Health

Continuing trends begun in recent years, SMHAs in 2009 are very different agencies than they were even a few years ago (Mazade & Glover, 2006; Hogan, 2008b). Most states are now operating much smaller and shrinking state psychiatric hospitals that are increasingly limited to forensic status clients. As a result, SMHAs are working to develop and coordinate comprehensive community mental health systems that are recovery focused and provide evidence-based services while becoming a smaller and smaller portion of the funding source for these systems.

SMHAs are likely to move toward becoming a mental health advocate and expert within state government where the SMHA reaches out to work with sister agencies such as Medicaid, corrections, education, housing, Veterans Affairs, and others to ensure quality services.

SMHAs today are being asked to assume responsibilities that were not part of their role years ago, including addressing the housing, employment, and physical health needs of mental health consumers and providing suicide prevention and mental health early intervention services. In addition, SMHAs are now being asked to help keep persons with mental illnesses out of jails and prisons by funding criminal justice diversion programs, using outpatient commitment statutes, and operating services for sex offenders.

A major challenge for SMHAs will be determining what approaches, organizational structures, and functions they should embrace as they become less of a direct mental health service provider and instead become mental health planning, monitoring, and advocacy organizations in the future.

References

Atay, J., Crider, R., Foley, D. (2007). *Additions and Resident Patients at End of Year, State and County Hospitals, by Age and Diagnosis, by State, United States 2005.* Rockville, MD: Center for Mental Health Services.

Colton, C. W., & Manderscheid, R. W. (2006). Congruencies in increased mortality rates, years of potential life lost, and causes of death among public mental health clients in eight states. *Preventing Chronic Disease, 3*(2), A42. Available online at http://www.cdc.gov/pcd/issues/2006/apr/05_0180.htm. Accessed August 8, 2009.

Deutsch, A. (1948). *The Shame of the States.* New York: Harcourt Brace.

Dixon v. Barry, 967 F. Supp. 535 D.D.C. (1997).

Frank, R. G., & Glied, S. A. (2006). *Better But Not Well: Mental Health Policy in the United States since 1950.* Baltimore: Johns Hopkins University Press.

Grob, G. N. (2008). *Mental Institutions in America: Social Policy to 1875.* New Brunswick, NJ: Transaction Publishers.

Hepburn, B. M., & Sederer, L. I. (2009). The state hospital. In S. S. Sharfstein, F. B. Dickerson, & J. Oldham (Eds.), *Textbook of Hospital Psychiatry* (pp. 197–210). Washington, DC: American Psychiatric Publishing.

Hogan, M. (2008a). *2008–2009 Executive Budget Recommendations Highlights Testimony, January 29, 2008.* Available online at http://www.omh.state.ny.us/omhweb/budget/2008%2D2009/testimony.html. Accessed August 6, 2009.

Hogan, M. (2008b). Transforming mental health care: Realities, priorities, and prospects. *Psychiatric Clinics of North America, 31*(1), 1–9.

Lamb, H. R. (1998). Community psychiatry and prevention. In J. A. Talbott, R. E. Hales, & S. C. Yudofsky (Eds.), *The American Psychiatric Press Textbook of Psychiatry* (pp 1141–1160). Washington, DC: American Psychiatric Press.

Lutterman, T., Ganju, V., Schacht, L., Shaw, R., Monihan, K., & Huddle, M. (2003). *Sixteen State Study on Mental Health Performance Measures.* DHHS Publication No. (SMA) 03-3835. Rockville, MD: Center for Mental Health Services, Substance Abuse and Mental Health Services Administration.

Lutterman, T., & Gonzalez, O. (2006). The CMHS Uniform Reporting System. In Center for Mental Health Services (with R. W. Manderscheid & J. T. Berry [Eds.]), *Mental Health, United States, 2004.* DHHS Pub No (SMA)-06-4195. Rockville, MD: Substance Abuse and Mental Health Services Administration.

Lutterman, T., Mayberg, M., & Emmet, W. (2006). State mental health agency implementation of the New Freedom Commission on Mental Health Goals: 2004. In Center for Mental Health Services (with R. W. Manderscheid & J. T. Berry [Eds.]), *Mental Health, United States, 2004.* DHHS Pub No (SMA)-06-4195. Rockville, MD: Substance Abuse and Mental Health Services Administration.

Mark, T. L., Levit, K. R., Coffey, R. M., McKusick, D. R., Harwood, H. J., King, E. C., et al. (2007). *National Estimates of Expenditures for Mental Health Services and Substance Abuse Treatment, 1993–2003.* Rockville, MD: Substance Abuse and Mental Health Services Administration.

Mauer, B. (2006, October) *Morbidity and Mortality in People with Serious Mental Illness.* Alexandria, VA: National Association of State Mental Health Program Directors, Medical Directors Council.

Mauer, B. (2008, October) *Measurement of Health Status for People with Serious Mental Illnesses.* Alexandria, VA: National Association of State Mental Health Program Directors, Medical Directors Council.

Mazade, N. A., & Glover, R. (2006). Critical priorities confronting state mental health agencies. *Psychiatric Services, 58*(9), 1148–1150.

National Association of State Mental Health Program Directors Research Institute (NRI). (2007). *The FY 2005 State Mental Health Revenue and Expenditure Study Results.* Available online at www.nri-inc.org/projects/profiles/revenuesexpenditures.cfm

National Association of State Mental Health Program Directors Research Institute. (2008). *2007 State Mental Health Agency Profiling System Results.* Available online at http://www.nri-inc.org/projects/Profiles/data_search.cfm. Accessed August 6, 2009.

National Association of State Mental Health Program Directors State MH Agency Commissioner Tenure Files. (2008). [Internal NASMHPD membership records]. Unpublished raw data.

National Conference on State Legislatures. (2008). *State Budget Update: November 2008.* Available online at http://www.ncsl.org/default.aspx?tabid=12574. Accessed August 5, 2009.

New Freedom Commission on Mental Health. (2003). *Achieving the Promise: Transforming Mental Health Care in America; Final Report.* DHHS Pub. No. SMA-03-3832. Rockville, MD: Author.

O'Connor v. Donaldson, 422 U.S. 563 (1975).

Roberts, K., & Lutterman, T. (2008). *SMHA Budget Shortfalls.* Alexandria, VA: National Association of State Mental Health Program Directors Research Institute. Available online at http://www.nri-inc.org/reports_pubs/2009/BudgetShortfalls.pdf. Accessed August 5, 2009.

Souder et al. v. Brennan et al., 367 F. Supp. 80 DC (1973).

Stinger, K. (2008). *Overview of Mental Health in New York and the Nation.* Kathi's Mental Health Review. Available online at http://www.toddlertime.com/interest/ny-history.htm. Accessed August 5, 2009.

U.S. Department of Health and Human Services (USDHHS). (1980). *Toward a National Plan for the Chronically Mentally Ill: Report to the Secretary.* Washington, DC: Author.

U.S. Department of Health and Human Services. (1999). *Mental Health: A Report of the Surgeon General.* Rockville, MD: U.S. Department of Health and Human Services, Substance Abuse and Mental Health Services Administration, Center for Mental Health Services, National Institutes of Health, National Institute of Mental Health.

U.S. Department of Health and Human Services. (2008). *Center for Mental Health Services Uniform Reporting System (URS) 2007.* Available online at http://mentalhealth.samhsa.gov/cmhs/MentalHealthStatistics/UniformReport.asp. Accessed August 5, 2009.

U.S. Department of Health and Human Services. (2009). *Online Glossary* [Electronic version]. Bethesda, MD: Author. Available online at http://www.cms.hhs.gov/apps/glossary/search.asp?Term=HMO&Language=English&SubmitTermSrch=Search#Terms. Accessed March 14, 2009.

Virginia Department of Mental Health, Mental Retardation, and Substance Abuse Services. (n.d.). *History of Eastern State Hospital.* Available online at http://www.esh.dmhmrsas.virginia.gov/history.html. Accessed August 5, 2009.

Wyatt v. Stickney, 503 F. 2d 1305 5th Cir. (1974).

Chapter 14

COMMUNITY MENTAL
HEALTH CENTERS

Thomas W. Doub, PhD; Dennis P. Morrison, PhD; and Jan Goodson, BS

THIS CHAPTER reviews the community mental health system in the United States, specifically some of the key issues facing the field and how it has evolved over the decades since President John F. Kennedy signed the Community Mental Health Centers Construction Act in 1963. The array of services offered in community mental health settings today is varied and diverse, not unlike the needs of consumers who receive community-based care. In recent years, traditional models of mental health care have been criticized as unresponsive to consumer and family needs, and often lacking research evidence of effectiveness. There has been a strong call, not just for incremental change, but for *transformation*, so that consumers and their families can easily access services that are culturally appropriate, evidence-based, and tailored to their individual recovery needs and preferences. In the coming years, community mental health is facing a number of challenges and opportunities: there is a need to work more effectively with other public systems, such as primary care and criminal justice; the mental health workforce is aging; and financing is extraordinarily complex. Despite these challenges, there are great new opportunities to make dramatic improvements to services by involving consumers and families more directly in their care and by shortening the gap between research and practice through broad systems change and improved support from information technology.

Overview

Community mental health care has changed dramatically since the origins of the community mental health movement in the 1940s and 1950s. Collective understanding of the brain, genetics, and the impact of the environment on psycho-pathology has made dramatic contributions to the development of new psychoso-cial and pharmacological approaches to care. The advent of antidepressant and antipsychotic medications more than 50 years ago had a tremendous impact on the ability of consumers to move from institutions to the community. Significant phar-macological breakthroughs since those initial medications have continued to improve symptom management, reduce side-effects, and support improved func-tioning in the community. While much of the research has been focused on under-standing the biological origins of mental illness, the community mental health movement has shifted from symptom control in the 1960s and 1970s, to rehabilita-tion in the 1980s, and to self-determination and recovery in the 1990s and beyond (Drake, Green, Mueser, & Goldman, 2003).

Perhaps the most important influence within the community mental health environment today is the concept of recovery—that people with mental illness can get well and pursue their individual goals (also see Chapter 20 in this volume on the recovery movement). Recovery does not have the same meaning for everyone, but instead holds unique meaning for each individual. Recurring themes often arise when people describe what recovery means to them, including hope, personal responsibility, education, self-advocacy, support, and self-determination (Copeland, 2004; Liberman & Kopelowicz, 2002). Recovery values represent a significant departure from previous attitudes about mental illness that have been common across a mental health system that has historically been oriented more toward relief from debilitating symptoms than pursuit of individual goals such as employment, better social relationships, and/or living independently. Realization of recovery-based services means achievement of a true partnership between service providers, consumers, and families, where decisions regarding treatment are fully informed and made in a shared fashion (Center for Substance Abuse Treatment [CSAT], 2007).

A significant barrier to achieving recovery is the length of time it takes for research-based treatments to move from the laboratory into the community, known as the "Science to Service Gap." The Institute of Medicine's *Crossing the Quality Chasm* report (2001) estimated that it takes an average of 15–20 years for research findings to make their way into common practice. For example, Aaron T. Beck published the book *Cognitive Therapy of Depression* in 1979, and while it is firmly established as an effective treatment for a range of psychological disorders (Butler, Chapman, Forman, & Beck, 2006), it is rarely practiced with fidelity in community mental health settings. In fact, in a review of studies assessing quality of care for serious conditions such as depression, anxiety, bipolar disorder, and schizophrenia, Bauer (2002) found that only 27% of these studies found provider compliance with evidence-based treatment guidelines. Treatment for alcohol dependence was even worse, with only 10.5% of individuals receiving evidence-based care (McGlynn et al., 2003).

Over the last 10 years, these quality problems have received significant atten-tion from policymakers, researchers, government officials, and care providers, and new strategies are being developed to help deliver treatments that are evidence-based and practical in community settings. Perhaps the most significant advance is the development of evidence-based treatment manuals, or toolkits, that are intended to help policymakers, managers, and clinicians adopt new and effective practices. In addition to the use of treatment manuals, a comprehensive strategy to minimize the science-to-service gap will include improved technology and diagnostic tools, use of outcome data from consumers, improved dissemination strategies, expansion of the national quality improvement and reporting infrastructure, and stronger quality improvement methods at the point of care, such as those promoted by the Institute for Healthcare Improvement and the Network for the Improvement of Addiction Treatment (NIATx) (Institute of Medicine [IOM], 2006).

Historical Perspective

The origins of the community mental health movement began in earnest following World War II, as troops returned home with "shell shock" from the war, new advances in medication began to reduce hospital stays, and growing opposition to institutionalization precipitated the need for a broad network of community-based mental health services. Mental institutions were viewed as inhumane, and advocates called for their elimination. In 1961, the Joint Commission on Mental Health and Illness published *Action for Mental Health*, recommending the development of an extensive network of community clinics and other treatment services, new research, greater public education, and improved identification and treatment for mental illness. This report articulated a revolutionary vision for treating mental illness in the community, culminating in the Community Mental Health Centers Construction Act passed by Congress and signed by President John F. Kennedy in 1963.

With growing de-institutionalization, community mental health centers (CMHCs) adopted a treatment paradigm that integrated public health philosophies of prevention and acute treatment with a more comprehensive approach promoting continuity of care in the community (Foley & Sharfstein, 1983). In the 1960s, many CMHCs received federal grant funding to serve new consumers, which did little to meet the needs of those people discharged from hospitals with chronic care needs. State hospital systems often perceived CMHCs as direct competitors, which hampered cooperation and collaboration. At the same time, many staff in CMHCs were more interested in delivering insight-oriented psychotherapy than in the rehabilitation of people with serious mental illness (Cutler, Bevilacqua, & McFarland, 2003). The CMHC system was subsequently criticized for its failure to meet the needs of people with chronic mental health conditions (Goldman & Morrissey, 1985).

Following rapid de-institutionalization, it became apparent in the 1970s that the network of community supports was inadequate to meet the needs of people with mental illness. In particular, supports for housing and income were very limited, resulting in rampant homelessness, poverty, and criminalization (Goldman & Morrissey, 1985). Awareness of these problems led to a President's Commission for Mental Health (1978), which concluded that many people across the country, particularly racial and ethnic minorities, women, veterans, people with physical disabilities, the poor, and children were not well served by the CMHC system. People had been discharged from institutional care without adequate housing, without sufficient food or clothing, and without medical care (Cutler et al., 2003).

The Commission's work led to the Mental Health Systems Act of 1980, which emphasized the expansion of services to vulnerable populations, gave more control and responsibility to states, and improved linkages to other health care services. This Act had no budgetary appropriation, however, and was never implemented by the Reagan administration.

With federal budget cuts to CMHC grant funding in the early 1980s, states and CMHCs began to access fee-for-service funds available through Medicaid, which provided federal matching dollars to help support service provision. As states and CMHCs figured out how to effectively leverage these funds, Medicaid costs grew rapidly, fueling fiscal concerns and prompting new strategies for cost containment using various managed care models in the 1990s (Mark et al., 2000).

Managed care is a health insurance model intended to reduce unnecessary costs by providing close oversight of services and ensuring that services are provided within strict limits and only as medically necessary (Sabin, 2000). Managed care has been a controversial issue. Advocates claim that such oversight is beneficial to minimize fraud and abuse, ensure quality, and promote continuity of care. Meanwhile, critics have contended that for-profit managed care companies have little long-term investment in local communities and ultimately maximize short-term profits by de-professionalizing the field and damaging service infrastructure.

Types of Services

From the early days of the community mental health movement over a half century ago, to today's vast array of CMHC services, much of the severely mentally ill (SMI) population has transitioned from institutionalization into a variety of less restrictive settings where clinical services complement those found in inpatient facilities. This ever-evolving mental health services environment is now consistently pulling away from traditional, isolated services to emphasize community collaboration, evidence-based practices, consumer/family member choice and satisfaction, child/family-centered care, primary and mental health services integration, and research with interdisciplinary partnerships designed to achieve improved outcomes via multiple avenues. The comprehensive components of today's mental health services are moving mental illness and mental health from their history of stigma and prejudice into a twenty-first century where brain disorders are appropriately addressed as, and considered synonymous with, biological and treatable medical illnesses.

TRADITIONAL MENTAL HEALTH SERVICES

Traditional mental health services, which are effectively detailed by Drake et al. (2003), primarily encompass psychosocial, somatic, and pharmacological treatments that target illness control and rehabilitative interventions that are designed to improve functioning. In the 1950s, the treatment of choice was often psychoanalysis, which was grounded in theories suggesting that most forms of severe mental illness were induced by bad parental bonds (Fromm-Reichmann, 1949;

Bellak, 1958). Today, psychosocial therapies focus on relationship-building between consumers and care providers, such that the consumer trusts the clinician to assist with personal goal development and accomplishment (Herz & Marder, 2002; Hogarty, 2002), all of which target "maximizing self control of symptoms and minimizing interference from the illness" (Drake et al., 2003). These services can take diverse forms including cognitive behavioral, motivational enhancement, and behavioral marital therapies, as well as relapse prevention, psychoeducation, case management, and social skills training.

Pharmacologic Services

Pharmacological interventions have also greatly evolved over the years from primarily sedating patients in the early days to currently alleviating symptoms and improving functioning. Medications play a significant role in treatment, helping manage symptoms and improving outcomes for people diagnosed with a range of mental health and addictive disorders, including those with schizophrenia, bipolar disorder, depression, and/or anxiety disorders (Mellman et al., 2001). Such medications include antipsychotic, antidepressant, mood-stabilizing, and anti-anxiety drugs (see Chapter 21 in this volume for additional information on psychotropic medication use).

Rehabilitative Services

Rehabilitative services shift the focus from symptom reduction to developing individual skills and supports needed to enable individuals with mental illness to live and function as independently as possible. Such interventions address activities of daily living, housing, social functioning, family relationships, work, education, and leisure (Drake et al., 2003) by maintaining a focus on community integration, normalization, and inclusion, while engaging consumers in activities to build skills and supports.

Over the past two to three decades, research has supported the efficacy and sparked the expansion of specialty services rooted in the above-mentioned traditional elements of care and designed to increase accessibility, improve outcomes, and support a greater likelihood of recovery for the SMI population, as well as for children with serious emotional disturbance (SED). A few examples of such specialty services are outlined in the following paragraphs (also see Chapter 20 in this volume on recovery).

Examples of Specialty Mental Health Services

Integrated Primary and Mental Health Care

Historically, primary and mental health care providers have operated in isolation. While both fields serve overlapping populations, care has been offered separately, with limited interdisciplinary communication. However, many more people with mental disorders receive treatment in general medical settings than in mental health clinics (Wang et al., 2006), suggesting the need to integrate primary care with mental health services. Integrated care promotes early and appropriate diagnosis and treatment of diverse health problems and has been shown to reduce costly and harmful polypharmacy (National Association of State Mental Health Program Directors [NASMHPD], 2005), reduce hospitalizations (NASMHPD, 2005; IOM, 2006), and reduce stigma and transportation barriers (New Freedom Commission on Mental Health, 2003). In recent years, implementing integrated services has become a priority for many government agencies, community primary care practices, CMHCs, public policy organizations, and other stakeholders involved with improving the nation's health care systems.

Diverse integrated care models have formed across disciplines. However, typical services involve co-location of medical and mental health staff; onsite mental health service provision (e.g., therapy and medication management); patient consent to share information between providers; individual treatment plans addressing primary, mental health, and support service needs; interdisciplinary consultations; linkages with community services to improve or sustain health status; and ongoing open communication between care providers (see Chapter 16 in this volume on the integration of primary care with specialty mental health care).

Telemedicine

Telemedicine is the use of audio and video telecommunications equipment to deliver psychiatric care when the consumer and care provider are at different locations. This technology offers a clinically and cost-effective method for clinicians to provide treatment for individuals who have limited access to service sites and enables consumer-to-provider interaction that closely mirrors face-to-face contact. Telemedicine is especially beneficial in increasing service access for rural areas, where medical provider shortages exist and qualified practitioners can be more than 100 miles away (Pignatiello et al., 2008). In rural areas, CMHCs may offer services via satellite sites, where the main office and the bulk of providers are located in urban areas. Telemedicine equipment can also be placed in hospital emergency departments, health clinics, or private practice offices and offer emergency or scheduled access to CMHC or specialty care clinicians. Telemedicine is also used in both rural and urban jails and prisons, where individuals with severe mental illness are significantly over-represented (two to three times the rate compared to the general population; Lamb & Weinberger, 1998) and accessing care would otherwise involve transportation away from a secured facility or onsite delivery of services. Early efforts in this area were expensive and technologically challenging, often resulting in poor video quality. Today, these challenges have been nearly eliminated, but telemedicine is yet to attain "routine" status as a method of service delivery.

School-Based Mental Health Services

School-based mental health services typically address the mental health needs of children and youth (grades K-12) who are experiencing serious emotional and behavioral problems (see Chapter 17 in this volume on school mental health). Such issues can range from attention deficits to violent outbursts, and school-based services can be appropriately offered in mainstream as well as alternative educational environments. These services are delivered confidentially within school settings, often comprising counseling (individual, family, and group), and are designed to strengthen and empower youth and families to be self-sufficient.

Within such service settings, parents are treated as the experts regarding their child, and mental health professionals (MHP) provide supports and services that build upon family strengths, helping parents manage behavioral problems. In addition to counseling, MHPs may provide case management services to ensure that each individual child's needs are comprehensively addressed. They also often provide classroom observations, consultations, and trainings in order to assist school personnel in supporting continued achievement of individual student counseling goals, as well as to support widespread integration of behavior modification tools and techniques that promote mental health for the overall student body. School-based mental health services focus on decreasing behavioral incidents and problem severity, as well as improving behavioral functioning and enhancing personal growth, educational development, and emotional well-being for students.

PREVENTION SERVICES

The first and arguably most effective stage on the mental health intervention spectrum (see Figure 14.1), prevention services primarily focus on positively influencing individual choices and behavior in order to protect children's mental health. Universal, selective, and indicated interventions are used to accomplish the more

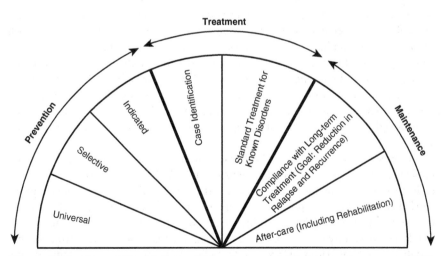

Figure 14.1 Mental Health Intervention Spectrum (Mrazek & Haggerty in IOM, 1994). (Mrazek, P.J., & Haggerty, R. J. *Reducing Risk for Mental Disorders: Frontiers for Preventive Intervention Research.* Committee on Prevention of Mental Disorders, Institute of Medicine. Copyright © 1994, National Academy of Sciences. Reprinted with permission from Rightslink.)

traditional public health approach of primary, secondary, and tertiary prevention, which respectively serve to reduce incidences of new cases of a disorder, rates of established cases of a disorder, and the amount of disability associated with a disorder (IOM, 1994). Universal interventions are population-focused and, in an educational setting, are offered to an entire school or school system. Selective interventions target groups of children who are perceived to be at high risk, and indicated interventions target intensive prevention services for specific children who are at especially high risk or may be displaying early warning signs of mental illness.

Some of the more successful prevention programs target serious problems such as suicide, substance use, sexually transmitted infections, and human immunodeficiency virus (HIV/AIDS) by focusing on reducing risk factors and increasing protective factors in order to strengthen resiliency in children and families. Prevention services may be offered in a variety of clinic and community settings; however, they are often provided in schools due to the ready accessibility of a primary target population: children and youth.

Systems of Care

"A system of care is a comprehensive spectrum of mental health and other necessary services which are organized into a coordinated network to meet the multiple and changing needs of children and adolescents with severe emotional disturbances and their families" (Stroul & Friedmen, 1986, p. iv). Systems of care began forming in the 1960s in order to address the needs of children with SED, and in the early twenty-first century, these systems continue to evolve. National estimates suggest approximately 9% to 13% of U.S. children have SED (Mark & Buck, 2006), and systems of care help envelop this population and their families with a comprehensive array of services to support individual recovery.

Systems of care comprise of partnerships between many child-serving public and private community agencies (see Figure 14.2). Associated efforts are the result of a collective agreement among these agencies acknowledging that children with SED and their families require child-centered, family-driven, multiple, coordinated, specialized treatments and services in order to be fully productive within the home, school, and community. These systems of care have been shown to be able to reduce hospitalization expenses, juvenile justice costs, child welfare placement costs, and special education costs while improving child and family functioning (Stambough et al., 2007; Grimes, Kapunan, & Mullin, 2006; Foster & Conner, 2005).

In recent years CMHCs and other community organizations have also begun implementing recovery-oriented systems of care (ROSC), which somewhat mirror child-focused systems but address the needs of adults with substance abuse problems. These ROSCs "support person-centered and self-directed approaches to care that build on the strengths and resilience of individuals, families, and communities to take responsibility for their sustained health, wellness, and recovery from alcohol and drug problems" (Kaplan, 2008, p. 6). In line with child-focused systems of care, ROSCs are culturally competent and consumer/family-focused. They involve diverse community collaborations and encircle individuals and their families with supports and services that help them achieve their highest possible level of recovery.

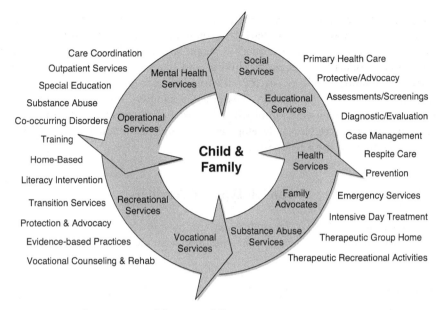

Figure 14.2   Components of Systems of Care.

Specialty Services and Stigma

A primary benefit of specialty services, like those described in the previous paragraphs, is that most combat stigma, a long-standing barrier to identification, treatment, and recovery for individuals with mental disorders. Many specialty services have developed a direct response to this barrier and are designed to consistently reduce and/or overcome the negative impact of stigma for individuals battling treatable disorders. Historically, mental health issues have been categorized as everything from demonic possession to character flaws that could be easily dispelled with a little willpower. Consequently, although a vast array of effective treatments are available, many individuals refuse to accept diagnosis and/or care provided in traditional clinic settings. Specialty services break down this barrier via multiple avenues, including:

- Offering services in nontraditional settings where individuals and their families are comfortable receiving care;
- Educating individuals, families, and communities about mental health disorders and treatments; and
- Providing training, consultation, and support for other health care and service providers (including physicians, teachers, and social service workers).

As mental health issues for individuals across the lifespan and socioeconomic continuum have been identified and continue to evolve and as the national human and fiscal costs associated with behavioral health disorders rise—approximately $193 billion in lost earnings each year (Kessler et al., 2008)—CMHCs have adapted to meet the changing demands. Partnerships at all community and government levels have formed to expand, evaluate, and improve care. These include collaborations between CMHCs, social service and government agencies, schools, criminal justice systems, the primary care community, and other service providers dedicated to meeting the diverse needs of people with mental illness and their families. Systems of care encompassing children and adults continue to be established across the country, as do research endeavors dedicated to improving associated implementation and sustainability measures. In addition, ongoing research and evaluation efforts, focused on improving all aspects of the mental health care continuum, are informing service development and implementation activities, as well as working to close the science-to-service gap.

Personnel/Types of Providers

Personnel found at CMHCs include many clinical staff responsible for direct service provision and administrative staff who provide all levels of support for operations. Positions often include:

- Executive Leadership (e.g., CEO or Executive Director, Chief Financial Officer);
- Senior Management (e.g., directors to manage clinical programs);
- Clinical Service Providers (i.e., psychiatrists, therapists, case managers, etc.); and
- Support Staff (e.g., receptionists, facilities managers, information systems specialists).

Clinical staff who provide direct services within CMHCs have a wide range of training and experience, from peer-support specialists with high school diplomas to psychologists and psychiatrists with many years of education and training. However, the majority of staff making up CMHC personnel fall between these two ends of the continuum. The bulk of services are provided via positions requiring bachelor's or master's degrees, often with licenses substantiating the knowledge and experience necessary to provide clinical services. More specialized care is often provided by psychologists or psychiatrists with advanced training in areas such as child, geriatric, and addiction services. In addition to educational credentials and professional licensure, staffing requirements for some positions can also include that the individual be in recovery or be the family member of someone in recovery. This can uniquely position them to understand the needs of consumers seeking mental health services, supporting treatment engagement and adherence.

As traditional treatments evolve and evidence-based practices become the standard of care, staff education, experience, and job requirements will also continue to be redefined. A few decades ago, staff would have been primarily or wholly clinic-based, delivering services in isolation. Today, CMHCs offer a comprehensive array of services delivered by multidisciplinary teams of professionals who work in concert to help consumers pursue their individual goals. While technology, research, funding streams, and the focus on recovery have changed staffing patterns, the following disciplines continue to represent the most common clinical service staffing areas (see Chapter 5 in this volume on the mental health workforce).

PSYCHIATRY

Psychiatrists, medical doctors who have completed psychiatric residency and often specialty training, number approximately 34,462 nationwide with 30% of psychiatrists working in mental health clinics (Ellis et al., 2007; Duffy et al., 2006). Specializing in diagnosing and treating mental illnesses, psychiatrists most often manage psychopharmacological and other therapies, conduct clinical and diagnostic evaluations, and provide leadership, supervision, and consultation to clinical treatment teams.

PSYCHOLOGY

In the early days of psychology, psychologists primarily worked in academic settings. However, over the decades, this profession has transitioned heavily into direct service, particularly following World War II and throughout the 1970s, when statutory recognition by state regulatory agencies supported the shift (DeLeon, Vanden Bos, & Kraut, 1984).

Of the nearly 85,000 psychologists in the United States, 51,354 are clinically trained (Duffy et al., 2006). Of those, 90% provide direct health services, with 38% operating in private practice and 6% providing care in outpatient clinic settings (Duffy et al., 2006). This includes doctoral level professionals who provide a variety of treatment services such as diagnosis of mental health and addictive disorders, psychotherapy, and psychological testing. A growing focus area for CMHC psychologists is also program management and evaluation, where psychologists oversee programs and evaluate the efficacy and efficiency of treatment services.

SOCIAL WORK

More than 99,559 clinically trained social workers make up one of the nation's largest segment of mental health service providers (Ellis et al., 2007). Over 200 accredited graduate and over 400 undergraduate programs continue to increase the availability of skilled bachelor's, master's, and doctoral level social workers, a workforce that grew by more than 21,000 between 1989 and 2004 (Duffy et al., 2006). Social workers offer a broad range of services with a core focus on meeting basic human needs. This often includes individual and group therapy addressing mental and addiction disorders, as well as case management, outreach, crisis intervention, social rehabilitation, and life- and social skills training.

COUNSELING

Counseling, as defined by the American Counseling Association and the National Board of Certified Counselors, is: "The application of mental health, psychological, or human development principles, through cognitive, affective, behavioral or systematic intervention strategies, that address wellness, personal growth, or career development, as well as pathology." Counselors generally acquire either a master's or doctoral degree and provide traditional therapies as well as consultation, outreach, and psychoeducation. Numbering more than 100,000, clinically trained counselors make up a significant and growing segment of the mental health workforce (Ellis et al., 2007). Of this total, 73.4% provide direct services, with 22.5% providing services in mental health clinics (Duffy et al., 2006).

PSYCHIATRIC NURSING

Approximately 80,000 Psychiatric Registered Nurses provide mental health services nationwide, and half of those are estimated to be practicing in community-based rather than hospital settings (Manderscheid & Henderson, 2006). In 2006, advanced practice registered nurses working in outpatient mental health and substance abuse clinics totaled nearly 6,000, a number projected to increase by 14% by 2016 (Bureau of Labor Statistics, 2006). Registered nurses with a psychiatric specialty and working in CMHCs treat, educate, and advise consumers concerning mental and physical health, as well as addiction-related, conditions, concerns, and risks. They offer services that range from individual and public psychoeducation to basic health screenings to intravenous injections and medication assistance. They maintain consumer health records and medical histories, assist with diagnostic tests and analysis, administer treatment and medications, as well as provide follow-up to monitor and support treatment adherence and health status.

Advance Practice Psychiatric Nurses are registered nurses with advanced degrees (minimum of master's degree) and clinical experience. These nurses diagnose and treat mental and physical health conditions, as well as addictive disorders. Typically, in collaboration with a physician, they may prescribe and monitor medications, as well as provide psychoeducation and other services to support health improvements and maintenance. There were 8,741 Advance Practice Psychiatric Nurses in 2007 (Ellis et al., 2007). Around 80.7% provided direct services and at least 5% worked in mental health clinics (Duffy et al., 2006).

INFORMATION TECHNOLOGY

In addition to individuals with clinical and consumer expertise, information systems experts are key to effective care, as well as efficient administrative operations, and are growing in prominence on CMHC staffing patterns nationwide. Such staff are supporting integration of electronic health records, clinical decision support systems (electronic decision trees for diagnosis and treatment), and Web-based clinical and administrative tools that are equipping clinicians to provide effective and efficient care (see Chapter 22 in this volume on accessing mental health information).

UTILIZATION DATA

CMHCs serve culturally, ethnically, and socioeconomically diverse populations and address a range of mental health issues, including serious diagnoses such as

schizophrenia, bipolar disorder, depression, anxiety disorders, substance dependence, and attention deficit hyperactivity disorder (see Chapters 6–12 in this volume on the epidemiology of mental disorders, substance use disorders, and
co-occurring disorders). Mental illness cuts across every demographic group in the
United States, with approximately 26.2% of the population meeting criteria for a
DSM-IV disorder in a given 12-month period (Kessler et al., 2004). In addition,
more than 28 million adults (12.9% of the population) received inpatient or outpatient treatment for a mental health problem during 2006 (Substance Abuse and
Mental Health Services Administration [SAMHSA], 2007). Of all adults, 0.7% were
hospitalized, 6.7% received outpatient treatment, and 10.9% received medication.
During the same time period, 21.3% of youth aged 12–17 received treatment or
counseling for mental health problems (SAMHSA, 2007).

While the numbers show that many people seek treatment for mental illness
each year, only 44% of the total population with a serious mental illness received
any form of treatment (SAMHSA, 2007), suggesting a significant gap in the need
for services and their accessibility and availability. Of those people reporting a need
for treatment, but failing to access treatment, a number of reasons are frequently
cited (see Figure 14.3), with "cost" being the most common (41%).

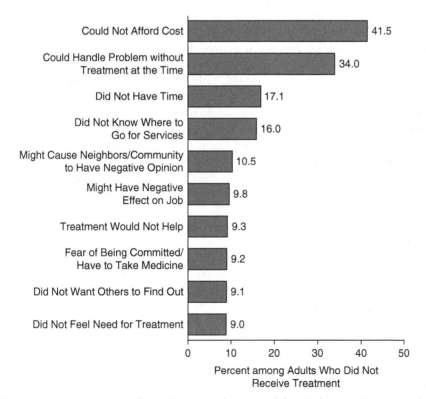

Figure 14.3 Reasons Why Substance Abusing Adults Did Not Receive Help
(SAMHSA, 2007).

Many more people with a DSM-IV diagnosis received treatment in a general medical setting (36.0%) compared to a mental health specialty setting (21.7%) (Wang et al., 2006). Of those people receiving treatment for a serious mental illness, 12.3% received treatment from a psychiatrist, 16.0% from a non-psychiatrist mental health specialist, and 22.8% from a general medical provider. In addition, demographic findings from the National Comorbidity Survey Replication (NCS-R) (see Chapter 7 in this volume) suggest that people who are young, female, low income, poorly educated, and/or unemployed-disabled are more likely to meet criteria for a DSM-IV diagnosis (Kessler & Merikangas, 2004). Accessibility of care varies substantially by race and ethnicity, with 15.2% of White adults seeking treatment in 2006, 11.9% of American Indians or Alaska Natives, 7.4% of Blacks, 7.0% of Native Hawaiians or Pacific Islanders, 7.0% of Hispanics, and 5.6% of Asians (SAMHSA, 2007).

Policy Issues

In 2001, the World Health Organization (WHO) established that mental illness is the leading cause of disability across the world, with depression, bipolar disorder, and schizophrenia accounting for approximately 25% of days lost to disability in industrialized countries (World Health Organization [WHO], 2001). Alcohol and drug use disorders account for an additional 12% of disability. More than 20% of U.S. adults between the ages of 18 and 54 receive care for a mental health or substance use problem in a given 12-month period (Kessler et al., 2005) (see Chapter 7 in this volume).

Despite the prevalence of mental health problems, the community mental health system has been continually challenged in meeting the needs of individuals with serious mental illness due to systemic barriers that result in limited service accessibility, inconsistent quality, and poor outcomes. Policymakers, providers, consumers, and advocates have identified a number of barriers that must be addressed to improve the quality of community-based care for mental illness (New Freedom Commission, 2003; IOM, 2006), including stigma, complex financing, co-occurring mental health and substance use disorders, employment, and housing.

Stigma

While much progress has been made regarding the public understanding of mental illness as a brain disease, stigma and discrimination continue to impede progress toward a community mental health system that is accessible and available to everyone. This is perhaps most evidenced by the reluctance of people to seek treatment when they experience symptoms of mental illness due to fears about how they will be perceived by their family, friends, coworkers, or employers. The lack of education about mental illness also reduces the likelihood that people will properly recognize signs and symptoms of mental illness and seek appropriate treatment. As research continues to enhance understanding of the biological underpinnings of mental illness, the public is gradually beginning to view mental illness as comparable to a physical illness. Unfortunately, stigma tends to be even more rampant among populations who have been historically underserved, particularly ethnic and racial minorities, older adults, and people in rural areas (U.S. Department of Health and Human Services, 2001). In recent years, government and community agencies have implemented large anti-stigma campaigns, which are gradually changing attitudes and reducing barriers to care.

COMPLEX FINANCING

Community mental health services are primarily funded by Medicaid, which has been growing rapidly in recent years and is now under significant pressure to contain costs and control growth. In addition to Medicaid, mental health services receive funding from a vast array of other sources, including 1) federal block grants; 2) state and local funds; 3) Medicare; 4) criminal justice; 5) education; 6) Social Security; 7) child welfare; 8) private insurance; 9) private pay; 10) vocational rehabilitation; 11) Temporary Assistance for Needy Families; and 12) philanthropic donations. Given the array of payers with different funding objectives, reporting demands, and administrative mandates, it can be difficult to link consumers (sometimes with multiple eligibilities and conflicting payer requirements) with appropriate funding sources even when the clinical need is great. This hampers access to care and impedes the development of broad evidence-based clinical pathways, as programs are often developed to align primarily with payer specifications, which may not always align with evidence-based care or consumer needs and preferences (see Chapter 2 in this volume for more information on financing mental health services).

CO-OCCURRING MENTAL HEALTH AND SUBSTANCE USE DISORDERS

Nowhere is the negative impact of stigma and disparate financing more apparent than in the treatment of co-occurring mental health and substance use disorders. Co-occurring disorders are quite common, as approximately 25–50% of individuals diagnosed with a mental health disorder have also had a diagnosable substance use disorder in their lifetime (Regier et al., 1990; Kessler, Nelson, & McGonagle, 1996). The presence of co-occurring disorders dramatically complicates treatment because the interactive and episodic nature of both illnesses impairs sustained recovery, but effective treatments do exist (Drake et al., 2001). For community mental health, effective treatment programs have been difficult to implement due to the historic separation between administrative and funding sources at the federal, state, and community level. Despite these challenges, much progress has been made in recent years to encourage effective integration of mental health and substance abuse services (see Chapter 12 in this volume for more information on co-occurring addictive and mental disorders).

EMPLOYMENT

Often the most important factor in sustained recovery is whether someone can secure employment in a meaningful and fulfilling job. Approximately 60% of adults with a mental health disability are out of the labor force (Kaye, 2002), despite many studies supporting the beneficial effects of returning to work and the desire of many consumers to secure competitive employment (Drake, Becker, Clark, & Mueser, 1999). In particular, supported employment programs (Bond et al., 2001), with an emphasis on using dedicated employment specialists to facilitate a rapid return to the competitive workplace, have shown effectiveness, with more than half of unemployed consumers returning to work (Cook et al., 2005). Many individuals with mental health disabilities receive Supplemental Security Income (SSI) or Social Security Disability Insurance (SSDI) benefits, which provide modest income assistance for people who are disabled and unable to work. The benefit programs often dis-incentivize work, however, because consumers who return to work may lose medical coverage and other disability supplements, such as support for housing, transportation, utilities, and food (Cook, 2003). While efforts are under way to revise federal policy to encourage a return to work, change has been slow to come (see Chapter 20 in this volume on the recovery movement).

Housing

Lack of safe and affordable housing is a primary barrier to recovery, and homelessness is "the most visible manifestation of the housing and support services problems of people with mental illnesses" (New Freedom Commission on Mental Health, 2004). Securing housing is often difficult due to stigma and difficulties navigating the complex affordable housing system. Former models of congregate living with residential staff support are giving way to independent community living with supports that are more often preferred by consumers (Tanzman, 1993). Effective models have been developed to facilitate access to housing that typically involve partnerships between state mental health authorities, community mental health providers, and local housing agencies to better leverage federal Housing and Urban Development (HUD) funding for people with mental health disabilities.

Implications for Mental Health

In recent years, it has become clear that the community mental health system, as it has evolved over the decade, is failing in many ways to meet the changing needs of consumers and families (New Freedom Commission, 2003; IOM, 2006). Most consumers and families still do not receive services that are founded in recovery and scientific evidence, and change has been slow to occur. There are calls for "transformational" reform, suggesting that incremental changes to the existing infrastructure are insufficient to address the behavioral health needs of consumers and families (SAMHSA, 2005). While transformational change will impact all public mental health systems, community mental health is expected to undergo change in several ways, including increased integration with primary care, use of information technology, and greater involvement of consumers and families in care decisions.

Primary Care Integration

Research shows that people with serious mental illness die approximately 25 years earlier than the general population (Parks, Svendsen, Singer, Foti, & Mauer, 2006; NASMHPD, 2006). Sixty percent of the early deaths of people with schizophrenia are related to cardiovascular, pulmonary, or infectious diseases; 30–40% of these deaths are related to suicide or injury (Parks et al., 2006). The traditional structure of community mental health clinics often creates a barrier to effectively coordinating care with medical providers working in other settings. In addition, 40% of consumers with mental health problems initially seek treatment in primary care settings (Chapa, 2004), where mental health problems are often undiagnosed or undertreated. There are serious consequences to undiagnosed mental illness and comorbid physical illness, as people with depression are far more likely to experience complications related to physical illness, take poor care of themselves, and die earlier (Ford et al., 1998; Frasure-Smith, Lesperance, Juneau, Talajic, & Bourassa, 1999; DeGroot, Anderson, Freedland, Clouse, & Lustman, 2001). Models are currently evolving to increase the integration of primary care and mental health services at the community level, largely by co-locating mental health staff in medical clinics. Research has consistently shown that such integrated programs increase access to care, reduce costs, and improve clinical and functional outcomes (Unutzer, Schoenbaum, Druss, & Katon, 2006).

Information Technology

Despite dramatic technological advances in recent years, community mental health has lagged behind the rest of health care in its use of information technology (IOM, 2006). New technologies offer great opportunity to revolutionize traditional clinic-based care. For example, advances in telemedicine are making otherwise scarce mental health resources (e.g., child psychiatry) more available in rural or underserved settings. Also, broader adoption of Electronic Health Records (EHRs) will improve the quality and outcomes of care. Early EHR software generally translated a CMHC's paper forms and processes to the electronic environment, which produced significant benefits in care coordination, privacy, security, and disaster recovery capability. These early systems were hampered by the lack of common data standards, however, and could rarely exchange information effectively.

Much work is ongoing at the national level to establish common data standards to facilitate the secure exchange of health information among different health care providers with the consumer's consent (see Chapters 4 and 22 in this volume). In addition, newer generations of EHRs do not simply replicate old paper processes, but actually re-engineer clinical workflows to increase efficiency and quality. Perhaps the greatest potential benefit of EHRs may come from the integration of Clinical Decision Support logic into electronic systems, so that evidence-based guidelines and other research-based advice can actively inform practitioners during the process of providing clinical services, thus supporting the delivery of improved care.

PERSON-CENTERED CARE

Consumers and families have been difficult to engage and retain in traditional community-based services, often because they perceive the fragmented and bureaucratic system of community services as inflexible and unresponsive. In a recovery-oriented system, the consumer and family should be in control of their care, which would in turn strengthen their engagement in services and improve outcomes (New Freedom Commission on Mental Health, 2003). Historically, stigma has fueled beliefs that individuals with mental illness are not capable of making appropriate decisions regarding their care (Martin, Pescosolido, & Tuch, 2000). This has resulted in consumer disengagement and poor compliance with treatment plans developed by well-meaning clinical staff (Bodenheimer, Lorig, Holman, & Grumback, 2002).

Making the community mental health system person-centered will require greater involvement of consumers across all aspects of service design and delivery. Shared decision-making (Adams & Drake, 2006) strategies, where consumers are given a lot of information regarding their diagnosis and various treatment options via paper, computer, and video methodologies, are now starting to be tested in mental health environments. These strategies may help facilitate an improved partnership between consumers, families, and clinicians, resulting in greater self-determination, improved compliance with ones' chosen treatment, and perhaps better outcomes.

Future Challenges

Community mental health is at a critical point, struggling with chronic underfunding, system fragmentation, and challenges in bringing advances from science into service settings. Perhaps the primary challenge faced by community mental health is related to the aging workforce, challenging work conditions, and low salaries, which have made it difficult to attract new and talented people. In addition, the entire mental health field has resisted integration with general health care, which has had negative consequences to financing and political support for mental health (Drake et al., 2003). In the future, community mental health will need to incorporate treatment pathways already common in general health care, such as reliance on measurement and treatment algorithms (i.e., a decision-tree approach to treatment). In addition, following a drop in state hospital institutionalization from 558,239 in 1955 to 52,539 fifty years later in 2005, as well as insufficient funding, community mental health centers were unable to meet the growing demand for services (Bureau of the Census, 1956; NASMHPD Research Institute, 2007). Consequently, prisons and jails have become the de facto psychiatric institutions in the United States, currently housing approximately 350,000 people with serious mental illness (Ditton, 1999; Sabol, Minton, & Harrison, 2007).

WORKFORCE DEVELOPMENT

The community mental health workforce is facing a significant staff shortage in the coming years, as well as challenges in adapting to new treatment methods and shifts in population demographics (Annapolis Coalition, 2007). The general population's needs for community mental health services have increased much faster in recent years than the availability of professionals entering the fields of psychiatry, psychology, social work, and nursing (Manderscheid & Henderson, 2006). In addition, the community service environment has been chronically underfunded and is experiencing increasing financial pressure, which increases the workload on staff who receive low wages and have few opportunities for advancement, often resulting in poor morale (Blankertz & Robinson 1997; Gellis & Kim, 2004).

The leadership of CMHCs is also aging out of the workforce. It has been estimated that 50% of the nation's CMHC chief executives will retire by 2013. This will not only create a gap in leadership, it will usher in a new generation of leaders who were not present at the birth of the CMHC movement.

A number of strategies have been proposed (Annapolis Coalition, 2007) to address this looming workforce problem, specifically to 1) broaden the concept of the behavioral health workforce by involving consumers, communities, and promoting recovery; 2) strengthen the workforce through recruitment, improved training and education, and active leadership development; and 3) support the workforce through improved national infrastructure and research (for additional material on workforce development, see Chapter 5 in this volume).

MEASUREMENT-BASED CARE

Unlike most other health care professions, where measurement of height and weight are routine and blood tests are commonly used to manage illnesses such as diabetes, objective measurement or assessment is infrequently used in community mental health settings. Measurement-based care requires the routine collection of standardized assessments (e.g., symptoms, side-effects, or other key indicators such as therapeutic alliance) at each treatment visit and provides guidelines for how treatment should proceed based on the results of each assessment (Trivedi et al., 2006). This approach to clinical care integrates assessment information with clinical decision-making using brief practical tools that can be used by clinical decision support systems to inform treatment decisions. While this approach holds much promise, community mental health agencies have rarely used ongoing assessment due to the many competing demands for time during clinical sessions. Implementation of measurement-based care approaches will require careful reworking of clinical processes and workflow in order for measurement in a mental health center to become as routine as it is in a primary care office. In addition, graduate training programs will need to adapt to this new way of doing business by training clinicians to integrate measurement into their clinical processes.

CRIMINAL JUSTICE

As detailed in Chapter 18 of this volume, individuals with mental illness have been incarcerated at a disproportionate rate, as people in jail or prison have approximately three times the prevalence of serious mental illness (16%) compared to the general population (5%) (Kessler et al., 1999; Ditton, 1999). Three-fourths of those also have a co-occurring substance use disorder (Abram & Teplin, 1991). The three largest psychiatric institutions in the United States are now jails: Rikers Island (New York City), Los Angeles County Jail, and Cook County Jail (Chicago) (Council of State Governments, 2002). This problem necessitates greater involvement from the community mental health system, as well as coordination with other social services to increase engagement of people with mental illness in effective care. Expanded partnerships between CMHCs and criminal justice systems can increase use of cost effective and socially beneficial practices such as jail diversion, mental health courts, drug courts, and re-entry programs. However, funding must be increased and streamlined. Philosophies of care between the justice community and the CMHC community must be integrated.

The Evolution of Community Mental Health Services

In 47 years since the establishment of the Community Mental Health Centers Construction Act in 1963, the community system has undergone continuous change. These changes include facing the influx of people seeking community-based supports in the aftermath of de-institutionalization, dramatic shifts in how health care is regulated and financed, adoption of new medicines and therapeutic advances, and the incorporation of new values emphasizing consumer self-determination and recovery. Despite the continuous evolution of community mental health, the system faces many new challenges and opportunities and has been characterized by the New Freedom Commission (2003) as in need of "transformational" change to improve the quality and accessibility of mental health care. While much remains to be done, the need for a strong community mental health system is greater than ever in order to ensure that consumers and families with mental illness have the diverse range of supports they need to live fully in the community.

With a nationwide network of service providers deeply rooted in both rural and urban settings, community mental health centers are an essential part of the nation's safety net for individuals with behavioral health needs. Many of the psychiatrists, therapists, case managers, and others employed by CMHCs bridge many disconnected systems, and they are able to work with consumers in all of the settings that they encounter—from hospitals and schools to courts and housing authorities. Well positioned for transformation, if CMHCs receive suitable funding to implement the needed changes to integrate on-site physical health services and implement electronic health record and clinical decision support technologies, they will be able to offer excellent care that is appropriate for the unique needs of adults with serious mental illnesses and children with severe emotional disturbance.

Signs of Hope

When evidence-based care that combines both patient-centered principles with access to the most recent research is available to consumers, recovery is a distinct and real possibility. With the current advances in the field, even individuals with disorders that ten years ago were only addressed with sedation and hospitalization are now able to reach remission from their symptoms. Some community mental health centers are now integrating research and practice to improve care through partnerships with academic researchers involved in the development of new treatment strategies. One example of the potential successes that can come from such partnerships is exemplified in the story of "George," an individual who was reached through one such partnership in 2008.

George, a 51-year-old man living with schizoaffective disorder, had hallucinations that left him homeless, wandering the streets, shouting at unseen forces out to destroy him. George was unable to physically care for himself, refusing showers and fresh clothing. After walking off the street into a community mental health clinic, George was invited to participate in a research study conducted by a researcher investigating whether higher doses of a long-acting injectable medication could help people with psychosis who were previously unresponsive to treatment. After six weeks in the study, George's delusions dramatically diminished. The accusing voices in his head hushed to the point where he had to strain to hear them, and most days they were simply gone. The once wild-eyed, unshaven man is now transformed, and George now smiles easily and lights up any room he enters.

This is but one example of the significant progress now being made to bridge the science-to-service gap and transform care provision nationwide. Much work remains to be done, but as this gap further narrows, more individuals with serious mental illness like George will be able to reach the recovery that they have been seeking and reclaim lives of promise and potential.

References

Abram, K. M., & Teplin, L. A. (1991). Co-occurring disorders among mentally ill jail detainees: Implications for public policy. *American Psychologist, 46*(10), 1036–1045.

Adams, J. R., & Drake, R. E. (2006). Shared decisionmaking and evidence-based practice. *Community Mental Health Journal, 21*, 1–19.

Annapolis Coalition. (2007). *An Action Plan for Behavioral Health Workforce Development: A Framework for Discussion.* SAMHSA/DHHS Publication No. 280-02-0302. Rockville, MD: Department of Health and Human Services.

Bauer, M. S. (2002). A review of quantitative studies of adherence to mental health clinical practice guidelines. *Harvard Review of Psychiatry, 10*(3), 138–153.

Beck, A. T., Rush, A. J., Shaw, B. F., & Emery, G. (1979). *Cognitive Therapy of Depression.* New York: Guilford Press.

Bellak, L. (1958). *Schizophrenia: A Review of the Syndrome.* New York: Logos Press.

Blankertz, L. E., & Robinson, S. E. (1997). Turnover intentions of community mental health workers in psychosocial rehabilitation services. *Journal of Community Mental Health, 33*(6), 517–529.

Bodenheimer, T., Lorig, K., Holman, H., & Grumbach, K. (2002). Patient self-management of chronic disease in primary care. *Journal of the American Medical Association, 288*(19), 2469–2475.

Bond, G. R., Becker, D. R., Drake, R. E., Rapp, C. A., Meisler, N., Lehman, A. F., et al. (2001). Implementing supported employment as an evidence-based practice. *Psychiatric Services, 52*, 313–322.

Bureau of Labor Statistics, U.S. Department of Labor. (2006). *Occupational Outlook Handbook, 2008–09 Edition, Bulletin 2700.* Washington, DC: Superintendent of Documents, U.S. Government Printing Office. Available online at http://www.bls.gov/oco/. Accessed August 21, 2008.

Bureau of the Census, U.S. Department of Commerce. (1956). *Statistical Abstract of the United States, 1956.* Washington, DC: U.S. Government Printing Office.

Butler, A. C., Chapman, J. E., Forman, E. M., & Beck, A. T. (2006). The empirical status of cognitive-behavioral therapy: A review of meta-analyses. *Clinical Psychology Review, 26*(1), 17–31.

Center for Substance Abuse Treatment. (2007). *National Summit on Recovery: Conference Report.* DHHS Publication No. SMA 07-4276. Rockville, MD: Substance Abuse and Mental Health Services Administration.

Chapa, T. (2004). *Mental Health Services in Primary Care Settings for Racial and Ethnic Minority Populations* [Draft issue brief; Rockville, MD: Office of Minority Health]. In C. Kautz, D. Mauch, & S. A. Smith, (2008), *Reimbursement of Mental Health Services in Primary Care Settings.* HHS Pub. No. SMA-08-4324. Rockville, MD: Center for Mental Health Services, Substance Abuse, and Mental Health Services Administration.

Cook, J. A. (2003). One-year follow-up of Illinois state vocational rehabilitation clients with psychiatric disabilities following successful closure into community employment. *Journal of Vocational Rehabilitation, 18,* 25–32.

Cook, J. A., Leff, H. S., Blyler, C. R., Gold, P. B., Goldberg, R. W., Mueser, K. T., et al. (2005). Results of a multisite randomized trial of supported employment interventions for individuals with severe mental illness. *Archives of General Psychiatry, 62,* 505–512.

Copeland, M. E. (2004). Self-determination in mental health recovery: Taking back our lives. In J. Jonikas & J. Cook (Eds.), *UIC NRTC's National Self-Determination and Psychiatric Disability Invitational Conference: Conference Papers* (pp. 68–82). Chicago: UIC National Research and Training Center on Psychiatric Disability.

Council of State Governments. (2002). *Criminal Justice/Mental Health Consensus Project: Fact Sheet; Mental Illness and Jails.* New York: Council of State Governments. Available online at http://consensusproject.org/downloads/fact_jails.pdf. Accessed June 22, 2009.

Cutler, D. L., Bevilacqua, J., & McFarland, B. H. (2003). Four decades of community mental health: A symphony in four movements. *Community Mental Health Journal, 39,* 381–398.

DeGroot, M., Anderson, R., Freedland, K. E., Clouse, R. E., & Lustman, P. J. (2001). Association of depression and diabetes complications: A meta-analysis. *Psychosomatic Medicine, 63,* 619–630.

DeLeon, P., Vanden Bos, G., & Kraut, A. (1984). Federal legislation recognizing psychology. *American Psychologist, 39,* 933–946.

Ditton, P. M. (1999). *Mental Health and Treatment of Inmates and Probationers.* Special report NCJ 174463. Washington, DC: U.S. Department of Justice, Office of Justice Programs, Bureau of Justice Statistics.

Drake, R. E., Becker, D. R., Clark, R. E., & Mueser, K. T. (1999). Research on the individual placement and support model of supported employment. *Psychiatric Quarterly, 70,* 289–301.

Drake, R. E., Essock, S. M., Shaner, A., Carey, K. B., Minkoff, K., Kola, L., et al. (2001). Implementing dual diagnosis services for clients with severe mental illness. *Psychiatric Services, 52,* 469–476.

Drake, R. E., Green, A. I., Mueser, K. T., & Goldman, H. H. (2003). The history of community mental health treatment and rehabilitation for persons with severe mental illness. *Community Mental Health Journal, 39*(5), 427–440.

Duffy, F. F, Wilk, J., West, J. C., Narrow, W. E., Rae, D. S., Hall, R., et al. (2006). Mental health practitioners and trainees. In R. W. Manderscheid & J. T. Berry (Eds.), *Mental Health, United States, 2004* (pp. 256–302). Rockville, MD: Substance Abuse and Mental Health Services Administration.

Ellis, A. R., Thomas, K., Konrad, T. R., & Morrissey, J. P. (2007, November). *Supply and Co-location of Mental Health Providers Across the U.S.* Paper presented at the American Public Health Association Annual Meeting, Washington, DC.

Foley, H. A., & Sharfstein, S. S. (1983). *Madness and Government: Who Cares for the Mentally Ill?* Washington, DC: American Psychiatric Press.

Foster, E. M., & Conner, T. (2005). Public costs of better mental health services for children and adolescents. *Psychiatric Services, 56*(1), 50–55.

Ford, D. E., Mead, L. A., Chang, P. P., Cooper-Patrick, L., Wang, N. Y., & Klag, M. J. (1998). Depression is a risk factor for coronary artery disease in men: The precursors study. *Archives of Internal Medicine, 158*, 1422–1426.

Frasure-Smith, N., Lesperance, F., Juneau, M., Talajic, M., & Bourassa, M. G. (1999). Gender, depression, and one-year prognosis after myocardial infarction. *Psychosomatic Medicine, 61*, 26–37.

Fromm-Reichmann, F. (1949). Notes on the development of treatment of schizophrenics by psychoanalytic psychotherapy. *Psychiatry, 11*, 263–273.

Gellis, Z. D., & Kim, J. C. (2004). Predictors of depressive mood, occupational stress, and propensity to leave in older and younger mental health case managers. *Community Mental Health Journal, 40*(5), 407–421.

Goldman, H. H., & Morrissey, J. P. (1985). The alchemy of mental health policy: Homelessness and the fourth cycle of reform. *American Journal of Public Health, 75*, 727–731.

Grimes, K. E., Kapunan, P. E., & Mullin, B. (2006). Children's health services in a "system of care": Patterns of mental health, primary, and specialty use. *Public Health Reports, 121*(3), 311–323.

Herz, M. I., & Marder, S. R. (2002). *Schizophrenia: Comprehensive Treatment and Management.* Baltimore: Lippincott Williams & Wilkins.

Hogarty, G. E. (2002). *Personal Therapy for Schizophrenia & Related Disorders: A Guide to Individualized Treatment.* New York: Guilford Publications.

Lamb, H. R., & Weinberger, L. E. (1998). Persons with severe mental illness in jails and prisons: A review. *Psychiatric Services, 49*(4), 483–492.

Institute of Medicine (with P. J. Mrazek & R. J. Haggerty [Eds.]). (1994). *Reducing Risks for Mental Disorders: Frontiers for Preventive Intervention Research.* Washington, DC: National Academy Press.

Institute of Medicine. (2001). *Crossing the Quality Chasm: A New Health System for the 21st Century.* Washington, DC: National Academy Press.

Institute of Medicine. (2006). *Improving the Quality of Health Care of Mental and Substance-Use Conditions.* Washington, DC: National Academies Press.

Joint Commission on Mental Illness and Health. (1961). *Action for Mental Health.* New York: Basic Books.

Kaplan, L. (2008). *The Role of Recovery Support Services in Recovery-Oriented Systems of Care.* DHHS Publication No. (SMA) 08-4315. Rockville, MD: Center for Substance Abuse Treatment, Substance Abuse and Mental Health Services Administration.

Kaye, H. S. (2002). *Employment and Social Participation among People with Mental Health Disabilities.* San Francisco: National Disability Statistics & Policy Forum.

Kessler, R. C., Berglund, P., Chiu, W. T., Demler, O., Heeringa, S., Hiripi, E., et al. (2004). The US National Comorbidity Survey Replication (NCS-R): Design and field procedures. *International Journal of Methods in Psychiatric Research, 13*, 69–92.

Kessler, R. C., Berglund, P. A., Walters, E. E., Leaf, P. J., Kouzis, A. C., Bruce, M. L., et al. (1999). Population-based analyses: A methodology for estimating the 12-month prevalence of serious mental illness. In R. W. Manderscheid & M. J. Henderson (Eds.), *Mental Health, United States, 1998* (pp. 99–109). Washington, DC: U.S. Government Printing Office.

Kessler, R. C., Demler, O., Frank R. G., Olfson, M., Pincus, H. A., Walters, E. E., et al. (2005). Prevalence and treatment of mental disorders, 1990 to 2003. *New England Journal of Medicine, 352*(24), 2515–2523.

Kessler, R. C., Heeringa, S., Lakoma, M. D., Petukhova, M., Rupp, A. E., Schoenbaum, M., et al. (2008). The individual-level and societal-level effects of mental disorders on earnings in the United States: Results from the National Comorbidity Survey Replication. *American Journal of Psychiatry, 165*, 703–711.

Kessler, R. C., & Merikangas, K. R. (2004). The National Comorbidity Survey Replication (NCS-R). *International Journal of Methods in Psychiatric Research, 13*, 60–68.

Kessler, R. C., Nelson, C., & McGonagle, K. (1996) The epidemiology of co-occurring addictive and mental disorders: Implications of prevention and service utilization. *American Journal of Orthopsychiatry, 66*, 17–31.

Liberman, R. P., & Kopelowicz, A. (2002). Recovery from schizophrenia: A challenge for the 21st century. *International Review of Psychiatry, 14*, 245–255.

Manderscheid, R. W., & Henderson, M. J. (Eds.). (2006). *Mental Health, United States, 2004.* DHHS Pub. No. SMA-06-4195. Rockville, MD: U.S. Department of Health and Human Services, Substance Abuse and Mental Health Services Administration, Center for Mental Health Services.

Mark, T. L., & Buck, J. A. (2006). Characteristics of U.S. youths with serious emotional disturbance: Data from the National Health Interview Survey. *Psychiatric Services, 57*(11), 1573–1578.

Mark, T. L., Coffey, R. M., King, E., Harwood, H., McKusick, D., Genurdi, J., et al. (2000). Spending on mental health and substance abuse treatment, 1987–1997. *Health Affairs, 19*, 108–120.

Martin, J. K., Pescosolido, B. A., & Tuch, S. A. (2000). Of fear and loathing: The role of "disturbing behavior," labels, and causal attributions in shaping public attitudes toward people with mental illness. *Journal of Health and Social Behavior, 41*(2), 208–223.

McGlynn, E. A., Asch, S. M., Adams, J., Keesey, J., Hicks, J., DeCristofaro, A., et al. (2003). The quality of health care delivered to adults in the United States. *New England Journal of Medicine, 348*(26), 2635–2645.

Mellman, T. A., Miller, A. L., Weissman, E. M., Crismon, M. L., Essock, S. M., & Marder, S. R. (2001). Evidence-based pharmacologic treatment for people with severe mental illness: A focus on guidelines and algorithms. *Psychiatric Services, 52*, 619–625.

National Association of State Mental Health Program Directors (NASMHPD) Medical Directors Council. (2005, January). *Integrating Behavioral Health and Primary Care Services: Opportunities and Challenges for State Mental Health Authorities.* Washington, DC: Author.

National Association of State Mental Health Program Directors (NASMHPD) Medical Directors Council. (2006, October). *Morbidity and Mortality in People with Serious Mental Illness.* Washington, DC: Author.

NASMHPD Research Institute (NRI). (2007). *2006 State Mental Health Agency Profiles.* Alexandria, VA: Author.

New Freedom Commission on Mental Health. (2003). *Achieving the Promise: Transforming Mental Health Care in America; Final Report.* DHHS Pub. No. SMA-03-3832. Rockville, MD: Author.

New Freedom Commission on Mental Health. (2004). *Subcommittee on Housing and Homelessness: Background Paper.* DHHS Pub. No. SMA-04-3884. Rockville, MD: Author.

Parks, J., Svendsen, D., Singer, P., Foti, M., & Mauer, B. (2006, October). *Technical Report: Morbidity and Mortality in People with Serious Mental Illness.* Washington, DC: National Association of State Mental Health Program Directors, Medical Directors Council.

Pignatiello, A., Boydell, K., Teshima, K., & Volpe, T. (2008). Supporting primary care through pediatric telepsychiatry. *Canadian Journal of Community Mental Health, 27*(2), 139–151.

President's Commission on Mental Health. (1978). *Report to the President from the President's Commission on Mental Health* (vol. 1). Stock Number 040-000-00390-8. Washington, DC: U.S. Government Printing Office.

Regier, D. A., Farmer, M. E., Rae, D. S., Locke, B. Z., Keith, S. J., Judd, L. L., et al. (1990). Comorbidity of mental disorders with alcohol and other drug abuse: Results from the Epidemiologic Catchment Area (ECA) Study. *Journal of the American Medical Association, 264*(19), 2511–2518.

Sabin J. (2000). Managed care and health care reform: Comedy, tragedy, and lessons. *Psychiatric Services, 51,* 1392–1396.

Sabol, W. J., Minton, T. D., & Harrison, P. M. (2007). *Prisons and Jail Inmates at Midyear 2006.* Bureau of Justice Statistics Special Report No. NCJ 217675. Washington, DC: U.S. Department of Justice.

Stambough, L. F., Mustillo, S. A., Burns, B. J., Stephens, R. L., Baxter, B., Edwards, D., et al. (2007). Outcomes from wraparound and multisystemic therapy in a center for mental health services system-of-care demonstration site. *Journal of Emotional and Behavioral Disorders, 15*(3), 143–155.

Stroul, B. A., & Friedman, R. M. (1986). *A System of Care for Children and Youth with Severe Emotional Disturbances* (rev. ed.). Washington, DC: Georgetown University Child Development Center, CASSP Technical Assistance Center.

Substance Abuse and Mental Health Services Administration. (2005). *Transforming Mental Health Care in America: The Federal Action Agenda.* Rockville, MD: DHHS.

Substance Abuse and Mental Health Services Administration. (2007). *Results from the 2006 National Survey on Drug Use and Health: National Findings.* Office of Applied Studies, NSDUH Series H-32, DHHS Publication No. SMA 07-4293. Rockville, MD: Author.

Tanzman, B. (1993). An overview of surveys of mental health consumers' preferences for housing and support services. *Hospital and Community Psychiatry, 44*(5), 450–455.

Trivedi, M. H., Rush, A. J., Wisniewski, S. R., Nierenberg, A. A., Warden, D., Ritz, L., et al. (2006). Evaluation of outcomes with citalopram for depression using measurement-based care in STAR*D: Implications for clinical practice. *American Journal of Psychiatry, 163,* 28–40.

U.S. Department of Health and Human Services. (2001). *Mental Health: Culture, Race, and Ethnicity—A Supplement to Mental Health; A Report of the Surgeon General.* Rockville, MD: U.S. Department of Health and Human Services, Substance Abuse and Mental Health Services Administration, Center for Mental Health Services.

Unutzer, J., Schoenbaum, M., Druss, B., & Katon, W. (2006). Transforming mental health care at the interface with general medicine: Report for the President's Commission. *Psychiatric Services, 57*(1), 37–47.

Wang, P. S., Lane, M., Olfson, M., Pincus, H.A., Schwenk, T. L., Wells, K. B., et al. (2006). The primary care of mental disorders in the United States. In R. W. Manderscheid & J. T. Berry (Eds.), *Mental Health, United States, 2004* (pp. 117–133). Rockville, MD: Substance Abuse and Mental Health Services Administration.

World Health Organization. (2001). *The World Health Report 2001: Mental Health; New Understanding, New Hope.* Geneva: World Health Organization.

Chapter 15

SPECIALTY HOSPITALS AND PSYCHIATRIC UNITS

Faith B. Dickerson, PhD, MPH; and Steven S. Sharfstein, MD, MPA

PSYCHIATRIC HOSPITALS have been a core component of mental health care systems in the United States since the mid-nineteenth century and Dorothea Dix's crusade to provide humane care in asylums for the insane who were housed in jails, almshouses, attics, and basements throughout America. Today, long-term hospitalization in large institutions has been replaced by community-based care, which includes specialty hospitals and specialty units within general hospitals. This chapter will review the history of hospital care, de-institutionalization, and the current configuration and role of the hospital from a public mental health perspective. Challenges to the future of hospitalization and the role of the acute inpatient stay within a comprehensive mental health care system will be discussed.

Historical Perspective

Until the second half of the twentieth century, most mental health services consisted of long-term custodial care provided in state or county inpatient hospitals. That pattern has changed dramatically. Today, the primary goal of hospital psychiatric care is to treat an acute illness episode in a brief time period; hospital care constitutes only one piece, albeit a crucial one, in an array of mental health services. Also, today inpatient psychiatric care is more likely to be delivered in a psychiatric unit of a general hospital or a private psychiatric care setting rather than in a state or county public hospital.

The single most major change over the past 50 years has been the massive downsizing of state- and county-operated psychiatric hospitals. In 1955, there were

340 state or county beds per 100,000 U.S. population; in 2005, there were 17 per 100,000 population, a 95% reduction (Torrey et al., 2008). At the same time as the number of beds in public mental health hospitals was declining, the proportion of persons treated in public vs. private hospital settings also was shifting. In 1970, there were 525,000 psychiatric beds in the United States, of which 80% were in state or county mental hospitals, while in 2002, there were of a total of 211,000 beds, of which over 68% were provided within the private sectors (Foley et al., 2004). The increase in capacity in private psychiatric hospitals and psychiatric units in general hospitals rose most sharply between 1980 and 1990, but has declined since then (Salinsky & Loftis, 2007), though psychiatric units in general hospitals have generally replaced state and county mental hospitals as the settings caring for publicly funded patients (Mechanic, McAlpine, & Olfson, 1998).

The dramatic shifts that have occurred over the past 50 years in the number and setting of psychiatric hospital beds have been dictated largely by economic and political forces, rather than by advances in medical science. Starting after World War II, and fueled by public revelations that most state mental hospitals were grossly overcrowded and that patients were living there in squalid conditions (see Albert Deutsch's 1948 exposé, *Shame of the States*), there began a broad social movement to reduce reliance on public institutional settings. As part of this trend, in the 1960s, a group of civil libertarian lawyers emerged who believed that mental patients were incarcerated in state institutions and who championed laws to force state hospitals to discharge patients and to make re-hospitalization very difficult. Related to this trend was the presence of influential writers such as Thomas Szasz, who argued that mental illness was a myth (see *The Myth of Mental Illness*, 1961) and other authors whose works contributed to the belief that persons were "made worse" in hospitals (Ken Kesey, *One Flew over the Cuckoo's Nest*, 1962 and Erving Goffman, *Asylums*, 1961). These books were widely read, especially on college campuses, and their message about psychiatric patients was seen as akin to the struggle for civil rights on the part of Blacks, women, and other oppressed groups.

Equally powerful was the development and initial usage of effective psychotropic medications starting with chlorpromazine (Thorazine) in 1954, enabling some patients with acute psychosis to be effectively treated and discharged from hospitals. Synergistic with the preceding factors was an effort by the states to reduce the burden of costs for mental health treatment. The creation in the 1960s of federal programs such as SSI (Supplemental Security Income), SSDI (Social Security Disability Insurance), Medicaid, and Medicare provided fiscal support, with federal funds for individuals with mental illness living in the community; patients in state hospitals were not eligible for these benefits for the most part. Hence, there was a broad financial incentive to move patients from state expense in state and county hospitals to federal expense in Medicaid-funded and other federally supported programs such as SSI.

Within the private sector, the upturn in psychiatric beds that took place, starting in 1970, was due to several factors, including the inclusion of psychiatric benefits in private health insurance coverage. By 1974, 95% of the health insurance plans surveyed provided some coverage for hospital care of mental conditions (Reed, 1975). There was also a relaxation of certificate of need requirements in some states. In addition, the federal government changed their policy so that Medicaid funds could be used for the care of patients under the age of 21 in psychiatric hospitals. Also, psychiatric services in psychiatric hospitals and in general hospitals were exempted from the Medicare prospective payment that was instituted in 1983, making the provision of these services more attractive in specialty hospitals and units.[1] Finally, starting in the 1970s, general hospitals saw a marked reduction in the length of stay and therefore bed utilization for medical and surgical patients. As a result, many community hospitals had empty beds available and saw opening a psychiatric unit as a way to fill some of those beds and recoup revenue.

By the 1990s, the pendulum in private psychiatric beds had swung in the other direction, due largely to the increasing penetrance of managed care practices. Managed care refers to the use by insurance companies of specialist managed behavioral health companies to manage psychiatric insurance benefits and reduce costs (Liptzin & Summergrad, 2008). Managed care companies developed programs of pre-admission review and continued care certification to control the utilization of psychiatric services, particularly on inpatient units. The companies developed review criteria and hired reviewers to apply these criteria to approve or disallow inpatient admissions. The effect on lengths of stay and on hospital admission decisions was dramatic and effectively eliminated long-term psychiatric hospitalization in the private sector. Insurance companies also negotiated lower reimbursement rates, which further lowered the profitability of providing inpatient services in private sector hospital settings.

In 1990, just over 50,000 beds were provided through psychiatric units in general hospitals and 45,000 in private psychiatric hospitals. Since that time, primarily due to managed care utilization review, these beds have also declined so that in 2004 they numbered about 40,000 in general hospital units and 21,000 in psychiatric hospitals (Manderscheid, personal communication, March, 2008). In terms of the number of inpatient admissions, these rose from 235,000 in 1986 to 529,000 in 2000 and to 577,000 in 2004 in private psychiatric hospitals (Foley et al., 2004; Manderscheid, personal communication, March, 2008). In contrast, there was a decline in annual inpatient admissions to state and county psychiatric hospitals: 330,000 in 1986 to 218,000 in 2000 (Manderscheid et al., 2002). Despite the overall long-term trend of bed reductions in state psychiatric hospitals, there was a 21% increase in admissions to these settings from 2002 to 2005; this increase was due primarily to forensic patients (Manderscheid, Atay, & Crider, 2009).

Expenditure trends for mental health care, and for hospital care within mental health, have also shifted. There has been a decrease in the proportion of health care dollars that are spent on mental health services and, within the mental health sector, there has been a decline in the proportion of spending on hospital vs. other services, especially medications. Mental health fell from 8% of all health expenditures in 1986 to 6% in 2003. During this same time period, inpatient spending within mental health treatment fell from 41% to 24%, and the proportion of spending on retail psychotropic drugs grew from 7% to 23% (National Association of State Mental Health Program Directors Medical Directors Council, 2006).

---

[1] Of note, in January 2005 Medicare began paying for inpatient psychiatric services on a prospective basis with a complicated methodology. It is considered uncertain how the prospective payment will affect the future funding and availability of inpatient beds (Liptzin & Summergrad, 2008).

Types of Services

HOSPITAL INPATIENT UNITS

Hospital inpatient units are the most expensive, restrictive, and regulated of mental health treatment settings. In the first decade of the twenty-first century, the typical psychiatric unit is located in a general hospital and is an acute unit with a mean length of stay of less than one week. The most common objective is crisis stabilization, with crisis defined as the danger of suicide or homicide, harmful acts to self or others, and/or impaired self-care, and the fact that this "dangerousness" is due to a mental disorder. Admission criteria vary among inpatient settings, but all criteria include some focus on safety/dangerousness and the absence of less restrictive treatment alternatives.

Acute inpatient units treat patients with a range of psychiatric disorders. In 2004, there were more than 1.8 million stays in psychiatric units of general hospitals. Of these, 38% were for mood disorders; 25% for substance abuse; 22% for schizophrenia and other psychotic disorders; 8% for delirium and dementia; and 7% for other disorders (Salinsky & Loftis, 2007). While only 25% of inpatients were admitted with a primary diagnosis of a substance abuse problem, it is noteworthy that over one-half of patients hospitalized for care in general hospitals have a substance abuse problem (Salinsky & Loftis, 2007).

The mode of practice on acute psychiatric inpatient units is driven in large part by constraints imposed by insurance payers; for an individual patient, the duration of the inpatient stay is typically short, usually one week or less. The goals of treatment on the acute unit are safety, diagnosis and triage, treatment, and respite (Glick, Carter, & Tandon, 2003). Components of acute inpatient care include stabilizing acute symptoms, making a comprehensive diagnosis, instituting effective psychopharmacologic treatment, and planning for discharge. While the focus of treatment on the unit is typically instituting pharmacotherapy, another objective is to develop a psychosocial treatment plan that includes appropriate psychotherapy and rehabilitation.

There is a need to develop a discrete set of objectives that are endorsed by the patient whose primary wish may simply be to be discharged and to get out of the hospital as soon as possible, while the perspective of the treating psychiatrist is likely more focused on specific signs and symptoms. One crucial task of the psychiatrist is to rule out a medical condition that could account for the patient's psychiatric symptoms, especially those conditions that could lead to brain failure such as a recent head injury, specific intoxication, or acute and chronic medical conditions that could lead to delirium. It is also crucial to identify, address, and alleviate the stressors that precipitated the crisis that led to the hospitalization. Another objective is to begin the process of educating the patient and the family about the nature of the illness, helping them to recognize signs and symptoms, and discussing what can be done to prevent further inpatient stays.

Apart from general acute units, many psychiatric units are highly specialized, with well-developed guidelines for medication treatment and psychosocial interventions for specific clinical disorders and/or age subpopulations. In the section that follows are examples of specialty units that are found in private sector psychiatric settings.

GERIATRIC UNIT

Compared to persons in other age ranges, persons aged 64 and older are almost twice as likely to be treated in a hospital psychiatric setting (Colenda et al., 2002). Among geriatric patients, the most common psychiatric disorders treated in the hospital are severe depressive disorders and cognitive disorders (Blank et al., 2005). The assessment of suicidality is a major concern, as the elderly have the highest suicide risk of any age subpopulation; the suicide rate for those 75 years and older is 1.5–2 times that of persons in the general population (Arias et al., 2003). Geriatric psychiatric inpatients have an average of five to six active medical problems, comparable to geriatric medical inpatients. The psychiatric disorders that occur in this context involve a complex interplay of these medical/neurological problems with the psychiatric condition. The psychiatric unit for geriatric patients also must attend to the needs of patients' community caregivers (Schulz, Martire, & Klinger, 2005). Discharge planning also must focus on the complex array of community social services for geriatric patients and planning the patient's interface with these services. The mean length of stay for older adults is almost twice as long as that of non-geriatric adults in inpatient psychiatric programs (National Association of Psychiatric Health Systems [NAPHS], 2009) (for further discussion on older adults, please see Chapter 10 in this volume).

EATING DISORDERS UNIT

Patients with eating disorders, typically adolescent and young adult women, present with both severe physical and psychological problems. Morbidity and mortality are high among patients with these disorders, arguably higher than for any other category of psychiatric disorders (Hoek, 2006). The indication for hospital admission is typically body weight that is less than 85% of healthy weight for age and height in an individual with an eating disorder or rapid weight decline secondary to marked food restriction or refusal (Halmi & Brandt, 2008). Reversing the weight loss, stabilizing the patient's medical status, and reducing the suicidality of the patient are all goals of the eating disorder unit (Commerford, Licinio, & Halmi, 1997). Limitations in the insurance benefit for inpatient treatment may present a problem if the mental health benefit is for only 30 days inpatient care per year and the patient remains severely emaciated at the end of that time period. An intensive day treatment program may be offered to patients, discharging them from inpatient care, given the long-term trajectory of eating disorder behavioral problems and the need to continue the supervision of eating and weight after the end of the inpatient stay.

SUBSTANCE ABUSE, DUAL DIAGNOSIS UNIT

The main treatment goal on this type of "co-occurring" unit is to effectively treat patients who have both psychiatric and substance use disorders in an integrative fashion. Careful assessment is needed to determine the interaction between the psychiatric and the substance abuse problems. Detoxification from the substance of abuse may be complicated, especially for patients with a history of delirium tremors or seizures (Kosten & O'Connor, 2003). Additional problematic clinical issues with this population include excess risk of violent behavior, violent victimization, criminal legal problems, and the risk of blood-borne infections such as HIV (Scott et al., 1998; Laudet, Magura, & Vogel, 2000). In addition, patients may have limited motivation to change their substance use and may be additionally stigmatized by their substance abuse, in addition to their psychiatric problems. Barriers in the service delivery systems may include separate funding streams for the two types of disorders and limited availability of integrated treatment (see Chapter 12 in this volume for additional material regarding co-occurring addictive and mental disorders).

CHILD AND ADOLESCENT UNITS

Child and adolescent units typically fall within the crisis stabilization model. Such units aim to provide short-term acute inpatient care for patients with dangerous or alarming psychiatric symptoms that cannot be managed elsewhere. There is a strong ethos of not separating children or adolescents from their families and communities for lengthy periods, and treatment is focused on discharge to home-based services. In the early years of this decade, the average length of stay in child inpatient programs was 11.7 days, and 8.8 days for adolescent inpatient programs (NAPHS, 2003); by 2007 these mean lengths of stay had increased to 12.2 days for child and 10.2 days for adolescent inpatient programs (NAPHS, 2009). One problem with a short hospital stay may be the unavailability of intensive outpatient services to complement inpatient services (Pottick et al., 2001).

Most children are admitted to a child unit because of aggressive and combative behavior that is escalating and out of control and cannot be managed by parents or other caregivers (Blader & Jensen, 2007). One major difference between the specialty child unit and other kinds of psychiatric units is that referrals to the child unit may be made by family courts or child welfare authorities in order to address questions related to children's disposition or special care needs. On child units, a developmental perspective must be taken into account and an assessment made of the child's psychiatric problems in the context of expected cognitive and social growth.

On the adolescent unit, special issues arise related to confidentiality that involve a delicate balancing of the adolescent's privacy interests with the parents' right to know about diagnosis and treatment. Suicide risk must be assessed in every admission. Controversy exists about the possible increased risk of suicidality secondary to treatment with antidepressant selective serotonin reuptake inhibitors (SSRIs) medications. This issue has not been fully resolved within the clinical and regulatory community (Gibbons, Hur, Bhaumik, & Mann, 2006). For additional discussion of children and adolescents, please see Chapter 8 in this volume.

PSYCHOTIC DISORDERS UNIT

Patients with schizophrenia and other psychotic disorders were historically the focus of inpatient psychiatry. During the last several decades as de-institutionalization coalesced with managed care, the care of patients with persistent psychotic disorders has largely moved to community settings. Hospitalization is reserved for acute exacerbations of symptoms with accompanying problems related to dangerousness or neglect of self-care. The goal of a hospital stay is crisis stabilization with the aim of providing optimal treatments with an understanding of the patient's illness in the community context to which the patient will return (Boronow, 2008). That context includes social (family, friends, care providers, outpatient treatment team members), historical (precipitators of relapse or noncompliance, motivators of positive change, response to past treatments), economic (available therapeutics of all sorts, from medications to Programs of Assertive Community Treatment, or PACT teams), and legal (restraining orders, criminal charges, mandated treatment orders) considerations.

TRAUMA DISORDERS UNIT

This type of specialized unit is predominantly focused on persons with psychiatric problems and post-traumatic stress disorder (PTSD) secondary to severe childhood maltreatment. Such specialty units are rare. The therapeutic work is directed toward the emotionally intense recollection and processing of trauma memories so that these memories are relegated to the status of the past rather than being re-lived in flashbacks, re-experiencing phenomena, or dissociative states (Loewenstein, 2006). These patients tend to be among the most difficult encountered in the inpatient setting.

Services Closely Affiliated with Psychiatric Hospitals/Units

EMERGENCY DEPARTMENTS

Patients with primary psychiatric disorders now comprise at least 8% of all emergency department visits (Larkin et al., 2005). Increased utilization of emergency services has followed from reductions in the number of inpatient psychiatric beds and the barriers to gaining admission to such beds through managed care authorization and review (McAlpine & Mechanic, 2000). At the same time that hospital psychiatric beds decreased in number, emergency department visits for mental disorders increased from 1.4 million visits in 1992 to nearly 2.5 million in 2003 (Salinsky & Loftis, 2007).

In the emergency department, assessment of the patient is aimed at determining if the person should be admitted to the hospital or discharged; appropriate determination is crucial and may have far-reaching consequences (Allen et al., 2003). There are many accounts of emergency rooms that are backed up with patients waiting sometimes for days for inpatient placement. On average, psychiatric patients remain in hospital emergency departments more than twice as long as other patients and staff have to spend twice as long looking for beds for psychiatric patients (Salinsky & Loftis, 2007). The problem is particularly acute for children given the few specialty psychiatric beds available for them (NAPHS, 2003). The surge in emergency department visits for mental illness affects access to emergency medical care for all patients, not just those with a mental illness.

Partial or Day Hospitals

These settings serve as alternatives to or "step-downs" from inpatient care. While in principle alternatives to inpatient care are attractive to patients and to payers, such settings have been affected by the same economic forces as inpatient beds. Many partial hospital programs have closed or have had to limit the number of patients they can accept. This trend is attributable to administrative costs due to Medicare regulations, fewer payers for partial hospital services, and pressures from managed care organizations to find lower-cost alternatives (NAPHS, 2003).

Long-Term Residential Treatment Programs

Long-term residential facilities include nursing homes and large group homes. A recent federal report noted 63 different types of facilities in 34 states (Torrey et al., 2008). There are a lack of good data on these types of facilities, so the extent to which they serve as alternatives to hospital settings is difficult to determine (Ireys, Achman, & Takyi, 2006). One recent survey indicated that the number of residents in nursing homes with a primary diagnosis of mental illness has been declining, especially for those under age 65 (Mark et al., 2007).

Policy Issues

Evidence-based practice (EBP) or evidence-based medicine (EBM) refers to a decision-making process in which the clinician endeavors to determine the best treatment for an individual patient or group of patients by reviewing the available research; expert clinician opinion may also be informative. While seemingly straightforward, interpretation of the evidence may be complicated when the body of evidence includes findings that are inconsistent, does not apply all to the exact parameters of clinical practice, or contains studies that may be biased. A second principle of evidence-based practice, and one which has been promulgated more recently, is that clinical decisions must attend not only to the best available evidence, but also to the values and preferences of the informed patient. Values and preferences refer not only to patients' beliefs and wishes, but also to the processes individuals use to consider treatment options. Progress in the field of shared decision making, the evolution of the patient rights movement, and the wide availability of information on the Internet have contributed to the implementation of this principle (Montori & Guyatt, 2008).

In contrast with evidence-based practice, the term evidence-based treatment (EBT) or empirically supported treatment (EST) refers to preferential use of mental and behavioral health interventions for which systematic empirical research has provided evidence of statistically significant effectiveness as treatments for specific problems. In psychiatry, practice guidelines have been published which contain the compilation of available evidence for specific treatments for specific disorders. For example, the American Psychiatric Association has published guidelines about schizophrenia, Alzheimer's disease and other dementias, bipolar disorder, and other conditions that are often treated in hospital settings (American Psychiatric Association [APA], 2009). It is important to note that these guidelines are not focused on treatment in the hospital or any other specific treatment setting, but of the psychiatric condition. Pressure toward EBT has also come from health insurance providers, which have sometimes refused coverage of practices that are not deemed to be evidence-based.

Apart from considerations of evidence-based treatment, constraints imposed by third-party payers remain a major policy issue in the provision of inpatient psychiatric care. Authorization review and utilization management are necessary for access to hospital care, and the objective of these practices is cost containment (Sharfstein, 1990). The effect has resulted in a limitation in the number of, and access to, psychiatric beds. A 2006 survey of state mental health authorities revealed that over 80% of the states reported a shortage of psychiatric beds; 34 states reported a shortage of acute care beds; and 16 states reported a shortage of long-term care beds (Salinsky & Loftis, 2007).

Efforts at cost containment on the part of the third-party payers have also led to reductions in the payment for hospital services to the point that third-party reimbursement for health care costs is not keeping up with hospital costs (Liptzin, Gottlieb, & Summergrad, 2007). There is a concern about what inpatient psychiatric services can do to survive. If reimbursement is not available to support the existing beds, then more will be expected to close and there may be a further reduction in the number of beds (as has been the case since 1990). Unless there are sufficient alternatives in the community to hospital stays, at some point the decrease in supply will fall below the demand for these services and reimbursement rates will have to rise to encourage an expansion in the number of beds. Without adequate alternatives for acutely ill patients in crisis, the demand for beds will escalate.

Costs shifting from local/state to federal monies also continue more than 50 years after the start of de-institutionalization. In recent years, there have been further closures of state hospitals leading to an all-time low in the number of public psychiatric beds (Torrey et al., 2008). Reductions in state hospital beds also create more pressure on the private sector to provide these sought-after services.

An increase in homelessness is one consequence of the massive emptying of the state hospitals that has taken place over the past 50 years. In 2005, it was estimated that approximately 500,000 persons were homeless in the United States at any one time (Brubaker, 2007); at least one-third of these individuals have severe mental illness. It is noteworthy that at any given time, there are many more people with severe mental illness living on America's streets than are receiving care in hospitals. These individuals are at heightened risk for violent victimization and for premature death due to both natural and unnatural causes (Torrey, 1988).

Another consequence of de-institutionalization and the shortage of psychiatric hospital beds is the trans-institutionalization of individuals with mental illness from the psychiatric to the criminal justice systems (Torrey et al., 2008). At least 7–10% of inmates in jails and prisons have severe mental illness, with estimates as high as 20%. The three largest de facto psychiatric institutions in the United States are jails: the Los Angeles County Jail; Chicago's Cook County Jail; and New York City's Rikers Island Jail. While some efforts may be made to provide treatment of individuals with mental disorders in criminal justice settings, the available resources for such treatment are limited, and in addition, prisons and jails are very poor treatment settings. In response to this disturbing trend, mental health courts have been developed to provide specialized adjudication for persons with mental illness who commit relatively minor crimes and may be persuaded to accept outpatient psychiatric treatment in the context of the court sentencing process (McNiel & Binder, 2007). However, there are few such specialized court programs in the United States. The problem of persons with mental illness in jails and prisons has also led to advocacy for more public psychiatric beds, although an overall increase has not occurred.

Although President Bush's New Freedom Commission on Mental Health focused primarily on outpatient community-based services that are needed to provide access to quality care, the report did recognize that acute care inpatient services are an essential part of the mental health care continuum (New Freedom Commission on Mental Health, 2003). Hospital psychiatric treatment does not necessarily represent a clinical failure; in fact, an acute hospital stay may provide an opportunity for the patient to receive intensive services that can change the course of treatment and the trajectory of the disorder (Glick et al., 2003). The need for inpatient psychiatric care is clear and compelling. Hospitalization with 24-hour nursing care provides the opportunity to evaluate, diagnose, and stabilize complex mental illnesses that are often comorbid with other psychiatric and medical problems. Such treatment is needed by a small but significant number of patients.

Implications and Future Challenges for Mental Health

Economic problems and barriers remain major challenges to the provision of hospital psychiatric treatment. Persons in need of inpatient care are disproportionately poor and under- or un-insured, and when such individuals have insurance coverage, it tends to be highly managed. The federal parity legislation (Paul Wellstone and Pete Domenici Mental Health Parity and Addiction Equity Act, 2008) which went into effect in January 2010 may reduce some barriers to hospital treatment in that it requires group health plans to provide mental health and substance abuse coverage on par with medical and surgical benefits. However, these plans will likely use medical management techniques to restrict inpatient stays to the narrowest definition of "medical necessity."

Even with the passage of parity legislation, the trends to lower reimbursement rates and shorter lengths of hospital stay are likely to continue, which makes it difficult to deliver high quality care (NAPHS, 2003). In addition, the costs of care continue to increase while payments often fail to keep pace. Major factors that contribute to the increased costs of care include workforce shortages and the need for more doctors and nurses; skyrocketing professional liability insurance; pharmaceutical costs; and increasingly complex regulatory requirements.

Another major challenge to the delivery of care in specialty hospitals and psychiatric units is the ongoing stigma associated with mental health care, especially in the hospital setting. In the past, individuals and families often have been ashamed to admit to psychiatric problems, and their treatment has been seen as somehow less deserving than for other medical conditions. However, brief inpatient psychiatric stays that are similar to stays for other medical or surgical conditions, or are provided in a general hospital setting, contribute to the lessening of stigma (Verhaeghe, Bracke, & Bruynooghe, 2007). Modern psychiatric units have private rooms and baths and other amenities that normalize a psychiatric admission, similar to other medical admissions. However, there are reminders that psychiatric units are different from other medical units, and such factors may contribute to stigma. For example, psychiatric units are invariably locked; sometimes persons on psychiatric units require seclusion or restraint; some persons coming into psychiatric units are admitted involuntarily, against their wishes, or on the basis of an emergency petition or other court order.

All of the U.S. states have statutes permitting persons to be civilly committed based upon their posing a danger to self or others and having a diagnosable mental illness. The definition of dangerousness varies among the states and may include the inability to care for oneself (Treatment Advocacy Center, 2008). Civil commitment statutes require a court hearing and specified review procedures if the person is to be hospitalized more than briefly. These legal safeguards have been instituted to help balance the deprivation of personal liberty and the prevention of harm to self or others.

Another major challenge for hospital psychiatric care is assessing and reducing the risk of patients' harming themselves in the hospital setting. "Dangerousness to self" is among the most common precipitants of urgent psychiatric evaluation, and many inpatients are hospitalized because of a recent suicide attempt or current suicidal ideation and intent. Once patients are hospitalized, the risk of suicide often persists (Busch, Fawcett, & Jacobs, 2003; Powell et al., 2000). Of the 30,000 suicides that occur annually in the United States, it is estimated that 1,500 occur in the hospital (APA, 2003), in some instances while patients are on the highest level of suicide observation (Busch et al., 2003). Of the "sentinel events" reported to the Joint Commission since 1995, only "wrong site surgery" has been reported more frequently than inpatient suicide (Joint Commission, 2007). Thus, it is extremely important that steps be taken to minimize the risk of suicide in the hospital. This requires building physical environments that are safe yet interpersonally warm; creating therapeutic milieus that provide support and restore hope; and performing suicide risk assessments to identify individuals at particularly high risk for suicide in the hospital so that special preventive measures can be instituted.

A final consideration for hospital units concerns a renewed emphasis on the role of the patient, known as "the consumer" in this context, in the delivery of mental health services (Halpern et al., 2008). This renewed emphasis is consistent with the principle of attending to patient preferences in evidence-based practice. Psychiatric hospitals serve a crucial role in the lives of individuals with psychiatric crises; yet until recently, these specialized hospitals and hospital units rarely involved their patients' experience and feedback in conceptualizing, designing, or improving care. The second goal of the President's New Freedom Commission on Mental Health (2003) defines an exemplary mental health system as one in which input and participation from consumers and family members inform clinical care at all levels of the mental health service system, including psychiatric hospital units. As the culture of welcoming consumer input and promoting a recovery orientation takes hold, material progress can be made toward the Freedom Commission's vision.

Another part of the paradigm shift to recovery is the fact that hospitals that rely solely on the medical model tend to focus primarily on pathology and disease (Mead, Hilton, & Curtis, 2001) and define outcomes in terms of symptom elimination and a return to pre-morbid functioning. This model of illness may be self-defeating because it may undermine hope, which has been described by advocates and consumer-leaders as a cornerstone of recovery (Deegan, 1988). Consumers of mental health services face many challenges in terms of social attitudes, low social status, and prejudice. However, attitudes are improving along with the knowledge that major mental illness is highly prevalent and that persons from all walks of life can have a mental illness at any time in their lives. The challenge is to integrate the best of the consumer recovery movement into the medical service model. The resulting synthesis can continue to improve the quality and experience of care at psychiatric hospitals/units.

References

Allen, M. H., Currier, G. W., Hughes, D. H., Docherty, J. P., Carpenter, D., Ross, R., (2003). Treatment of behavioral emergencies: A summary of the expert consensus guidelines. *Journal of Psychiatric Practice, 9*, 16–38.

American Psychiatric Association. (2003). *Practice Guideline for the Assessment and Treatment of Patients with Suicidal Behaviors* (p. 12). Washington, DC: APA Press.

American Psychiatric Association. (2009). *Practice Guidelines.* Available online at http://www.psych. org/psych_pract/treatg/pg/prac_guide.cfm. Accessed April 22, 2009.

Arias, E., Anderson, R. N., Kung, H. C., Murphy, S.,L., Kochanek, K., D. (2003). Deaths: Final data for 2001. *National Vital Statistics Reports, 52*, 1–115.

Blader, J. C., & Jensen, P. S. (2007). Aggression in children: An integrative approach. In A. Martin & F. R. Volkmar (Eds.), *Lewis' Child and Adolescent Psychiatry: A Comprehensive Textbook* (4th ed.). Baltimore, MD: Lippincott, Williams, & Wilkins.

Blank, K., Hixon, L., Gruman, C., Robison, J., Schwartz, H,I. (2005). Determinants of geropsychiatric inpatient length of stay. *Psychiatric Quarterly, 76*, 195–212.

Boronow, J. (2008). The psychotic disorders unit. In S. S. Sharfstein, F. B. Dickerson, & J. M. Oldham (Eds.), *Textbook of Hospital Psychiatry* (pp. 119–134). Washington, DC: American Psychiatric Publishing.

Brubaker, B. (2007, March 1). HUD study of homeless quantifies the problem. *Washington Post.*

Busch, K. A., Fawcett, J., & Jacobs, D. G. (2003). Clinical correlates of inpatient suicide. *Journal of Clinical Psychiatry, 64*, 14–19.

Colenda, C. C., Mickus, M. A., Marcus, S. C., Tanielian, T. L., Pincus, H. A. (2002). Comparison of adult and geriatric psychiatric practice patterns: Findings from the American Psychiatric Association's practice research network. *American Journal of Geriatric Psychiatry, 10*, 609–617.

Commerford, M. C., Licinio, J., & Halmi, K. A. (1997). Guidelines for discharging eating disorder patients. *Eating Disorders, 5*, 69–74.

Deegan, P. E. (1988). Recovery: The lived experience of rehabilitation. *Psychosocial Rehabilitation Journal, 11*, 11–19.

Deutsch, A. (1948). *The Shame of the States: Mental Illness and Social Policy; The American Experience.* New York: Harcourt Brace & Co.

Foley, D. J., Manderscheid, R. W., Atay, J. E., Maedke, J., Sussman, J., Cribbs, S. (2004). Highlights of organized mental health services in 2002 and major national and state trends. In R. W. Manderscheid & J. T. Berry (Eds.), *Mental Health, United States, 2004.* Rockville, MD: Substance Abuse and Mental Health Services Administration, Center for Mental Health Services.

Gibbons, R. D., Hur, K., Bhaumik, D. K., & Mann, J. J. (2006). The relationship between antidepressant prescription rates and rate of early adolescent suicide. *American Journal of Psychiatry*, *163*, 1898–1904.

Glick, I. D., Carter, W. G., & Tandon, R. (2003). A paradigm for treatment of inpatient psychiatric disorders: From asylum to intensive care. *Journal of Psychiatric Practice*, *9*, 395–402.

Goffman, E. (1961). *Asylums: Essays on the Social Situation of Mental Patients and Other Inmates.* New York: Doubleday.

Halmi, K., & Brandt, H. A. (2008). The eating disorder unit. In S. S. Sharfstein, F. B. Dickerson, & J. M. Oldham (Eds.), *Textbook of Hospital Psychiatry* (pp. 89–101). Washington, DC: American Psychiatric Publishing.

Halpern, L., Trachtman, H. D., & Duckworth, K. (2008). From within: A consumer perspective on psychiatric hospitals. In S. S. Sharfstein, F. B. Dickerson, & J. M. Oldham (Eds.), *Textbook of Hospital Psychiatry* (pp. 237–244). Washington, DC: American Psychiatric Publishing.

Hoek, H. W. (2006). Incidence, prevalence, and mortality of anorexia nervosa and other eating disorders. *Current Opinion in Psychiatry*, *19*, 389–394.

Ireys, H., Achman, L., & Takyi, A. (2006). *State Regulations of Residential Facilities for Adults with Mental Illness.* Rockville, MD: Center for Mental Health Services, Substance Abuse and Mental Health Services Administration.

Joint Commission. (2007). *Sentinel Event Statistics*. Available online at http://www.jointcommission.org/SentinelEvents/Statistics/. Accessed September 18, 2009.

Kesey, K. (1962). *One Flew over the Cuckoo's Nest.* New York: Viking.

Kosten, T. R., & O'Connor, P. G. (2003). Management of drug and alcohol withdrawal. *New England Journal of Medicine*, *348*, 1786–1795.

Larkin, G. L., Claassen, C. A., Emond, J. A., Pelletier, A. J., Camargo, C. A. (2005). Trends in U.S. emergency department visits for mental health conditions, 1992 to 2001. *Psychiatric Services*, *56*, 671–677.

Laudet, A. B., Magura, S., & Vogel, H. S. (2000). Recovery challenges among dually diagnosed individuals. *Journal of Substance Abuse Treatment*, *18*, 321–329.

Liptzin, B., Gottlieb, G. L., & Summergrad, P. (2007). The future of psychiatric services in general hospitals. *American Journal of Psychiatry*, *164*, 1468–1472.

Liptzin, B., & Summergrad, P. (2008). Financing of care. In S. S. Sharfstein, F. B. Dickerson, & J. M. Oldham (Eds.), *Textbook of Hospital Psychiatry* (pp. 403–409). Washington, DC: American Psychiatric Publishing.

Loewenstein, R. J. (2006). A hands-on clinical guide to the stabilization phase of dissociative identity disorder treatment. *Psychiatric Clinics of North America*, *29*, 305–332.

Manderscheid, R. W., Atay, J. E., & Crider, R. A. (2009). Changing trends in state psychiatric hospital use from 2002 to 2005. *Psychiatric Services*, *60*(1), 29–34.

Manderscheid, R., Atay, J. E., Male, A., Blacklow, B., Forest, C., Ingram, L., et al. (2002). Highlights of organized mental health services in 2000 and major national and state tends. In R. J. Manderscheid & M. Henderson (Eds.). *Mental Health, United States, 2002*. Rockville, MD: Substance Abuse and Mental Health Services Administration.

Mark, T. L., Levit, K. R., Buck, J. A., Coffey, R. M., Vandivort-Warren, R. (2007). Mental health treatment expenditure trends, 1986–2003. *Psychiatric Services*, *58*, 1041–1048.

McAlpine, D. D., & Mechanic, D. (2000). Utilization of specialty mental health care among persons with severe mental illness: The roles of demographics, need, insurance, and risk. *Health Services Research*, *35*, 277–292.

McNiel, D. E., & Binder, R. L. (2007). Effectiveness of a mental health court in reducing criminal recidivism and violence. *American Journal of Psychiatry*, *164*, 1395–1403.

Mead, S., Hilton, D., & Curtis, L. (2001). Peer support: A theoretical perspective. *Psychiatric Rehabilitation Journal*, *25*, 134–141.

Mechanic, D., McAlpine, D., & Olfson, M. (1998). Changing patterns of psychiatric inpatient care in the United States, 1988–1994. *Archives of General Psychiatry*, *55*, 785–791.

Montori, V. M., & Guyatt, G. H. (2008). Progress in evidence-based medicine. *Journal of the American Medical Association, 300*(15), 1814–1816.

National Association of Psychiatric Health Systems. (2003). *Challenges Facing Behavioral Health Care.* Washington, DC: Author.

National Association of Psychiatric Health Systems. (2009). *2008 Annual Survey: Behavioral Healthcare Today.* Washington, DC: Author.

National Association of State Mental Health Program Directors Medical Directors Council (with J. Parks, D. Svendsen, & P. Singer et al. [Eds.]). (2006). *Morbidity and Mortality in People with Serious Mental Illness, 13th Technical Report.* Alexandria, VA: National Association of State Mental Health Program Directors Medical Directors Council.

New Freedom Commission on Mental Health. (2003). *Achieving the Promise: Transforming the Mental Health Care in America, Final Report.* DHHS Pub. No. SMA–03-3832. Rockville MD: Author.

Paul Wellstone and Pete Domenici Mental Health Parity and Addiction Equity Act, PL–110-343, Title V, Subtitle B (2008). Available online at http://frwebgate.access.gpo.gov/cgi-bin/getdoc. cgi?dbname=110_cong_public_laws&docid=f:publ343.110.pdf. Accessed February 24, 2009.

Pottick, K. J., Barber, C. C., Hansell, S., Coyne, L. (2001). Changing patterns of inpatient care for children and adolescents at the Menninger Clinic, 1988–1994. *Journal of Consulting and Clinical Psychology, 69,* 573–577.

Powell, J., Geddes, J., Deeks, J., Goldacre, M., Hawton, K. (2000). Suicide in psychiatric hospital in-patients. *British Journal of Psychiatry, 176,* 266–272.

Reed, L. S. (1975). *Coverage and Utilization of Care for Mental Conditions under Health Insurance— Various Studies, 1973–74.* Washington, DC: American Psychiatric Association.

Salinsky, E., & Loftis, C. (2007). Shrinking inpatient psychiatric capacity: Cause for celebration or concern? *National Health Policy Forum, 823,* 1–21.

Schulz, R., Martire, L. M., & Klinger, J. N. (2005). Evidence-based caregiver interventions in geriatric psychiatry. *Psychiatric Clinics of North America, 28,* 1007–1038.

Scott, H., Johnson, S., Menezes, P., Thornicroft, G., Marshall, J., Bindman, J., et al. (1998). Substance misuse and risk of aggression and offending among the severely mentally ill. *British Journal of Psychiatry, 172,* 345–350.

Sharfstein, S. S. (1990). Utilization management: Managed or mangled psychiatric care? *American Journal of Psychiatry, 147,* 965–966.

Szasz, T. (1961). *The Myth of Mental Illness: Foundations of a Theory of Personal Conduct.* New York: Paul B. Hoeber.

Torrey, E. F. (1988). *Nowhere to Go: The Tragic Odyssey of the Homeless Mentally Ill.* New York: Harper & Row.

Torrey, E. F., Entsminger, K., Geller, J., Stanley, J., Jaffe, D. J. (2008). *The Shortage of Public Hospital Beds for Mentally Ill Persons.* Arlington, VA: Treatment Advocacy Center.

Treatment Advocacy Center. (2008). *Standards for Assisted Treatment: State by State Summary.* Available online at http://www.treatmentadvocacycenter.org/LegalResources/statechart.htm. Accessed April 24, 2008.

Verhaeghe, M., Bracke, P., & Bruynooghe, K. (2007). Stigmatization in different mental health services: A comparison of psychiatric and general hospitals. *Journal of Behavioral Health Services Research, 34,* 186–197.

Chapter 16

EVOLUTION AND INTEGRATION OF PRIMARY CARE SERVICES WITH SPECIALTY SERVICES

Ronald W. Manderscheid, PhD

Introduction

American mental health care is currently in a period of rapid change that is moving the field ever so slowly toward effective integration with primary care services (Druss et al., 2007, especially the detailed citations; Wang et al., 2007). This change is occurring within a 250-year context of isolation in which the mental health field operated independently of primary care.

Beginning in the colonial period, mental health care was considered to be a local responsibility (see Grob, 1994, 2008). Subsequent to the American Revolution, it was considered to be a state responsibility. Primary care, by contrast, was never considered to be either a local or a state responsibility. As such, these patterns fostered the evolution of a separately organized state mental hospital system and separate disciplines to care for the patients who were sent there. It is fair to say that, until the founding of the National Institute of Mental Health (NIMH) in 1949, the major mental health leaders in the United States came from this separately organized state mental hospital system.

At the time of the founding of NIMH, many in the field expressed the need for a separate Institute and separate services (Grob, 1991). They feared that the mental health field would not be able to survive and compete with a more robust primary care field. In subsequent years, this same rationale was used to justify a growing budget for a separately organized NIMH, as well as for new programs created by the U.S. Congress, such as community mental health centers, which themselves were envisioned and implemented as separately organized services. When the service and training components of NIMH were transferred to a new Substance Abuse and Mental Health Services Administration (SAMHSA), one of the units of the

U.S. Department of Health and Human Services, in 1992, the pattern of separately organized federal functions was retained and reinforced through a separate Community Mental Health Services Block Grant. To the present day, federal, state, and local mental health functions are separately organized and operate in parallel with primary care services.

There are two essential reasons to seek integration of mental health and primary care services at the present time. First, many public mental health consumers need, but do not receive, primary care services for their physical health problems. Second, many primary care providers are not trained appropriately to deliver high quality specialty mental health services. Each of these reasons will be explained further in the next section of this chapter.

The purpose of this chapter is to explore the growth of mental health service delivery in the primary care sector in recent years, as well as the process of integration that has begun between the mental health and primary care fields. Throughout the chapter, the author will also consider substance use care services. The fields of mental health and substance use care have worked much more closely together during the past two to three years (Manderscheid, 2008; also note the activities of the Whole Health Campaign at www.wholehealthcampaign.org).

Developing a Perspective on Primary Care Services

Because national data on primary care services for mental health and substance use conditions are incomplete at best, it is necessary to rely on national community epidemiological survey data to set an overall context on the use of primary care services. Once this overall perspective is presented, then it will also be useful to add additional detail from national data on some of the key service settings where primary care services are offered.

The National Comorbidity Survey Replication (NCS-R), conducted in 2003, shows that about 9.3% of the adult population age 18 and older received primary care services in a one-year period for mental and substance use conditions (Wang et al., 2007). This rate translates into about 20.6 million adults. By contrast, specialty services were received by 8.8% of the adult population, or 19.5 million persons. Hence, the primary care sector served 1.1 million more adults for mental and substance use conditions in 2003 than did the specialty sector.

The NCS-R findings also show that, of those who received primary care services for mental and substance use conditions, about 12.6 million had a mental or substance use diagnosis in the year in which they received services, while the remainder did not. By contrast, the parallel figure for specialty services was 12.0 million adults with diagnoses in the year during which services were received. The rate of those with diagnoses served in the two settings was equivalent, approximately 61%. These findings do not suggest however, that those without diagnoses should not have received care. Some had symptoms that were becoming more severe, but did not yet meet diagnostic criteria. Others had symptoms that were becoming less severe and had fallen below diagnostic criteria. Nevertheless, this group without diagnoses is very large, more than 15.1 million adults across the specialty and primary care sectors. It will not be possible to track this phenomenon into the national service databases because diagnostic data in the NCS-R are based upon research diagnostic criteria, while those in treatment settings are based upon the professional judgment of individual clinicians. Obviously, the two are not always likely to agree. Although it is badly needed, very little research has examined the care of persons without diagnoses of mental or substance use conditions (see Chapter 7 in this volume for additional information on the epidemiology of mental disorders).

The critical trend to remember from these data is that the primary care sector is currently serving a larger number of persons with mental and substance use conditions than is the specialty sector. There are several reasons why this is the case. Many people prefer the primary care sector over the specialty sector because of the stigma associated with use of the latter, or simply because they like to see "their doctor." Further, in many rural and poverty areas, specialists are simply not available to provide services.

Primary care services are offered in a range of settings. The National Center on Health Statistics (NCHS) (see www.cdc.gov/nchs/), Centers for Disease Control and Prevention (CDC), one of the units of the U.S. Department of Health and Human Services, collects data from all types of ambulatory care settings: individual and group practices; hospital outpatient departments; and hospital emergency departments. Although a small portion of the care provided in these settings may be given by specialists, the vast majority of care is provided by primary care physicians.

Two Cases for Better Integration between Primary Care and Specialty Services

The first reason for integrating mental health and primary care services is exceptionally compelling and particularly heart wrenching. In April 2006, Colton and Manderscheid (2006) published a study which shows clearly that public mental health clients on average die 25 years younger than other Americans. Previous research suggests that this health disparity has increased rather than decreased over the past 15 to 20 years (McCarrick, Manderscheid, Bertolucci, Goldman, & Tessler, 1986). Between 15 to 20 years of the disparity are attributable to heart and circulatory disorders, diabetes, or other chronic diseases which are very prevalent in the elderly. Some second generation antipsychotic medications can lead to metabolic effects that can trigger these chronic diseases. Often these problems are aggravated by co-occurring substance use conditions. Frequently, these disorders can be controlled or even prevented with quality health care. Yet many public mental health care recipients do not receive appropriate physical health care for such disorders. By contrast, only 5 to 10 years of the disparity can be attributed to mental disorders per se, such as suicide.

The findings on premature death have led to a broad range of actions across the mental health care field. The National Association of State Mental Health Program Directors (NASMHPD) issued a policy paper on steps that state agencies can take to address this severe problem (available at www.nasmhpd.org). Central to these state efforts are basic screening and treatment for the chronic diseases and their precursors: high blood pressure; obesity; diabetes; and heart disease. NASMHPD has more recently issued additional papers on smoking, psychotropic medications, suicide, and screening (all of which are also available at the NASMHPD web site).

The Center for Mental Health Services (CMHS) at SAMHSA also is focusing attention on this crisis. In 2007, the CMHS Consumer Affairs Program hosted a Wellness Summit specifically to address this problem (see the overview of the Summit at www.bu.edu/cpr/). At the suggestion of the federal center, the assembled group issued a national call to action: reduce the disparity in life expectancy by 10 years within the next 10 years ("10 by 10"). Participants also pledged to improve consumer wellness through major field initiatives.

Papers from this Summit have already been published (Manderscheid & Delvecchio, 2008). In the first of these papers, Everett, Mahler, Biblin, Ganguli, and Mauer (2008) found that practice improvement can be addressed by examining the risk factors associated with early death that, if managed appropriately, could make the biggest impact on the health of mental health care recipients.

In a second paper, Swarbrick, Hutchinson, and Gill (2008) examine the need for training to promote optimal health for mental health care recipients. Effective health promotion and wellness strategies must be made an integral part of treatment so that care recipients and family members can access necessary knowledge and technology to ensure a normal lifespan. To accomplish this goal, curriculum redesign is needed in all mental health disciplines and in the allied health professions.

Finally, Manderscheid, Druss, and Freeman (2008) examine data availability and deficits surrounding the crisis of premature death. The fundamental need is for the federal government to collect mortality data on a continuing basis through the state mental health agencies. Beyond this basic need, no available datasets include longitudinal designs or combine high-quality data including psychiatric diagnosis, health risk behaviors, medical comorbidity, medical and mental health service use, and quality of care.

The Primary Care–Behavioral Health Learning Community initiative of the National Council for Community Behavioral Healthcare (NCCBH) is designed to implement healthy lifestyle approaches in local community mental health centers (see www.nccbh.org). Also, consumer self-help and peer-support programs across the nation are enlisting in the CMHS effort (see the Web site of the National Coalition of Mental Health Consumer/Survivor Organizations at www.ncmhcso. org). Primary care partners need to be identified who will work with the mental health field to address public mental health care recipients' chronic health problems through integrated care that embraces these fields.

The second reason for integrating mental health, substance use, and primary care services is equally compelling. Frequently, mental health and substance use services delivered by primary care physicians lack necessary quality because primary care physicians and their nursing assistants are not adequately trained to recognize or treat mental health and substance use conditions appropriately. For many primary care providers, this training deficiency extends to lack of knowledge about appropriate psychotropic medications and dosages for particular disorders. Many primary care physicians receive at most three to five hours of training in mental health or substance use care throughout their residencies.

The findings regarding the quality of primary care services are particularly compelling. A good summary of these findings, with detailed references, has been presented by deGruy (1996). Multiple studies cited by deGruy (1996) document that from one-third to two-thirds of care recipients meeting the criteria for a mental disorder are unrecognized in primary care settings. Part of this problem is due to the fact that many mental health and substance use care recipients present with somatic problems. In some instances, this miscoding is deliberate to meet reimbursement requirements or to avoid the stigma associated with a diagnosis of a mental disorder. Multiple studies cited by deGruy (1996) also document that many persons with mental disorders, even when recognized, are not offered appropriate care that would meet the requirements of an evidence-based practice. This may involve wrong medications, wrong dosages, or wrong durations of medication. A related factor leading to these problems is the pace of primary care practice. Most care recipients are seen for no longer than 10 to 15 minutes, which is minimally sufficient to establish rapport, but inadequate to delve into complex problems. Finally, the structure of services delivery and reimbursement systems can inhibit good quality care.

Integration of Specialty and Primary Care

It is now almost 60 years since the decision was reconfirmed nationally and enshrined in the structure of the new NIMH to promote mental health care and later substance use care as fields that operate separately from primary care. This decision may have been quite appropriate during the early years of NIMH in order to foster the full development of fields that were struggling at the time. However, as early as 1999, *Mental Health: A Report of the Surgeon General* (U.S. Department of Health and Human Services, 1999) called for the integration of specialty and primary care services. This call to action was echoed in rapid succession by the report of the President's New Freedom Commission on Mental Health, *Achieving the Promise* (New Freedom Commission on Mental Health, 2003), and by the Institute of Medicine (IOM) report, *Improving the Quality of Health Care for Mental and Substance Use Conditions* (Committee on Crossing the Quality Chasm, 2006). Each of these major reports argues that good mental health and good health are mutually essential and that good health care must treat the whole person, both mind and body.

The Surgeon General's report was concerned with the scientific underpinnings of the mental health care field. This report found that mental health care has a good scientific basis, with evidence-based practices rooted in scientific research, and that the next step that needs to be taken by the mental health field is the integration of specialty and primary care.

In December 2000, the Surgeon General hosted a Working Meeting on the Integration of Mental Health Services and Primary Health Care at the Carter Center. This meeting of leaders from the mental health and substance use care fields resulted in a Working Meeting Report that details a set of principles to guide action on moving the field forward and a set of action steps to be carried out by the federal government (this report is available at www.surgeongeneral.gov, click on Surgeon General Collection at the National Library of Medicine, then The Reports of the Surgeon General, then Workshops (seminars)). Many of the recommendations from this meeting anticipated the content and recommendations of the subsequent reports discussed below.

The report of the President's New Freedom Commission focused principally on the problems of fragmentation and the resultant lack of quality in the delivery of mental health care. The very first recommendation in this blue-ribbon report was the integration of specialty and primary care. Subsequently, the IOM report presented a blueprint for addressing the fragmentation in care, especially at the mental health, substance use, and primary care interface. Overall, the IOM blueprint was intended to improve the quality of health care for mental and substance use conditions.

Since its release in 2006, the IOM report has had a growing impact upon the mental health and substance use care fields. At the time of its release, an informal national leadership group was developed to promote reforms leading to care integration. This work has led to proposed federal legislation to remove financial and human resource barriers collaboration with the American Academy of Family Practitioners and the creation of the Whole Health Campaign, in which the mental health and substance use care fields have agreed to pursue common joint goals (see www.wholehealthcampaign.org). Also, in 2006, 2007, and 2008, the American College of Mental Health Administration featured integration issues and strategies in its annual Santa Fe Summit (see www.acmha.org, click on Summit Reports).

Models of Care Integration

Several models predominate among the types of integration between mental health, substance use, and primary care. These models are 1) integration of specialty services into primary care programs; 2) a consumer directed medical home; 3) integration of primary care services into specialty programs; and 4) collaborative care models. Below, the author will describe these models further and provide some concrete examples. An excellent summary of developments in this area, *Making the Case for Collaboration: Improving Care at the Behavioral and Primary Healthcare Interface*, by Mauer and Druss (2007), is available at www.acmha.org under Summit Reports for 2007.

INTEGRATION OF SPECIALTY SERVICES INTO PRIMARY CARE PROGRAMS

In this model, specialty providers, services, and programs are incorporated into primary care programs. A very large-scale example of this is the incorporation of specialty services into the Federally Qualified Health Centers (FQHCs). Since 2000, FQHCs have been at the forefront of building specialty services by including specialty providers into ongoing primary care clinical operations.

FQHCs are funded through the Health Resources and Services Administration (HRSA), a unit of the U.S. Department of Health and Human Services. They have emerged as one of the principal primary care settings in which specialty services are offered (Druss et al., 2006). In approximate terms, the federal funding for the FQHCs has grown from about $1 billion in 2000 to more than $2 billion in 2007 (www.hrsa.gov, and click on Primary Health Care).

The author has provided a separate analysis of FQHCs in this chapter because of their growing importance as a primary care service site for treating mental health and substance use conditions, their growth as a primary care site in which most specialty care is provided by mental health or substance use care specialists, their growing importance as a service site for persons without health insurance, and the remarkable overall growth of the program since 2000.

Data from HRSA (presented in Figure 16.1) show that the prevalence of depression in FQHCs increased dramatically between 1995 and 2002 (Feetham, McCombs, Daly, & Engram, 2004). The smallest increase observed was 6% for all care recipients age 18+, while the largest increase was 16% for males. These growth rates assume even more importance when coupled with the fact that mental health and substance use encounters in FQHCs nearly doubled during this period.

A related observation is also important. In 2003, more than 2.8 million visits to FQHCs were related to mental or substance use conditions. Of this number, slightly more than 2.3 million visits, or about 81%, were seen by a specialist. Background data on FQHCs show that these numbers grew dramatically between 1996 and 2003. The FQHCs are the most pointed national example of the movement of specialty services and providers into a primary care setting.

Another frequently cited example of the integration of specialty services into primary care is that of Intermountain Health Care (IHC) in Utah (Reiss-Brennan, Briot, Cannon, & James, 2006). IHC serves as the care provider for more than half of the population of Utah.

Approximately a decade ago, IHC recognized that a significant number of care recipients who came to IHC primary care clinics were suffering from depression. This recognition was accompanied by another realization untreated depression also had a negative impact upon the effectiveness of other primary care treatments. Subsequently, IHC began a sequenced process of integrating specialty services into all of its primary care clinics. Results have been exceptional: Care has been shown to be effective and cost has been controlled (Reiss-Brennan et al., 2006).

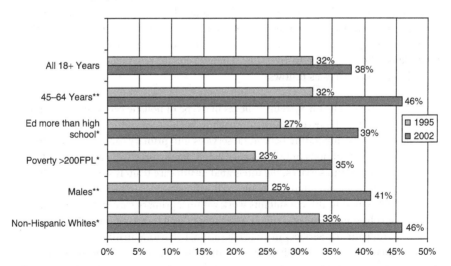

Figure 16.1 Percent of Federally Qualified Health Center Patients with Selected Characteristics Reporting Depression, 1995 and 2002, from FQHC User Visit Surveys. (Adapted from Feetham, McCombs, Daly, and Engram (2004).)

Consumer-Directed Medical Home

The recovery movement in mental health and substance use care has led to several exciting developments that can collectively be called a consumer-directed medical home. The essence of this model can be summarized in a few words: person centered and consumer directed. Person centered means that care is focused on all of the person's needs, without consideration of artificial disciplinary or program boundaries. Hence, the care can focus on all of a person's health conditions. Consumer directed means that the care is controlled and guided by the consumer, in collaboration with a provider. Specific features may include joint planning of care and shared decision-making between consumer and provider, as well as consumer directed payment for care (Alakeson, 2007; Manderscheid, 2007).

Just a little reflection will show how person-centered and consumer-directed care permits integration of mental health, substance use, and primary care. Stated simply, care integration occurs uniquely for each person depending upon that person's health care needs. Viewed in this way, the question of integration within a program becomes secondary. Thus, it should also be clear that a consumer-directed medical home can be operated in a virtual or a programmatic environment. Good conceptual background pieces on this model have been published by CMHS (2005) and by Cook and Jonikas (2002). The latter document includes a broad range of specific examples (also see Chapter 20 in this volume on the recovery movement).

Integration of Primary Care Services into Specialty Programs

At one level, this model can be viewed as the recreation in a community-based ambulatory program of the integrated mental health, substance use, and primary care services of a traditional state mental hospital. The most obvious way this integration can occur is when a community mental health center also becomes a FQHC, so that both types of services are available to center care recipients. A very good example is Cherokee Health Systems. Their Web site (www.cherokeehealth.com) describes their services as follows:

> Cherokee Health Systems believes in a type of holistic care called Integrated Care. This biopsychosocial approach to health care addresses the whole person by integrating behavioral services into primary care. By combining the best traditions of primary care (adult, family practice, pediatric) and mental health services, the integrated health care team is able to treat the whole person—mind and body so all patient needs are met.
> Behavioral health consultants work within a primary care setting and are involved in on site and timely assessment, brief intervention and consultation with patients. Services include education, behavioral management and treatment for mental health disorders. After meeting with a physician or nurse, a psychologist may assess and treat patients with behavioral concerns and work with the medical provider regarding referral questions and follow-up.
> (Cherokee Health Systems, 2007, p. 1)

COLLABORATIVE CARE PROGRAMS

As their name implies, the collaborative care model involves programs that remain separate, yet work together. In this model, specialty services and primary care services may be operated by different entities and may be located at different sites. Frequently, a care coordinator is available to assure that care recipients actually receive the specialty and primary care services that are needed. Of the four models, this one is the closest to the traditional pattern of separated specialty services prevalent at the present time. Research shows that collaborative care programs may be more appropriate for some types of care recipients than for others (Terry & Taylor, 1999).

The Wellness Model: A Conceptual Framework for Integrated Care

A Wellness Model, developed more than a quarter-century ago, provides a conceptual framework for helping to understand the need for integration of mental health, substance use, and primary care services (Ng, Davis, Manderscheid, & Elkes, 1981; Manderscheid, 2006). The Wellness Model is presented in Figure 16.2. In this model, illness and wellness are conceptualized as two separate, independent dimensions of health. Illness refers to disease, while wellness refers to one's outlook, social supports, and self-care activities. When combined, these two dimensions frame two strategies for achieving recovery and good health: traditional biopsychosocial interventions and lifestyle changes through improved self-help. Two separate paths are

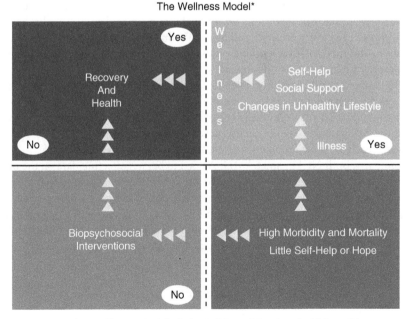

Figure 16.2   The Wellness Model. (Adapted from Manderscheid [2006].)

required to address these two dimensions—one directed toward physical health problems and the other directed toward wellness problems. Good health and well-being demand that attention be given to both. This joint approach can be achieved by integrating primary care and specialty services.

Implications for Mental Health

Several major implications emerge from this review of the specialty care–primary care interface.

- The specialty care–primary care interface is in rapid flux. Because of the problem of premature death of public mental health care recipients, specialty providers are under intense pressure to make primary care services available. On the other hand, primary care providers have witnessed a very rapid increase in the number of mental health care recipients, particularly persons with depression. In many instances, these providers are not fully equipped to deal with these clients. Hence, a need exists for primary care providers to work much more closely with specialty providers.
- New operational approaches are emerging about how the specialty and primary care fields can work together more closely. These new approaches express every possible relationship between the fields: integration in both directions, virtual integration, and collaboration without integration. Hence, it is probably a mistake to assume that a single approach will emerge and predominate. In the future, it is likely that the full range of approaches will be used.
- Mental health and substance use care recipients have yet to fully express their opinion about integration of specialty care and primary care. As they do, it seems clear that they will favor and promote the consumer directed medical home approach. Recovery efforts based on the Wellness Model that combines psychosocial and medical interventions with strategies that promote hope are likely to become a major part of this approach.
- To plan effectively, behavioral health care needs improved data on the care that persons with mental health and substance use conditions receive in primary care settings. Such data are gradually beginning to emerge through NCHS. However, more comparable data are needed across settings on record diagnoses, specific care received, including medications, and disposition after initial care.
- Similarly, both NCHS and SAMHSA need to begin collecting data on the organizational arrangements between specialty care and primary care organizations, their staffing patterns, and their referral patterns. Very little of these organizational data currently exist. Collection of such data would promote both increased understanding about the current dynamics of care and increased understanding about the new organizational forms that are currently emerging.

Conclusion

Overall, it seems very clear that integration between mental health, substance use, and primary care services can address important service needs of care recipients.

For this reason alone, expect major growth in efforts to offer integrated services in the future. Undoubtedly, these efforts not only reflect recipients' needs but also partially reflect the coming of age of mental health and substance use care as full and equal partners in the health care world. This partnership is to be welcomed because it also signals an increased focus on quality and outcome of care. Care recipients can only benefit from these important developments.

References

Alakeson, V. (2007). *Putting Patients in Control: The Case for Extending Self*-Direction *into the NHS.* London: Social Market Foundation.

Center for Mental Health Services. (2005). *Transforming Behavioral Health Care to Self Direction: Report of the 2004 Consumer Direction Initiative Summit.* Available online at www.samhsa.gov. Accessed August 11, 2009.

Cherokee Health Systems. (2007). *Integrated Care.* Available online at http://www.cherokeehealth. com/index.php?page=About-Us-Integrated-Care. Accessed August 11, 2009.

Colton, C. W., & Manderscheid, R. W. (2006) Congruencies in increased mortality rates, years of potential life lost, and causes of death among public mental health clients in eight states. *Preventing Chronic Disease, 3*(2). Available online at http://www.cdc.gov/pcd/issues/2006/apr/05_0180.htm. Accessed August 11, 2009.

Committee on Crossing the Quality Chasm: Adaptation to Mental Health and Addictive Disorders. (2006). *Improving the Quality of Healthcare for Mental and Substance Use Conditions.* Washington, DC: Institute of Medicine.

Cook, J. A., & Jonikas, J. A. (2002). Self determination among mental health consumers/survivors. *Journal of Disability Policy Studies, 13*(2), 88–96.

deGruy, F. (1996). Mental health care in the primary care setting. In M. S. Donaldson, K. D. Yordy, K. N. Lohr, & N. A. Vanselow (Eds.), *Primary Care: America's Health in a New Era* (pp. 285–311). Washington, DC: Institute of Medicine.

Druss, B. G., Bornemann, T., Daniels, E., Fry-Johnson, Y. Manderscheid, R. W., Rust, G., et al. (2007). The primary care/behavioral health interface. In R. W. Manderscheid & J. T. Berry (Eds.), *Mental Health, United States, 2004* (pp. 106–116). Rockville, MD: U.S. Department of Health and Human Services.

Druss, B. G., Bornemann, T., Fry-Johnson, Y. W., McCombs, H. G., Politzer, R. M., & Rust, G. (2006). Trends in mental health and substance abuse services at the nation's community health centers. *American Journal of Public Health, 96*(10), 1779–1784.

Everett, A., Mahler, J., Biblin, J., Ganguli, R., & Mauer, B. (2008). Improving the health of mental health consumers. *International Journal of Mental Health, 37*(2), 8–48.

Feetham, S., McCombs, H., Daly, C., & Engram, L. (2004, November 9). *Expanding and Improving Mental Health, Drug, and Alcohol Services in Primary Care Health Centers.* Presentation at the BPHC Invited Panel, American Public Health Association Annual Meeting.

Grob, G. N. (1991). *From Asylum to Community: Mental Health Policy in Modern America.* Princeton, NJ: Princeton University Press.

Grob, G. N. (1994). *The Mad among Us: A History of the Care of America's Mentally Ill.* New York: Free Press.

Grob, G. N. (2008). *Mental Institutions in America: Social Policy to 1875.* New York: Transaction Books.

Manderscheid, R. W. (2006). Saving lives and restoring hope. *Behavioral Healthcare, 26*(9), 58–59.

Manderscheid, R. W. (2007). Asking Peter to empower Paul. *Behavioral Healthcare, 27*(7), 46–47.

Manderscheid, R. W. (2008). Join the whole health campaign. *Behavioral Healthcare, 28*(4), 68.

Manderscheid, R. W., & Delvecchio, P. (Eds.). (2008). Mortality and wellness. *International Journal of Mental Health, 37*(2), 88.

Manderscheid, R. W., Druss, B., & Freeman, E. (2008). Data to manage the mortality crisis. *International Journal of Mental Health, 37*(2), 49–68.

Mauer, B. J., & Druss, B. G. (2007). *Making the Case for Collaboration: Improving Care at the Behavioral and Primary Healthcare Interface.* Background paper commissioned for the 2007 American College of Mental Health Administration Summit, Mind and Body Reunited. Available online at www.acmha.org. Accessed August 11, 2009.

McCarrick, A. K., Manderscheid, R. W., Bertolucci, D. E., Goldman, H. H., & Tessler, R. C. (1986). Chronic medical problems in the chronically mentally ill. *Hospital and Community Psychiatry, 37*(3), 289–291.

New Freedom Commission on Mental Health. (2003). *Achieving the Promise: Transforming Mental Health Care in America: Final Report.* DHHS Pub. No. SMA-03-3832. Rockville, MD: Author.

Ng, L. K. Y., Davis, D. L., Manderscheid, R. W., & Elkes, J. (1981). Toward a conceptual formulation of health and wellbeing. In L. K. Y. Ng & D. L. Davis (Eds.), *Strategies for Public Health: Promoting Health and Preventing Disease* (pp. 44–58). New York: Van Nostrand Reinhold.

Reiss-Brennan, B., Briot, P., Cannon, W., & James, B. (2006). Mental health integration: Rethinking practitioner roles in the treatment of depression; The specialist, primary care physicians, and the practice nurse. *Ethnicity and Disease, 16*(2, Suppl. 3), 37–43.

Swarbrick, P., Hutchinson, D. S., & Gill, K. (2008). The quest for optimal health: Can education and training cure what ails us? *International Journal of Mental Health, 37*(2), 69–88.

Terry, S. P., & Taylor, D. A. (1999). The effectiveness of collaborative care between primary care providers and mental health providers on distressed high utilizers. *Abstract Book, Association of Health Services Research Meeting, 16,* 185.

U.S. Department of Health and Human Services. (1999). *Mental Health: A Report of the Surgeon General, Executive Summary.* Rockville, MD: U.S. Department of Health and Human Services, Substance Abuse and Mental Health Services Administration, Center for Mental Health Services, National Institutes of Health, National Institute of Mental Health.

Wang, P. S., Lane, M., Olfson, M., Pincus, H. A., Schwent, T. L., Wells, K. B., et al. (2007). The primary care of mental disorders in the United States. In R. W. Manderscheid & J. T. Berry (Eds.), *Mental Health, United States, 2004* (pp. 117–133). Rockville, MD: U.S. Department of Health and Human Services.

Chapter 17

SCHOOL MENTAL HEALTH

Mark D. Weist, PhD; Robert W. Burke, PhD; Carl E. Paternite, PhD; Julie Goldstein Grumet, PhD; and Paul Flaspohler, PhD

Overview

Based on perceptions of mutual benefit and a commitment to reform, education and mental health (along with other child-serving delivery) systems are joining together to build more comprehensive school mental health services. These "expanded" programs involve provision of a full continuum of mental health promotion and intervention in schools for youth in general and special education toward the achievement of outcomes valued by families and schools. There has been considerable development in the school mental health (SMH) field over the past few decades, with a major emphasis on a public health approach that also resonates with priorities of schools. This chapter reviews key themes in the SMH national (and international) movement, in dimensions of background, current status, challenges, and implications for mental health systems, with conclusions and recommendations.

Background

Innovations in education and in child and adolescent mental health are occurring at an increasing rate, which relates in part to enhanced linkages between these two systems as in school mental health programs and services (Burke & Paternite, 2007). Services are more likely to connect to the evidence base of what actually leads to enhanced outcomes, and interventions are expanding to places where children and youth are located: in their homes, schools, and communities (Greenberg et al., 2003; Ringeisen, Henderson, & Hoagwood, 2003).

However, in spite of this progress, epidemiologic data continue to suggest a very large gap between children and adolescents who need and receive effective mental health services (U.S. Department of Health and Human Services [USDHHS], 1999; U.S. Public Health Service [USPHS], 2000; President's New Freedom Commission on Mental Health [PNFC], 2003). For example, at least 20% of youth present emotional/behavioral disorders at levels that could lead to diagnosis, but less than one-third receive any services (Marsh, 2004; Leaf, Schultz, Kiser, & Pruitt, 2003). Further, for the small percentage of youth who do receive mental health services, most receive them within schools (Rones & Hoagwood, 2000; USDHHS, 1999) (see Chapters 6 and 7 in this volume for additional information on the epidemiology of mental disorders and Chapter 8 in this volume on children and adolescents).

In response to this large gap between children's unmet mental health needs and the provision of effective services to address them, increasing numbers of mental health programs and services are being developed and implemented in schools across the United States and around the world (Foster, Rollefson, Doksum, Noonan, & Robinson, 2005; Rowling & Weist, 2004; see the International Alliance for Child and Adolescent Mental Health and Schools, www.intercamhs.org). These programs have emerged from increasing recognition that 1) traditional community systems (e.g., community mental health centers and private practices) are not reaching enough youth in need; and 2) schools are typically under-resourced to effectively promote the mental health of students and to address the full spectrum of their needs (Weist, 1997).

The importance of school mental health is supported by major policy initiatives in the United States, including the reports of the Surgeon General (USDHHS, 1999; USPHS, 2000) and the Achieving the Promise Initiative (PNFC, 2003), the second presidential commission on mental health and the first in 30 years. In fact, the Achieving the Promise Initiative has as one of its 19 recommendations to "improve and expand school mental health programs" (recommendation 4.2).

In the remainder of the chapter, three salient themes critical to advancing SMH are presented: 1) description of the current state of school mental health, including approaches and evidence for effectiveness; 2) review of challenges to SMH, including those related to ideology, implementing preventive and evidence-based services, policy development, and financing; and 3) implications and recommendations for mental health in the United States, with concluding comments and recommendations.

Current Status of School Mental Health

This section includes the following themes related to school mental health: 1) overview of program and service characteristics; 2) key national study on service characteristics; and 3) empirical support.

Overview of Program and Service Characteristics

There are many approaches to SMH, with a large proportion of programs and services being offered by school-employed staff such as school psychologists, counselors, and social workers, as well as other staff including school nurses, and educators focused on behavioral issues (Flaherty et al., 1998). In addition, prominent developments within education systems are increasing emphasis on mental health issues. For example, Response to Intervention (RTI) is a major movement focusing on making decisions about student learning and placement needs based upon ongoing assessment of learning rate and level of performance (as compared to an approach involving periodic "testing"). It emphasizes screening for problems, data-based decision making and problem-solving, ongoing progress monitoring, and evidence-based practices (National Center on Response to Intervention, 2009; Sugai, 2009), as well as within-school collaboration between different service agents, including educators, family members, and mental health staff (Ehren, Montgomery, Rudebusch, & Whitmire, 2006). Another example is provided by the No Child Left Behind legislation (2002), which provides a number of opportunities to build mental health promotion and intervention in schools, including provisions related to early identification and intervention, using evidence-based practices, and providing training and support to teachers as promoters of positive student behavior (Anglin, 2003; Daly et al., 2006).

The term *expanded school mental health* (Weist, 1997; Weist, Paternite, & Adelsheim, 2005) refers to those programs and services that incorporate recognized best practices that include the following elements: 1) authentic partnerships among families, schools, and community agencies; 2) effective collaborative relationships among school-employed mental health staff and community-employed mental health professionals working in schools; 3) dedicated commitment to a public health model that includes mental health education, promotion, assessment, prevention, early intervention, and treatment; and 4) provision of services for *all* students, including those enrolled in general and special education classrooms. Thus, expanded school mental health (ESMH) implies an *augmentation* of the programs and services typically found in most schools (e.g., the roles and responsibilities assumed by school-employed staff such as psychologists, social workers, counselors, and school nurses).

Further, within ESMH, attention is directed toward establishing effective collaboration among schools and community entities (e.g., mental health centers, health departments, and university-affiliated centers). This is related to the recognition that K-12 public schools should not be expected to be the sole providers of comprehensive mental health and other social services. Indeed, it is often the case that schools are overburdened with demands that would be more appropriately addressed by other community delivery systems. Strong connections between schools and community organizations also help communities move toward establishing a comprehensive system of care (Leaf et al., 2003). An additional advantage of the ESMH framework is that it facilitates other essential elements such as interdisciplinary collaboration, engagement of families and other stakeholders, continuous quality assessment and improvement, and assurance of culturally competent practices and services that are empirically supported (Weist, Paternite et al., 2005).

In addition to mental health services delivered by school-employed staff and these "expanded" programs, there are many other programs in schools involving mental health. A very prominent approach is Positive Behavior Support, a framework that uses a systems approach to promote positive school climate and student behavior, which is broadly being used in schools across the country (Sugai et al., 2000; see www.pbis.org). In addition, programs training students in social emotional learning (SEL) skills, often integrated into education curricula, are growing substantially (Greenberg et al., 2003; Zins, Weissberg, Wang, & Walberg, 2004; see www.casel.org).

Further, some schools are able to implement more formal research supported programs, such as Promoting Alternative Thinking Strategies (a very notable SEL program; Kusché & Greenberg, 1994), the Good Behavior Game (Dolan, Jaylen, Werthamer, & Kellam, 1989), and Anger Coping (Lochman, Lampron, Gemmer, & Harris, 1987). Many of these programs are listed on the National Registry of Evidence-Based Practices and Programs (NREPP) Web site of the Substance Abuse and Mental Health Services Administration (http://www.nrepp.samhsa.gov). However, implementation of these programs requires a range of supports, including strong training, technical assistance, on- and off-site coaching, fidelity monitoring and feedback, and administrative support, elements commonly not available in schools or in SMH programs unless there is connection to a grant or special initiative (see Fixsen, Naoom, Blase, Friedman, & Wallace, 2005).

Another mechanism for the delivery of mental health services is through school-based health centers (SBHCs), which offer a range of health services to students (e.g., treatment of acute illnesses and accidents, management of some chronic illnesses, immunizations, and sports physicals). School-based health centers operate in over 1,700 schools across 44 states and Puerto Rico, serving approximately 1.7 million enrolled students annually (Brown & Bolen, 2003; National Assembly on School-Based Health Care, 2006), and they are increasingly providing comprehensive mental health care (Weist, Goldstein, Morris, & Bryant, 2003). Studies of SBHC service utilization demonstrate that mental health counseling has been identified as the leading reason for visits by students, representing approximately one-third to one-half of all visits (Center for Health and Health Care in Schools, 2001). In many ways, embedding SMH within SBHCs is an ideal arrangement involving interdisciplinary collaboration between health and mental health staff to address mental health issues, including those that often co-occur with health issues (e.g., increased anxiety among students with asthma) (Hacker & Wessel, 1998; Papa, Rector, & Stone, 1998).

Student Assistance Programs (SAPs) also represent a method to provide mental health services to students in schools. Student Assistance Programs (SAPs) provide school-based services to students displaying academic, behavior, and/or attendance concerns as a result of substance abuse, mental health, and/or social issues (California Student Assistance Program Resource Center, 2009). Initial models of SAPs mirrored their professional counterparts, Employee Assistance Programs, with an emphasis on targeting students at-risk for or affected by substance abuse (Texas Student Assistance Program Initiative, 2009). In response to growing mental health concerns, the model was expanded to include services for student substance abuse and mental health needs (Commonwealth Student Assistance Program Interagency Committee, 2004). These programs often have a focus on helping students contending with substance abuse issues, but increasingly are also addressing mental health concerns.

KEY NATIONAL STUDY ON SERVICE CHARACTERISTICS

In 2002–2003, the Center for Mental Health Services of the Substance Abuse and Mental Health Services Administration (SAMHSA) conducted a landmark study on characteristics of school mental health programs and services in the United States. During this study, 1,147 schools and 1,064 districts across the country responded to a survey that included a comprehensive array of questions about SMH services (Foster et al., 2005). Specifically, schools and districts were asked to respond to questions about presenting problems of students and the availability of school mental health services to help address those concerns, administrative arrangements and coordination for providing services, characteristics of school mental health providers, and funding strategies and challenges. Findings indicated the most prevalent problems facing both male and female students were social, interpersonal, and family problems. For males, aggression and disruptive behavior and behavior problems followed closely behind, whereas for females, these were anxiety and adjustment issues. The most common services provided by schools included assessment for mental health problems, behavioral management consultation, crisis intervention, and referrals to specialized programs. Further, more than two-thirds of schools reported providing individual counseling, case management, and group counseling. Schools reported curriculum and classroom-based social/emotional skills interventions as being the most successful strategies in providing mental health services to their students, with family support services being among the most difficult to deliver. School counselors, nurses, school psychologists, and social workers were the most common personnel providing school mental health services, and close to half of the districts reported having collaborated with an outside agency to provide these services. The most frequently reported funding sources for mental health services in schools were the Individuals with Disabilities Education Act (IDEA) and state special education funds. Funding sources for prevention services specifically were Title IV, local funds, and state general funds. It is important to note that although 69% of districts reported a greater need for mental health services from the previous year, only 29% reported having increased their mental health staff (Foster et al., 2005). While the survey documented a comprehensive array of mental health services offered in U.S. schools, clearly the depth of services could be enhanced in almost all schools (see Teich, Robinson, & Weist, 2007).

EMPIRICAL SUPPORT

The "evidence base" of SMH programs and services includes dimensions of service quality, such as access, stigma, and burden. Along these dimensions, there is supportive evidence. For example, supporting *access*, Catron, Harris, and Weiss (1998) found that 96% of youth started SMH services as compared to only 13% whose families were offered services in more traditional community settings such as community mental health centers (CMHCs). The World Health Organization (1995) concluded that schools may be the most "sensible point of intervention" for mental health services. Burns et al. (1995) noted that schools are *the only source* of mental health services for two-thirds of youth with diagnosable disorders and for nearly half of students with severe emotional disabilities (also see Rones & Hoagwood, 2000).

Nabors and Reynolds (2000), in a qualitative study of high school students receiving SMH, found that they perceived less stigma for school-based versus other community services. Atkins and colleagues pointed to the many benefits of an "ecological approach" to delivering mental health to youth in the natural setting of schools (e.g., Atkins, Adil, Jackson, McKay, & Bell, 2001).

There is some evidence that SMH programs also increase the likelihood of early problem identification. For example, Weist, Myers, Hastings, Ghuman, and Han (1999) found that youth with internalizing problems (such as depression and anxiety) receiving SMH services were less likely to have had prior mental health treatment than youth with these disorders receiving services within community mental health centers.

Other evidence supports advantages of SMH in enabling prevention programs (Elias, Gager, & Leon, 1997; Weare, 2000), enhancing interdisciplinary collaboration and the coordination of programs and services (American Academy of Pediatrics, 2004), and increasing the likelihood of generalization of intervention impacts across settings (Evans, Langberg, & Williams, 2003).

Note that all of the above reflects findings on *advantages of SMH as a service delivery approach*. A related agenda is the implementation of formal, evidence-based practices or research supported programs in schools. In the National Registry of Evidence-Based Programs and Practices (NREPP), the Substance Abuse and Mental Health Services Administration (SAMHSA) provides a "searchable database of interventions for the prevention and treatment of mental health and substance use disorders" (www.nrepp.samhsa.gov). All listed interventions have documented empirical support including an intensive review process by SAMHSA staff. Currently, 137 interventions are listed, with 48 appearing when the search term "schools" is used. Most of these interventions involve some level of cost, significant training, and ongoing coaching and support for their effective implementation, a significant level of infrastructure support that most SMH programs lack (see previous discussion, and Fixsen et al., 2005).

Thus, in discussing the "evidence base" for SMH, the most accurate summary is evidence that schools provide many advantages for the delivery of mental health promotion and intervention, and there are a number of evidence-based programs that are being implemented in schools. In addition, when services are done well across the above dimensions, it likely sets the stage for the implementation of research-supported interventions. While the authors have noticed a trend for some to do this, it is not substantiated to refer to SMH as an evidence-based approach. This theme of integrating evidence-based practice in schools is explored in more detail in the next section of this chapter.

Challenges

This section reviews critical challenges in the SMH field in the areas of 1) ideology; 2) implementing more preventive services; 3) implementing evidence-based practices; and 4) advancing supportive policy and expanded funding.

Ideology

An issue that constrains the scope of daily work for school-based providers stems from long-standing tenets underpinning theory and practice of "mental health" in the United States. In brief, professional training programs, service delivery approaches, and funding mechanisms built upon a fee-for-service model are based upon a practice perspective focused primarily on treating disorders that are presumed to exist within individuals (Weist & Paternite, 2006). Terms such as "psychopathology" perpetuate this view, suggesting that causality in problems lies within students.

Another set of conceptual challenges relates to the tenuousness of the relationships between school mental health service providers and educators reflecting competing political ideologies and agendas dating back to the creation of the first "common schools" in the United States (see Burke & Paternite, 2007). One unfortunate, long-standing consequence of the contentious political debate about public education is that the services of mental health professionals (e.g., social workers, psychologists, and counselors) have come to be thought of by educators as "add-ons" that are not central to the academic mission of schools (Sedlak, 1997; Paternite & Johnston, 2005; School Mental Health Alliance, 2005). From the perspectives of many stakeholders in school mental health and public education, there is an incompatibility between the "nonacademic" interests of mental health providers and the "academic" interests of educators (Staup, 1999). On a positive note, this trend seems to be changing, with more and more support for SMH from major child-serving delivery systems including education, mental health, juvenile services, and child welfare, as well as growing local, state, national, and international interest in the field (see Weist & Murray, 2007).

Implementing More Preventive Services

School mental health is increasingly embracing the triangular public health approach involving environmental enhancement at the base and progressing up with universal prevention, prevention, early intervention, intervention, and intensive treatment for highly challenged youth at the apex (see also the positive behavioral support model in Sugai et al., 2000). While this is the vision for the work, many programs encounter pressures to provide services to the most needy of students, which in many cases mitigates directly against promotion and prevention programs and services. A related challenge is that funding for SMH is tenuous, and existing funding mechanisms, such as public mental health services, often rely on fee-for-service mechanisms for youth with diagnoses (see discussion on funding that follows). Thus, related to unmet need and poor capacity in child mental health and the resultant press on SMH clinicians to provide intensive and often crisis services to high needs youth, as well as funding contingencies, the focus on promotion and prevention can be diminished or lost. Without diligence about dedicating time for preventive and mental health promotion efforts, school-based practitioners can easily drift toward the traditional model of providing primarily individual services for students with severe and/or chronic problems (Weist et al., 2005). In many cases, this is not a model of effective services. For example, active family involvement in services is generally associated with better outcomes for youth (Lowie, Lever, Ambrose, Tager, & Hill, 2003), and there are some circumstances where individual therapies are of limited or no benefit, such as with younger children who are presenting disruptive behaviors (see Weisz, Jensen-Doss, & Hawley, 2006).

IMPLEMENTING EVIDENCE-BASED PRACTICES (EBPs)

Despite recent advancements in promoting expanded mental health practices in schools, the field's research base lacks breadth and depth (DuPaul, 2007; Rones & Hoagwood, 2000). Currently, the development and delivery of evidence-based child mental health services stands out as the dominant research focus. Still limited, however, is research examining the effects of evidence-based services on everyday practice in school and community settings (Evans & Weist, 2004).

The promotion of effective mental health practices in schools extends beyond grand proclamations about the selection of specific "evidence-based" approaches, in part because most programs and services have not been examined for their effectiveness, palatability, durability, affordability, sustainability, and transportability for use in particular schools or clinics (Jensen, Hoagwood, & Trickett, 1999; Schoenwald & Hoagwood, 2001; Hoagwood, Burns, & Weisz, 2002; Weisz, 2004; Weisz, Chu, & Polo, 2004). Also contributing to the uncertainty about evidence-based practices is the dearth of research on diffusion, dissemination, and processes endemic to the widespread implementation of effective mental health practices (Silverman, Kurtines, & Hoagwood, 2004). Shirk (2004) observed that even the most studied mental health treatments for children and adolescents are "not quite ready for prime time" because they lack a knowledge base of effectiveness trials under clinically representative conditions. Shirk (2004) and others have suggested that treatments undergoing efficacy trials will need to be stretched, modified, or comprehensively reworked to achieve effectiveness in real-world clinics and schools. This point was emphasized by Ringeisen, Henderson, and Hoagwood (2003) who concluded that "unfortunately, the literature on 'evidence-based practices' in children's mental health pays insufficient attention to features of the school context that might influence intervention delivery" (p. 154). Thus, while strengthening SMH by infusing a public health policy and evidence-based practice framework has garnered considerable support among school mental health professionals (e.g., Duchnowski & Kutash, 2007; Forness, 2003; Friedman, 2003; Pianta, 2003), obvious by its absence is substantial support by teachers and school administrators, or, perhaps more importantly, parents and other patrons of local school districts across the United States.

Resolution of these issues may be achieved by incorporation of the community science model proposed by Wandersman (2003) and the deployment-focused model of intervention development and testing proposed by Weisz and colleagues (Weisz, 2004; Weisz et al., 2004). Because of the significant variability present in everyday clinical practice settings, both of these models suggest that *practice-based evidence* is an under-utilized resource in developing and delivering effective school- and community-based mental health services (Flaspohler, Anderson-Butcher, Paternite,

Weist, & Wandersman, 2006; Wandersman, 2003). The relevance of practice-based evidence emerged from suggestions that current models for implementing "evidence-based best practices" were not working as intended. Although there are several "evidence-based" programs available that address a wide range of problems and/or seek to prevent risk and/or promote protective factors, these programs often fail to deliver anticipated outcomes when widely implemented (e.g., Biglan & Taylor, 2000).

Successful implementation of evidence-based school mental health practices depends upon many factors including school (and community) support, resources, strong training of staff, technical assistance and coaching of staff, and "fidelity monitoring" of their efforts (see Graczyk, Domitrovich, & Zins, 2003; Domitrovich et al., 2008), supports that are found in research supported studies, but not usually found in schools. In this context, there is increasing emphasis on "achievable" EBPs in schools; an example of this is the work of Chorpita and colleagues (Chorpita, 2006; Chorpita & Daleiden, 2007; Chorpita, Taylor, Francis, Moffitt, & Austin, 2004) in empirically identifying and implementing the "common elements" associated with successful intervention and often found in manualized interventions.

Further, the promotion of EBP in SMH should not be done in isolation, but within a broader context and commitment to ongoing quality assessment and improvement (QAI). However, QAI research has been limited in the school mental health field (Weist et al., 2007). Although QAI approaches typically focus on bureaucratic processes (e.g., credentialing and paperwork) and/or liability protection, more substantive dimensions of quality have been articulated (Ambrose, Weist, Schaeffer, Nabors, & Hill, 2002; Evans, Sapia, Axelrod, & Glomb, 2002). A particular emphasis has been placed on articulating principles for best practice in the field, along dimensions such as active stakeholder involvement, cultural and developmental competence, strong planning and coordination of efforts, implementing a full continuum of promotion and intervention, emphasizing EBPs, and having strong program evaluation. Weist, Sander, and colleagues (2005) formalized these principles for SMH through a mixed methods (survey and key informant interviews) study (see Table 17.1) and also developed a measure for ongoing QAI: the School Mental Health Quality Assessment Questionnaire (SMHQAQ; see www.schoolmentalhealth.org).

Some critical dimensions of effectiveness in SMH involve achievable strategies for EBP, as above, and an emphasis on quality. Two other dimensions are family engagement and empowerment and implementation support. Hoagwood (2005), in a review of empirically supported approaches to working with families, presented four critical domains: 1) *Engagement*: establishing a connection with the family, addressing any concerns about services, and problem-solving on ways to overcome barriers for working together; 2) *Collaboration*: maintaining a collaborative, working together approach in developing and implementing services, and honoring the family's knowledge and voice; 3) *Support*: helping the family connect to supportive resources in the school and community (e.g., tutoring, job training, child care); and 4) *Empowerment*: helping the family to take control of challenges and to experience hope for positive outcomes.

Implementation support involves moving past limited "supervision" models in SMH (see Stephan, Davis, Burke, & Weist, 2006) toward models involving

Table 17.1   Ten Principles for Best Practice in School Mental Health

1. All youth and families are able to access appropriate care regardless of their ability to pay.
2. Programs are implemented to address needs and strengthen assets for students, families, schools, and communities.
3. Programs and services focus on reducing barriers to development and learning, are student- and family-friendly, and are based on evidence of positive impact.
4. Students, families, teachers, and other important groups are actively involved in the program's development, oversight, evaluation, and continuous improvement.
5. Quality assessment and improvement activities continually guide and provide feedback to the program.
6. A continuum of care is provided, including school-wide mental health promotion, early intervention, and treatment.
7. Staff hold to high ethical standards, are committed to children, adolescents, and families, and display an energetic, flexible, responsive, and proactive style in delivering services.
8. Staffs are respectful of and competently address developmental, cultural, and personal differences among students, families, and fellow staff.
9. Staffs build and maintain strong relationships with other mental health and health providers and educators in the school, and a theme of interdisciplinary collaboration characterizes all efforts.
10. Mental health programs in the school are coordinated with related programs in other community settings.

Source: Weist et al., 2005b.

strong training, ongoing behavioral rehearsal and feedback, technical assistance and administrative support, and emotional support (see Fixsen et al., 2005). A critical challenge in the field is to integrate these supports, often necessary to achieve valued outcomes, into schools (see Domitrovich et al., 2008).

Advancing Supportive Policy and Expanding Funding Mechanisms

Given that SMH is an emerging field with a general lack of depth in services across U.S. schools (Teich et al., 2007) and "patchy" progress related to federalism, or states' rights and local control that results in tremendous variability in progress from community to community (Weist, Paternite et al., 2005), there is a clear need to systematically improve and expand programs and services (PNFC, 2003). The federal government is playing a critical role in this improvement and expansion, with prominent federal grant initiatives that support SMH including Safe Schools/ Healthy Students, Coordinated School Health, Mental Health—Education System Integration, and School Mental Health Capacity Building (see Anglin, 2003; www. schoolmentalhealth.org).

In addition, states are increasingly investing in SMH. For example, 12 states supported by the IDEA Partnership (funded by the Office of Special Education Programs and housed at the National Association of State Directors of Special

Education; www.ideapartnership.org) and the University of Maryland, Center for School Mental Health (http://csmh.umaryland.edu) are purposefully building a shared school-family-community system partnership model for these programs and services. These states are a part of a National Community of Practice on Collaborative School Behavioral Health (see Wenger, McDermott, & Snyder, 2002) that also includes 12 practice groups promoting deeper involvement and interaction in key knowledge domains in the field (e.g., on SMH and systems of care, quality and evidence-based practice, family partnerships, positive behavior support, and youth leadership). The National Community meets annually in conjunction with the Center for School Mental Health's *Annual National Conference on Advancing SMH*, and community participants stay connected throughout the year via state and practice group teleconferences, e-mail, and an interactive Web site (www.sharedwork.org). The goal is to provide supportive and convening functions to promote multiscale learning (e.g., sharing among national organizations, federal agencies, states, and communities) and progression from discussion to dialogue to collaborative action and policy enhancement (Wenger et al., 2002).

While increasing federal support and national developments (noted above) are encouraging, the true challenge for building capacity for SMH is at the local and school building level. Here, programs are encountering a "catch-22" of increased demand for school-based services with insufficient funding and infrastructure support, which results in the tendency toward superficial, crisis driven services (Weist et al., 2007). As presented earlier in this chapter, in SAMHSA's comprehensive assessment of school mental health services in the United States over the 2002–2003 school year, demand for SMH was increasing, but funding was reported to be a particular challenge (Foster et al., 2005).

School mental health programs are funded by a range of resources, including federal and state special education funds, Title I (for economically challenged families), Safe and Drug Free Schools, allocations from school budgets, variable local and state dollars, funding from collaborating community systems such as fee-for-service for youth from the mental health system, and rare allocations from other delivery systems, such as juvenile services and child welfare (see Evans et al., 2003). It can be very difficult to navigate this patchwork of funding opportunities, and as a result, SMH programs potentially remain in a highly marginalized and tenuous status.

Often, the way forward is to provide high quality services that lead to outcomes that are valued by schools, families, community systems, and members. This presents another dimension of the "catch-22": to achieve these outcomes, a certain level of infrastructure support for recruiting the right staff, training them well, and providing ongoing coaching and support for high quality and evidence-based programs and services is required (Domitrovich et al., 2008; Fixsen et al., 2005; Weist et al., 2007). The authors have observed that when this infrastructure support is in place, programs can indeed grow and achieve sustainable, even expanding funding.

For example, SMH programs in Talbot County, Maryland, and Palm Beach County, Florida, have emphasized high quality, evidence-based services, have demonstrated improvements in valued outcomes, and now have strong community support, a stable funding base, and momentum to grow into additional schools (Weist et al., 2007). This reflects a critical need for the field: investing in fewer programs at a level where they can achieve valued outcomes, and then publicizing the experiences of these exemplary programs to build policy support for improvement (including deepening services) and expansion.

Implications for Mental Health

This final section briefly discusses the implications for mental health systems as they increasingly embrace the SMH agenda. This discussion is framed in relation to a community mental health system that is not connected to the schools but desires this connection. Progress would be driven by asking and answering a number of questions such as the following within planning meetings involving mental health system staff and with families and youth, schools, and other child-serving systems. Examples of questions would include:

1. What SMH programs and services are currently being implemented in the schools in this community and how could they be augmented?
2. What are the pressing needs of youth and families in the community and how can SMH best address these needs?
3. What are the perspectives of youth and families, child-serving systems staff educators, and others, and how can these perspectives genuinely shape the work that will follow?
4. How do we assure a full continuum of promotion and intervention and avoid a "co-located" arrangement of providing only intensive services for students with diagnoses?
5. How will we provide strong training for mental health staff on working effectively in schools, and how can we build interdisciplinary training to include educators, other school personnel, and family members?
6. How can we utilize professional development opportunities within schools to build this training agenda?
7. Which EBPs will we emphasize and how will we provide implementation support to assure their fidelity in implementation?
8. Which funding mechanisms will we use, and how will we balance demands of fee-for-service funding with other resources to allow staff to be in more preventive roles?
9. How will we continuously assess and improve the quality of services?
10. What strategies will be used to evaluate services on outcomes valued by schools, families, and community members, and how will outcome findings be used to improve and expand programs and services?

These are some of the major questions for community mental health systems to consider as they seek to collaborate with school systems in the development, improvement, and expansion of SMH programs and services. Context for this work is provided by the community science framework of Wandersman (2003) and colleagues (Chinman et al., 2005; Flaspohler et al., 2006). Community science is an interdisciplinary approach designed to strengthen community functioning by examining ways to realize the interrelated goals of a public health model (health promotion, education, prevention, and treatment) when programs and services are implemented in real-world settings. The community science approach moves beyond the dominant research-to-practice model of developing best practices (Mrazek & Haggerty, 1994) toward community-centered models. Community-centered models "begin with the community and ask what it needs in terms of scientific information and capacity-building to produce effective interventions" (Wandersman, 2003, p. 203). Community-centered models focus attention on local needs; regard "best practice" programs as process-oriented rather than problem-oriented; and prioritize local control and decision making by the community, its leaders, and stakeholders. It emphasizes local evaluation and self-monitoring and fluid adjustment of interventions in order to better respond to local needs and contexts (Flaspohler et al., 2006; Green, 2001; Backer, 2002).

Importantly, community science approaches involve key stakeholders (e.g., families, youth, education and other child-serving system leaders and staff, faith, and business leaders) in all phases of community innovation. Such an inclusive planning agenda, from early needs assessment and resource mapping to program evaluation and use of findings for policy impact, is fundamental to the growth of SMH initiatives. An illustrative example is presented below (from Weist et al., 2007).

Based upon a local needs assessment, a community decides to prioritize bullying prevention in the schools. A planning team, including all key stakeholder groups (education and mental health staff, families and youth, staff from other child-serving systems), conducts needs assessments and researches program options based upon the science base. As a result, the planning team chooses the Olweus program (Olweus, Limber, & Mihalic, 1999) and plans to implement the program in two local middle schools. Efforts are taken to tailor the program to the local community (a community-centered approach). As the program takes shape, there are ongoing quality assessment and improvement efforts, as well as meta-cognitive analyses ("thinking about thinking") of processes. For example, analyses of processes include attention to how meetings are held, leadership, genuine involvement of stakeholders, "take" of the intervention in the two schools, and engagement of youth participants. When processes appear to be moving in a negative direction, adjustments are made and processes are improved, in an iterative and continuously evolving manner (see Chinman et al., 2005).

Currently, the Center for School-Based Mental Health Programs at Miami University (Ohio; http://www.units.muohio.edu/csbmhp) and the Center for School Mental Health at the University of Maryland (http://csmh.umaryland.edu) are pursuing the interface between community science and school mental health, including the tracking of programs using this framework. Early experience suggests that this framework facilitates collaboration among the mental health system, schools, families, and other child-serving systems in the advancement of school mental health.

Conclusion and Recommendations

In most communities, traditional fee-for-service reimbursement mechanisms for mental health services can be rapidly applied within schools, and mental health systems are moving to provide treatment to youth in schools through the fee-for-service approach (Evans et al., 2003). However, doing the work well, as included in the dimensions reviewed above, is complicated and challenging. Thus, community systems may fail to take on this agenda because of either the complex challenges involved or the lure of maintaining the status quo by doing what is commonly done. Nevertheless, many community mental health delivery systems are successfully joining with their colleagues in schools to augment programs and services to create a full continuum of mental health promotion and intervention for youth in general and special education, framed in relation to the promotion of school success. There are many resources for this work (see Adelman & Taylor, 2000; Evans, Weist, & Serpell, 2007; Kutash, Duchnowski, & Lynn, 2006; Malti & Nome, 2008; Robinson, 2004; Weist, Evans, & Lever, 2003). As mentioned, there are also many relevant federal grant programs and pending legislation to expand federal support for SMH (e.g., the Mental Health in Schools Act, which would dramatically expand the Safe Schools/Healthy Students federal grant program).

What is needed at the community level is for a group of committed systems leaders and family advocates to step forward and be willing to convene planning meetings, following the community science framework. This initial step is often the most difficult, and the work of developing SMH is hardest in its early phases. However, progressive and even compelling progress is being made. For example, Baltimore has moved from four schools providing expanded SMH in 1989 to over 100 in 2009, and this is now a prioritized city initiative with stable and growing funding, a committed advisory group of city system leaders and stakeholders, a strategic plan, and a growing pool of braided funding from over six child-serving systems and philanthropic groups. Similar progress is being made in other communities (e.g., Charlotte, Chicago, and Cincinnati).

As mentioned, states, communities, national organizations, and practice groups are coming together in a National Community of Practice on Collaborative School Behavioral Health, and any organization or interested person can get involved through IDEA Partnership Communities of Practice (www.sharedwork.org).

School mental health is also an emerging international theme. For example, Australia, New Zealand, and many nations in Western Europe have established, as a priority in schools, mental health promotion strategies for all youth (Mrazek & Hosman, 2002; Rajala, 2001; Rowling, 2002). Further evidence of international interest in school mental health promotion can be found in the current work of groups such as the Clifford Beers Foundation, the World Federation for Mental Health, the International Union for Health Promotion and Education, and the Society for Prevention Research (Weist, Paternite et al., 2005). The International Alliance for Child and Adolescent Mental Health and Schools (www.intercamhs. org) is gaining strength, and global forums related to SMH have taken place in Minneapolis, Geneva, and Washington, DC.

Education and mental health systems have been working together for decades to build school mental health. The hope is that the promise of this work, as reviewed in this chapter, compels even greater mental health system involvement.

Acknowledgments

Please direct correspondence to Mark Weist, Center for School Mental Health, University of Maryland School of Medicine; mweist@psych.umaryland.edu.

Correspondence for co-authors: Robert Burke, burkerw@muohio.edu; Carl Paternite, paternce@muohio.edu; Julie Goldstein Grumet, julie.goldstein@dc.gov; and Paul Flaspohler, flaspopd@muohio.edu. We extend our sincere appreciation to Kerri Stiegler, Christianna Andrews, and Matthew Page of the Center for School Mental Health for help in conducting background research for this chapter.

References

Adelman, H. S., & Taylor, L. (2000). Promoting mental health in schools in the midst of school reform. *Journal of School Health, 70,* 171–178.

Ambrose, M. G., Weist, M. D., Schaeffer, C., Nabors, L. A., & Hill, S. (2002). Evaluation and quality improvement in school mental health. In H. Ghuman, M. D. Weist, & R. Sarles (Eds.), *Providing Mental Health Services to Youth Where They Are: School- and Community-Based Approaches* (pp. 95–110). New York: Brunner-Routledge.

American Academy of Pediatrics Committee on School Health. (2004). Policy statement: School-based mental health services. *Pediatrics, 113,* 1839–1845.

Anglin, T. (2003). Mental health in schools: Programs of the federal government. In M. D. Weist, S. W. Evans, & N. A. Lever (Eds.), *Handbook of School Mental Health Programs: Advancing Practice and Research* (pp. 89–106). New York: Springer.

Atkins, M., Adil, J., Jackson, M., McKay, M., & Bell, C. (2001). An ecological model for school-based mental health services. In *13th Annual Conference Proceedings: A System of Care for Children's Mental Health; Expanding the Research Base.* Tampa: University of South Florida.

Backer, T. (2002). *Evaluating Community Collaborations for Serving Youth at Risk: A Handbook for Mental Health, School, and Youth Violence Prevention Organizations.* Rockville, MD: Center for Mental Health Services.

Biglan, A., & Taylor, T. K. (2000). Why have we been more successful in reducing tobacco use than violent crime? *American Journal of Community Psychology, 28,* 269–302.

Brown, M. B., & Bolen, L. M. (2003). School-based health centers: Strategies for meeting the physical and mental health needs of children and families. *Psychology in the Schools, 40,* 279–287.

Burke, R. W., & Paternite, C. E. (2007). Teacher engagement in expanded school mental health. In S. Evans, Z. Serpell, & M. D. Weist (Eds.), *Advances in School-Based Mental Health* (vol. 2, pp. 21.1–21.15). Kingston, NJ: Civic Research Institute.

Burns, B. J., Costello, E. J., Angold, A., Tweed, D., Stangl, D., Farmer, E. M. Z., et al. (1995). Children's mental health service use across service sectors. *Health Affairs, 14*(3), 147–159.

California Student Assistance Program Resource Center. (2009). What is a student assistance program? Available online at http://casapresources.org/about/. Accessed August 24, 2009.

Catron, T., Harris, V. S., & Weiss, B. (1998). Post-treatment results after 2 years of services in the Vanderbilt school-based counseling project. In M. H. Epstein, K. Kutash, & A. Ducknowski (Eds.), *Outcomes for Children and Youth with Behavioral and Emotional Disorders and Their Familes: Programs and Evaluation Best Practices* (pp. 633–656). Austin, TX: Pro-Ed.

Center for Health and Health Care in Schools. (2001). *School-Based Health Centers: Results from a 50 State Survey; School Year 1999–2000.* Washington, DC: George Washington University.

Chinman, M., Hannah, G., Wandersman, A., Ebener, P., Hunter, S. B., Imm, P., et al. (2005). Developing a community science research agenda for building community capacity for effective preventive interventions. *American Journal of Community Psychology, 35*(3/4), 143–158.

Chorpita, B. (2006). *Modular Cognitive-Behavioral Therapy for Childhood Anxiety Disorders.* New York: Guilford Press.

Chorpita, B. F., & Daleiden, E. L. (2007). *2007 Biennial Report: Effective Psychosocial Intervention for Youth with Behavioral and Emotional Needs.* Child and Mental Health Division, Hawaii

Department of Health. Available online at http://hawaii.gov/health/mental-health/camhd/library/pdf/ebs/ebs012.pdf. Accessed on August, 2009.

Chorpita, B. F., Taylor, A. A., Francis, S. E., Moffitt, C. E., & Austin, A. A. (2004). Efficacy of modular cognitive behavior therapy for childhood anxiety disorders. *Behavior Therapy, 35*, 263–287.

Commonwealth Student Assistance Program Interagency Committee. (2004). *History of Secondary Student Assistance Programs in Pennsylvania*. Available online at http://www.sap.state.pa.us/UploadedFiles/historyofsap.pdf. Accessed August 26, 2009.

Daly, B. P., Burke, R., Hare, I., Mills, C., Owens, C., Moore, E., et al. (2006). Enhancing No Child Left Behind: School mental health connections. *Journal of School Health, 76*, 446–451.

Dolan, L. J., Jaylan, T., Werthamer, L., & Kellam, S. (1989). *The Good Behavior Game Manual*. Baltimore, MD: Johns Hopkins Prevention Research Center.

Domitrovich, C. E., Bradshaw, C. P., Poduska, J. M., Hoagwood, K., Buckley, J. A., Olin, S., et al. (2008). Maximizing the implementation quality of evidence-based preventive interventions in schools: A conceptual framework. *Advances in School Mental Health Promotion, 1*(3), 6–28.

Duchnowski, A., & Kutash, K. (2007). School-based mental health services: Meeting the challenge, realizing the potential. In S. Evans, M. Weist, & Z. Serpell (Eds.), *Advances in School-Based Mental Health Interventions: Best Practices and Program Models* (vol. 2, pp. 24.1–24.13). New York: Civic Research Institute.

DuPaul, G. (2007). School-based mental health: Current status and future directions. In S. Evans, M. Weist, & Z. Serpell (Eds.), *Advances in School-Based Mental Health Interventions: Best Practices and Program Models* (vol. 2, pp. 25.1–25.8). New York: Civic Research Institute.

Elias, M. J., Gager, P., & Leon, S. (1997). Spreading a warm blanket of prevention over all children: Guidelines for selecting substance abuse and related prevention curricula for use in the schools. *Journal of Primary Prevention, 18*, 41–69.

Evans, S. W., Glass-Siegel, M., Frank, A., Van Treuren, R., Lever, N. A., & Weist, M. D. (2003). Overcoming the challenges of funding school mental health programs. In M. D. Weist, S. W. Evans, & N. A. Lever (Eds.), *Handbook of School Mental Health: Advancing Practice and Research* (pp. 73–86). New York: Springer.

Evans, S. W., Langberg, J., & Williams, J. (2003). Achieving generalization in school-based mental health. In M. D. Weist, S. W. Evans, & N. A. Lever (Eds.), *Handbook of School Mental Health: Advancing Practice and Research* (pp. 335–348). New York: Springer.

Evans, S. W., Sapia, J. L., Axelrod, J., & Glomb, N. K. (2002). Practical issues in school mental health: Referral procedures, negotiating special education, and confidentiality. In H. Ghuman, M. Weist, & R. Sarles (Eds.), *Providing Mental Health Services to Youth Where They Are* (pp. 75–94). New York: Brunner-Routledge.

Evans, S. W., & Weist, M. D. (2004). Implementing empirically supported treatments in the schools: What are we asking? *Clinical Child and Family Psychology Review, 7*, 263–267.

Evans, S. W., Weist, M. D., & Serpell, Z. (2007). *Advances in School-Based Mental Health* (vol. 2). Kingston, NJ: Civic Research Institute.

Fixsen, D. L., Naoom, S. F., Blase, K. A., Friedman, R. M., & Wallace, F. (2005). *Implementation Research: A Synthesis of the Literature*. FMHI Publication #231. Tampa: University of South Florida, Louis de la Parte Florida Mental Health Institute, The National Implementation Research Network.

Flaherty, L. T., Garrison, E., Waxman, R., Uris, P., Keyes, S., Siegel, M. G., et al. (1998). Optimizing the roles of school mental health professionals. *Journal of School Health, 68*, 420–424.

Flaspohler, P. D., Anderson-Butcher, D., Paternite, C. E., Weist, M. D., & Wandersman, A. (2006). Community science and expanded school mental health: Bridging the research to practice gap to promote child well being and academic success. *Educational and Child Psychology, 23*(1), 27–41.

Forness, S. R. (2003). Barriers to evidence-based treatment: Developmental psychopathology and the interdisciplinary disconnect in school mental health practice. *Journal of School Psychology, 41*(1), 61–67.

Foster, S., Rollefson, M., Doksum, T., Noonan, D., & Robinson, G. (2005). *School Mental Health Services in the United States, 2002–2003.* DHHS Pub. No. (SMA) 05-4068. Rockville, MD: Center for Mental Health Services, Substance Abuse and Mental Health Services Administration.

Friedman, R. M. (2003). Improving outcomes for students through the application of a public health model to school psychology: A commentary. *Journal of School Psychology, 41*(1), 69–75.

Graczyk, P. A., Domitrovich, C. E., & Zins, J. E. (2003). Facilitating the implementation of evidence-based prevention and mental health promotion efforts on schools. In M. D. Weist, S. W. Evans, & N. A. Lever (Eds.), *Handbook of School Mental Health Programs: Advancing Practice and Research* (pp. 301–318). New York: Kluwer Academic/Plenum Publisher.

Green, L. W. (2001). From research to "best practices" in other settings and populations. *American Journal of Public Health, 25,* 165–178.

Greenberg, M. T., Weissberg, R. P., O'Brien, M. U., Zins, J. E., Fredericks, L., Resnik, H., et al. (2003). Enhancing school-based prevention and youth development through coordinated social, emotional, and academic learning. *American Psychologist, 58,* 466–474.

Hacker, K., & Wessel, G. L. (1998). School-based health centers and school nurses: Cementing the collaboration. *Journal of School Health, 68,* 409–414.

Hoagwood, K. E. (2005). Family-based services in children's mental health: A research review and synthesis. *Journal of Child Psychology and Psychiatry, 46*(7), 690–713.

Hoagwood, K., Burns, B., & Weisz, J. (2002). A profitable conjunction: From science to service in children's mental health. In B. Burns & K. Hoagwood (Eds.), *Community Treatment for Youth: Evidence-Based Interventions for Severe Emotional and Behavioral Disorders* (pp. 327–338). New York: Oxford University Press.

Jensen, P. S., Hoagwood, K., & Trickett, E. J. (1999). Ivory towers or earthen trenches? Community collaboration to foster real-world research. *Applied Developmental Science, 3,* 206–212.

Kusché, J. L., & Greenberg, M. (1994). *The PATHS Curriculum.* Seattle, WA: Development Research and Programs.

Kutash, K., Duchnowski, A. J., & Lynn, N. (2006). *School-Based Mental Health: An Empirical Guide for Decision Makers.* Tampa: University of South Florida, The Louis de la Parte Florida Mental Health Institute, Department of Child & Family Studies, Research and Training Center for Children's Mental Health.

Leaf, P. J., Schultz, D., Kiser, L. J., & Pruitt, D. B. (2003) School mental health in systems of care. In M. D. Weist, S. W. Evans, & N. A. Lever (Eds.), *Handbook of School Mental Health Programs: Advancing Practice and Research* (pp. 239–256). New York: Springer.

Lochman, J. E., Lampron, L. B., Gemmer, T. C., & Harris, S. R. (1987). Anger coping intervention with aggressive children: A guide to implementation in school settings. In P. Keller & S. Heyman (Eds.), *Innovations in Clinical Practice: A Sourcebook* (vol. 6, pp. 339–356). Sarasota, FL: Professional Resource Exchange.

Lowie, J. A., Lever, N. A., Ambrose, M. G., Tager, S. B., & Hill, S. (2003). Partnering with families in expanded school mental health programs. In M. D. Weist, S. W. Evans, & N. A. Lever (Eds.), *Handbook of School Mental Health Programs: Advancing Practice and Research* (pp. 135–148). New York: Springer.

Malti, T., & Noam, G. (2008). *Where Youth Development Meets Mental Health and Education: The Rally Approach.* Hoboken, NJ: Wiley.

Marsh, D. (2004). Serious emotional disturbance in children and adolescents: Opportunities and challenges for psychologists. *Professional Psychology: Research and Practice, 35,* 443–448.

Mrazek, P. J., & Haggerty, R. (Eds.). (1994). *Reducing Risks for Mental Disorders.* Washington, DC: National Academy Press.

Mrazek, P. J., & Hosman, C. M. (Eds.) (2002). *Toward a Strategy for Worldwide Action to Promote Mental Health and Prevent Mental and Behavioral Disorders.* Alexandria, VA: World Federation for Mental Health.

Nabors, L. A., & Reynolds, M. W. (2000). Program evaluation activities: Outcomes related to treatment for adolescents receiving school-based mental health services. *Children's Services: Social Policy, Research, and Practice, 3*, 175–189.

National Assembly on School-Based Health Care. *National Census Data, 2006.* Washington, DC: Author. 2007.

National Center on Response to Intervention. (2009). *National Center on Response to Intervention, Definition of RTI.* Available online at http://www.rti4success.org/index.php?option=com_content&task=view&id=4&Itemid=24. Accessed August 24, 2009.

No Child Left Behind Act of 2001, Pub.L. 107-110, 115 Stat. 1425 (2002). Available online at http://www.ed.gov/policy/elsec/leg/esea02/index.html. Accessed August 24, 2009.

Olweus, D., Limber, S. P., & Mihalic, S. (1999). *The Bullying Prevention Program: Blueprints for Violence Prevention* (vol. 10). Boulder, CO: Center for the Study and Prevention of Violence.

Papa, P. A., Rector, C., & Stone, C. (1998). Interdisciplinary collaborative training for school-based health professionals. *Journal of School Health, 68,* 415–419.

Paternite, C. E., & Johnston, T. C. (2005). Rationale and strategies for central involvement of educators in effective school-based mental health programs. *Journal of Youth and Adolescence, 34,* 41–49.

Pianta, R. C. (2003). Editorial. *Journal of School Psychology, 41*(1), 1–2.

President's New Freedom Commission on Mental Health. (2003). *Achieving the Promise: Transforming Mental Health Care in America; Final Report for the President's New Freedom Commission on Mental Health.* SMA Publication No. 03-3832. Rockville, MD: Author.

Rajala, M. (2001). European developments in health promotion. *Promotion and Education,* (Suppl.), 5–6.

Ringeisen, H., Henderson, K., & Hoagwood, K. (2003). Context matters: Schools and the "research to practice gap" in children's mental health. *School Psychology Review, 32,* 153–168.

Robinson, K. E. (2004). *Advances in School-Based Mental Health Interventions: Best Practices and Program Models.* Kingston, NJ: Civic Research Institute.

Rones, M., & Hoagwood, K. (2000). School-based mental health services: A research review. *Clinical Child and Family Psychology Review, 3,* 223–241.

Rowling, L. (2002). Mental health promotion. In L. Rowling, G. Martin, & L. Walker (Eds.), *Mental Health Promotion and Young People* (pp. 10–23). London: McGraw-Hill.

Rowling, L., & Weist, M. D. (2004). Promoting the growth, improvement, and sustainability of school mental health programs worldwide. *International Journal of Mental Health Promotion, 6*(2), 3–11.

Schoenwald, S. K., & Hoagwood, K. (2001). Effectiveness, transportability, and dissemination of interventions: What matters when? *Psychiatric Services, 52,* 1190–1197.

School Mental Health Alliance. (2005). *Working Together to Promote Learning, Social-Emotional Competence, and Mental Health for all Children.* New York: Columbia University Center for the Advancement of Children's Mental Health.

Sedlak, M. W. (1997). The uneasy alliance of mental health services and the school: An historical perspective. *American Journal of Orthopsychiatry, 67,* 349–362.

Shirk, S. R. (2004). Dissemination of youth ESTs: Ready for prime time? *Clinical Psychology: Science and Practice, 11,* 308–312.

Silverman, W. K., Kurtines, W. M., & Hoagwood, K. (2004). Research progress on effectiveness, transportability, and dissemination of empirically supported treatments: Integrating theory and research. *Clinical Psychology: Science and Practice, 11,* 295–299.

Staup, J. (1999, September). *The Integration of Mental Health and Education Systems.* Workshop presented at the Fourth National Conference on Advancing School-Based Mental Health Programs, Denver, CO.

Stephan, S. H., Davis, E., Burke, P. C., & Weist, M. D. (2006). Supervision in school mental health. In T. K. Neill (Ed.), *Helping Others Help Children: Clinical Supervision of Child Psychotherapy* (pp. 209–222). Washington, DC: American Psychological Association.

Sugai, G. (2009). *School-Wide Positive Behavior Support and Response to Intervention*. RTI Action Network. Available online at http://www.rtinetwork.org/Learn/Behavior/ar/Schoolwide Behavior. Accessed August 24, 2009.

Sugai, G., Horner, R. H., Dunlap, G., Hieneman, M., Nelson, M. C., Scott, T., et al. (2000). Applying positive behavior support and functional behavioral assessment in schools. *Journal of Positive Behavior Intervention, 2*(3), 131–143.

Teich, J. L., Robinson, G., & Weist, M. (2007). What kinds of mental health services do public schools in the United State provide? *Advances in School Mental Health Promotion, 1,* 13–22.

Texas Student Assistance Program Initiative. (2009). History of the SAP. Available online at http://www.studentassistance.org/frameabout.html. Accessed August 24, 2009.

U.S. Department of Health and Human Services. (1999). *Mental Health: A Report of the Surgeon General—Executive Summary*. Rockville, MD: U.S. Department of Health and Human Services, Substance Abuse and Mental Health Services Administration, Center for Mental Health Services, National Institute of Health, National Institute of Mental Health.

U.S. Public Health Service. (2000). *Report on the Surgeon General's Conference on Children's Mental Health: A National Action Agenda*. Washington, DC: U.S. Government Printing Office.

Wandersman, A. (2003). Community science: Bridging the gap between science and practice with community-centered models. *American Journal of Community Psychology, 31,* 227–242.

Weare, K. (2000). *Promoting Mental, Emotional, and Social Health: A Whole School Approach*. London: Routledge.

Weist, M. D. (1997). Expanded school mental health services: A national movement in progress. In T. Ollendick & R. J. Prinz (Eds.), *Advances in Clinical Child Psychology* (vol. 19, pp. 319–352). New York: Plenum Press.

Weist, M. D., Evans, S. W., & Lever, N. A. (2003). *Handbook of School Mental Health: Advancing Practice and Research*. New York: Kluwer Academic/Plenum Publishers.

Weist, M. D., Goldstein, A., Morris, L., & Bryant, T. (2003). Integrating expanded school mental health and school-based health centers. *Psychology in the Schools, 15,* 297–308.

Weist, M. D., & Murray, M. (2007). Advancing school mental health promotion globally. *Advances in School Mental Health Promotion, 1,* 2–12.

Weist, M. D., Myers, C. P., Hastings, E., Ghuman, H., & Han, Y. (1999). Psychosocial functioning of youth receiving mental health services in the schools vs. community mental health centers. *Community Mental Health Journal, 35,* 69–81.

Weist, M. D., & Paternite, C. E. (2006). Building an interconnected policy-training-practice-research agenda to advance school mental health. *Education and Treatment of Children, 29*(1), 173–196.

Weist, M. D., Paternite, C. E., & Adelsheim, S. (2005). *School-Based Mental Health Services*. Commissioned report for the Institute of Medicine, Board of Health Care Services, Crossing the Quality Chasm: Adaptation to Mental Health and Addictive Disorders Committee.

Weist, M. D., Sander, M. A., Walrath, C., Link, B., Nabors, L., Adelsheim, S., et al. (2005). Developing principles for best practice in expanded school mental health. *Journal of Youth and Adolescence, 34,* 7–13.

Weist, M. D., Stephan, S., Lever, N., Moore, E., Flaspohler, P., Maras, M., et al. (2007). Quality and school mental health. In S. Evans, M. Weist, & Z. Serpell (Eds.), *Advances in School-Based Mental Health Interventions* (pp. 4.1–4.14). New York: Civic Research Institute.

Wenger, E., McDermott, R., & Snyder, W. M. (2002). *Cultivating Communities of Practice: A Guide to Managing Knowledge*. Boston: Harvard Business School Press.

Weisz, J. (2004). *Psychotherapy for Children and Adolescents: Evidence-Based Treatments and Case Examples*. New York: Cambridge University Press.

Weisz, J. R., Chu, B. C., & Polo, A. J. (2004). Treatment dissemination and evidence-based practice: Strengthening intervention through clinician-research collaboration. *Clinical Psychology: Science and Practice, 11,* 300–307.

Weisz, J. R., Jensen-Doss, A., & Hawley, K. M. (2006). Evidence-based youth psychotherapies versus usual clinical care: A meta-analysis of direct comparisons. *American Psychologist, 61*(7), 671–689.

World Health Organization. (1995). *The Health Promoting School: A Framework for Action in the WHO Western Pacific Region.* Manilla, Phillippines, Regional Office for the Western Pacific.

Zins, J. E., Weissberg, R. P., Wang, M. C., & Walberg, H. J. (Eds.). (2004). *Building Academic Success on Social and Emotional Learning: What Does the Research Say?* New York: Teachers College Press.

Chapter 18

MENTAL HEALTH TREATMENT IN CRIMINAL JUSTICE SETTINGS

Allison D. Redlich, PhD; and Karen J. Cusack, PhD

IN ANY comprehensive discussion of persons with mental illness, criminal justice involvement is a necessary and defining issue. Over the past three decades, there is a clear and consistent body of evidence demonstrating that persons with serious mental illness (SMI) are over-represented in the criminal justice system (e.g., James & Glaze, 2006; Lamb & Weinberger, 1998; Teplin, 1984, 2000; but see Engel & Silver, 2001). Both the number of individuals and the frequency with which they come into contact with the system is disproportionate. Compared to rates of serious mental illness in the general population, rates of SMI in the criminal justice system are at least two to five times higher (e.g., James & Glaze, 2006; Lamb & Weinberger, 1998; Munetz, Grande, & Chambers, 2001). In addition, the high volume of offenders involved in the criminal justice system with SMI issues often cycle repeatedly through the system earning them the title of "frequent flyers." To further compound the problem, the majority (75–80%) of offenders with mental illness have co-occurring substance abuse or dependence disorders (Abram, Teplin, & McClelland, 2003; GAINS, 2005).

In this chapter, the authors provide an overview of the prevalence of individuals with SMI in the legal system, and then discuss the treatment and related issues of individuals with SMI at various intercept points along the criminal justice system continuum. The focus in this chapter is on individuals with SMI as offenders, not as victims of or witnesses to crimes (see Silver, Arseneault, Langley, Caspi, & Moffitt, 2005; Teplin, McClelland, Abram, & Weiner, 2005 for more on the victimization of persons with SMI). Using a theoretically driven framework, the authors discuss five main intercept points: 1) law enforcement and emergency services; 2) initial detention and initial court hearing; 3) jails and courts; 4) prisons and re-entry; and 5) community corrections and community support. In addition to reviewing the historical and "usual" treatment at these points of contact, the authors review innovative and more recent efforts aimed at reducing the recidivism cycle among this population. Finally, the authors discuss policy issues, implications for mental health, and future challenges facing the field.

Prevalence of Persons with Serious Mental Illness in the Criminal Justice System

Today there are more than seven million people in the U.S. correctional system. Two point three million people are incarcerated in local jails and state and federal prisons, and five million people are in the community being supervised by probation and parole agencies (Pew Center on the States, 2009). These numbers represent an astounding 500% increase in the last 35 years (Glaze & Bonczar, 2006). State spending on corrections has risen faster than spending on nearly every other state budget item, increasing from $9 billion to $48.6 billion a year from 1984 to 2007 (National Association of State Budget Officers, 1987, 2008).

Recent estimates are that annually about 1.1 million jail admissions are persons with SMI (see Steadman, Robbins, Islam, & Osher, 2007). In 1978, at a national workshop on mental health services in the jails, Brodsky described jails as a "public health outpost." Thirty years later, the same sentiment applies despite a steady acknowledgement of, and attention to, this problem. Today, urban jails, such as jails in Los Angeles, New York City, and Chicago, are the largest provider of inpatient mental health services, encountering more persons with SMI than any hospital nationwide. Simply put, the presence of persons with SMI in our nation's criminal justice system overwhelms an already overburdened fragile system, from contact with law enforcement to community supervision, and all points in between, making this problem one of the major public health issues of our time. The President's New Freedom Commission on Mental Health (2003) recognized that the combination of mental illness and substance use is a major public health problem. The addition of criminal justice involvement only intensifies the severity of the problems.

Because five of the seven million U.S. citizens under correctional supervision are in the community under probation or parole supervision (Glaze & Bonczar, 2006), and because when in the community, persons with mental illness have no constitutional right to treatment as they do when they are incarcerated, arguably the largest set of issues for justice-involved persons with mental illness is the generic problem of accessing appropriate community-based services. The accessing of services is often exacerbated by fear, stigma, and exclusionary policies associated with their criminal justice histories. In the discussion below, the authors review traditional and newer innovative interventions for offenders with mental illness in the community and in confinement.

Mental Health Issues and Treatment in the Criminal Justice System

The criminal justice system, at a basic level, is made up of three prongs: 1) law enforcement; 2) the courts; and 3) corrections (jails and prisons as well as probation

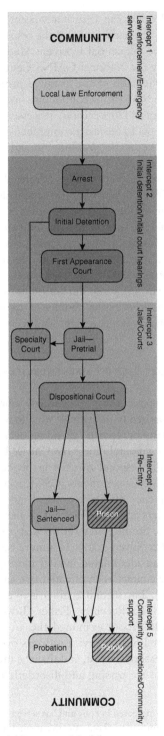

Figure 18.1 The Sequential Intercept Model

and parole). Mental health issues can arise at any point in the criminal justice process. To frame a discussion of these issues and the responses that have been developed, the authors utilize the Sequential Intercept Model (SIM). The SIM, which was originally developed by the National GAINS Center[1] and refined by Munetz and Griffin (2006), is a schematic of the criminal justice system's processing of cases. At each point in the SIM (from community law enforcement involvement through community re-entry and supervision), it is essential to design interventions that attend to these intercepts to ensure a comprehensive, systematic approach to problems associated with the over-representation and treatment of persons with SMI in the criminal justice system.

At each intercept point, there are a range of related problems that can greatly affect individuals with SMI and affect the professionals and larger systems that process them. Thus, interventions can be designed or refined at each point to address these issues to avoid the basic issue of an individual with SMI unnecessarily penetrating deeper into the criminal justice system. As discussed by Munetz and Griffin (2006), best clinical practices are the "ultimate intercept." This is the core goal of all interventions: to prevent people from penetrating more deeply at much higher costs (fiscally and with regard to human rights) simply because they have a mental disorder and because there is an absence of appropriate community-based supports for their maintenance, improvement, and recovery.

INTERCEPT 1: LAW ENFORCEMENT/EMERGENCY SERVICES

In the community, police spend a disproportionate amount of time dealing with individuals with SMI as opposed to individuals who do not have SMI. For example, Los Angeles Police Department reported spending over 28,000 hours a month on calls involving people with a mental illness (DeCuir & Lamb, 1996), and the New York City police reportedly respond to calls involving people with SMI every 6.5 minutes (Council of State Governments [CSG], 2002). There are two primary ways to examine the frequency of interactions of individuals with SMI and law enforcement. First is to determine the percent of persons with SMI among all police-suspect interactions. Studies have shown that approximately 3% to 6% of suspects have SMI (Engel & Silver, 2001). In a more recent study in Canada, less than 1% of suspects had an identifiable mental illness, although having a SMI increased the risk of police contact as an offender two and one half times (Crocker, Hartford, & Heslop, 2009). The second manner is to examine arrest rates among cohorts of people with SMI. Recently, Fisher, Roy-Bujnowski, Grudzinskas, Clayfield, Banks, and Wolff (2006) examined the arrest histories of more than 13,000 Massachusetts mental health service utilizers over a 10-year period. They reported that 28% had at least one arrest, and that the most common charges were public order crimes, such as trespassing and disorderly conduct. They also found

---

[1] The National GAINS Center originated in 1995 and has served as the national locus for the collection and dissemination of information about effective mental health and substance abuse services for people with co-occurring disorders in contact with the criminal justice system (see www.gainscenter.samhsa.gov).

that a small subset of individuals, 1.5% of the total sample or 5% of those with any arrest, accounted for 17% of all arrests.

When police officers interact with persons with SMI who are suspected of committing crimes, they generally have two discretionary options, depending upon the severity and circumstances of the crime: 1) a mental health option (e.g., hospitalization); or 2) a criminal justice option (arrest). Research has demonstrated that police are much more likely to utilize the criminal justice option, as this is often the only viable and most convenient option from the police officer's perspective (sometimes referred to as "mercy booking"; Lamb, Weinberger, & DeCuir, 2002; Green, 1997). Pursuing a mental health option can be frustrating and time-consuming, with long (e.g., eight-hour) waiting periods until the person is seen at a hospital which may or may not result in an admission. In communities that have instituted 24-hour crisis drop-off centers, police officers perceived their specialized response to mental disturbance calls as two to eight times more effective than officers without such centers (Borum, Deane, Steadman, & Morrissey, 1998). However, currently most communities do not have such resources, and thus law enforcement often utilize their discretion to arrest (Lamb et al., 2002). Interestingly, Green (1997) found that more experienced officers (compared to less experienced officers) were less likely to arrest persons with mental illness, particularly when there was no evidence of a crime, or when the person was homeless.

Many law enforcement agencies, recognizing the over-abundance of resources and potential for harm when officers deal with persons with SMI, have sought out solutions to the problem. The most notable solution is pre-arrest diversion, of which there are typically three models: 1) police-based specialized police response; 2) police-based specialized mental health response; and 3) mental health–based specialized mental health response (Deane, Steadman, Borum, Veysey, & Morrissey, 1999; Steadman, Deane, Borum, & Morrissey, 2000). In the first model, police officers are specially trained in crisis intervention and act as liaisons to the mental health system. In the second model, mental health professionals work collaboratively with police to provide on-site or telephone consultation. In the third model, mental health professionals provide on-site help to the police in situations involving persons with a mental illness (see Reuland & Cheney, 2005).

A growing and successful pre-arrest diversion program is Crisis Intervention Teams, or CIT, which conforms to the first model described above. CIT originated in Memphis, Tennessee, in 1988 and is focused on de-escalating crisis situations between law enforcement and individuals with SMI. A primary element of CIT is officer training. The Memphis CIT model prides itself on its initial 40-hour (plus refresher courses) intensive training. The curriculum includes information on mental illness, crisis skills, and a heavy concentration on interactive role playing. A second element of CIT is community outreach and collaboration, including forging mental health partnerships. A third element of CIT is re-conceptualizing police roles for the specialized diversion officers. That is, under the CIT model, officers volunteer or are specially selected (i.e., not randomly assigned), and the agency promotes bonding among them (Reuland & Cheney, 2005). In addition to these elements, Steadman et al. (2001) stressed that legal foundations and linkages to community services are important aspects of pre-booking diversion. Legal foundations in the form of statutes, codes, or policies can help ensure that it is legally permissible for crisis facilities to accept and detain persons who may or may not have criminal charges pending.

In general, the research on the effectiveness of CIT and other specialized responses to PSMI is positive. Steadman, Deane, Borum, and Morrissey (2000) examined three such programs and reported 46% of mental disturbance calls resulted in the individuals' being taken to treatment, 35% were resolved at the scene, and 13% were referred to treatment. Perhaps more importantly, only 7% of calls resulted in an arrest. Moreover, jurisdictions with specialized responses have seen decreases in the number of injuries to officers and citizens (Dupont & Cochran, 2000; Reuland, 2004).

INTERCEPT 2: INITIAL DETENTION/INITIAL COURT HEARING

Partly due to the lack of appropriate alternatives discussed above, individuals with SMI are more likely to be arrested compared to persons without mental illness. In fact, the odds of a person with SMI being jailed are *significantly greater* than the odds of being hospitalized (Morrissey, Meyer, & Cuddeback, 2005). In one study, individuals displaying symptoms characteristic of mental illness were found to have a 67% higher probability of being arrested than individuals not displaying such symptoms (Teplin, 1984, 2000). Moreover, after this initial arrest, individuals with SMI are more likely to be detained in jail (as opposed to being released on their own recognizance or having cases dismissed), and once jailed, stay incarcerated two and a half to eight times longer in comparison to their non–mentally ill counterparts (CSG, 2002). The rate of mental illness in jail is substantially higher for women than for men (James & Glaze, 2006; Teplin, Abram, & McClelland, 1996), and women detainees generally present with more complex issues in jail, such as child care, histories of violence, physical and sexual abuse, and post-traumatic stress disorder (PTSD) (Steadman & Naples, 2005). Although jails are required by law to provide mental health services, most have inadequate mental health staffing to provide even the most basic services of screening and crisis intervention (see below). Further, some have suggested that the primary cause of criminal justice involvement is de-institutionalization and fragmented community mental health systems (Abramson, 1972; Teplin, 1983; see Morabito, 2007, for a recent discussion), further pointing to the need to address the problem *not in jails* but in specialized community programs.

Recommendations for diversion programs date back at least to the 1970s, when the National Coalition for Jail Reform began advocating for new methods of addressing individuals with SMI in jail. More recently, the National Alliance on Mental Illness (NAMI) reported on the misuse of jails as mental hospitals and called for the development of jail diversion programs (Torrey et al., 1992). Methods of reducing the numbers of persons with SMI in the criminal justice system require collaboration between two systems with a long history of little or no collaboration. Criminal justice and mental health systems have different goals (punishment vs. treatment) and funding streams, as well as training backgrounds and expectations of personnel (Fagan, Morrissey, & Cocozza, 2007). However, despite these obstacles, jail diversion programs have proliferated since the 1990s in order to address the problem of persons with SMI cycling in and out of jail without proper mental health care. Currently, there are approximately 300 non-specialty court diversion programs in the United States (GAINS, 2007).

The term "jail diversion" is actually made up of two distinct processes: 1) eliminating or reducing jail time by diverting the individual from the criminal justice system; and 2) linking these individuals with community-based treatment. Jail diversion programs are considered "pre-booking" diversion if the intervention occurs before an arrest is made (e.g., see CIT above) or "post-booking" diversion if the intervention occurs after arrest but before prosecution or sentencing. At this stage in the Sequential Intercept Model, the goal is to reduce the length of time under criminal justice supervision. Potential legal outcomes of post-booking diversion include alternative sentencing, conditional release, or dropped charges based on the assumption that well-supervised mental health treatment will be initiated and maintained in the community (Morrissey & Cuddeback, 2007). Steadman, Barbera, and Dennis (1994) identified what they consider the core elements of a post-booking jail diversion program. These include 1) screening for the presence of a mental disorder; 2) evaluation by a mental health professional of those who screen positive; and 3) negotiation between the diversion program, prosecutors, defense attorneys, and the courts to produce a disposition outside the jail with charges either dropped or reduced.

The proliferation of jail diversion programs across the country has significantly outpaced the research, such that many basic questions about jail diversion remain unanswered. For instance, it is unclear who is best served by jail diversion programs. However, in practice, studies have identified older age, female gender, and non-felony, non-violent charges as predictors of referral for diversion (Naples, Morris, & Steadman, 2007; Steadman, Cocozza, & Veysey, 1999).

Steadman, Morris, and Dennis (1995) conducted on-site interviews with 18 programs that met the definition of a jail diversion program in order to determine characteristics associated with effective programs. Through these interviews they identified six central themes that appear to characterize effective programs. The first was providing *integrated services* for mental health, substance abuse, and housing within the auspices of a single entity. The second included involving key stakeholders from multiple agencies early in the process and holding *regular meetings* to facilitate information sharing and discussion of concerns. The third included the presence of "boundary spanners," individuals who serve as a liaison between the behavioral health and criminal justice systems. Fourth, effective programs were also defined by *strong leadership* for the program. Fifth, *early identification* of possible mental illness (i.e., screening within the first 24–48 hours) was seen as a critical component to effective programs. Finally, *intensive, culturally diverse case management* was considered one of the most critical factors.

Only a handful of studies have been conducted on outcomes associated with jail diversion programs, and most have utilized pre-post designs (Lamberti et al., 2001; GAINS, 2002) or compared outcomes of diverted vs. non-diverted individuals in quasi-experimental designs (Lamb, Weinberger, & Reston-Parham, 1996; Steadman et al.,1999; Steadman & Naples, 2005). Overall, findings from these studies indicate that participants in jail diversion spend less time in jail, do not have an increase in re-arrest rates, and are more likely to be linked to community-based services. However, little or no improvement was noted in the areas of mental health symptoms and functioning, suggesting that participants may not be receiving the type and/or amount of services necessary. Finally, jail diversion programs appear to result in lower criminal justice costs and greater behavioral health costs (Steadman & Naples, 2005).

INTERCEPT 3: JAILS AND COURTS

Despite the popularity of jail diversion programs, these programs serve only a fraction of individuals with SMI. There are many reasons why offenders with serious mental health problems are not diverted. For one, diversion programs often have maximum capacities and to our knowledge, there is no one program that could meet the need of the community. Further, not all offenders are eligible (e.g., committed a violent crime) and not all offenders are recognized and referred to programs even when eligible. As such, large urban jails necessarily must house and provide some treatment for offenders identified as having mental illnesses. While in jail (which are distinguishable from prisons in that they are most often county-operated, short-term placements focusing on processing detainees and sentencing serving misdemeanants), PSMI often have behavioral problems, decompensate, and generally do not fare well in these settings. For example, James and Glaze (2006) found that 19% of jail inmates with mental illness had been charged with breaking jail rules, in comparison to only 9% of jail inmates without mental illness. Violations of rules and other disciplinary infractions can lead to longer stays because of increased sanctions and/or, sadly enough, for the purposes of treatment.

Traditionally, treatment services provided by jails have varied widely, and they are often dependent on the size of the jail, whether the jail is pre-trial detention only or houses sentenced inmates as well, and relations between outside treatment providers and jails. Morris, Steadman, and Veysey (1997) surveyed 1,036 small and large jails about their mental health treatment services. They found that only 33% provided any counseling or therapy, 20% had inpatient care inside the jail (45% had the capacity for inpatient care outside the jail), and 45% had special housing areas for offenders with mental illness. On average, jails provided four different types of mental health services, though the larger jails provided an average of seven or eight services.

Similarly, Anno (2001) reported that of eight large county jails, 50% had programs for aggressive mentally ill offenders; 38% had programs for offenders with co-occurring disorders; 75% had inpatient beds for offenders with mental illness; and 88% had different levels of care for offenders with mental illness. In James and Glaze's (2006) report on the mental health and treatment of offenders, they noted that only 17% of persons with SMI in jail had received any treatment since being admitted in contrast to 34% of individuals with SMI in prison.

Inadequate accommodations and access to treatment in jail pre-trial can also have implications for court proceedings, particularly adjudicative competence issues. Competency to stand trial (CST) has been a primary issue among forensic researchers and forensic practitioners for decades. The American Bar Association's Criminal Justice Mental Health Standards noted that "the issue of present mental incompetence, qualitatively speaking, is the single most important issue in the criminal mental health field" (1994). Further, more resources are spent on competency evaluations and treatment than any other forensic service (Zapf, Hubbard, Cooper, Whelles, & Ronan, 2004). Estimates of competency evaluations in the United States range from approximately 50,000 to 60,000 yearly (Mossman et al., 2007; Poythress, Bonnie, & Oberlander, 1994).

There is a comprehensive research base indicating that, in comparison to persons without mental illness, persons with SMI are more likely to have deficits in adjudicative competence, such that they may not understand and appreciate the plea/trial process (Poythress et al., 1994; Poythress et al., 1998; Rosenfeld & Wall, 1998). This lack of understanding and appreciation, which is constitutionally afforded to all defendants, can lead to increased lengths of incarceration, especially if defendants do not have access to effective defense counsel.

An important policy and legal issue that has emerged from this problem is the inability to evaluate (and potentially restore if necessary) competence in a timely manner, leaving many suspected incompetent offenders to languish in jail until an assessment can be conducted, often times longer than if they had simply pled out on "time served" (Pinals, 2005). After a finding of incompetence to stand trial, it is incumbent for the state to treat the defendant in order to restore competency. This treatment has almost always been in high-cost, maximum security state forensic mental hospitals. Whereas competency evaluations underwent significant change in the late 1970s and 1980s from inpatient to outpatient settings, competency restorations did not follow suit (Miller, 2003). Most states have established outpatient pre-trial evaluation systems for court ordered defendants (Grisso, Cocozza, Steadman, Fisher, & Greer, 1994; Miller, 2003; Pinals, 2005).

Above, the authors discussed pre-and post-booking jail diversion programs. Mental health courts (MHCs) are another form of post-booking jail diversion. A main difference between MHCs and other post-booking programs is that participants are required to return for status review hearings before the MHC judge. The first two courts appeared in 1997, and today there are estimated to be more than 150 courts (GAINS, 2007). As addressed by Redlich (2005), there are five characteristics that operationally define the courts. First, the courts are part of the criminal justice system and are for offenders with mental health problems. All courts focus on non-violent offenders, though the gap between misdemeanant and felony offenders is closing (Redlich, Steadman, Monahan, Petrila, & Griffin, 2005; Redlich, Steadman, Monahan, Robbins, & Petrila, 2006), and many handle only persons with serious mental illnesses. Second, as mentioned, the courts are a form of diversion. Third, the courts mandate and monitor treatment in the community. Fourth, the courts tend to follow a therapeutic jurisprudence model, in that they are lenient (e.g., understand and expect relapses, have gradated sanctions) and informal (non-adversarial). Finally, all mental health courts are intended to be voluntary.

There are several notable research studies indicating that MHCs are effective in reducing recidivism and accessing treatment. For example, McNiel and Binder (2007) found that, in comparison to a treatment-as-usual group, clients in the San Francisco MHC were less likely to re-offend over 18 months; rates of re-offense were 56% for the comparison and 34% for the MHC samples (see also Moore & Hiday, 2006). Effectiveness has also been noted in regard to treatment. In a study of the MHC in Broward County, Florida, Boothroyd, Poythress, McGaha, and Petrila (2003) found that, when compared to non-MHC defendants in another county, participants in the MHC were more likely to access services and, when services had been accessed, have a higher volume of service encounters. Lastly, a recent study by Redlich, Hoover, Summers, and Steadman (in press) found that a significant minority of MHC clients from two courts lacked sufficient general legal knowledge (adjudicative competence) and MHC-specific knowledge about court procedures and requirements. Whether knowledge is important for MHC success has not yet been addressed.

Intercept 4: Prisons and Re-entry

State prisons face many of the same challenges as county jails regarding offenders with mental health problems. The data on the prevalence of mental illness in prisons are similar to those discussed in jails. James and Glaze (2006) reported a 56% prevalence rate of inmates with at least one mental problem in state prisons. Using a much more conservative definition of serious mental illness, Steadman, Fabisiak, Dvoskin, and Holohean (1987) discovered an 8% rate among New York state prison inmates.

In comparison to similar data on jails reported above, prisons are seemingly more likely to have mental health treatments in place, however. In light of the fact that jails are usually more temporary settings, it is not surprising that prisons were more likely to have these services available. In a survey concerning correctional health care (see Anno, 2001), state prisons were asked about the special services they provide to inmates. Data from 28 prisons were collected: 79% had programs for aggressive mentally ill inmates; 75% had programs for inmates with co-occurring disorders; 100% had inpatient beds for offenders with mental illness; and 96% had different levels of care for offenders with mental illness. However, the adequacy and effectiveness of services provided has received less scrutiny.

The continuity of care upon release from confinement settings has been a major area of concern and recent reform. After jail or prison terms, many PSMI are left on their own to determine how to successfully re-enter society. More than 7 million individuals will be released from jails and prisons annually, with the majority coming out of local and county jails (Hammett, Roberts, & Kennedy, 2001). It has been suggested that many of these inmates with mental illness and other serious health problems will likely return to jail without appropriate services to help them reintegrate into communities (Osher, 2007).

Inadequate transition planning puts people with mental and substance use disorders who were incarcerated in a state of crisis back on the streets in the middle of the same crisis. The outcomes of inadequate transition planning include the compromise of public safety, an increased incidence of psychiatric symptoms, relapse to substance abuse, hospitalization, suicide, homelessness, and re-arrest (Osher, Steadman, & Barr, 2002). Because of these known potential consequences and their high risk, re-entry of justice-involved persons with SMI is a pressing policy topic, one nearly devoid of theoretically driven outcome research. Although the President's New Freedom Commission highlighted the issue of re-entry as a priority, few

U.S. jails and prisons have adequate plans in place (Austin, 2001; Veysey, Steadman, Morrissey, & Johnsen, 1997). Without proper re-entry planning and subsequent community supervision and community support, the likelihood of individuals with SMI re-entering the criminal justice system is high. How infrequently these issues are addressed is apparent in the major federal re-entry initiative (Serious and Violent Offender Re-entry Initiative, SVORI) in which 88 programs were funded, but only six focused on inmates with mental illness (GAINS, 2006).

In an effort to provide guidance on community re-entry of offenders with mental illness from jails, the National GAINS Center held meetings with jail administrators and reviewed programmatic re-entry efforts around the country. As a result, a best practice approach to managing the early release and re-entry of jail detainees known as the APIC (Assess, Plan, Identify, Coordinate) Model was developed (Osher, Steadman, & Barr, 2002). An important tenet of the APIC model is that jail staff, jail-based mental health and substance abuse treatment providers, and community-based treatment providers must each play an important role in transition planning. At the *Assess* stage it is recommended that the detainee's psychosocial, medical, and behavioral needs as well as public safety risks be assessed. The *Plan* stage suggests making plans for critical periods, such as the first few hours or days post-release, plans for medication until follow-up appointments take place, and plans for benefits application or reinstatement. The *Identify* stage is concerned with specific service referrals that are appropriate to the detainee's needs. Finally, the *Coordinate* stage involves coordinating the transition plan to ensure implementation and avoid gaps in care with community-based services.

The *Identify* and *Coordinate* stages pose some of the biggest challenges for communities attempting to divert persons with SMI away from jail and into effective mental health and substance abuse treatment. This is because despite the fact that approximately 500 diversion programs (pre- and post-booking and MHCs combined) exist in the United States today, there is little empirical guidance regarding effective treatment to address the complex needs of this population.

INTERCEPT 5: COMMUNITY CORRECTIONS/COMMUNITY SUPPORT

As noted above, approximately five million U.S. citizens are currently under community correctional supervision, of whom about 1 million are estimated to have mental illnesses (Crilly, Caine, Lamberti, Brown, & Friedman, 2009; Glaze & Bonczar, 2006). Compared with probationers or parolees without mental illness, those with mental illness are much more likely to fail supervision (i.e., have probation revoked for violating terms or for committing a new offense). These problems have widespread public health and public safety implications. One study found the re-arrest rate of probationers with mental illness was nearly double that of probationers without mental illness (54% vs. 30%) (Dauphinot, 1997). Similarly, in a study that matched pairs of parolees with and without mental illness on age, offense, and sentence, parolees with mental illness were twice as likely to have their parole suspended (65% vs. 30%) (Porporino & Motiuk, 1995).

The extent of this problem has led to explicit recommendations for probationers and parolees with mental illness to be assigned to specialized mental health probation agencies in order to provide assistance complying with the conditions of probation and parole (CSG, 2002). Specialty probation has been characterized by a number of features that distinguish it from traditional departments (Skeem, Emke-Francis, & Eno Louden, 2006). First, specialty probation officers have exclusive mental health caseloads. Another important feature is meaningfully reduced caseloads. Specialty probation officers carry caseloads that are roughly one-third that of traditional probation. Sustained officer training is another defining feature, where officers receive 20 to 40 hours of mental health training each year. Specialty probation also integrates internal and external resources, meaning that probation officers work directly with probationers and coordinate with probationers' treatment providers. Finally, specialty probation is characterized by the use of problem-solving strategies in working with probationers to remedy non-compliance issues (Skeem & Eno Louden, 2006). Not only are specialty probation agencies perceived as more effective by stakeholders (Skeem et al., 2006), but there is also some evidence to suggest their potential effectiveness in linking probationers with services, reducing risk of probation violation, and improving overall functioning (Skeem & Eno Louden, 2006). Recently, Skeem and colleagues found that probationers with co-occurring problems were less likely to receive future (eight months later) probation violations when they had a good, rather than poor relationship with their probation officer (Skeem, Eno Louden, Manchak, Vidal, & Haddad, 2009), leading to their conclusion that relationship quality, in addition to traditional probation strategies, is important in understanding why probationers with mental disorders may fail on probation.

Community-based interventions for mentally ill offenders have generally fallen into three types: 1) services-as-usual; 2) evidence-based programs such as Assertive Community Treatment (ACT) or Integrated Dual Disorders Treatment (IDDT); and 3) forensic adaptations of evidence-based programs. Forensic adaptations of programs such as ACT include many of the same elements, yet have the added criteria of prior arrests, referrals from criminal justice, use of criminal justice partners, court sanctions, probation officers as members of the treatment team, and the explicit goal of preventing re-arrest (Lamberti, Weisman, & Faden, 2004).

Outcomes associated with diverting persons with SMI into services-as-usual come from the SAMHSA-funded jail diversion study (Broner, Lattimore, Cowell, & Schlenger, 2004; Steadman & Naples, 2005). Using a quasi-experimental design, individuals with SMI who were diverted were compared with those not selected for diversion. Diverted individuals spent more days in the community (as opposed to jail, hospital, or residential care), had fewer days in jail, and reported more behavioral health service use. However, no clear improvements were noted for mental health symptoms or quality of life.

ACT is a well-established evidence-based practice for PSMI in the community, with over 40 randomized controlled trials conducted to date (Bond, Drake, Mueser, & Latimer, 2001; Marshall, Gray, Lockwood, & Green, 1998). ACT has been widely disseminated in order to help PSMI who are at high risk for repeated psychiatric hospitalization. However, despite the success of ACT in reducing hospitalization, there is considerable evidence that ACT is not effective in keeping

PSMI who are involved in the criminal justice system out of jail (Bond et al., 2001; Calsyn, Yonker, Lemming, Morse, & Klinkenberg, 2005; Marshall & Lockwood, 2004). As a result, forensic adaptations of ACT (FACT) and other Intensive Case Management (FICM) programs have developed. While the concept of FACT is rapidly catching on, there is no standardization of FACT in terms of program elements, client eligibility, or staffing (Cuddeback, Morrissey, & Cusack, 2007; Cuddeback, Morrissey, Cusack, & Meyer, 2009).

The evidence base for these forensic adaptations (FACT or FICM) can be described as preliminary at best. In two separate pre-post studies of FACT, significant reductions in arrests, jail days, hospitalizations, and hospital days were found (McCoy, Roberts, Hanrahan, Clay, & Luchins, 2004; Weisman, Lamberti, & Price, 2004). The California statewide Mentally Ill Offender Crime Reduction Grant (MIOCRG) program used randomized clinical trials to evaluate 20 programs (either FACT or FICM) designed to reduce the criminal justice involvement of PSMI (California Board of Corrections, 2004). Data were aggregated across the 20 sites. According to the statewide summary report, the intervention groups resulted in small but significant differences on bookings, convictions, and jail days, as well as some quality of life measures. The report further noted that programs with higher fidelity to the ACT model achieved better outcomes. A limitation of the aggregated statewide report is that there were many differences in the types of programs and how they were implemented, and no statistical controls were used to adjust for potential confounding variables.

Two randomized clinical trials of FICM programs have been reported. Solomon and Draine (1995) found no differences between FACT, FICM, and usual care with regard to clinical or social outcomes. There was no benefit of the interventions on criminal justice outcomes. Interestingly, the FACT group actually had a *higher* re-arrest rate, although this was attributed to more intense supervision of clients via a probation officer on the team. Cosden, Ellens, Schnell, and Yamini-Diouf (2005) evaluated a mental health court combined with a FICM-model versus usual care. Improvements were seen at 24 months post-treatment for mental health symptoms, quality of life, and drug and alcohol problems. Regarding criminal justice outcomes, this study also found an increase in bookings for the intervention condition (perhaps for the same reason as the Solomon & Draine [1995] study), but no other criminal justice findings.

Overall, it is unclear to what extent intensive treatment programs such as FACT are needed, and whether FACT or the less intensive FICM is capable of achieving positive mental health and criminal justice outcomes. More research is needed to evaluate these interventions to determine their effectiveness in reducing criminal justice involvement and improving mental health functioning of PSMI.

In sum, at each intercept along the criminal justice system, there are multiple and inter-related ways for a person with mental health problems to enter and remain in the web of the criminal justice system. Above, we attempted to demonstrate at each intercept how the relevant systems make it easier for people to enter than exit. Whereas the pathways into the system have been well researched and are generally now well understood, the factors associated with keeping people out of the system are much less clear.

Policy Issues

There are numerous policy issues at each point along the Sequential Intercept Model, many of which were alluded to above. In large part, theories on the criminalization of persons with mental illness surmise the problem began with the closings of and significant reductions in state mental hospitals (i.e., de-institutionalization), as well as changes in civil commitment statutes (see Patch & Arrigo, 1999). The problem is further exacerbated by the numerous barriers to accessible and affordable mental health treatment in the community (see Chapter 14 in this volume). Morgan, Steffan, Shaw, and Wilson (2007) surveyed over 400 adult male inmates about the reasons for and against seeking mental health services in secure settings. They found four main types of barriers to willingness to seek help: 1) self-preservation concerns (confidentiality risks and perceptions of weakness); 2) procedural concerns (not knowing how to access services); 3) self-reliance (reliance on self or close others for help); and 4) professional service provider concerns (staff qualifications and prior dissatisfaction). Inmates with and without past community mental health treatment experiences did not significantly differ in regard to reported barriers. Many of these barriers overlap with barriers found in the community. Further, once released from confinement, individuals with SMI with criminal histories face additional barriers, including limited access to housing and treatment programs. For example, convictions on drug charges can make one ineligible for government-supported housing.

Another policy issue concerns Medicaid benefits and offenders with serious mental illness, particularly as it relates to confinement. Across a series of studies, Morrissey and colleagues have found several interesting trends and outcomes. First, although many states have written policy to terminate Medicaid benefits upon incarceration, Morrissey, Dalton, Steadman, Cuddeback, Haynes, and Cuellar (2006) discovered in two counties (one in Florida and one in Washington) that Medicaid disenrollment was rare, occurring only 3% of the time. Second, using data from the same two counties, Morrissey and colleagues (Morrissey, Steadman et al., 2006b; Morrissey, Cuddeback, Cuellar, & Steadman, 2007) examined the impact of Medicaid benefits on future arrests and access to community services on jail detainees with severe mental illness. They found that in comparison to persons who had their benefits taken away, persons with intact Medicaid benefits had 16% fewer jail stays over 12 months, longer stays in the community before detention (Morrissey et al., 2007), and were more likely to utilize treatment services, and when used, accessed services more quickly and more often (Morrissey, Steadman et al., 2006). Thus, though disenrollment because of incarceration appears to be rare (at least in two counties), disenrollment has negative consequences associated with it.

Implications for Mental Health

Given the high rates of involvement of persons with SMI in the criminal justice system, communities will continue to be faced with finding new methods to address the problem. As noted by Morrissey and colleagues, "the interface between criminal justice and mental health is the new frontier for innovative services and research in the community mental health field" (2007, p. 540). Developing programs that are effective and sustainable will require careful planning as well as early and strong collaboration from all key stakeholders within the behavioral health and criminal justice systems. Effective programming should include multiple points along the Sequential Intercept Model, including law enforcement, the courts, jail, and the community.

Studies of jail diversion programs indicate that such programs appear to be at least modestly successful in diverting people *away from* the criminal justice system (Steadman & Naples, 2005). However, given the lack of theoretically driven and evidence-based interventions for this population, the ability to divert people *into* appropriate treatment for their mental illness, substance abuse, and other psychosocial needs is currently lacking. Despite the pressing need to quickly identify effective interventions to address people with SMI in the criminal justice system, the authors suggest that there are a number of basic questions that should be addressed before interventions are rolled out. What are the main reasons that persons with SMI are first entering the criminal justice system and what factors are responsible for an individual with SMI further penetrating the system? Are there distinct subgroups that would suggest distinct interventions? In what ways are the mental health and substance abuse needs of this population different from persons with SMI who are not criminal justice involved? Once these questions are addressed, interventions can then be developed and/or adapted to the unique needs of this population. Only at this point should such interventions be disseminated to communities engaged in addressing the needs of mentally ill offenders.

Future Challenges

In 2004, the Subcommittee on Criminal Justice for the New Freedom Commission on Mental Health concluded that three major responses were needed regarding people with SMI in the criminal justice system. The first response was diversion programs, with an emphasis on distinguishing between people who do and do not need to be part of the criminal justice system. The second response was the provision of adequate treatment services in correctional institutions, and the third response was re-entry transition programs to better link people re-entering the community with appropriate services. Further, the Subcommittee endorsed nine policy options, many of which focused on evidence-based practices, such as supported housing and employment, as well as ensuring that treatment within jails and prisons is consistent with the current and best available evidence. A challenge related to implementing these policy options is the adaptation of evidence-based practices for forensic populations. Evidence-based practices that were devised on non-offender populations do not necessarily translate into effective interventions for offenders who may have similar mental health issues but different sets of surrounding issues. As described above, forensic adaptations, such as FACT and FICM, are not yet empirically supported.

An additional challenge echoed throughout this volume is the lack of adequate, accessible, and affordable mental health care in the community. Although the number of formal diversion programs continues to rise, the corresponding treatment in the community (the "to" in diversion) remains stagnant. Re-entry programs face a similar challenge. It is important to note that the majority of innovative solutions to handle the over-representation of PSMI in the criminal justice system, such as mental health courts and CIT, arise from, are created by, and operate out of the criminal justice system, not the mental health system. Without the criminal justice and mental health/substance abuse systems working in concert, persons with SMI are likely to continue to be arrested, confined, and convicted at disproportionate rates.

References

Abram, K. M., Teplin, L. A., & McClelland, G. M. (2003). Comorbidity of severe psychiatric disorders and substance use disorders among women in jail. *American Journal of Psychiatry*, *160*(5), 1007–1010.

Abramson, M. F. (1972). The criminalization of mentally disordered behavior: Possible side effect of a new commitment law. *Hospital and Community Psychiatry*, *23*, 101–107.

American Bar Association. (1994). *Criminal Justice Section Standards*. Available online at www.aba net.org. Accessed August 24, 2009.

Anno, B. J. (2001). *Correctional Health Care: Guidelines for the Management of an Adequate Delivery System*. Washington, DC: U.S. Department of Justice, National Institute of Corrections.

Austin, J. (2001). Prisoner reentry: Current trends, practices, and issues. *Crime and Delinquency*, *47*(3), 314–334.

Bond, G. R., Drake, R. E., Mueser, K. T., & Latimer, E. (2001). Assertive community treatment: Critical ingredients and impact on patients. *Disease Management and Health Outcomes*, *9*(3), 141–159.

Boothroyd, R., Poythress, N., McGaha, A., & Petrila, J. (2003). The Broward Mental Health Court: Process, outcomes, and service utilization. *International Journal of Law and Psychiatry*, *26*, 55–71.

Borum, R., Deane, M. W., Steadman, H. J., & Morrissey, J. (1998). Police perspectives on responding to mentally ill people in crisis: Perceptions of program effectiveness. *Behavioral Sciences and the Law*, *16*, 393–405.

Brodsky, S. L. (1978). *Intervention Models for Mental Health Services in Jails*. Presentation at Mental Health Services in Local Jails: Special National Workshop, Rockville, MD.

Broner, N., Lattimore, P., Cowell, A. J., & Schlenger, W. E. (2004). Effects of diversion on adults with co-occurring substance abuse and mental illness: Outcomes from a national multi-site study. *Behavioral Sciences and the Law*, *22*, 519–541.

California Board of Corrections. (2004). *Mentally Ill Offenders Crime Reduction Grant Program: Annual Report to the Legislature*. Available online at http://www.cdcr.ca.gov/Divisions_Boards/CSA/CPP/Grants/MIOCR/Docs/Final_MIOCRG_report.pdf. Accessed August 24, 2009.

Calsyn, R. J., Yonker, R. D., Lemming, M. R., Morse, G. A., & Klinkenberg, D. (2005). Impact of assertive community treatment and client characteristics on criminal justice outcomes in dual disorder homeless individuals. *Criminal Behaviour and Mental Health*, *15*(4), 236–248.

Cosden, M., Ellens, J., Schnell, J., & Yamini-Diouf, Y. (2005). Efficacy of a mental health treatment court with assertive community treatment. *Behavioral Sciences and the Law*, *23*, 199–214.

Council of State Governments. (2002). *Criminal Justice/Mental Health Consensus Project*. New York: Council of State Governments/Eastern Regional Conference.

CMHS National GAINS Center. (2009). *Developing a comprehensive plan for mental health and criminal justice collaboration: The sequential intercept model*. Delmar, NY: Author.

Crilly, J. F., Caine, E. D., Lamberti, J. S., Brown, T., & Friedman, B. (2009). Mental health services use and symptom prevalence in a cohort of adults on probation. *Psychiatric Services, 60,* 542–544.

Crocker, A. G., Hartford, K., & Heslop, L. (2009). Gender differences in police encounters among persons with and without serious mental illness. *Psychiatric Services, 60,* 86–93.

Cuddeback, G. S., Morrissey, J. P., & Cusack, K. J. (2007). How many forensic assertive community treatment teams do we need? *Psychiatric Services, 59*(2), 205–208.

Cuddeback, G. S., Morrissey, J. P., Cusack, K. J., & Meyer, P. S. (2009). Challenges to developing forensic assertive community treatment teams. *American Journal of Psychiatric Rehabilitation, 12,* 225–246.

Dauphinot, L. (1997). The efficacy of community correctional supervision for offenders with severe mental illness. Unpublished doctoral dissertation, Department of Psychology, University of Texas, Austin.

Deane, M. W., Steadman, H. J., Borum, R., Veysey, B. M., & Morrissey, J. P. (1999). Emerging partnerships between mental health and law enforcement. *Psychiatric Services, 50,* 99–101.

DeCuir, Jr., W., & Lamb, P. (1996, October). Police response to the dangerously mentally ill. *The Police Chief,* 99–106.

Dupont, R., & Cochran, S. (2000). Police response to mental health emergencies: Barriers to change. *Journal of the American Academy of Psychiatry and the Law, 28,* 338–344.

Engel, R. S., & Silver, E. (2001). Policing mentally disordered suspects: A re-examination of the criminalization hypothesis. *Criminology, 39,* 225–252.

Fagan, J. A., Morrissey, J. P., & Cocozza, J. J. (2007, September 21). *New Models of Collaboration between Criminal Justice and Mental Health Systems.* Prepared for John D. and Catherine T. MacArthur Foundation's Mental Health Policy Research Network.

Fisher, W. H., Roy-Bujnowski, K. M., Grudzinskas, A. J., Clayfield, J. C., Banks, S. M., & Wolff, N. (2006). Patterns and prevalence of arrest in a statewide cohort of mental health care consumers. *Psychiatric Services, 57,* 1623–1628.

Glaze, L. E., & Bonczar, T. P. (2006). *Probation and Parole in the United States, 2005.* Publication No. NCJ 215091. Washington, DC: U.S. Department of Justice, Office of Justice Programs, Bureau of Justice Statistics.

Green, T. M. (1997). Police as frontline mental health workers: The decision to arrest or refer to mental health agencies. *International Journal of Law and Psychiatry, 20,* 469–486.

Grisso, T., Cocozza, J. J., Steadman, H. J., Fisher, W. H., & Greer, A. (1994). The organization of pretrial forensic evaluation services. *Law and Human Behavior, 18*(4), 377–393.

Hammett, T. M., Roberts, C., & Kennedy, S. (2001). Health-related issues on prisoner reentry. *Crime and Delinquency, 47*(3), 390–409.

James, D. J., & Glaze, L. E. (2006). *Mental Health Problems of Prison and Jail Inmates.* Washington, DC: U.S. Dept of Justice, Office of Justice Programs, Bureau of Justice Statistics.

Lamb, H. R., & Weinberger, L. E. (1998). Persons with severe mental illness in jails and prisons: A review. *Psychiatric Services, 49,* 483–492.

Lamb, H. R., Weinberger, L. E., & DeCuir, W. J. (2002). The police and mental health. *Psychiatric Services, 53*(10), 1266–1271.

Lamb, R. L., Weinberger, L. E., & Reston-Parham, C. (1996). Court intervention to address the mental health needs of mentally ill offenders. *Psychiatric Services, 47,* 275–281.

Lamberti, J. S., Weisman, R., & Faden, D. I. (2004). Forensic assertive community treatment : Preventing incarceration of adults with severe mental illness. *Psychiatric Services, 55*(11), 1285–1293.

Lamberti, J. S., Weisman, R. L., Schwarzkopf, S. B., Mundondo-Ashton, R., Price, N., & Trompeter, J. (2001). The mentally ill in jails and prisons: Towards an integrated model of prevention. *Psychiatric Quarterly, 72,* 63–77.

Marshall, M., Gray, A. Lockwood, A., & Green, R. (1998). Case management for people with severe mental disorders. *Cochrane Database of Systematic Reviews*, 2(Art. CD000050).

Marshall, M., & Lockwood, A. (2004). Assertive community treatment for people with severe mental disorders (Cochrane Review). In The Cochrane Library Issue 3. Chichester, UK: Wiley.

McCoy, M. L., Roberts, D. L., Hanrahan, P., Clay, R., & Luchins, D. J. (2004). Jail linkage assertive community treatment services for individuals with mental illnesses. *Psychiatric Rehabilitation Journal*, 27(3), 243–250.

McNiel, D. E., & Binder, R. L. (2007). Effectiveness of a mental health court in reducing criminal recidivism and violence. *American Journal of Psychiatry*, *164*, 1395–1403.

Miller, R. D. (2003). Hospitalization of criminal defendants for evaluation of competence to stand trial or for restoration of competence: Clinical and legal issues. *Behavioral Sciences & the Law*, *21*(3), 369–391.

Moore, M. E., & Hiday, V. A. (2006). Mental health court outcomes: A comparison of re-arrest and re-arrest severity between mental health court and traditional court participants. *Law and Human Behavior*, *30*, 659–674.

Morabito, M. S. (2007). Horizons of context: Understanding the police decision to arrest people with mental illness. *Psychiatric Services*, *58*, 1582–1587.

Morgan, R. D., Steffan, J., Shaw, L. B., & Wilson, S. (2007). Needs for and barriers to correctional mental health services: Inmate perceptions. *Psychiatric Services*, *58*, 1181–1186.

Morris, S. M., Steadman, H. J., & Veysey, B. M. (1997). Mental health services in American jails: A survey of some innovative practices. *Criminal Justice & Behavior*, *24*, 3–19.

Morrissey, J. P., & Cuddeback, G. S. (2007). Jail diversion. In K. T. Mueser & D. Jeste (Eds.), *Clinical Handbook of Schizophrenia*. New York: Guilford Press.

Morrissey, J. P., Cuddeback, G. S, Cuellar, A., & Steadman, H. J. (2007). The role of Medicaid enrollment and outpatient service use in jail recidivism among persons with severe mental illness. *Psychiatric Services*, *58*, 794–801.

Morrissey, J. P., Dalton, K. M., Steadman, H. J., Cuddeback, G. S., Haynes, D., & Cuellar, A. (2006). Assessing gaps between policy and practice in Medicaid disenrollment of jail detainees with severe mental illness. *Psychiatric Services*, *57*, 803–808.

Morrissey, J. P., Meyer, P., & Cuddeback, G. (2005). Extending assertive community treatment to criminal justice settings: Origins, current evidence, and future directions. *Community Mental Health Journal*, *43*(5), 527–544.

Morrissey, J. P., Steadman, H. J., Dalton, K. M., Cuellar, A., Stiles, P., & Cuddeback, G. S. (2006). Medicaid enrollment and mental health service use following release of jail detainees with severe mental illness. *Psychiatric Services*, *57*, 809–815.

Mossman, D., Noffsinger, S. G., Ash, P., Frierson, R. L., Gerbasi, J., Hackett, M., et al. (2007). AAPL practice guideline for the forensic psychiatric evaluation of competence to stand trial. *Journal of the American Academy of Psychiatry and Law*, *35*(Suppl.), S3–S72.

Munetz, M. R., Grande, T., & Chambers, M. (2001). The incarceration of individuals with severe mental disorders. *Community Mental Health Journal*, *37*, 361–372.

Munetz, M. R., & Griffin, P. A. (2006). Use of the sequential intercept model as an approach to decriminalization of people with serious mental illness. *Psychiatric Services*, *57*(4), 544–549.

Naples, M., Morris, L. S., & Steadman, H. J. (2007). Factors in disproportionate representation among persons recommended by programs and accepted by courts for jail diversion. *Psychiatric Services*, *58*(8), 1095–1101.

National Association of State Budget Officers. (1987). *The State Expenditure Report*. Washington, DC: Author.

National Association of State Budget Officers. (2008). *State Expenditure Report, Fiscal Year 2007*. Washington, DC: Author.

National GAINS Center. (2002). *The Nathaniel Project: An Alternative to Incarceration Program for People with Serious Mental Illness Who Have Committed Felony Offenses*. Delmar, NY: Author.

National GAINS Center for People with Co-Occurring Disorders in the Justice System. (2005). *The Prevalence of Co-Occurring Mental Illness and Substance Use Disorders in Jails.* Fact Sheet Series. Delmar, NY: Author.

National GAINS Center for People with Co-Occurring Disorders in the Justice System. (2006). *Serious Violent Reentry Initiative (SVORI): Reentry Projects for Inmates with Serious Mental Illness.* Delmar, NY: Author.

National GAINS Center for People with Co-Occurring Disorders in the Justice System. (2007). *Practical Advice on Jail Diversion: Ten Years of Learnings on Jail Diversion from the CMHS National GAINS Center.* Delmar, NY: Author.

New Freedom Commission on Mental Health. (2003). *Achieving the Promise: Transforming Mental Health Care in America; Final Report.* DHHS Publication No. SMA-03-3832. Rockville, MD: Government Printing Office.

Osher, F. C. (2007, January/February). Short-term strategies to improve reentry of jail populations: Expanding and implementing the APIC model. *American Jails,* 9–18.

Osher, F., Steadman, H. J., & Barr, H. (2002). *A Best Practice Approach to Community Re-Entry from Jails for Inmates with Co-Occurring Disorders: The APIC Model.* Delmar, NY: National GAINS Center.

Patch, P. C., & Arrigo, B. A. (1999). Police officer attitudes and the use of discretion in situations involving the mentally ill: The need to narrow the focus. *International Journal of Law and Psychiatry, 22,* 23–55.

Pew Center on the States. (2009, March). *One in 31: The Long Reach of American Corrections.* Washington, DC: The Pew Charitable Trusts.

Pinals, D. A. (2005). Where two roads meet: Restoration of competence to stand trial from a clinical perspective. *New England School of Law, 31*(1), 81–108.

Porporino, F. J., & Motiuk, L. L. (1995). The prison careers of mentally disordered offenders. *International Journal of Law and Psychiatry, 18,* 29–44.

Poythress, N. G., Bonnie, R. J., & Oberlander, L. B. (1994). Client abilities to assist counsel and make decisions in criminal cases. *Law and Human Behavior, 18*(4), 437–452.

Poythress, N., Hoge, S., Bonnie, R., Monahan, J., Eisenberg, M., & Feucht-Haviar, T. (1998). The competence-related abilities of women criminal defendants. *Journal of the American Academy of Psychiatry and the Law, 26,* 215–222.

Redlich, A. D. (2005). Voluntary, but knowing and intelligent? Comprehension in mental health courts. *Psychology, Public Policy, and Law, 11,* 605–619.

Redlich, A. D., Hoover, S., Summers, A., & Steadman, H. J. (in press). Enrollment in mental health courts: Voluntariness, knowingness, and adjudicative competence. *Law and Human Behavior.*

Redlich, A. D., Steadman, H. J., Monahan, J., Petrila, J., & Griffin, P. (2005). The second generation of mental health courts. *Psychology, Public Policy, and Law, 11,* 527–538.

Redlich, A. D., Steadman, H. J., Monahan, J., Robbins, P. C., & Petrila, J. (2006). Patterns of practice in mental health courts: A national survey. *Law and Human Behavior, 30,* 347–362.

Reuland, M. (2004). *A Guide to Implementing Police-Based Diversion Programs for People with Mental Illness.* Delmar, NY: National GAINS Technical Assistance and Policy Analysis Center for Jail Diversion.

Reuland, M., & Cheney, J. (2005). *Enhancing Success of Police-Based Diversion Programs for People with Mental Illness.* Delmar, NY: National GAINS Technical Assistance and Policy Analysis Center for Jail Diversion.

Rosenfeld, B., & Wall, A. (1998). Psychopathology and competence to stand trial. *Criminal Justice and Behavior, 25*(4), 443–462.

Silver, E., Arseneault, L., Langley, J., Caspi, A., & Moffitt, T. E. (2005). Mental disorder and violent victimization in a total birth cohort. *American Journal of Public Health, 95,* 2015–2021.

Skeem, J. L., Emke-Francis, P., & Eno Louden, J. (2006). Probation, mental health, and mandated treatment: A national survey. *Criminal Justice and Behavior, 33*(2), 158–184.

Skeem, J., & Eno Louden, J. (2006). Toward evidence-based practice for probationers and parolees mandated to mental health treatment. *Psychiatric Services, 57*(3), 333–342.

Skeem, J., Eno Louden, J., Manchak, S., Vidal, S., & Haddad, E. (2009). Social networks and social control of probationers with co-occurring mental and substance abuse problems. *Law and Human Behavior, 33*(2), 122–135.

Solomon, P., & Draine, J. (1995). One-year outcomes of a randomized trial of case management with seriously mentally ill clients leaving jail. *Evaluation Review, 19*, 256–273.

Steadman, H. J., Barbera, S., & Dennis, D. L. (1994). A national survey of jail diversion programs for mentally ill detainees. *Hospital and Community Psychiatry, 45*, 1109–1113.

Steadman, H. J., Cocozza, J. J., & Veysey, B. M. (1999). Comparing outcomes for diverted and nondiverted jail detainees with mental illnesses. *Law and Human Behavior, 23*(6), 615–627.

Steadman, H. J., Deane, M. W., Borum, R., & Morrissey, J. P. (2000). Comparing outcomes of major models of police responses to mental health emergencies. *Psychiatric Services, 51*, 645–649.

Steadman, H. J., Fabisiak, S., Dvoskin, J., & Holohean, E. J. (1987). A survey of mental disability among state prison inmates. *Hospital and Community Psychiatry, 38*(10), 1086–1090.

Steadman, H. J., Morris, S. M., & Dennis, D. L. (1995). The diversion of mentally ill persons from jails to community-based services: A profile of programs. *American Journal of Public Health, 85*(12), 1630–1635.

Steadman, H. J., & Naples, M. (2005). Assessing the effectiveness of jail diversion programs for persons with serious mental illness and co-occurring substance use disorders. *Behavioral Sciences and the Law, 23*, 163–170.

Steadman, H. J., Robbins, P. C., Islam, T., & Osher, F. C. (2007). Re-validating the Brief Jail Mental Health Screen to increase accuracy for women. *Psychiatric Services, 58*, 1598–1601.

Steadman, H. J., Stainbrook. K. A., Griffin, P., Draine, J., Dupont, R., & Horey, C. (2001). A specialized crisis response as a core element of police-based diversion programs. *Psychiatric Services, 52*, 219–222.

Teplin, L. A. (1983). The criminalization of the mentally ill: Speculation in search of data. *Psychological Bulletin, 94*(1), 54–67.

Teplin, L. A. (1984). Criminalizing mental disorder: The comparative arrest rate of the mentally ill. *American Psychologist, 39*(7), 794–803.

Teplin, L. A. (2000). *Keeping the Peace: Police Discretion and Mentally Ill Persons*. Washington, DC: National Institute of Justice Journal.

Teplin, L. A., Abram, K. M., & McClelland, G. M. (1996). Prevalence of psychiatric disorders among incarcerated women: I, Pretrial jail detainees. *Archives of General Psychiatry, 53*, 505–512.

Teplin, L. A., McClelland, G. M., Abram, K. M., & Weiner, D. A. (2005). Crime victimization in adults with severe mental illness: Comparison with the National Crime Victimization Survey. *Archives of General Psychiatry, 62*, 911–921.

Torrey, E. F., Stieber, J., Ezekiel J., et al. (1992). *Criminalizing the Seriously Mentally Ill: The Abuse of Jails as Mental Hospitals*. Washington, DC: National Alliance for the Mentally Ill and Public Citizen's Health Research Group.

Veysey, B. M., Steadman, H. J., Morrissey, J. P., & Johnsen, M. (1997). In search of the missing linkages: Continuity of care in U.S. jails. *Behavioral Sciences and the Law 15*, 383–397.

Weisman, R. L., Lamberti, J. S., & Price, N. (2004). Integrating criminal justice, community healthcare, and support services for adults with severe mental disorders. *Psychiatric Quarterly, 75*(1), 71–85.

Zapf, P. A., Hubbard, K. L., Cooper, V. G., Whelles, M. C., & Ronan, K. A. (2004). Have the courts abdicated their responsibility for determination of competency to stand trial to clinicians? *Journal of Forensic Psychology Practice, 4*(1), 27–44.

Part III

Special Issues

Chapter 19

MENTAL HEALTH DISPARITIES

Junius J. Gonzales, MD, MBA; and Airia Sasser Papadopoulos, MPH

Introduction

Even before the Institute of Medicine released its critical report *Unequal Treatment: Confronting Racial and Ethnic Disparities in Health Care,* evidence was mounting on the differential rates of access to services, quality of care received, and improvement in health outcomes among different groups of people (Smedley, Stith, & Nelson, 2003). Since 2003, the Agency for Health Care Research and Quality (AHRQ) has released its annual *National Healthcare Disparities Report* (Agency for Healthcare Research and Quality [AHRQ], 2009), which "summarizes health care quality and access among various racial, ethnic, and income groups and other priority populations, such as children and older adults" (p. 1). As an example, the 2008 report includes residents of rural areas and individuals with disabilities and special health care needs as priority populations.

The evidence on mental health disparities is increasing. Studies from the 1980s show that minorities were more likely to delay or not seek mental health care, receive less adequate care, and terminate care earlier (McGuire & Miranda, 2008). More recent work denotes that disparities are found in access to and the provision and receipt of care, for example, for the treatment of depression (Miranda, McGuire, Williams, & Wang, 2008; Harman, Edlund, & Fortney, 2004), help-seeking behaviors of children and adolescents (Zimmerman, 2005), overall mental health care services use (Garland et al., 2005), and psychotropic drug use (Han & Liu, 2005). These mental health disparities data are important in light of the fact that although rates for most mental disorders are lower in Hispanics and Blacks than in Whites, the individuals receive poorer prognoses and their disorders are more chronic (Breslau et al., 2006; Williams et al., 2007).

The goals of this chapter are to 1) provide a background and definitions of key concepts in disparities; 2) describe useful conceptual frameworks and constructs for health disparities; 3) present an overview and examples of mental health disparities in selected populations; and 4) summarize findings and consider future directions.

Definitions of Racial and Ethnic Disparities, Inequalities, and Inequities in Health

The literature on racial and ethnic disparities, inequalities, and inequities in health is complex, ambiguous, and opens the door to wide interpretation of terminology. McGuire, Alegria, Cook, Wells, and Zaslavsky (2006) write:

> A consensus has emerged that eliminating disparities should be a major goal of health policy, but the empirical and policy literature fails to agree on what a "disparity" is, and how it should be measured. Empirical research often estimates coefficients of race/ethnicity variables without relating these coefficients to an explicit definition of disparity. (pp. 1979–1980)

Inconsistencies in the definitions and uses of the terms disparity, inequality, and inequity in health care allow for a shaping of meaning that may be specifically relevant to a discipline or even to an individual. Differences in the use of these terms have potential policy implications that affect measurements used to monitor health outcomes and also the priority setting for programs to receive financial support (Braveman, Starfield, & Geiger, 2001).

A disparity is defined as something "containing or made up of fundamentally different and often incongruous parts" (*Merriam-Webster Online Dictionary*, 2009a). Given this common definition, a disparity within a given category contains disagreement between two or more aspects of itself. Similarly, an inequality is defined as "the quality of being unequal or uneven" and as the "disparity of distribution or opportunity" (*Merriam-Webster Online Dictionary*, 2009b). As with these dictionary definitions, disparities and inequalities are used interchangeably within the public health literature to define differences with regard to health status and outcomes, services provided, and treatment received. Though not stated, implicit assumptions within these definitions are that "disparities" are inequalities that are potentially unexpected, undesirable, and even problematic.

Inequity, however, is defined as "injustice" or "unfairness" (*Merriam-Webster Online Dictionary*, 2009c). Unlike the objective definitions used to describe disparity and inequality, the definition of inequity carries within its scope an inherent moral claim (Whitehead, 1990). Close examination of the words "justice" and "fairness" reveals the explicitly contained belief that two or more of the compared aspects are different from one another and should not be. Thus, an inequity holds within its definition a stance that goes beyond simply recognizing an inherent imbalance. Inequity is the judgment of a disparity as being contemptible and in need of rebalance. In her 1990 paper, Margaret Whitehead provides distinctions between health disparities and health inequity describing populations in Europe. She adds to the above definition of inequity the dimension that such differences in health are also "unnecessary and avoidable" (p. 7).

Though not consistently applied, these above-noted definitions also are resonant within the scientific literature and particularly common in documenting racial and ethnic differences in health. Scientists agree that a seminal reference, buttressed by scientific data on racial and ethnic disparities, is *Unequal Treatment: Confronting Racial and Ethnic Disparities in Health Care* (Smedley et al., 2003). According to the report, disparities in health care are "racial and ethnic differences in the quality of healthcare that are not due to access-related factors or clinical needs, preferences and appropriateness of intervention" (Smedley et al., 2003, p. 4). This definition attempts to "control" for variability in the reasons why differences exist in the care a patient receives by removing financial factors and distinguishes health care use *differences* (unadjusted difference in rates or means between different groups, which may be accounted for by other factors such as age, baseline health, etc.) from disparities. The variation is also not related to patient preferences for care or any resistance to the treatment recommended or received. Rather, health disparities are defined here as different outcomes for patients who receive quality care but whose health status, regardless of the treatment received, remains worse than the comparative, healthier population. Specifically in the United States, health disparities afflict people of African, Hispanic, Asian, and Native American ancestry when health status, across a number of categories, is compared to the health of people of European ancestry (Smedley et al., 2003). Though the report provides no definition of inequities, it does indicate that the prevalence of health disparities keeps all Americans separate from the possibility of true equality, a core American value (Smedley et al., 2003).

Whitehead and Dahlgren (2007) define health inequities as the "unjust distribution" of health conditions while stating that health equity "is when everyone has the opportunity to 'attain their full health potential'" regardless of "social position or other socially determined circumstance" (pp. 5–6). Their definition of health inequities, used frequently at the international level, is echoed in a recent federal CDC report (e.g., Brennan Ramirez, Baker, & Metzler, 2008).

The existence of racial and ethnic disparities in health is inequitable and problematic, as evidenced by the attention to this issue by the federal government and other influential scientific bodies. Better defining health disparities and elucidating the nature of health inequity are beginning steps for moving beyond an objective examination of health status in the United States toward answering a larger policy issue to improve quality of life for all citizens. This overview of definitions is important to convey the complexity of racial and ethnic disparities.

Health Disparities Frameworks and Other Important Constructs

Conceptual models, developed by both federal agencies and independent researchers who study health disparities, provide diverse perspectives in attempts to describe the extent of the problem and understand how and why disparities occur. Early efforts include the Healthy People 2000 initiatives (U.S. Department of Health and Human Services [USDHHS], 2001) and the US-DHHS Office of Minority

Health (2003). In 1989, the Agency for Health Care Policy and Research was created within the U.S. Department of Health and Human Services. Its charge was to "improve the quality, safety, efficiency, and effectiveness of health care for all Americans" (AHRQ, 2008). In 1999, Congress mandated through the passage of the Healthcare Research and Quality Act that the agency, now renamed as the Agency for Healthcare Research and Quality (AHRQ), produce annual reports on health care quality and disparities in the United States (Poker, Hubbard, Sharp, & Collins, 2004).

Commissioned by the AHRQ, a special committee on quality and quality measurement produced two reports (Hurtado, Swift, Corrigan, & the Committee on the National Quality Report on Health Care Delivery, 2001; Swift & the Committee on Guidance for Designing a National Healthcare Disparities Report, 2002) that assisted in the creation of the *National Health Care Quality Report (NHQR)* and the *National Healthcare Disparities Report (NHDR)* in 2003.

The 2002 IOM report titled *Unequal Treatment: Confronting Racial and Ethnic Disparities in Health Care* (Smedley et al., 2003) was produced within a year of the AHRQ reports and denoted a slightly different framework. The report also studied factors that contribute to inequities and proposed recommended policies for eliminating the inequities (Smedley et al., 2003). IOM's model for health disparities emphasized the presentation of patient needs to providers as the central pathway for how racial and ethnic disparities emerge. According to the framework, three parties (clinicians, utilization managers who are slightly distanced but who participate in the treatment process, and patients) exercise discretion in influencing the health care received by patients in a clinical setting. The model begins with patient input, which leads to both the patient's contribution to a medical history and a physical examination of symptoms. The second step outlines social, economic, and cultural influences on interpretation and intervention, respectively, both of which are potentially subject to the outside influences of stereotyping, prejudice, and financial incentives. The third step and outcome of the first two steps is racially disparate clinical decisions.

The primary goal of the two AHRQ reports is to outline and monitor the status of the quality of health care provided to Americans with particular emphasis on subpopulations. The *NHQR* identifies gaps in the provision of quality health care in the United States. The *NHDR* is focused on racial, ethnic, and socioeconomic disparities in health care provided to vulnerable populations. It identifies where differences exist and has the potential to influence the development of new and improved interventions to ensure that the highest quality of care is delivered to subpopulations (AHRQ, 2009).

From the *NHQR* emerged an early conceptual framework that identified two aspects of treatment in a clinical setting that potentially influence health disparities. The first aspect of treatment addresses provider elements of treatment quality, such as the effectiveness of treatment and the quality of the interaction between clinician and patient. The second aspect of treatment identifies patient needs, such as staying healthy and living with illness/disability, which are potentially of primary concern to recipients of care. A slightly expanded framework appears in the *NHDR* that builds upon the initial *NHQR* framework with the addition of measures that address equity, including access to care, use of services, and costs. The dimensions of race, ethnicity, and socioeconomic status were incorporated into the framework with a focus on influencing health outcomes (Poker et al., 2004).

Interestingly, the AHRQ and the IOM reports situate key elements of responsibility for the occurrence of health disparities with both patients and clinicians. Neither report specifically condones or condemns the clinical structure/provider or the patient, but rather identifies that both parties play a key role. Most evident within these and other reports developed since that examine health disparities is the challenge to revamp health care systems in order to better meet patient needs and to reduce, rather than further widen, gaps in outcomes.

Individual researchers expanded upon old frameworks and created new ones for understanding disparities using the elements described above. Kilbourne, Switzer, Hyman, Crowley-Matoka, and Fine (2006) observed, in a review of the health disparities literature, that many researchers devoted their attention to documenting the occurrences of disparate treatment in clinical settings and less to understanding the underlying causes. In addition, little focus was placed upon how to address health disparities systematically. In response to this observation, they developed an epidemiologically based conceptual framework (see Figure 19.1) to guide health services researchers, clinicians, and policymakers in future health disparities research in health care settings.

The framework focuses on the health care system, precisely and uniquely extends the definition of vulnerable populations to include impoverished populations in addition to racial ethnic minorities, and provides a distinct plan for how to proceed with effecting change in disparities. It consists of three phases, the first of which is the detection of disparities and causes. The second phase is the understanding of social determinants of disparities at four levels: patient, provider, the clinical encounter, and the health care system. The third phase includes stages for reducing or eliminating health disparities, including developing interventions, evaluating the effectiveness of treatment, translating and disseminating the findings, and changing policy. The authors posit a possible addition to this framework, namely, reciprocal feedback between phases. For example, interventions to reduce disparities (phase 3) may yield information for new ways to measure disparities (phase 1).

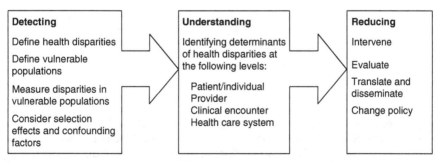

Figure 19.1   The Three Phases of the Disparities Research Agenda. (*Source*: Kilbourne, A. M., Switzer, G., Hyman, K., Crowley-Matoka, M., & Fine, M. J. [2006]. Advancing health disparities research within the health care system: A conceptual framework. *American Journal of Public Health*, 96[12], 2113–2121.)

A second component of Kilbourne et al.'s framework builds upon the elements outlined in the other conceptual frameworks for identifying and understanding the nature of health disparities. This framework examines four factors (health care system, patient, clinical encounter, and provider) with the inclusion of a final step for drawing the findings back into the overarching health care system in order to create changes in the delivery of care (see Figure 19.2).

Examining the patient experience in treatment settings has been a primary focus of conceptual frameworks on health disparities. Cooper, Hill, and Powe (2002) credit the IOM report as moving beyond a traditional examination of patient-provider interaction to examining issues that affect equity, and they state that it is "a useful starting point" (p. 478). They developed a new conceptual model, based upon Donabedian's traditional structure-process-outcomes model that merges elements of a 1993 IOM report on access to care and the ability for a provider to adequately address a patient's needs. In addition, they layer in personal and familial barriers that may intercede with a patient's ability to engage fully in treatment (see Figure 19.3). The model begins with the patient's financial and personal situation and progresses to use of services, mediators, and outcomes. One additional unique element of this framework is the importance of the patient's experience with the

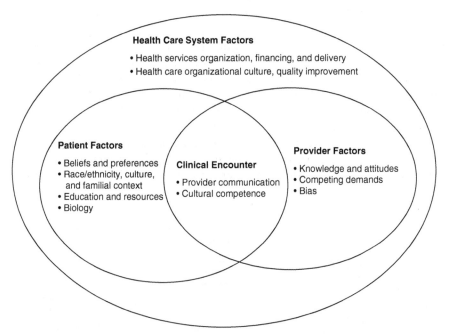

Figure 19.2 Understanding the Origins of Health and Health Care Disparities from a Health Services Research Perspective: Key Potential Determinants of Health Disparities within the Health Care System, Including Individual, Provider, and Health Care System Factors. (*Source*: Kilbourne, A. M., Switzer, G., Hyman, K., Crowley-Matoka, M., & Fine, M. J. [2006]. Advancing health disparities research within the health care system: A conceptual framework. *American Journal of Public Health*, 96[12], 2113–2121.)

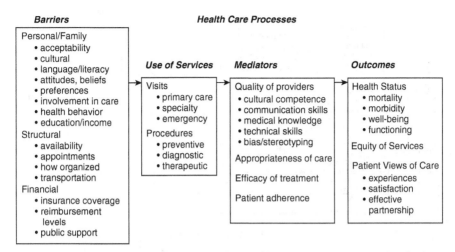

Figure 19.3 Barriers to and Mediators of Equitable Health Care for Racial and Ethnic Minorities. (*Source*: Adapted from Cooper, L. A., Hill, M. N., & Powe, N. R. [2002]. Designing and evaluating interventions to eliminate racial and ethnic disparities in health care. *Journal of General Internal Medicine*, 17[6], 477–486.)

encounter influencing multi-dimensional outcomes, ranging from physical and well-being endpoints to satisfaction and partnership. This framework allows for recognition of the natural elements that influence a person's health beyond clinical treatment. This includes the patient's perception of the provider and other structural interactions with the health care system before treatment even begins.

Other Models of Providers and Disparities

Since disparities exist in the process of care, from provision to receipt of services, two models addressing provision of care by clinicians are important to consider and illustrate other levels of complexity, such as attitudinal factors and decision-making paradigms. Van Ryn and colleagues (van Ryn & Fu, 2003; van Ryn, Burgess, Malat, & Griffin, 2006) focus on the unconscious biases and stereotypical reactions providers may have and how those may affect clinical decision making, from diagnosis to referral to treatment. Drawing from social cognitive and attitude theories, van Ryn and Fu (2003) describe potential mechanisms (e.g., social categorization and stereotyping) by which health and human service providers may contribute to racial and ethnic disparities. They suggest that these mechanisms are efficient ways for processing large amounts of complex information. However, they warn providers (and patients) not to "unconsciously and automatically assign the characteristics of that group to the individual in question, a process referred to as 'stereotype application'" (p. 250). The model, depicted in Figure 19.4, contains multiple possible targets for intervention to decrease automatically activated stereotypical and related thinking that might impinge upon the appropriate provision of care.

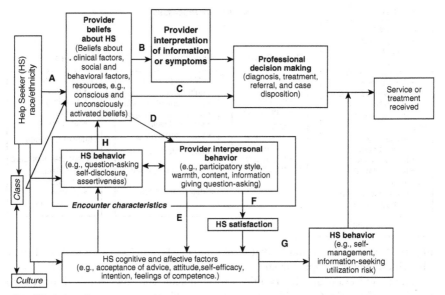

Note. HS = help seeker.

Figure 19.4 Proposed Mechanisms through which Health and Human Service Providers Can Influence Race/Ethnicity Disparities in Treatment. (*Source*: van Ryn, M., & Fu, S. S. [2003]. Paved with good intentions: Do public health and human service providers contribute to racial/ethnic disparities in health? *American Journal of Public Health*, *93*[2], 248–255.)

Recent work, using decision-making theories and Bayesian models to understand disparities, has resulted in the concept of "statistical discrimination." Borrowed from the labor literature, statistical discrimination in health care addresses how patient needs are *matched* to treatment by the provider based upon the quality of information. Poor communication between the patient and provider, for example, may result in a minority-group patient being worse off on average when compared to majority-group patients. Add to this the use of patient categorization, as mentioned above, and one can see how miscommunication may result in less-than-effective treatment, a stance supported in the empirical literature addressing patient-physician communication and improved patient outcomes (Balsa, McGuire, & Meredith, 2005; McGuire et al., 2006).

New statistical approaches (Duan, Meng, Lin, Chen, & Alegria, 2008) attempt to address the complexity of factors, at multiple levels, that may or may not contribute to health disparities. Complex methodological issues are of paramount importance and have even led to recommendations by the National Center for Health Statistics within the Federal Centers for Disease Control and Prevention (Keppel et al., 2005). The main six issues (with eleven ensuing guidelines) in that report on measuring disparities are:

1. The selection of a reference point from which to measure disparity;
2. Measurement of disparity in absolute or in relative terms;
3. Measurement of disparity in terms of favorable or adverse events;

4. Measurement of disparity focusing on individual groups in a pair-wise fashion or focusing on a summary measure for the domain that includes these groups;

5. Choosing whether to weight component groups when calculating summary measures of disparity; and,

6. Choosing whether or not to consider the order inherent in the domains with ordered categories when calculating summary measures of disparity. (Keppel et al., 2005, p. 1)

These recommendations are important in accurately describing the size and direction of a disparity, changes over time, and conclusions across different indicators, geographic locations, or groups. As the report notes "different choices can, and frequently do, lead to different conclusions about disparities" (Keppel et al., 2005, p. 1).

DISPARITIES AND STIGMA

Stigma may contribute to or even moderate intervention effects on disparities. The United Kingdom Government's Foresight Programme report on mental capital and well-being contains a thorough and exceptionally complex influence diagram that denotes relationships between the target (person with mental illness) and source of stigma using constructs from emotion, cognition, social policy, and other research (Jenkins et al., 2008). On the target side, the combination of behavior representing mental ill health, stress, and loss of socioeconomic opportunities can lead to complex emotional states, such as loss of self-confidence and anticipated discrimination. This side intersects with the "source" side where emotions, prejudice, culture, and ignorance can contribute to a multi-layered discrimination.

One important question is whether and how stigma may play a role in the various levels of putative mechanisms that can partially explain mental health disparities, such as the work by McGuire and colleagues on statistical discrimination discussed earlier (Balsa et al., 2005; McGuire et al., 2006). Does a provider, as a "source of stigma," possibly have "potential priors" about mental illness that exist because of stigma? Does a patient, because of prior experience with stigma, present (or not) certain things to the provider? Recent work on stigma in poor young immigrant and U.S.-born Black, Latina, and White depressed women offers some interesting insights. Nadeem et al. (2007) found that Black and Latina (U.S.-born and immigrant) women had more stigma-related concerns than White women and that stigma was correlated with less desire for treatment except in the case of immigrant Latina women. This work was extended to confirm, per previous studies, that different people from different backgrounds have different preferences for mental health care. Minorities are less favorably inclined toward antidepressant medication, but the stigma of mental illness reduced the preference for group counseling (Nadeem, Lange, & Miranda, 2008). Even work from large secondary data analyses using four years of data suggest that some disparities in mental health care use may result from different propensities to both interpret and report symptoms (Zuvekas & Fleishman, 2008).

Other recent work investigated whether racial and ethnic differences existed in attitudes about people with mental illness or stigma. Issues of perceived dangerousness and desire for segregation from people with mental illness were examined and found to differ. For example, while African Americans and Asian Americans perceived higher dangerousness and had more desire for segregation than Caucasians, Latinos perceived lower dangerousness and had less desire for segregation than Caucasians (Rao, Feinglass, & Corrigan, 2007).

MENTAL HEALTH DISPARITIES: SELECTED FINDINGS

The literature related to health disparities has exploded and includes mental health conditions. Much of the work is descriptive, limited by the nature of data and study designs, and thereby often unable to elucidate mechanisms of action or contribute to thinking about predictive causal models. While factors such as income and limited English proficiency are associated with poorer physical and mental health and services utilization (Bandiera, Pereira, Arif, Dodge, & Asal, 2008; Dobalian & Rivers, 2008; Sentell, Shumway, & Snowden, 2007), much less work has elucidated possible mediating or moderating factors, especially in regard to preventing or reducing disparities.

The 2001 Surgeon General's report titled *Mental Health: Culture, Race and Ethnicity* highlighted critical issues that special populations face. It also illuminated the complexity and difficulty involved in the development of evidence-based practices and the conducting of day-to-day practice and policy decision-making (USDHHS, 2001). That report cited evidence for the following: 1) minorities have less access to, and availability of, mental health services; 2) minorities are less likely to receive needed mental health services; 3) minorities in treatment often receive poorer quality care; and 4) minorities are under-represented in mental health research studies. The relationship of ethnicity to outcomes is often difficult to understand given not only the measurement of ethnicity, but also important factors such as acculturation, previous provision and receipt of services, discrimination, immigration experiences, cultural beliefs, environment, and social influences by other groups (Bernal, Bonilla, & Bellido, 1995).

The National Institute of Mental Health (NIMH) recently funded two large epidemiologic studies of racial and ethnic minorities, the National Latino and Asian American Survey (NLAAS) and the National Survey of American Life (NSAL), to augment the most recent survey of mental disorders known as the National Comorbidity Survey-Replication (Collaborative Psychiatric Epidemiology Surveys, n.d.). Known as the Collaborative Psychiatric Epidemiology Surveys (CPES), the CPES combined dataset is considered by many as a single, nationally representative study. Data are available on the prevalence of mental disorders, impairments associated with these disorders, and treatment patterns from representative samples of majority and minority U.S. adult populations. Additional data collected examined the ties between mental disorders and socio-cultural issues, such as language use, perception of disparities, support systems, discrimination, and assimilation.

The CPES and similar studies can help tease out the possible differences in mental health symptoms, disorders, and related functional status. Capturing all of these differences is beyond the scope of this chapter, but knowledge about these "clinical" differences is helpful in better understanding disparities. The CPES has found that for many mental disorders, either overall prevalence rates across racial and ethnic groups are similar, or, in fact, minorities may have lower prevalence rates (e.g., major depressive disorder or MDD). However, drill-down analyses across and within groups are critical to employ. For example, while Blacks may have lower rates of MDD, the course and severity of the disorder may be more serious and difficult. Even within the larger group of Blacks who have MDD, the long-standing notion of higher prevalence rates in women (e.g., 2/3) does not seem to hold among Caribbean Blacks, where men have rates of 50% (Williams et al., 2007). Other studies indicate such findings as lower rates of reported functional impairment in depressed Latinos versus other groups but no other differences related to race or ethnicity (that is, similar levels of functioning in the presence of depressive symptoms). Interestingly, the issue of how people express and report their functioning is critical, and similar findings for Latinos are seen in studies of diabetics and other chronic medical illnesses (Huang, Chung, Kroenke, & Spitzer, 2006).

New reports from one of the largest epidemiologic studies focusing on Latino mental health (using nationally representative samples) indicate that lifetime prevalence rates of mental disorders are nearly equal in Latino men (28.1%) and women (30.2%) (Alegria et al., 2007). Prevalence rates were higher overall for people who had migrated before the age of 13 or after age 34, while good or excellent language proficiency was associated with increased risk for past year disorders in both genders. The complex results suggest multi-factorial effects cutting across genetic, environmental, role, and nativity/origin constructs. The same study showed that cultural factors such as language, age of migration, nativity, years of U.S. residence, and generational status were associated with use (or lack) of mental health services for Latinos who did not meet full disorder status, but "who may need preventive services or who are symptomatic but not diagnosed with a disorder" (Alegria et al., 2007).

Access and Barriers to Care

The 1993 IOM report Access to Health Care in America noted:

> *Access* is a shorthand term used for a broad set of concerns that center on the degree to which individuals and groups are able to obtain needed services from the medical care system. Often because of difficulties in defining and measuring the term, people equate access with insurance coverage and having enough doctors and hospitals in the areas in which they live. But having insurance or nearby health care providers is no guarantee that people who need services will get them. Conversely, many who lack coverage or live in areas that appear to have shortages of health care facilities do, indeed, receive services. (Millman, 1993, p. 32)

The IOM committee took these concerns and predicated its final definition on both use and impact of services: access is "the timely use of personal health services

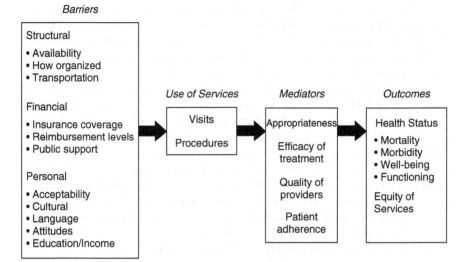

Barriers

Figure 19.5   Model of Access to Personal Health Care Services. (*Source*: Millman M, L. [1993]. A model for monitoring access. In *Access to Health Care in America* [pp. 31–45]. Washington, DC: Institute of Medicine, Committee on Monitoring Access to Personal Health Care Services. Washington, D.C.: The National Academies Press.)

to achieve the best possible health outcomes" (p. 33). The report depicted the following model and created indicators for utilization and outcomes, but noted the dynamic and complex relationships between these factors.

The authors describe this "'access' model in order to provide a straightforward framework for the many examples of mental health disparities in the literature. Another example is a recent review on Latino adults' access to mental health care (Cabassa, Zayas, & Hansen, 2006). It found existing studies to be helpful, but also fraught with limitations that might provide misleading conclusions.

Whether or not someone uses services is a complex phenomenon that touches issues at many levels, from an individual level—from knowledge to attitudes to preferences—to social level (e.g., stigma) to systems level (availability), as noted in the Barriers category in Figure 19.5. Furthermore, unique combinations between access factors may or may not sum up service utilization, quantity, and duration of the utilization, or appropriateness. The following simple example notes the complexity of factors that play into access such as the personal factor of attitudes. A person may personally acknowledge mental health concerns, such as depressive symptoms, but then not communicate those to the caregiver. This can certainly impact the provision and receipt of services.

Using a large national survey, Probst, Laditka, Moore, Harun, and Powell (2007) found that of those people who acknowledge depressive symptoms, only 51.8% reported those to a physician or other practitioner (e.g., social worker, counselor, nurse). For the Whites (54%), Hispanics (48%), and African Americans (35.7%) who did report depression concerns, other differences and interactions were found among individual characteristics, such as gender, age, marital status, health status, and health insurance. Another study using a large national survey with a baseline population of nearly 300,000 found complex interactions between race/ethnicity, income, and chronic medical disease (asthma) on the reporting of poor mental health (Bandiera et al., 2008). Sentell et al. (2007) found that language barriers were critical in mental health treatment in non-English speaking Asian/ Pacific Islander and Latino persons with mental disorders.

Finally, important factors such as family support (or lack thereof as a barrier) are not represented in the model, but are often described in studies. Ethnic and cultural differences in family involvement were associated with disparities in outpatient and inpatient mental health services (Snowden, 2007). Similarly, the role of spirituality (Williams et al., 2007) is an emerging area of inquiry.

The health services research literature is replete with descriptions of the structural and financial barriers to care, and the area of mental health services is not an exception. Both qualitative and quantitative approaches have provided data from multiple perspectives, and organizational characteristics (e.g., chaotic work environment; level of work control) of where minority patients receive care may offer some new insights for multi-level interventions (Barrio et al., 2008; Varkey et al., 2009).

Culture: A Barrier?

One important issue, linked to personal and social "barriers," that impacts access is culture. While beyond the scope of this chapter, a long-standing literature on the relationships between culture, illness, and help-seeking has provided understanding of their influence on mental health. A recent paper proposes a conceptual paradigm, the Cultural Influences on Mental Health (CIMH) model, to better understand "the dynamic and interactive nature of culture on interrelated mental health domains" (Hwang, Myers, Abe-Kim, & Ting, 2008). The authors define culture "broadly as not only including the set of attitudes, values, beliefs, and behaviors shared by a group of people, but also as inclusive of culture-related experiences such as those related to acculturation and being an ethnic minority" (p. 212). The figure below illustrates how culture might affect six domains of mental health: 1) the prevalence of mental illness; 2) etiology of disease; 3) phenomenology of distress; 4) diagnosis and assessment issues; 5) coping styles and help-seeking pathways; and 6) treatment and intervention issues.

The CIMH model can be used to understand recent work such as new data from audiotaped and videotaped clinical encounters, in both specialty mental health and primary care, which try to elucidate missing information in diagnoses and possible ensuing disparities for Latinos and about differences in visit duration for African Americans (Alegria, Nakash, Lapatin et al., 2008; Ghods et al., 2008; Olfson, Cherry, & Lewis-Fernandez, 2009). Again, though beyond the scope of this discussion, attention to culture and health care has led to developments and research on cultural competency including new measure development (Lucas, Michalopoulou, Falzarano, Menon, & Cunningham, 2008) to overcome thorny measurement issues that troubled the concept. In similar fashion, the recent development of sociocultural assessment protocols (SCAP), specifically for people who suffer from mental disorders, offers promise, but will need more testing and linking to consumer

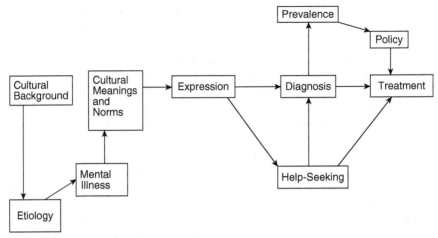

Figure 19.6   The Cultural Influences on Mental Health (CIMH) Model. (*Source*: Hwang, W.-C., Myers, H. F., Abe-Kim, J., & Ting, J. Y. [2008]. A conceptual paradigm for understanding culture's impact on mental health: The cultural influences on mental health [CIMH] model. *Clinical Psychology Review, 28*[2], 211–227.)

outcomes (Yamada & Brekke, 2008). More work is needed on understanding how culture is not a barrier but a facilitator to access care and perhaps reduce disparities.

Utilization of Services: The Provision and Receipt of Care

While the literature is rapidly accumulating studies of racial and ethnic disparities, one important empirical paper actually implemented the IOM definition of disparities regarding outpatient mental health care. The IOM definition was chosen for three key reasons: 1) high prevalence of mental disorders; 2) the role of social factors in the recognition and treatment of these disorders (status as mediators of disparities can be tested); and 3) data demonstrating disparities in mental health care (McGuire et al., 2006). Using a large national survey of nearly 10,000 persons, the study modeled expenditures for mental health care for Whites, Blacks and Latinos but asked the important guiding question to apply the IOM definition of disparity to the analytic strategies: "how much more (or less) treatment would minorities receive than whites if they had the same health status as whites?" (p. 1986). Analyses examined initial *differences*, computations based upon the estimated effect of race and ethnicity, and then adjustments of all other variables (e.g., SES), thereby making comparisons with other disparity "measures." Significant differences (disparities) in care for mental health problems were found between Whites and both Blacks and Latinos. McGuire and co-authors note that one key piece of the IOM definition, preferences, could not be examined with this data-set, but the rigorous methods used in this study set excellent standards given the variable application of definitions and conclusions drawn in other work. Other studies used the same approach to test for "statistical discrimination" with a different large national dataset, the Medical Expenditures Panel Survey, and data from a trial in primary care. Both of these studies found similar results (Cook, McGuire, & Miranda, 2007; McGuire et al., 2008).

In the National Comorbidity Survey-Replication (NCS-R), racial and ethnic minorities had higher rates of no initial treatment contact after onset of a mental disorder and longer delays to seek treatment, and they were less likely to use services that were capable of delivering adequate psychopharmacology and psychotherapy services (Wang et al., 2006). In a study of nearly 1,200 primary care patients, Latinos and Blacks were less than half as likely as Whites to receive any depression care, much less quality guideline-concordant care, even controlling for such factors as age, education, employment status, comorbid medical illness, or depression or anxiety diagnosis (Lagomasino et al., 2005). Several other studies continue to show similar racial and ethnic disparities in the use of mental health services (Dobalian & Rivers, 2008) even when co-occurring chronic medical diseases (e.g., diabetes and ischemic heart disease) (Glover et al., 2007; Waldman et al., 2009) or co-occurring substance use is present, which usually increases service utilization (Hatzenbuehler, Keyes, Narrow, Grant, & Hasin, 2008).

Disparities persist across age and subgroups from children (Howell & McFeeters, 2008; Snowden, 2007) to elders (Barrio et al., 2008; Dobalian & Rivers, 2008), and across service sectors such as primary care (Stockdale, Lagomasino, Siddique, McGuire, & Miranda, 2008), emergency room settings, and other public mental health settings (Snowden, 2005) and modalities of treatment (e.g., medication, counseling, referral [Miranda et al., 2008; Stockdale et al., 2008]). Disparities in receipt of medication exist even after controlling for actual access and utilization of specialty or tertiary services, yet some total psychotropic medication utilization differences are not accounted for by observable characteristics and may represent unobserved issues such as provider-patient relationships, trust, and socio-cultural factors (Zuckerman et al., 2008; Chen & Rizzo, 2008). A recent study (Alegria, Chatterji et al., 2008) using the CPES—with national samples, good diagnostic and quality indicators, and large numbers of non-English speaking people—found that in people with depression in the past year, 40.2% of Whites did not access mental health care, but that respectively 58.8% of African Americans, 63.7% of Latinos, and 68.7% of Asians did not access care. Furthermore, the three minority groups were on average nine to 23 percentage points less likely to access care and receive adequate treatment.

Outcomes

The literature is thin on longitudinal assessment of mental health disparities regarding outcomes and even thinner on intervention work specifically designed to target disparities reduction. However, data from large studies where the primary goal was improving outcomes, in general, for mental health problems are able to make a contribution. Using data from a large quality improvement trial, depressed Latinos who had initially much lower rates of care gained significant improvements at 6 and 12 months compared to Whites that did not differ from the controls (Miranda et al., 2003). Nine year follow-up data indicate that, although the minority groups are aggregated into one group for analysis, long-term benefits on outcomes for depressed minorities may come from psychotherapy interventions (Wells et al., 2007). Some recent work demonstrates that interventions aimed at structural barriers, integrating mental health into primary care, might overcome some racial and ethnic disparities in both access to and engagement in mental health treatments (Ayalon, Arean, Linkins, Lynch, & Estes, 2007) (see Chapter 16 for more information on integration of primary care and mental health care).

Finally, work has indicated that "control-oriented" strategies to improve functional disablement associated with depression may have differential and improved impact on depression in older African Americans than Whites and provides insight into the discrepancy between lower reported emotional distress and higher functional impairment in the former group (Gitlin, Hauck, Dennis, & Schultz, 2007). The literature is not lacking in calling for more inquiry into interventions to reduce disparities by cultural tailoring but also to consider low cost dissemination at the start (Chin, Walters, Cook, & Huang, 2007; Van Voorhees, Walters, Prochaska, & Quinn, 2007).

Federal entities, such as the National Institute of Mental Health, are concerned about disparities and supported two important workgroups—one in 2001 on psychosocial intervention development and one in 2005 on services and intervention research for Latinos. Both had relevant recommendations to this study (Hollon et al., 2002; Vega et al., 2007). The first one was the "development of user-friendly interventions and non-traditional delivery methods to increase access to evidence-based interventions, especially among underserved special populations" (Hollen et al., 2002, p. 615). The second group emphasized the importance of five research foci: diagnosis, quality of care and appropriate services, psychosocial intervention development, psychopharmacologic interventions, and access to care (Vega et al., 2007). The sparse literature on outcomes and intervention work must be augmented by new investments in these areas. Two disparities scholars (Rust & Cooper, 2007) delineated a dozen gaps in existing disparities research but offered recommendations to overcome those gaps using practice-based research-which can extend beyond primary care (Table 19.1).

Implications for Mental Health

A rapidly growing literature on mental health disparities and the enormous disease burden that mental disorders incur provide a call for action and for a comprehensive research agenda to tease out the complex factors that belie the findings and shed light on intervention development. Since resources to develop brand new agendas for all subgroups are not a reality, this is particularly critical for anti-stigma interventions and processes for cultural adaptation of existing interventions. Despite progress made through some policy and national initiatives, work demonstrates that the disparity gaps for mental health care in certain groups, like Latinos, are widening (Blanco et al., 2007). The title of a recent commentary (*Race and Mental Health: More Questions than Answers*) summarizes where the field is:

Table 19.1 A Dozen Gaps in Existing Disparities Research and How Practice-Based Research could meet the Need

Why Current Disparities Research Sometimes Falls Short	*How Practice-Based Research Could Meet the Need*
1. Research in academic or closed-panel settings	Conduct research in real-world, limited resource, high-disparity primary care practice settings
2. Nondiverse research teams	Develop diverse research teams that are proportionately representative of the disparity population being studied
3. Investigator-initiated research	True community partnership
4. Focus on changing provider behaviors	Research on systems change involving patients, teams, and processes of care
5. "Inside-the-practice" research	Blur the boundaries between practice-based research and community-based interventions
6. Focus on process measures	Measure health outcomes at the community population health level
7. Narrowly focused single disease interventions	Address complex mix of disparities in chronic disease outcomes, risk factors, and mental health comorbidities
8. Experiments test one intervention	Test multi-dimensional interventions that triangulate on improved outcomes from at least three directions—provider, patient, and community
9. Static interventions held constant throughout the study period	Test dynamic, constantly improving interventions
10. Academic cycle time	Rapid-change cycles, continuously revising intervention based on rapid-feedback health outcomes data loops
11. Randomized-controlled clinical trials	Alternative study designs to measure multi-dimensional, dynamic interventions repeatedly
12. Replicability without scalability	Test interventions that are both *replicable and scalable* in real-world, under-resourced settings that serve high-disparity populations

Source: Rust, G., & Cooper, L. (2007). How can practice-based research contribute to the elimination of health disparities? *Journal of the American Board of Family Medicine: JABFM, 20*(2), 105–114.

A researcher's understanding of what "race" captures can importantly affect the questions that are asked and the questions that remain unasked. Extant racial categories do not capture biological distinctiveness in human populations and single-gene disorder models are unlikely to account for racial differences in disease with a complex etiology. Race is an imprecise variable that captures differential exposure to the resources and rewards in society and SES is regarded as a proxy for the social and economic inequality that race historically and currently reflects. (Williams & Earl, 2007, p. 1)

Finally, not just researchers, but practitioners, policymakers, and communities must all take up the following:

> The challenge for disparities researchers in the 21st century will be to show, at the level of an entire zip code or county, and then an entire state, and ultimately for the nation, that we can substantially reduce disparities not just in quality of care but in health outcomes across all racial/ethnic groups and achieve health equity for all. (Rust & Cooper, 2007, p. 111)

Racial and ethnic disparities in health continue to be a complicated issue that cannot be reduced to either simple causes or resolutions. It has yet to be determined whether there are unique or special factors that distinguish disparities in mental health. Additional consideration is needed to understand the implications for developing, adopting, and implementing evidence-based practices for multicultural communities and for determining which factors facilitate or prevent a reduction in disparities. Knowledge of the potential causes and effects is one of many steps needed to reduce and eventually eliminate disparities.

References

Agency for Healthcare Research and Quality. (2009). *National Healthcare Disparities Report, 2008.* AHRQ Pub. No. 09-0002. Rockville, MD: U.S. Department of Health & Human Services.

Alegria, M., Chatterji, P., Wells, K., Cao, Z., Chen, C. N., Takeuchi, D., et al. (2008). Disparity in depression treatment among racial and ethnic minority populations in the United States. *Psychiatric Services, 59*(11), 1264–1272.

Alegria, M., Mulvaney-Day, N., Woo, M., Torres, M., Gao, S., & Oddo, V. (2007). Correlates of past-year mental health service use among Latinos: Results from the national Latino and Asian American study. *American Journal of Public Health, 97*(1), 76–83.

Alegria, M., Nakash, O., Lapatin, S., Oddo, V., Gao, S., Lin, J., et al. (2008). How missing information in diagnosis can lead to disparities in the clinical encounter. *Journal of Public Health Management & Practice, 14*(Suppl.), S26–S35.

Ayalon, L., Arean, P., Linkins, K., Lynch, M., & Estes, C. L. (2007). Integration of mental health services into primary care overcomes ethnic disparities in access to mental health services between black and white elderly. *American Journal of Geriatric Psychiatry, 15*(10), 906–912.

Balsa, A. I., McGuire, T. G., & Meredith L. S. (2005). Testing for statistical discrimination in health care. *Health Services Research, 40*(1), 227–252.

Bandiera, F. C., Pereira, D. B., Arif, A. A., Dodge, B., & Asal, N. (2008). Race/ethnicity, income, chronic asthma, and mental health: A cross-sectional study using the behavioral risk factor surveillance system. *Psychosomatic Medicine, 70*(1), 77–84.

Barrio, C., Palinkas, L., Yamada, A.-M., Fuentes, D., Criado, V., Garcia, P., et al. (2008). Unmet needs for mental health services for Latino older adults: Perspectives from consumers, family members, advocates, and service providers. *Community Mental Health Journal, 44*(1), 57–74.

Bernal, G., Bonilla, J., & Bellido, C. (1995). Ecological validity and cultural sensitivity for outcome research: Issues for the cultural adaptation and development of psychosocial treatments with Hispanics. *Journal of Abnormal Child Psychology, 23*(1), 67–82.

Blanco, C., Patel, S. R., Liu, L., Jiang, H., Lewis-Fernández, R., Schmidt, A. B., et al. (2007). National trends in ethnic disparities in mental health care. *Medical Care, 45*(11), 1012–1019.

Braveman, P., Starfield, B., & Geiger, H. J. (2001). World Health Report 2000: How it removes equity from the agenda for public health monitoring and policy. *British Medical Journal, 323*(7314), 678–681.

Brennan Ramirez, L. K., Baker, E. A., & Metzler, M. (2008). *Promoting Health Equity: A Resource to Help Communities Address Social Determinants of Health.* Atlanta, GA: U.S. Department of Health and Human Services, Centers for Disease Control and Prevention.

Breslau, J., Aguilar-Gaxiola, S., Kendler, K. S., Su, M., Williams, D., & Kessler, R. C. (2006). Specifying race-ethnic differences in risk for psychiatric disorder in a USA national sample. *Psychological Medicine, 36*(1), 57–68.

Cabassa, L. J., Zayas, L. H., & Hansen, M. C. (2006). Latino adults' access to mental health care: A review of epidemiological studies. *Administration and Policy in Mental Health and Mental Health Services Research, 33*(3), 316–330.

Chen, J., & Rizzo, J. A. (2008). Racial and ethnic disparities in antidepressant drug use. *Journal of Mental Health Policy & Economics, 11*(4), 155–165.

Chin, M. H., Walters, A. E., Cook, S. C., & Huang, E. S. (2007). Interventions to reduce racial and ethnic disparities in health care. *Medical Care Research and Review, 64*(Suppl. 5), 7S–28S.

Collaborative Psychiatric Epidemiology Surveys. (n.d.). Ann Arbor, MI: Inter-University Consortium for Political and Social Research and Institute for Social Research. Available online at http://www.icpsr.umich.edu/CPES/. Accessed June 22, 2009.

Cook, B. L., McGuire, T., & Miranda, J. (2007). Measuring trends in mental health care disparities, 2000–2004. *Psychiatric Services, 58*(12), 1533–1540.

Cooper, L. A., Hill, M. N., & Powe, N. R. (2002). Designing and evaluating interventions to eliminate racial and ethnic disparities in health care. *Journal of General Internal Medicine, 17*(6), 477–486.

Dobalian, A., & Rivers, P. (2008). Racial and ethnic disparities in the use of mental health services. *Journal of Behavioral Health Services and Research, 35*(2), 128–141.

Duan, N., Meng, X.-L., Lin, J. Y., Chen, C. N., & Alegria, M. (2008). Disparities in defining disparities: Statistical conceptual frameworks. *Statistics in Medicine, 27*(20), 3941–3956.

Garland, A. F., Lau, A. S., Yeh, M., McCabe, K. M., Hough, R. L., & Landsverk, J. A. (2005). Racial and ethnic differences in utilization of mental health services among high-risk youths. *American Journal of Psychiatry, 162*(7), 1336–1343.

Ghods, B. K., Roter, D. L., Ford, D. E., Larson, S., Arbelaez, J. J., & Cooper, L. A. (2008). Patient-physician communication in the primary care visits of African Americans and whites with depression. *Journal of General Internal Medicine, 23*(5), 600–606.

Gitlin, L. N., Hauck, W. W., Dennis, M. P., & Schultz, R. (2007). Depressive symptoms in older African American and white adults with functional difficulties: The role of strategies. *Journal of the American Geriatric Society, 55*(7), 1023–1030.

Glover, S., Elder, K., Xirasagar, S., Baek, J.-D., Piper, C., & Campbell, D. (2007). Disparities in mental health utilization among persons with chronic diseases. *Journal of Health Disparities Research and Practice, 1*(3), 45–65.

Han, E., & Liu, G. G. (2005). Racial disparities in prescription drug use for mental illness among population in US. *Journal of Mental Health Policy & Economics, 8*(3), 131–143.

Harman, J. S., Edlund, M. J., & Fortney, J. C. (2004). Disparities in the adequacy of depression treatment in the United States. *Psychiatric Services, 55*(3), 1379–1385.

Hatzenbuehler, M. L., Keyes, K. M., Narrow, W. E., Grant, B. F., & Hasin, D. S. (2008). Racial/ethnic disparities in service utilization for individuals with co-occurring mental health and substance use disorders in the general population: Results from the national epidemiologic survey on alcohol and related conditions. *Journal of Clinical Psychiatry, 69*(7), 1112–1121.

Hollon, S. D., Muñoz, R. F., Barlow, D. H., Beardslee, W. R., Bell, C. C., Bernal, G., et al. (2002). Psychosocial intervention development for the prevention and treatment of depression: Promoting innovation and increasing access. *Biological Psychiatry, 52*(6), 610–630.

Howell, E., & McFeeters, J. (2008). Children's mental health care: Differences by race/ethnicity in urban/rural areas. *Journal of Health Care for the Poor and Underserved, 19*(1), 237–247.

Huang, F. Y., Chung, H., Kroenke, K., & Spitzer, R. L. (2006). Racial and ethnic differences in the relationship between depression severity and functional status. *Psychiatric Services, 57*(4), 498–503.

Hurtado, M. P., Swift, E. K., Corrigan, J. M., & the Committee on the National Quality Report on Health Care Delivery. (2001). *Envisioning the National Health Care Quality Report.* Washington, DC: National Academy Press.

Hwang, W.-C., Myers, H. F., Abe-Kim, J., & Ting, J. Y. (2008). A conceptual paradigm for understanding culture's impact on mental health: The cultural influences on mental health (CIMH) model. *Clinical Psychology Review, 28*(2), 211–227.

Jenkins, R., Meltzer, H., Jones, P. B., Brugha, T., Bebbington, P., Farrell, M., et al. (2008). *Foresight Mental Capital and Wellbeing Project. Mental Health: Future Challenges.* London: Government Office for Science.

Keppel, K., Pamuk, E., Lynch, J., Carter-Pokras, O., Kim, I., Mays V., et al. (2005). Methodological issues in measuring health disparities. *Vital Health Statistics, 2*(141), 1–16.

Kilbourne, A. M., Switzer, G., Hyman, K., Crowley-Matoka, M., & Fine, M. J. (2006). Advancing health disparities research within the health care system: A conceptual framework. *American Journal of Public Health, 96*(12), 2113–2121.

Lagomasino, I. T., Dwight-Johnson, M., Miranda, J., Zhang, L., Liao, D., Duan, N., et al. (2005). Disparities in depression treatment for Latinos and site of care. *Psychiatric Services, 56*(12), 1517–1523.

Lucas, T., Michalopoulou, G., Falzarano, P., Menon, S., & Cunningham, W. (2008). Healthcare provider cultural competency: Development and initial validation of a patient report measure. *Health Psychology, 27*(2), 185–193.

McGuire, T. G., Alegria M., Cook B. L., Wells, K. B., & Zaslavsky, A. M. (2006). Implementing the Institute of Medicine definition of disparities: An application to mental health care. *Health Services Research, 41*(5), 1979–2005.

McGuire, T. G., Ayanian, J. Z., Ford, D. E., Henke, R. E., Rost, K. M., & Zaslavsky, A. M. (2008). Testing for statistical discrimination by race/ethnicity in panel data for depression treatment in primary care. *Health Services Research, 43*(2), 531–551.

McGuire, T. G., & Miranda, J. (2008). New evidence regarding racial and ethnic disparities in mental health: Policy implications. *Health Affairs, 27*(2), 393–403.

Merriam-Webster Online Dictionary. (2009a). Disparity. Available online at http://www.merriam-webster.com/dictionary/disparity. Accessed June 22, 2009.

Merriam-Webster Online Dictionary. (2009b). Inequality. Available online at http://www.merriam-webster.com/dictionary/inequality. Accessed June 22, 2009.

Merriam-Webster Online Dictionary. (2009c). Inequity. Available online at http://www.merriam-webster.com/dictionary/inequity. Accessed June 22, 2009.

Millman, M. L. (1993). A model for monitoring access. In *Access to Health Care in America* (pp. 31–45). Washington, DC: Institute of Medicine, Committee on Monitoring Access to Personal Health Care Services.

Miranda, J., Duan, N., Sherbourne, C., Schoenbaum, M., Lagomasino, I., Jackson-Triche, M., et al. (2003). Improving care for minorities: Can quality improvement interventions improve care and outcomes for depressed minorities? Results of a randomized, controlled trial. *Health Services Research, 38*(2), 613–630.

Miranda, J., McGuire, T. G., Williams, D. R., & Wang, P. (2008). Mental health in the context of health disparities. *American Journal of Psychiatry, 165*(9), 1102–1108.

Nadeem, E., Lange, J. M., Edge, D., Fongwa, M., Belin, T., & Miranda, J. (2007). Does stigma keep poor young immigrant and U.S.-born black and Latina women from seeking mental health care? *Psychiatric Services, 58*(12), 1547–1554.

Nadeem, E., Lange, J. M., & Miranda, J. (2008). Mental health care preferences among low-income and minority women. *Archives of Women's Mental Health, 11*(2), 93–102.

Olfson, M., Cherry, D. K., & Lewis-Fernandez, R. (2009). Racial differences in visit duration of outpatient psychiatric visits. *Archives of General Psychiatry, 66*(2), 214–221.

Poker, A., Hubbard, H., Sharp, B. A., & Collins, B. A. (2004). The first national reports on United States healthcare quality and disparities. *Journal of Nursing Care Quality, 19*(4), 316–321.

Probst, J., Laditka, S., Moore, C., Harun, N., & Powell, M. P. (2007). Race and ethnicity differences in reporting of depressive symptoms. *Administration and Policy in Mental Health and Mental Health Services Research, 34*(6), 519–529.

Rao, D., Feinglass, J., & Corrigan, P. (2007). Racial and ethnic disparities in mental illness stigma. *Journal of Nervous and Mental Disease, 195*(12), 1020–1023.

Rust, G., & Cooper, L. (2007). How can practice-based research contribute to the elimination of health disparities? *Journal of the American Board of Family Medicine, 20*(2), 105–114.

Sentell, T., Shumway, M., & Snowden, L. (2007). Access to mental health treatment by English language proficiency and race/ethnicity. *Journal of General Internal Medicine, 22*(Suppl. 2), 289–293.

Smedley, B. D., Stith, A. Y., & Nelson, A. R. (2003) *Unequal Treatment: Confronting Racial and Ethnic Disparities in Health Care*. Washington, DC: National Academies Press.

Snowden, L. (2007). Explaining mental health treatment disparities: Ethnic and cultural differences in family involvement. *Culture, Medicine, and Psychiatry, 31*(3), 389–402.

Snowden, L. R. (2005). Racial, cultural and ethnic disparities in health and mental health: Toward theory and research at community levels. *American Journal of Community Psychology, 35*(1-2), 1–8.

Stockdale, S. E., Lagomasino, I. T., Siddique, J., McGuire, T., & Miranda, J. (2008). Racial and ethnic disparities in detection and treatment of depression and anxiety among psychiatric and primary health care visits, 1995–2005. *Medical Care, 46*(7), 668–677.

Swift, E. K., & the Committee on Guidance for Designing a National Healthcare Disparities Report. (2002). *Guidance for the National Healthcare Disparities Report*. Washington, DC: National Academies Press.

U.S. Department of Health and Human Services. (2001). *Mental Health: Culture, Race, and Ethnicity: A Supplement to Mental Health: A Report of the Surgeon General*. Rockville, MD: U.S. Department of Health and Human Services, Substance Abuse and Mental Health Services Administration, Center for Mental Health Services.

U.S. Department of Health and Human Services, Office of Minority Health (2003). *Final Report: Developing a Self-Assessment Tool for Culturally and Linguistically Appropriate Services in Local Public Health Agencies*. Washington, DC: Author.

van Ryn, M., Burgess, D., Malat J., & Griffin, J. (2006). Physicians' perceptions of patients' social and behavioral characteristics and race disparities in treatment recommendations for men with coronary artery disease. *American Journal of Public Health, 96*(2), 351–357.

van Ryn, M., & Fu, S. S. (2003). Paved with good intentions: Do public health and human service providers contribute to racial/ethnic disparities in health? *American Journal of Public Health, 93*(2), 248–255.

Van Voorhees, B. W., Walters, A. E., Prochaska, M., & Quinn, M. T. (2007). Reducing health disparities in depressive disorders outcomes between non-Hispanic whites and ethnic minorities: A call for pragmatic strategies over the life course. *Medical Care Research and Review, 64*(Suppl. 5), 157S–194S.

Varkey, A. B., Manwell, L. B., Williams, E. S., Ibrahim, S. A., Brown, R. L., Bobula, J. A., et al. (2009). MEMO Investigators. Separate and unequal: Clinics where minority and nonminority patients receive primary care. *Archives of Internal Medicine, 169*(3), 243–250.

Vega, W. A., Karno, M., Alegria, M., Alvidrez, J., Bernal, G., Escamilla, M., et al. (2007). Research issues for improving treatment of U.S. Hispanics with persistent mental disorders. *Psychiatric Services, 58*(3), 385–394.

Waldman, S. V., Blumenthal, J. A., Babyak, M. A., Sherwood, A., Sketch, M., Davidson J., et al. (2009). Ethnic differences in the treatment of depression in patients with ischemic heart disease. *American Heart Journal, 157*(1), 76–83.

Wang, P. S., Demler, O., Olfson, M., Pincus, H. A., Wells, K. B., & Kessler, R. C. (2006). Changing profiles of service sectors used for mental health care in the United States. *American Journal of Psychiatry, 163*(9), 1187–1198.

Wells, K. B., Sherbourne, C. D., Miranda, J., Tang, L., Benjamin, B., & Duan, N. (2007). The cumulative effects of quality improvement for depression on outcome disparities over 9 years: Results from a randomized, controlled group-level trial. *Medical Care, 45*(11), 1052–1059.

Whitehead, M. (1990). *The Concepts and Principles of Equity and Health.* EUR/ICP/RPD 414. Copenhagen, Denmark: World Health Organization Regional Office for Europe.

Whitehead, M., & Dahlgren, G. (2007). *Concepts and Principles for Tackling Social Inequities in Health.* Liverpool, UK: WHO Collaborating Centre for Policy Research on Social Determinants of Health, University of Liverpool.

Williams, D. R., & Earl, T. R. (2007). Commentary: Race and mental health; More questions than answers. *International Journal of Epidemiology, 36*(4), 751–758.

Williams, D. R., Gonzalez, H. M., Neighbors, H., Nesse, R., Abelson, J. M., Sweetman, J., et al. (2007). Prevalence and distribution of major depressive disorder in African Americans, Caribbean blacks, and non-Hispanic whites: Results from the National Survey of American Life. *Archives of General Psychiatry, 64*(3), 305–315.

Yamada, A-M., & Brekke, J. S. (2008). Addressing mental health disparities through clinical competence not just cultural competence: The need for assessment of sociocultural issues in the delivery of evidence-based psychosocial rehabilitation services. *Clinical Psychology Review, 28*(8), 1368–1399.

Zimmerman, F. J. (2005). Social and economic determinants of disparities in professional help-seeking for child mental health problems: Evidence from a national sample. *Health Services Research, 40*(5, Pt. 1), 1514–1533.

Zuckerman, I. H., Ryder, P. T., Simoni-Wastila, L., Shaffer, T., Sato, M., Zhao, L., et al. (2008). Racial and ethnic disparities in the treatment of dementia among Medicare beneficiaries. *Journals of Gerontology: Series B Psychological Sciences and Social Sciences, 63*(5), S328–S333.

Zuvekas, S. H., & Fleishman, J. A. (2008). Self-rated mental health and racial/ethnic disparities in mental health service use. *Medical Care, 46*(9), 915–923.

Chapter 20

THE RECOVERY MOVEMENT

William A. Anthony, PhD; and Lori Ashcraft, PhD

THIS CHAPTER examines the mental health field prior to the recovery movement and then traces the origins of recovery from severe mental illnesses and how recovery became the guiding vision for the mental health field. The chapter notes emerging consensus as to the definition, components, and assumptions of recovery; identifies the research forming the evidence base for recovery; and advances a public health conceptual model of recovery, based upon the recovery research. It describes service delivery that is guided by the vision of recovery, and, lastly, discusses policy issues, including implications for mental health and future challenges.

Introduction and Overview

For most of the previous century, the notion of recovery from severe mental illnesses was certainly not a movement in the mental health field. Not only was recovery not a movement, it was not even a mental health concept. In actuality, the mental health system seemed to be designed to hinder recovery. The idea of recovery from severe mental illnesses was largely absent from the last century's diagnostic schemes (American Psychiatric Association [APA], 1987) and maintenance-type interventions (Bachrach, 1976; Grob, 1994a; New Freedom Commission on Mental Health [NFCMH], 2003). The Diagnostic and Statistical Manual of the American Psychiatric Association characterized schizophrenia in this way: "the most common outcome is one of acute exacerbations with increasing deterioration between episodes" (APA, 1980, p. 195). Even worse, for much of the previous century, throughout North America and Europe, not only were people with severe mental illnesses not expected to recover, they were often dehumanized and devalued by both society and treatment professionals alike (Braslow, 1997, 1995; Grob, 1994a, 1994b, 1996; Micale & Porter, 1994).

In contrast to most of the previous century, the recovery vision is now beginning to transform the field of mental health. Late in the twentieth century, Anthony (1992) wrote of the harbinger of the twenty-first century's focus on recovery:

> There is a revolution brewing in the field of severe mental illnesses. . . . It is a revolution in vision—in what is believed to be possible for people with severe mental illnesses. . . . For the past century it was believed that people with severe mental illnesses must suffer a lengthy duration of severe disability, with a deteriorating course over their lifetime. . . . I am more convinced than ever that recovery from severe mental illnesses is possible for many more people than was previously believed. I believe that much of the chronicity is due to the way the mental health system and society treat mental illnesses and not the nature of the illness itself. . . . A vision of the possibilities of recovery can change how we treat people with mental illnesses even if the illness itself hasn't changed. (Anthony, 1992, p. 1)

The recovery concept itself emerged from the writing and speeches of people with severe mental illnesses. While people with psychiatric disabilities have been experiencing recovery and now talking and writing about their own recovery, professionals are continuing to try to understand the implications of recovery for how they practice.

The 1990s have been called the "decade of recovery" (Anthony, 1993b). Two seminal events of the preceding decade paved the way for the concept of recovery from mental illnesses to take hold in the 1990s. One factor was the writing of consumers (e.g., Anonymous, 1989; Deegan, 1988; Houghton, 1982; Leete, 1989; McDermott, 1990; Unzicker, 1989). For the preceding decades, and culminating in the decade of the 1980s, consumers had been writing about their own and their colleagues' recovery. Now, of course, the writing of consumers about their own recovery is voluminous (e. g., Huntley, 2006; Legere, 2007; Mead & Copeland, 2000), as are qualitative studies of consumers' recovery experiences (Jacobson, 2001; Jenkins, Strauss, Carpenter et al., 2007; Ridgway, 2001; Spaniol, Gagne, & Koehler, 2003; Williams & Collins, 1999). The other major factor precipitating the acceptance of the recovery vision was the empirical work of Harding and her associates, whose research and analytic work initially impacted the field in the 1980s. Over the years, Harding (1994, 2003) and her colleagues have reviewed a number of long-term research studies, including their own (DeSisto, Harding, McCormick, Ashikaga, & Brooks, 1995a, 1995b; Harding, Brooks, Ashekaga, Strauss, & Breier, 1987a, 1987b), that suggested a deteriorating course for severe mental illnesses was not the norm.

What Is Meant by Recovery?

There are many definitions of recovery from severe mental illnesses (Onken, Craig, Ridgway, Ralph, & Cook, 2007; Ralph, 2000). An early, succinct, and straightforward definition of recovery was "the development of new meaning and purpose as one grows beyond the catastrophe of a severe mental illness" (Anthony, 1993a).

In December of 2005, in an attempt to develop more clarity concerning what is meant by recovery, the Center for Mental Health Services (within the United States Substance Abuse and Mental Health Services Administration) convened a National Consensus Conference on Mental Health Recovery. Conference participants included over 100 people: consumers, advocates, family members, practitioners, administrators, and researchers (del Vecchio & Fricks, 2007). The conference resulted in a national consensus statement defining recovery and 10 fundamental components of recovery.

Recovery was defined as a "journey of healing and transformation enabling a person with a mental health problem to live a meaningful life in a community of his or her choice while striving to achieve his or her full potential" (del Vecchio & Fricks, 2007, p. 7). Ten fundamental components of recovery were identified: 1) self-direction; 2) individualized and person centered; 3) empowerment; 4) holistic; 5) non-linear; 6) strengths-based; 7) peer support; 8) respect; 9) responsibility; and 10) hope. A complete statement of the conference results is available online (http://www.mentalhealth.samhsa.gov/publications/allpubs/sma05-4129).

The eight basic assumptions underlying the vision of recovery, which seem compatible with the consensus definition and fundamental components, had been advanced earlier (Anthony, 1993a; Anthony, Cohen, Farkas, & Gagne, 2002).

1. *Recovery can occur without professional intervention.* Professionals do not hold the key to recovery—the individual does. The task of professionals is to facilitate recovery; the task of people with a disability is to recover.
2. *A common denominator of recovery is the presence of people who believe in and stand by the person in need of recovery.* Seemingly universal in the recovery concept is the notion that critical to one's recovery is a person or persons one can trust to "be there" in times of need.
3. *A recovery vision is not related to one's theory about the causes of mental illnesses.* A recovery vision is applicable whether the causes of mental illnesses are viewed as biological and/or psychosocial.
4. *Recovery can occur even though symptoms re-occur.* The episodic nature of severe mental illnesses does not prevent recovery.
5. *Recovery changes the frequency and duration of symptoms.* As one recovers, the symptom frequency and duration appear to have been changed for the better. That is, symptoms interfere with functioning less often and for briefer periods of time, if at all.
6. *Recovery does not feel like a linear process.* Recovery involves growth and setbacks, periods of rapid change and little change. While the overall trend may be upward, the moment-to-moment experience does not feel so linear.
7. *Recovery from the consequences of the illness is sometimes more difficult than recovering from the illness itself.* Issues of dysfunction, disability, and disadvantage are often more difficult than impairment issues. An inability to perform valued tasks and roles, and the resultant loss of self-esteem, are significant barriers to recovery, as are prejudice and discrimination.
8. *Recovery from a mental illness does not mean that one was not "really ill."* At times, people who have recovered successfully from a severe mental illness have been discounted as not "really" ill. Their successful recovery must be seen as a model and as a beacon of hope for those beginning the recovery process.

In line with this emerging consensus on the definition of recovery, its ten fundamental components and eight basic assumptions, most state mental health systems no longer view the course of serious mental illnesses as necessarily deteriorative (Anthony & Huckshorn, 2008). This vision of recovery began to guide policies and practice in many individual states in the late 1990s (see for example, Beale & Lambric, 1995; Jacobson & Curtis, 2000; Legislative Summer Study Committee of the Vermont Division of Mental Health, 1996; State of Nebraska, 1997; State of Wisconsin, 1997), and even more recently, the recovery vision has guided the policy of the United States' federal government (New Freedom Commission on Mental Health, 2003) as well as other countries such as New Zealand (Lapsley, Nikora, & Black, 2002).

An Update on Recovery Research

The synthesis and dissemination of long-term outcome studies, which suggested that a significant percentage of people with serious mental illnesses were dramatically improving over time, has been accomplished most rigorously by Harding (e.g., Harding, 1994, 2003). In 2003, Harding reviewed 10 United States and international longitudinal studies of 20 to 30 years' duration, demonstrating the recovery and community integration of many people with schizophrenia and other serious mental illnesses (Bleuler, 1972; Ciompi & Muller, 1976; Desisto et al., 1995a, 1995b; Harding et al., 1987a, 1987b; Hinterhuber, 1973; Huber, Gross, & Schuttler, 1979; Kreditor, 1977; Marinow, 1974; Ogawa et al., 1987; Tsuang, Woolson, & Fleming, 1979).

More recently, Rogers, Farkas, and Anthony (2005) have examined the evidence base for recovery. These authors believe that three threads of research are most relevant to recovery: 1) the long-term follow-up studies reviewed by Harding and referenced previously; 2) the qualitative studies and first-person narratives (examples of which were also referenced previously); and 3) the services intervention research that demonstrates peoples' capacity to improve their living, learning, working, and/or social roles (see, e.g., Drake & Bond, 2008; Rogers, Anthony, & Farkas, 2006).

A Public Health Model of Recovery

Based upon the recovery research literature (Rogers et al., 2005), the authors propose a public health model of recovery (see Figure 20.1). Consistent with a public health approach, the proposed recovery model hypothesizes that recovery is affected by individual and environmental dimensions. Factors associated with mental health care systems and individual factors such as diagnosis, mental status, and genetics are only a part of the equation.

Future research on recovery from severe mental illnesses will determine how much of an influence on recovery they have vis-a-vis factors outside formal mental health systems (i.e., people, such as family and friends, and socio-cultural factors, such as educational opportunity, discrimination, and poverty). The outcomes

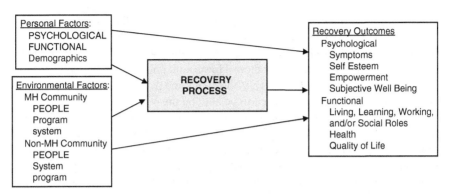

Note: Entire word capitalized = personal factors and environmental factors hypothesized to be most important to recovery outcomes; 1st letter capitalized = next most important; no capitals = least important.

Figure 20.1   Factors Associated with Recovery

suggested by this conceptual model are broader than psychiatric symptoms, including, for example, employment, housing, self-esteem, and empowerment.

Furthermore, concepts of wellness and its complement, health promotion, have advanced the notion that mental health itself is more than simply the absence of a disorder. Aligned with a public health perspective, the wellness concept in the mental health field has furthered the idea of the importance of engaging in certain health-promoting behaviors within healthy environments, not simply for the purpose of preventing or better managing a disorder, but also to enhance one's well-being and quality of life (Hutchinson et al., 2006).

In essence, the recovery model, as depicted in Figure 20.1, hypothesizes the dynamics of the relationship between recovery antecedents, processes, and outcomes, drawing from theory and research on adaptation and psychosocial adjustment to physical disability (Livneh, 2001) and its conceptual and empirical extension to the psychiatric rehabilitation field (Anthony, Cohen, Farkas, & Gagne, 2002). This model of recovery suggests a complexity and comprehensiveness that facilitates discussion and future research. As a heuristic model, it suggests possible contributing factors to recovery that might seem extraneous to previous mental health research on the pathology of severe mental illnesses, such as alternative health care, informal supports, and contingencies of self-worth.

Services Delivery

As mentioned earlier, mental health programs were built upon the assumption that people did not recover, and that assumption became a self-fulfilling prophecy. Now that the basic assumption has changed, care systems need to change radically in order to support the recovery process. Systemic changes have happened, but at a slow and disappointing pace. Since the process of recovery can be accelerated and proliferated in settings where policies promote the use of recovery oriented principles and practice, the first critical path to mobilizing the recovery vision is system transformation. Often the effort that could be invested in promoting recovery becomes misdirected into complying with regulations that actually stall the recovery process. Thankfully, the hope for recovery lives and breathes within each person who is trying to achieve it and the staffs who believe it is possible, so the process is not wholly dependent upon systemic circumstances. However, if one truly were committed to a "world where everyone will recover" (NFCMH, 2003), acceleration and proliferation of recovery systems would need to be high on the priority list.

The second critical path for moving the vision of recovery forward expeditiously is equipping staff with skills that inspire people to become self-determining and to begin and continue their recovery journey. These are "higher order" skills, not geared to care-taking, stabilizing, or controlling behaviors, but imparting the enthusiasm and vision that inspire people to recognize and actualize their potential. These skills need to be delivered in the context of positive empowering relationships that establish a safe place for people to learn and grow.

Closely examining the personal recovery experience can provide us with glimpses of what the new skills are and how they can be applied. When people reflect upon their recovery process, they describe "moments" of insights and choice when they realize they can respond in new ways to familiar experiences. The "moment" is a *split* second when they can either surrender to the symptom, reacting in habitual ways, or they can choose a new path, leading to further recovery and personal growth. When asked how they felt in that moment, people often said, "I don't know, I've never been here before" (Spaniol, 2007). The "moment" allows them to make a conscious choice: follow the familiar path or choose new options that lead to self-determination and personal growth. Spaniol (2007) refers to these latter times as "upward turning points," which, as they accumulate over time, represent an awakening sense of self and efficacy and a growing awareness of one's own ability to develop a satisfying and contributing life. This process is not unique to people with mental illnesses. It is the process by which most of us learn and grow. Perhaps those pursuing recovery are more acutely aware of it because they are usually highly motivated to regain parts of themselves temporarily lost during their illness.

The "higher order" staff skills and approaches that set the stage for "moments of recovery" and the "upward turning points" can have an extremely positive impact on the process of recovery. Paradoxically, these advanced helping skills are conceptually relatively uncomplicated. They usually involve the provision of hope, understanding, choices, empowerment, and meaning and purpose. They are not schemes or techniques, but are simply the truth delivered in the context of an intentionally sincere relationship. While this sounds like an obvious approach, it is actually more challenging than the traditional methods of "care-taking and stabilizing" and requires a great deal more sophistication and creativity. It can be argued that these skills are included in much of the academic training most professionals receive. However, the sequence of delivery and the emphasis and focus are significantly different. *A meaningful shift must occur in approach, application, and attitude if professional staffs are going to be able to facilitate a recovery response from those they serve.*

A Shift in Definition

The framework in which services are delivered has been focused upon illness. The framework then has defined everything within its context as illness-related.

For example, if people are brought into a crisis program on an involuntary deten-tion, they were undoubtedly transported by law enforcement in handcuffs. They are probably angry, confused, disoriented, and lashing out. Within the illness framework, one would define this behavior as evidence of illness that validated the decision to force these individuals into the facility and perhaps restrain and sedate them with medications. The recovery framework is distinctly different; it assumes people's reactions are reasonable and understandable given the devastating and frightening nature of the involuntary admission. Assuring people that their reac-tions are understandable often elicits reasonable behavior and can initiate self-management. What may have been labeled as illness in the earlier model is now seen as understandable and even normal in the recovery model.

A SHIFT IN POWER DYNAMICS

Shifting the dynamics in the "treatment" relationship is essential to promoting recovery. In a traditional "treatment" relationship, the power has been with the staff and the assumption has been that they know what is best for the person; the staff's job was to manage and control people who receive services. More often than not, people have been agreeable to this, and in fact, have given whatever power they may have to the "treaters" and waited to be "fixed." In the recovery relation-ship, the staff intentionally reverses this dynamic by facilitating the empowerment of the person. Since the person is the one who is recovering, the person is the one who needs the power. The necessary skill set includes shifting the power back to the person so he or she can begin or continue their recovery journey under their own power.

A SHIFT IN FOCUS

Shifting the focus from what is *wrong* to what is *strong* is fundamental to promoting recovery. Prior to knowing that people could recover, the focus was on what was wrong with them. Consistent with the public health model, in order to build enough strength for people to recover, the focus needs to shift to the whole person: their strengths, abilities, accomplishments, and also their challenges. Focusing on strengths has proven to be an effective way to empower people so they can take the lead in their recovery, which is an essential part of the process. The skill set in this case includes recognizing the issues, but viewing them through the lens of a solu-tion instead of a problem.

A SHIFT IN CONVERSATION

The recovery conversation has distinct characteristics that distinguish it from past practices. The language is non-clinical and optimistic. The flow is geared more toward listening than directing; more toward inspiring than controlling; more about choices and options than direction and coercion; more about recovery than stabilization. Language and attitude are keys to successfully making this shift.

A Shift in Practice

One of the assumptions that has driven treatment practices is that those with a mental illness often make irrational decisions and must be controlled. In "crisis" situations, people are often coerced, threatened, and even physically forced to comply with established rules. Forcing people into seclusion and restraining them are primitive practices that require no sophistication on the part of staff: no brilliance, creativity, or other "higher order" skills (Anthony, 2006; Ashcraft & Anthony, 2008). After resorting to these practices for thousands of years, a more humane approach can be used, one that will further recovery instead of set it back. Force does not elicit the recovery response from anyone, whether or not mental illness is present. The message it conveys to the person is not about their strengths and potential and does not promote self-determination. Instead, it reinforces the notion that they are dangerous and to be feared, not trustworthy and, in fact, criminal in nature.

The recovery approach requires skilled staff who can create healing partnerships that promote self-management and focus on potential for using a negative situation for learning better ways of responding to stressful life situations. There are many excuses used to continue the use of force, most of which are not legitimate. Perhaps we have become accustomed to resorting to it because we have not understood the importance of inspiring people to recover.

A Shift in Planning

A significant amount of time and effort goes into the development of treatment plans in most mental health programs. Plans are usually required by a variety of funding sources and provide the foundation used by auditors to assess medical necessity and progress toward treatment goals. While they have played a significant role in most treatment or case management approaches, these plans have not been of much interest to the people for whom they were written. It has not been their plan, and in fact, they often do not even get copies of it. An effective plan gives a person a way to guide their own ship, become self-determining, and chart a course toward goals that have meaning for them. It can provide ways of measuring and celebrating progress, which allows for the building of resilience and self-esteem. Ownership is the key to creating an effective plan that can become a meaningful resource to a person on the road to recovery. The plan needs to be conceived by the persons who are using it, and it must be their plan and reflect their values and goals. An effective plan creates opportunities for choice, followed by deliberate action. Choice is the process that promotes self-discovery and builds a personal identity and provides an avenue of self-expression and originality. This lays the groundwork for actions that can lead to a meaningful and fulfilling life with hopes and dreams. The acquisition of "higher order" skills is required, since supporting a person to develop such a plan is much more involved than simply filling in the blanks on a form and asking the person to sign it.

Policy Issues

Policies attempt to translate the vision of recovery into practice. Depending upon who and what is the focus of the policy, policies may be implemented in procedures, legislation, rules and/or regulations. Recovery oriented policies are needed at the system, program, and practitioner level, so that systems provide funding for recovery practices, programs provide access to recovery practices, and practitioners deliver recovery practices (Anthony, 2000; Farkas, 2007).

Presently, there is policy failure at each of these system, program, and practitioner levels. Current system funding still leans toward financing more traditional diagnostic and treatment procedures that have not focused on recovery as a treatment goal. As a result, access to these more traditional programs (e.g., inpatient and day treatment) is simpler to obtain than access to programs that support more recovery oriented goals (e.g., employment, independent living, and supported education). Practitioners still tend to be heavily trained on the assessment and treatment of symptoms rather than the assessment and rehabilitation of a person's strengths and supports relevant to their own self-determined goals.

More funding, more access to recovery programs, and a better trained workforce are more obvious in their listing than in their implementation. To the current authors, these and other policy needs are not going to be fully implemented until the recovery vision is accepted into the very fabric of the mental health field. Currently, its acceptance remains at the margins. The transformation of the field, based upon the vision of recovery, has not yet happened, and until it does, policy changes will not be dramatic.

Most critical to policy implementation at a system, program, or practitioner level is the commitment to a recovery oriented mission, the values underlying the mission, and the processes, procedures, and practices necessary to achieve the mission. To ensure this commitment to recovery, each level of mental health systems must be guided by recovery values in order for the processes, procedures, and practices to be relevant. Consensus recovery values include growth, choice, person centeredness, and partnership (Farkas, Gagne, Anthony, & Chamberlin, 2005). Every mental health activity at every system, program, or practitioner level must be run through a values check to determine if the activity reflects one or more recovery values. At the system level, the system functions of planning, funding, management, program development, coordination, evaluation, and advocacy must support and not contradict the values of recovery. For example, in the system level activity of evaluation, consumer and family measures might be included in the evaluation in order to make the evaluation function consistent with the recovery value of partnership. An example at the program level activity, which is consistent with the recovery value of growth, might be that records are designed to capture indices of consumer growth and not simply service utilization. A practitioner level example might be that practitioners are taught the skill of collaborative goal-setting, which is consistent with the recovery value of choice.

Future Challenges

While the challenges in transforming the system to a recovery orientation are many and have been mentioned in this chapter's sections on service delivery and policy, the authors choose to focus on three challenges that can be immediately addressed. These three challenges are peer services, supported housing, and case management.

Peer Support Services

Services provided by people who have had a diagnosis of a severe mental illness have emerged over the past ten years as a powerful antidote to the traditional methods of service delivery. The greatest impact peer support employees have is simply in being themselves: persons who are recovering from mental illnesses. When the persons being served realize that the peer supporter was in the same circumstance they are in and has made major improvements, they say "if you could do it, maybe I can, too." This insight around a new level of being has a tremendous impact on how people see themselves and their potential. To assure the fidelity of this peer workforce, high quality training is imperative, as is continuing education and advanced training in recovery, as peers learn from their work experience. The training should focus on helping peers understand how to use their personal experience in ways that promote recovery in others. In this regard, both their training and their contribution are quite unique.

Supported Housing

The way people with mental illnesses have been housed has shifted significantly over the past 40 years, but still has a long way to go. When de-institutionalization began in the mid-sixties, people were placed in nursing homes, halfway houses, boarding homes, and shelters; many became homeless, jailed, or victims of criminal intent. In an attempt to organize the few services that were available, "continuums of care" were planned so that people could be moved up and down the various types of housing, depending upon their service and support needs. It later became apparent that moving people around had an adverse effect upon their wellness and that it would be better to move staff instead of the people who were being served. Thus, the concept of supported housing was born (Ridgway & Zipple, 1990). The implementation time lag regarding this insight was fueled by economics and convenience, since it was more lucrative and comfortable for programs to move people and to assume their lack of wellness was the result of illness instead of service methodology. People were trapped in disempowered roles and in settings that did not know how to promote recovery. In actuality, few communities developed a full continuum of care due to the expense. However, the continuum of care concept remained the standard toward which community living programs were designed, and the notion of moving people without their choice became an accepted practice.

Once the principles of recovery infiltrated the literature, it became clear that the "continuum of care" concept was fatally flawed in many ways and was counterproductive. The two most glaring flaws were 1) moving people around did not allow them to develop supportive relationships that could help them sustain recovery; and 2) decisions were made by staff who were "placing" people instead of maximizing choices that could promote recovery.

Now that we know people can recover, we can mobilize their desire for decent housing by helping them explore their own ideas about "home" and what we can do together to help them get "home." This lays the groundwork for successful housing outcomes because the person takes the lead in setting goals and developing self-management skills. This is very different from earlier approaches where "placing" became a way of distributing people to various residential places. The recovery approach begins with asking people what they want in a housing setting and what would help them be successful in living independently (see, for example, Shern et al., 2000).

CASE MANAGEMENT

Case management is a popular practice used to manage people diagnosed with mental illnesses. Significant changes need to take place in order to reconstruct this service to align with recovery principles and practices. The term "case management" is, in actuality, an accurate description of what currently happens to people using case management services. They become cases, and they are managed. Not only does this approach not promote recovery, it gets in the way of the recovery process. Ironically enough, case management staff are probably in the most influential position to promote recovery, since they tend to have regular contact and are in a key role to support the recovery process. For the most part, however, they are not trained in recovery practices and often set the recovery process back instead of moving it forward. Regulations tend to prompt them to "take care of" and "control," which does not allow them to be inspiring and creative or to allow them learn and grow themselves as professionals.

When the authors have asked people using case management what an effective case manager does, most said something to the effect, "they were a real person to me" (Anthony et al., 2002). In other words, they established a relationship on a person-to-person basis rather than a practitioner-to-sick-person status.

Implications for Mental Health

The vision of recovery necessitates the adoption of a public health perspective for the mental health field. The proposed recovery model (Figure 20.1) is compatible with a public health approach and is consistent with the public health perspective of this book. For example, the preliminary conceptual model of recovery (Figure 20.1) mandates that we look beyond established measures of pathology and mental health treatment to examine what recovery means, why some people recover and under what circumstances, as well as characteristics of those who recover. Directed by this evolving model, which is based upon the extant literature, the outcomes studied include both psychological dimensions (e.g., subjective well-being) and functional dimensions (e.g., instrumental role functioning) and not merely symptom maintenance and stabilization. The central direction for the mental health field is that there are environmental and individual factors that affect both the processes and outcomes of recovery. Features of formal mental health systems as well as features outside mental health systems are relevant in the recovery model, such as the treatment environment, the interpersonal relationships between the person with a mental illness and family and friends, and other societal and community dimensions.

This model of recovery, its assumptions and implications, will continue to be revised using a multidisciplinary perspective, incorporating research conducted both inside and outside the field of severe mental illnesses, as well as research conducted in other behavioral health fields. Historically, people with psychiatric disabilities were not considered "normal" people, but rather "the mentally ill." Thus, factors that influenced the behavior of "the mentally ill" were studied primarily with respect to disease-specific variables, rather than factors common to all people, disabled or not.

With respect to the historical distinction between mental health and substance abuse services (often collectively referred to as "behavioral health" services), Gagne, White, and Anthony (2007) described how the recovery vision applies to both the mental health and addiction services fields. The values underlying all recovery oriented mental health and addiction systems are based upon the notion that each person is the agent of his or her own recovery and that all services can be organized to support recovery. Compatible with a public health perspective, the recovery vision requires that the mental health and addictions systems collaborate with people in recovery as well as the communities in which they live in order to develop effective services and supports.

Conclusions

The concept of recovery and the recovery movement, spurred by this concept, have the potential to revolutionize how we think about and treat people with severe mental illnesses. While people with severe mental illnesses have been experiencing recovery and are now writing and speaking about recovery, professionals are now just beginning to understand the implications of recovery oriented, public mental health systems. The next several decades will reveal the notion of systems built upon a vision of recovery, which will take its place as a vision commensurate with the public health vision of preventing and curing mental illnesses. Recovery is a vision that will pull us, prod us, and direct us in the twenty-first century. It is the authors' hope that this analysis of the recovery movement will inform and stimulate the field's thinking about recovery and its implications for mental health practice and policy.

References

American Psychiatric Association. (1980). *Diagnostic and Statistical Manual of Mental Disorders DSM-III* (3rd ed.). Washington, DC: Author.

American Psychiatric Association. (1987). *Diagnostic and Statistical Manual of Mental Disorders* (3rd ed.). Washington, DC: Author.

Anonymous. (1989). How I've managed chronic mental illness. *Schizophrenia Bulletin, 15*, 635–640.

Anthony, W. A. (1992). Psychiatric rehabilitation: Key issues and future policy. *Health Affairs, 11*(3), 164–171.

Anthony, W. A. (1993a). Recovery from mental illness: The guiding vision of the mental health service system in the 1990s. *Psychosocial Rehabilitation Journal, 16*(4), 11–23.

Anthony, W. A. (1993b). Editorial: The decade of recovery. *Psychosocial Rehabilitation Journal, 16*(4), 1.

Anthony, W. A. (2000). A recovery oriented service system: Setting some system level standards. *Psychiatric Rehabilitation Journal, 24*(2), 159–168.

Anthony, W. A. (2006). What my MS has taught me about the field of severe mental illness. *Psychiatric Services, 57*(8), 1080–1082.

Anthony, W. A., Cohen, M. R., Farkas, M. D., & Gagne, C. (2002). *Psychiatric Rehabilitation* (2nd ed.). Boston: Boston University, Center for Psychiatric Rehabilitation.

Anthony, W. A., & Huckshorn, K. A. (2008). *Principled Leadership in Mental Health Systems and Programs*. Boston: Boston University Center for Psychiatric Rehabilitation.

Ashcraft, L., & Anthony, W. A. (2008) Eliminating seclusion/restraint in recovery oriented crisis services. *Psychiatric Services, 59*, 1198–1202.

Bachrach, L. L. (1976). A note on some recent studies of released mental hospital patients in the community. *American Journal of Psychiatry, 133*(1), 73–75.

Beale, V., & Lambric, T. (1995). *The Recovery Concept: Implementation in the Mental Health System (Report by the Community Support Program Advisory Committee)*. Columbus: Ohio Department of Mental Health.

Bleuler, M. (1972). *Die schizophrenen Geistesstorungen im Lichte langjahriger Kranken und Familiengeschichten*. Stuttgart: Georg Thieme. Translated by S. M. Clemens as *The Schizophrenic Disorders: Long-term Patient and Family Studies*. New Haven, CT: Yale University Press, 1972.

Braslow, J. T. (1995). Effect of therapeutic innovation on perception of disease and the doctor-patient relationship: A history of general paralysis of the insane and malaria fever therapy. *American Journal of Psychiatry, 152*, 660–665.

Braslow, J. T. (1997). *Mental Ills and Bodily Cures: Psychiatric Treatment in the First Half of the Twentieth Century*. Berkeley: University of California Press.

Ciompi, L., & Muller, C. (1976). *Lebensweg und Alter der Schizophrenen: Eine katamnestische Longzeitstudie bis ins senium*. Berlin: Springer-Verlag.

Deegan, P. E. (1988). Recovery: The lived experience of rehabilitation. *Psychosocial Rehabilitation Journal, 11*(4), 11–19.

Del Vecchio, P., & Fricks, L. (2007). Guest editorial. *Psychiatric Rehabilitation Journal, 31*, 7–8.

DeSisto, M. J., Harding, C. M., McCormick, R. V., Ashikaga, T., & Brooks, G. W. (1995a). The Maine and Vermont three-decade studies of serious mental illness: I, Matched comparisons of cross-sectional outcome. *British Journal of Psychiatry, 167*, 331–338.

DeSisto, M. J., Harding, C. M., McCormick, R. V., Ashikaga, T., & Brooks, G. W. (1995b). The Maine and Vermont three-decade studies of serious mental illness: II, Longitudinal course comparisons. *British Journal of Psychiatry, 167*, 338–341.

Drake, R. E., & Bond, G. R. (2008). Supported employment: 1998–2008. *Psychiatric Rehabilitation Journal, 31*, 274–276.

Farkas, M. (2007). The vision of recovery today: What it is and what it means for services. *World Psychiatry, 6*(2), 1–7.

Farkas, M., Gagne, C., Anthony, W., & Chamberlin, J. (2005). Implementing recovery oriented evidence based programs: Identifying the critical dimensions. *Community Mental Health Journal, 41*(2), 141–158.

Gagne, C. A., White, W., & Anthony, W. A. (2007). Recovery: A common vision for the fields of mental health and addtictions. *Psychatric Rehabilitation Journal, 31*(4), 32–37.

Grob, G. N. (1994a). *The Mad among Us: A History of the Care of America's Mentally Ill*. New York: Maxwell Macmillan International.

Grob, G. N. (1994b). Mad, homeless, and unwanted: A history of the care of the chronic mentally ill in America. *Psychiatric Clinics of North America, 17*, 541–558.

Grob, G. N. (1996). The severely and chronically mentally ill in America: A historical perspective. In S. M. Soreff (Ed.), *Handbook for the Treatment of the Seriousy Mentally Ill*. Ashland, OH: Hogrefe & Huber Publishers.

Harding, C. M. (1994). An examination of the complexities in the measurement of recovery in severe psychiatric disorders. In R. J. Ancill, D. Holliday, & G. W. MacEwan (Eds.), *Schizophrenia: Exporing the Spectrum of Psychosis* (pp. 153–169). Chichester, UK: J. Wiley & Sons.

Harding, C. M. (2003). Changes in schizophrenia across time: Paradoxes, patterns, and predictors. In C. Cohen (Ed.), *Schizophrenia into Later Life* (pp. 19–41). Washington, DC: APA Press.

Harding, C. M., Brooks, G. W., Ashikaga, T., Strauss, J. S., & Breier, A. (1987a). The Vermont longitudinal study of persons with severe mental illness: I, Methodology, study sample, and overall status 32 years later. *American Journal of Psychiatry, 144*(6), 718–726.

Harding, C. M., Brooks, G. W., Ashikaga, T., Strauss, J. S., & Breier, A. (1987b). The Vermont longitudinal study of persons with severe mental illness: II, Long-term outcome of subjects who retrospectively met DSM-III criteria for schizophrenia. *American Journal of Psychiatry, 144*(6), 727–735.

Hinterhuber, H. (1973). Zur Katamnese der Schizophrenien. *Fortschritte der Neurologie Psychiatrie, 41*, 527–588.

Houghton, J. F. (1982). Maintaining mental health in a turbulent world. *Schizophrenia Bulletin, 8*, 548–552.

Huber, G., Gross, G., & Schuttler, R. (1979). *Schizophrenie: Verlaufs und sozialpsychiatrische Langzeit unter suchugen an den 1945 bis 1959 in Bonn hospitalisierten schizophrenen Kranken.* Monographien aus dem Gesamtgebiete der Psychiatrie Bd. 21 Berlin: Springer-Verlag.

Huntley, R. (2006). Lawyering, psychiatric treatment, and schizophrenia: A healing interaction. *Psychiatric Services, 57*, 1387–1389.

Hutchinson, D. S., Gagne, C., Bowers, A., Russinova, Z., Skrinar, G. S., & Anthony, W. A. (2006). A framework for health promotion services for people with psychiatric disabilities. *Psychiatric Rehabilitation Journal, 29*(4), 241–250.

Jacobson, N. (2001). Experiencing recovery: A dimensional analysis of consumers' recovery narratives. *Psychiatric Rehabilitation Journal, 24*(3), 248–256.

Jacobson, N., & Curtis, L. (2000). Recovery as policy in mental health services: Strategies emerging from the states. *Psychiatric Rehabilitation Journal, 23*(4), 333–341.

Jenkins, J. H., Strauss, M. E., Carpenter, E. A., Miller, D., Floersch, J., & Sajatovic, M. (2007). Subjective experience of recovery from schizophrenia-related disorders and atypical antipsychotics. *International Journal of Social Psychiatry, 51*, 211–227.

Kreditor, D. K. (1977). Late catamnesis of recurrent schizophrenia with prolonged remissions (according to an unselected study). *Zh Nevropatol Psikiatr Im S.S. Korsakova, 77*(1), 110–113.

Lapsley, H., Nikora, L. W., & Black, R. (2002). *"Kia Mauri Tau!" Narratives of recovery from disabling mental health problems.* Wellington, New Zealand: Mental Health Commission.

Leete, E. (1989). How I perceive and manage my illness. *Schizophrenia Bulletin, 15*(2), 197–200.

Legere, L. (2007). The importance of rehabilitation. *Psychiatric Rehabilitation Journal, 30*(3), 227–229.

Legislative Summer Study Committee of the Vermont Division of Mental Health. (1996). *A Position Paper on Recovery and Psychiatric Disability.* Waterbury, VT: Vermont Development Disability & Mental Health Services.

Livneh, H. (2001). Psychosocial adaptation to chronic illness and disability: A conceptual framework. *Rehabilitation Counseling Bulletin, 44*(3), 151–160.

Marinow, A. (1974). Klinisch-statische und katamnestische Untersuchungen und chronisch Schizophrenen 1951-1960 und 1961-1970. *Archiv fur Psychiatrie und Nervenkrankheiten, 218*, 115–124.

McDermott, B. (1990). Transforming depression. *The Journal, 1*(4), 13–14.

Mead, S., & Copeland, M. E. (2000). What recovery means to us: Consumers' perspectives. *Community Mental Health Journal, 36*(3), 315–328.

Micale, M. S., & Porter, R. (1994). *Discovering the History of Psychiatry*. New York: Oxford University Press.

New Freedom Commission on Mental Health. (2003). *Achieving the Promise: Transforming Mental Health Care in America; Final Report*. DHHS Pub. No. SMA-03-3832. Rockville, MD: Author.

Ogawa, K., Miya, M., Watarai, A., Nakazawa, M., Yuasa, S., & Utena, H. (1987). A long-term follow-up study of schizophrenia in Japan: With special reference to the course of social adjustment. *British Journal of Psychiatry, 151*, 758–765.

Onken, S. J., Craig, C. M., Ridgway, P., Ralph, R. O., & Cook, J. A. (2007). An analysis of the definitions and elements of recovery: A review of the literature. *Psychiatric Rehabilitation Journal, 31*, 9–22.

Ralph, R. O. (2000). Recovery. *Psychiatric Rehabilitation Skills, 4*(3), 480–517.

Ridgway, P. A. (2001). Re-storying psychiatric disability: Learning from first person recovery narratives. *Psychiatric Rehabilitation Journal, 24*(4), 335–343.

Ridgway, P., & Zipple, A. M. (1990). Challenges and strategies for implementing supported housing. *Psychosocial Rehabilitation Journal, 13*, 115–120.

Rogers, E., Anthony, W., & Farkas, M. (2006). The Choose-Get-Keep Approach to psychiatric rehabilitation. *Rehabilitation Psychology, 51*(3), 247–256.

Rogers, E., Farkas, M., & Anthony, W. A. (2005). Recovery and evidence based practices. In C. Stout & R. Hayes (Eds.), *The Evidence Based Practice: Methods, Models, and Tools for Mental Health Professionals* (pp. 199–219). New Jersey: John Wiley & Sons, Inc.

Shern, D. L., Tsemberis, S., Anthony, W., Lovell, A. M., Richmond, L., Felton, C. J., et al. (2000). Serving street-dwelling individuals with psychiatric disabilities: Outcomes of a psychiatric rehabilitation clinical trial. *American Journal of Public Health, 90*, 1873–1878.

Spaniol, L. (2007). *Phases of the Recovery Process from Psychiatric Disabilities*. Unpublished manuscript, Boston University Center for Psychiatric Rehabilitation.

Spaniol, L., Gagne, C., & Koehler, M. (2003). The recovery framework in rehabilitation and mental health. In D. Moxley & J. R. Finch (Eds.), *Sourcebook of Rehabilitation and Mental Health Practice* (pp. 37–50). New York: Kluwer Academic/Plenum Publishers.

State of Nebraska. (1997). *Recovery: A Guiding Vision for Consumers and Providers of Mental Health Services in Nebraska*. Omaha, NE: Recovery Work Team.

State of Wisconsin. (1997). *Final Report*. Madison, WI: Department of Health and Family Services, Blue Ribbon Commission on Mental Health.

Tsuang, M. T., Woolson, R. F., & Fleming, J. A. (1979). Long-term outcome of major psychoses: 1, Schizophrenia and affective disorders compared with psychiatrically symptom free surgical conditions. *Archives of General Psychiatry, 36*, 1295–1131.

Unzicker, R. (1989). On my own: A personal journey through madness & re-emergence. *Psychosocial Rehabilitation Journal, 13*(1), 71–77.

Williams, C. C., & Collins, A. A. (1999). Defining frameworks for psychosocial intervention. *Interpersonal and Biological Processes, 62*, 61–78.

Chapter 21

ECONOMIC ISSUES IN PSYCHOTROPIC MEDICATION USE

Marisa Elena Domino, PhD; and Joel F. Farley, RPh, PhD

Chapter Objectives

While the term *pharmacoeconomics* often carries with it a narrower context of economic evaluations, in this chapter the authors will consider many of the broader issues of pharmaceutical use, supply, and policy that are of interest to economists. Specifically, the authors will explain economic concepts and issues relating to the use of psychotropic products, review the literature in these areas, explain their implications for mental health, and point out many of the gaps in the literature and other challenges.

Introduction and Overview

One of the most rapidly changing areas in mental health services is the use of prescription medications. The technology surrounding psychotropic medication treatments has changed enormously in the recent past as whole new classes of psychotropic medications have appeared on the market, with new innovations expected in the future as well. The size and composition of the population using psychotropic medications has changed dramatically, as have the incentives and policies regarding their use.

Health economics, through its focus on the incentives in health care systems and the process of changing health, can provide an important framework to studying issues surrounding psychotropic medications. Health economics relies on behavioral models, and pharmacoeconomics is no different in this regard. Most health economic analyses can be categorized as studies of *efficiency*, the optimal use of a constrained set of resources, or *equity*, a focus on the distribution of those resources across individuals or institutions. Pharmacoeconomics addresses questions of importance to policymakers and decision makers in these areas, such as whether newer medications are worth their higher costs due to market exclusivity, how sensitive is demand for medication to changes in price, what affects the diffusion of new medications, how well constraints such as prior authorization or medication limits affect the use of pharmaceuticals and among which populations and types of medications.

This chapter presents material that is of interest to non-economists as well as economists. The authors admittedly focus more on the consumption of psychotropic medications and leave many of the production issues to others, since the authors suspect that there are a greater number of peculiarities in the consumption of these medications than in the production. For an excellent overview of the pharmaceutical industry in general, see Scherer (2000).

Services Delivery and Policy Issues

PREVALENCE OF PSYCHOTROPIC MEDICATION USE

Medications are an increasingly important part of behavioral health treatments. The probability of receiving a psychotropic medication has increased dramatically over the past decades, from an estimated 5.9% of the U.S. population in 1996 to 9.7% in 2006[1] (Paulose-Ram, Safran, Jonas, Gu, & Orwig, 2007; Zuvekas, 2005).

Developed in the late 1980s, selective serotonin reuptake inhibitors (SSRIs) and second generation, or atypical, antipsychotics, are two of the newer classes of psychotropic medications. These two classes alone are responsible for a remarkable 80% of the growth in use and spending of psychotropic medications (Zuvekas, 2005). These new technologies are not only replacing the older technologies, such as tricyclic antidepressants and first generation antipsychotics, but the presence, marketing, and ease of use of these new products that have diffused into general practices have substantially increased the number of psychotropic medication users.

Despite the increasing incidence of psychotropic drug use, psychotropic drugs and other mental health treatments are still underused in mental health care (Frank, Conti, & Goldman, 2005; Kessler et al., 2005) due to barriers to treatment, such as cost and stigma. The National Comorbidity Survey Replication study, a large population-based survey of mental illness and treatments in the United States, found that while treatment rates for mental illness had increased in the early 2000s over the prior decade despite a constant prevalence rate, only one-third of those with a diagnosable mental health disorder had received any treatment (Kessler et al., 2005) (see Chapter 7 in this volume for additional information on the epidemiology of mental disorders).

In contrast to the low treatment rates among those with a psychiatric disorder, the off-label use of psychotropic medication, or the use of medications for conditions other than those approved by the U.S. Food and Drug Administration, has also been increasing. Almost a third of psychotropic medication use has been

---

[1] Authors' calculation on the 2006 MEPS data, the most recent year available.

estimated to be off-label in one recent analysis (Radley, Finkelstein, & Stafford, 2006). Off-label use may represent innovative behavior by physicians and pharmaceutical companies extending the knowledge base on the current set of approved medications into their use in conditions for which fewer treatment options may be available. Off-label use also means the use of medications for symptoms or diseases without an evidence base. In many cases, off-label medication use is dangerous at worst and a waste of resources at best. In the exploration of off-label use of psychotropic medications cited above, only 6% of the off-label use of these medications was determined to have strong scientific support, leaving the remaining 94% of off-label uses for diseases and symptoms for which little or no such evidence exists (Radley et al., 2006).

The use of psychotropic medications, especially antipsychotics in institutional settings, is also an important issue (Briesacher et al., 2005; Semla, Palla, Poddig, & Brauner, 1994). Although the appropriate use of antipsychotics can improve the quality of life for those with clinical psychotic disorders, the overuse of this class of medications in institutions, such as nursing homes, has long been suspected. Although it is increasingly monitored, quality improvements have not been seen (Briesacher et al., 2005).

Spending

Almost $19 billion was spent on outpatient prescriptions of psychotropic medications in 2005 (Medical Expenditure Panel Survey, 2008). This level of spending placed psychotropic medications as the fourth most expensive medication class in 2005, just behind metabolic agents, cardiovascular agents, and central nervous system agents, respectively.

Psychotropic medications are a significant expense in the Medicaid program. Psychotropic medications accounted for more than $4 billion in the Medicaid program in 2001–2002, prior to the implementation of Medicare Part D (Banthin & Miller, 2006). In 2006, the first year of Medicare Part D, Medicaid expenditures on psychotropic medications decreased to $2.7 billion, while Medicare's expenditures on psychotropic medications were $3.6 billion.[2] Antidepressants and antipsychotics were the largest two categories of psychotropic medications in the Medicaid program, accounting for $1.7 and $1.9 billion, respectively. Spending on psychotropic medications is increasing rapidly, with an estimated annual increase of 17.1%, in contrast to other medication categories, which are growing at a rate of 12.1% (Coffey et al., 2000; Mark et al., 2005).

Spending on psychotropic medications comprises a substantial portion of total behavioral health dollars. In 2003, psychotropic medications accounted for an estimated 19% of total mental health expenditures, up from 13% of expenditures in 1997 (Coffey et al., 2000; Mark, Levit, Buck, Coffey, & Vandivort-Warren, 2007). Per person spending on behavioral health benefits has been shrinking while spending on pharmaceutical products has increased (Mark et al., 2005; Mark et al., 2007), indicating that the psychotropic portion of mental health expenditures is increasing and will likely continue to do so in the future.

---

[2] Psychotropic medications are a significant

The Diffusion of Psychotropic Medications

Once a drug is approved, what factors affect whether it becomes widely used and in what populations? Research is only beginning to examine the diffusion or rate of use of psychotropic medications over time since introduction. Whether the drug represents a significant breakthrough in technology over currently available competitors, the level of marketing efforts, the generosity of coverage, the evidence on its clinical effectiveness, and adverse effect profile all affect the diffusion of new medications. Other factors, such as insurance arrangements, mental health carve-outs, or the more broad use of managed care tools, have also been shown to affect the diffusion level (Ling, Berndt, & Frank, 2008) and diffusion path (Domino, 2008) of psychotropic medications.

In markets where under-use is thought to be an inefficient solution, such as most psychotropic drug markets, the greater diffusion of drug products could be more efficient if drug expenditures are concentrated on individuals who have the greatest net benefit from use. Diffusion curves per se cannot provide a value judgment as to whether more use is better in every case, or even whether use is at a rate clinically determined to improve health outcomes. Greater use of psychotropic medications may indicate increases at the *intensive margin*, or level of use among a constant group of users, or increases at the *extensive margin*, or number of users. For example, a recent examination of the growth of outpatient antipsychotic medications (Domino & Swartz, 2008) found that the substantial increase in antipsychotic diffusion from 1996 to 2005 was almost exclusively from increases in the extensive margin, through greater rates of use among children and those with diagnoses other than schizophrenia.

The Value of Psychotropic Medications

The greater use of psychotropic medications begs the question of whether these new expensive treatments are worth their cost. That is, is society seeing gains from greater investments in psychotropic medication treatments through symptom reduction, lower rates of hospitalization, and greater quality of life, which may translate to greater employment and wages and increased participation in all aspects of society? There seems to be clear consensus that there is value in the appropriate treatment of most psychiatric disorders (U.S. Public Health Service, 1999), but at issue is whether the newer, more expensive medications add sufficient value through greater benefits net of price to justify their use over older, cheaper alternatives.

The substantial diversity in benefits from specific drugs, tolerance and preferences for side-effects, and mix of patient histories and comorbidities indicate that the answer is not a simple one, but depends upon a combination of factors (Huskamp, 2006). One recent study quantified the savings in reduced use of hospitals and other types of health services for those on Medicaid using the newer second generation antipsychotic agents (Duggan, 2005). The greater drug spending on the newer agents in this study was not offset by equivalent reductions in health care use, indicating that from a Medicaid program perspective, the newer antipsychotics were not worth the additional investment. However, potentially greater improvements in health from symptom reduction or fewer side-effects were not separately incorporated in this analysis unless they resulted in a change in health care use. Results from the Clinical Antipsychotic Trials of Intervention Effectiveness (CATIE), the largest federally funded antipsychotic clinical trial to date, the Cost Utility of the Latest Antipsychotic Drugs in Schizophrenia Study (CUtLASS), and other recent antipsychotic trials have also recently called into question the cost-effectiveness of second generation antipsychotics as compared to their less-expensive first generation antipsychotic alternatives (Jones et al., 2006; Rosenheck et al., 2006).

These studies underscore an important distinction in pharmacoeconomic studies of value: that costs and benefits can be defined from a number of different perspectives. Individual consumers make decisions based upon their out-of-pocket costs and time spent for treatment and potential benefits, such as symptom reduction or overall increases in quality of life. Health plans, in contrast, consider a different set of costs and benefits. Costs from a health plan perspective include the price paid to a pharmacy or pharmacy benefits manager for a medication, as well as the costs of follow-up care or ancillary care. Benefits of treatment to a health plan include decreases in other types of service use. For example, consumers who demonstrate clinical responses to pharmaceutical treatment may use fewer hospital days or emergency room visits, which represents a savings from a health plan perspective. Health plans, however, may not adequately absorb some of the benefits and costs that consumers care about, such as their time spent traveling to service sites or in waiting rooms, or benefits that improve health but do not result in changes in health care expenditures. These distinctions have led to suggestions that researchers take a societal perspective that encompasses the perspective of all relevant parties when conducting economic evaluations, such as cost-benefit or cost-effectiveness analyses (Gold, 1996). Decisions around pharmaceutical coverage or use, however, may still be decided according to narrower perspectives, so consideration of each party's costs and benefits is still important.

For off-label uses, the story is less clear. By definition, not enough evidence exists on the off-label use of most psychotropic medications to determine whether these uses have value over more established treatments. In many cases, off-label use is associated with greater risks and costs, but few expected gains. For example, the use of antipsychotic medications in elderly patients with dementia-related psychosis is one such case where the greater risk of death and minimal clinical improvement seem to indicate that use is not justified for most individuals (Wang et al., 2005).

Drug Selection: The Influence of Multiple Parties

The process by which a specific drug is chosen points out many of the complexities in undertaking pharmacoeconomic analysis. Informational asymmetries lead a consumer with a health concern to seek care from a physician. The physician generally provides both a diagnosis and a recommendation for a course of treatment to the patient. The patient, however, is unable to effectively evaluate the treatment choice of the physician and must rely on trust, accreditation, and/or licensing, and in extreme cases, the legal system to monitor the performance of the physician.

Under traditional fee-for-service arrangements, the physician has little financial incentive to promote cost-effective treatments and may even profit if further care is required. This is especially apparent in the case of medication prescribing. The physician must select a product from several medication options, but receives no financial reward for careful selection and even receives additional revenues if the patient must return for a prescription adjustment. This effect is at least partially distorted by the presence of managed care insurance, whereby the insurer can exercise some amount of control over the treatment choices made by the physician, either through direct restrictions or incentive schemes.

Simplistic economic models assume that physicians act as *perfect agents* for patients, internalizing relevant prices, preferences across side-effects, and the value of treatment outcomes, recommending the prescription product that maximizes the patient's well-being, or *utility*. This premise has been discredited by studies showing that physicians are influenced by professional norms and pharmaceutical marketing, demonstrate individual prescribing patterns, and have little knowledge of the prices of various pharmaceutical products (Frank & Zeckhauser, 2007). It is estimated that 9–30% of prescriptions written are never filled (Shah et al., 2009; Bazargan, Barbre, & Hamm, 1993; Henry, 1993; Lash & Harding, 1995; Shulman, 1991), indicating serious flaws in the success of the physician as a perfect and independent agent. It is clear that patients, pharmacists, and insurers may all play an important role in the prescription decision.

Insurance

The evolution of health insurance over the last several decades has had significant implications for the use of prescription drug use. Prescription drugs used to be an inconsequential portion of health care budgets and were largely paid for out of pocket by U.S. consumers. The growth of prescription drug coverage has been phenomenal, and presently just over a third of prescription drug expenditures for people under age 65 are paid for out of pocket (Sommers, 2008). Many seniors and persons with disabilities participating in the Medicare program are newly covered for prescription drug expenditures through the Medicare Part D program, which began in January 2006.

Prescription Managed Care for Psychotropic Medications

As psychopharmacological expenditures continue to grow, many insurers have turned to prescription managed care policies in an effort to control pharmaceutical spending. Insurers have a wide range of tools available to curb growth in psychopharmacological expenditures and utilization. Prescription managed care policies are known to influence prescription expenditures. However, there is evidence to suggest that managed care policies may not be as effective when applied to psychotropic medications. This is the result of substantial biological heterogeneity associated with treating most mental health conditions (Huskamp, 2003; Soumerai, 2004). This heterogeneity means that the same medication may not be suitable for all patients, requiring providers to individualize medication therapy for a given patient. Therefore, once a patient is stabilized on medication, changes in medications or other psychosocial treatments associated with the introduction of managed care policies may have unintended consequences for patients, providers, and insurers. Below, the authors describe four main tools used by managed care insurers to manage pharmaceutical expenditures.

Formularies

One of the more common methods to control mental health medication use is the drug formulary. Formularies are a listing of drugs preferred by health care organizations for use in treating patients with a given condition. In the case of a *closed formulary*, drugs not listed on the formulary are excluded from health plan coverage, leaving patients responsible for any charges incurred as a result of filling a non-formulary medication. In the case of an *open formulary* (sometimes referred to as a *preferred drug list*), the formulary simply provides a recommendation for prescribing, allowing providers the final decision on treatment.

Preferred drug lists are commonly used in Medicaid because of federal stipulations that preclude Medicaid from excluding any medication for which a manufacturer agrees to provide a rebate. Therefore, preferred drug lists are in combination with prior authorization procedures to allow beneficiaries to have access to non-preferred drugs. For private insurers, formularies are commonly tied to patient cost sharing amounts. Under a tiered formulary, preferred drugs carry less out-of-pocket costs for a patient than non-preferred drugs. Under these examples, managed care policies often act in concert with one another.

The purpose of a formulary is both to obtain discounts from pharmaceutical manufacturers in exchange for the increased use of the manufacturer's products in lieu of competing products, and to provide information to physicians on the relative costs of the various treatment options (although this function is limited with the "silo" treatment of drugs in these plans). The Congressional Budget Office found that discounts to health maintenance organization (HMO) plans average as much as 18% off the average retail price of drugs and vary with the degree of competition in the therapeutic class (Congressional Budget Office [CBO], 1998).

The net effect of formularies on the use of new drug products is difficult to determine (CBO, 1998). While brand name drug manufacturers that successfully negotiate admittance to an insurer's formulary can expect to receive an increase in the utilization of their products over other products that are excluded from the formulary, these brand name products also receive intense competition from lower priced generic products that are members of the same therapeutic class.

In addition, formularies are updated on a periodic rather than continual basis, delaying the introduction of new drug products to insured persons subject to a formulary. Often formulary committee members rely on drug information obtained from peer-reviewed literature (CBO, 1998) which further increases this delay due to the long process involved in peer reviewed publications. For example, one survey found that only 20% of HMOs included new drugs in their formularies immediately after FDA approval (Novartis, 1998). However, formularies may increase the flow of information to physicians in participating plans and thus serve to speed changes in prescribing behavior.

A concern behind restricting access to the types of medications that are covered by a health plan is the potential for patients to be denied access to a treatment they may otherwise benefit from using. This has the potential to reduce efficiencies in treatment and cause unintended clinical or economic consequences. Most health plans recognize these problems and allow patient access to non-formulary medications through a prior authorization process. Therefore, few plans utilize a true closed formulary design and there are few examinations of their impact upon psychotropic medication use in patients with mental illness.

An early example documenting unintended consequences from a restrictive formulary is seen in a study by Bloom and Jacobs (1985). As a result of restricting access to peptic ulcer medications in the West Virginia Medicaid program, this study suggested that prescription savings were substantially offset by an increase in the use of expensive inpatient hospital treatment. Other studies have suggested that closed formularies may result in sub-optimal medication use. Motheral and Henderson (1999–2000) noted a substantial reduction in the use of essential medications for chronic medical conditions such as hypertension following the introduction of a closed formulary in a managed care organization. This study examined 20 common prescription drug classes, including antidepressant medications. Although there was no evidence of a reduction in antidepressant medication use in this study, the researchers did not limit their examination to patients with depression.

Prior Authorization

Many insurers implement *prior authorization* procedures in tandem with medication formularies. Prior authorization requirements allow access to medications otherwise excluded from a formulary only after certain pre-approved criteria have been met and cleared with a patient's insurer. A criterion that must be met for reimbursement commonly includes confirmation of a pre-approved medical condition. For example, atypical antipsychotic medications may be restricted to patients confirmed to have schizophrenia to limit potentially dangerous prescribing for conditions such as dementia. Prior authorization may also be used to restrict questionable prescribing practices for medications. One example is a requirement of pre-approval for the use of multiple atypical antipsychotic medications for a single patient. In the case of step-therapy or fail-first prior authorization policies, patients may be required to prove prior treatment failure with a preferred medication before being allowed to receive non-preferred alternatives. For example, atypical antipsychotic medications may only be reimbursed following treatment failure on less expensive typical antipsychotic medications.

Recent studies have examined the impact of implementing prior authorization policies for psychotropic medications in state Medicaid programs. One study, by Soumerai and colleagues (2008), examined a step-therapy prior authorization policy implemented in the Maine Medicaid program in 2003. This policy required patients to first fail treatment on Risperidone and then either Ziprasidone or Quetiapine before being allowed reimbursement for one of two non-preferred medications (Olanzapine or Aripiprazole). The study showed a slight reduction in atypical antipsychotic spending ($18.63 per patient over an 8 month policy period). However, it also suggested significant treatment discontinuation among Medicaid enrollees with schizophrenia.

Another recent study examined an older fail-first prior authorization policy implemented in the Georgia Medicaid program in 1996 (Farley, Cline, Schommer, Hadsall, & Nyman, 2008). This policy required patients to fail at least two therapies of an older typical antipsychotic before being reimbursed to receive an atypical antipsychotic. Again, significant prescription savings were shown from the policy. However, there was also evidence of a significant monthly ($31.59) increase in outpatient expenditures per person. This suggests that cost savings resulting from restricting psychotropic medication use is potentially offset by increased spending in other health sectors.

Dispensing Limits

One policy that is not limited to a specific type of medication, but may disproportionately influence patients with mental illness is the use of a dispensing limit or a prescription "cap." Dispensing limits refer to restrictions placed upon the quantity of medication that is reimbursable by an insurer. Most insurers place dispensing limits on the amount of medication that is reimbursable per prescription claim (i.e., limiting prescription claims to a 30-days supply). However, a more aggressive means of limiting medication is by capping the number of prescriptions an insurer will reimburse over a defined interval or limiting the dollar amount an insurer will reimburse.

The best-known example to detail the influence of using dispensing limits in patients with severe mental disorders is an examination of a prescription cap introduced in the New Hampshire Medicaid program in 1981 (Soumerai, McLaughlin, Ross-Degnan, Casteris, & Bollini, 1994). This restriction capped the number of prescriptions reimbursable per month at 3. The policy resulted in a substantial 15.4% decrease in antipsychotic medication utilization and a 23% decline in prescription expenditures. However, the authors also showed evidence of significant increases in community mental health center visits, emergency mental health visits, and partial hospitalizations among patients with schizophrenia. These increases exceed prescription savings, suggesting their ineffectiveness in managing drug costs for patients with severe mental illness.

Cost Sharing

Cost sharing refers to health plan policies that require patients to share in the cost of their treatment by paying either a percentage of their medication cost or a fixed co-payment amount. Cost sharing policies are designed, in part, to reduce the potential for moral hazard (i.e., to minimize the potential for changes in medical consumption as a result of not bearing the total market cost of receiving that care). In theory, requiring patients to pay a portion of the market cost of a medication should make them more likely to consider whether to use a medication with little expected benefit than they would be if they did not share in the cost of that care. While co-payments are designed, in part, to reduce potentially unnecessary medication use, their application to all drugs has implications for essential medication use as well and depends upon how responsive consumers are to prices (details described below).

Although most health plans use some form of cost sharing, the amount and type of cost sharing differs across health plans. In Medicaid, most cost sharing requirements are set as a fixed co-payment, with amounts ranging from $1 to $3 per prescription, with a cap on the total amount a patient is responsible for paying per month. By contrast, private health plans have moved toward tiered cost sharing arrangements that reflect health plan preference for a medication on the plan's formulary (Huskamp et al., 2003). For example, a four-tier cost sharing structure may require co-payments of $5 for generic drugs, $15 for preferred brand name drugs, $30 for non-preferred brand name drugs, and $50 for specialty drugs. This structure is designed to steer patients toward preferred medications that are typically less expensive than non-preferred agents.

The Influence of Drug Prices

Understanding how sensitive consumers of psychotropic medication are to price is important to policymakers in both public and private insurance policies, since it indicates how out-of-pocket price will affect medication purchases and adherence. *Price elasticity* is an expression of price sensitivity widely used by economists. It is a ratio of the percent change of a good quantity over the percent change in price. The price elasticity of demand related to cost sharing policies has been estimated at -0.2 to -0.6. In other words, a 10% increase in cost sharing would be expected to reduce medication consumption 2% to 6% (Goldman, Joyce, & Zheng, 2007). For antidepressants, the elasticity has been estimated at 0 to -11.0 (Domino & Salkever, 2003; Landsman, Yu, Liu, Teutsch, & Berger, 2005). In another study, it was estimated that by doubling medication co-payments, there would be a resulting 8% reduction in antidepressant medication use among patients seeing a provider for depression (Goldman et al., 2004). Aggregate demand for prescription medication has been shown to be negatively related to price, with price elasticity estimates ranging from -17.27 to -0.316 (Baye, Maness, & Wiggins, 1997; Reekie, 1978; Stern, 1995). Combined, these results suggest a potential for co-payments to adversely affect essential medication use for severe mental illness.

Co-payment increases also have been shown to influence antipsychotic prescription filling behavior. One study, which examined the effect of increasing co-payments from $2 to $5 in the Department of Veterans Affairs (VA), showed a 25% decline in antipsychotic prescription refills among patients with schizophrenia following introduction of the policy (Zeber, Grazier, Valenstein, Blow, & Lantz, 2007). This led to a minimal, although significant, 3% increase in psychiatric admissions 20 months following implementation of the policy. Similar antipsychotic medication utilization reductions are also seen in patients with schizophrenia following the introduction of co-payments in Medicaid (Hartung et al., 2008).

There are several levels at which prices may affect the demand for prescription medications. Physicians may change their choice of a prescription medication to recommend according to the cost of a product and of its competitors. However, the *cost* of pharmaceuticals is somewhat of an ambiguous concept and may be interpreted as the cost to consumers of filling a medication (or the co-payment), the cost to the health plan or insurance company of reimbursing a medication prescription, or even the total societal cost of a medication, which includes any needed ancillary tests and follow-up visits. The cost of a medication from a health plan perspective may vary from plan to plan according to the discounts negotiated with the drug manufacturers. Since physicians generally contract with multiple payers, it may be seemingly impossible for them to make an informed decision based upon the actual cost of a medication.

Safavi and Hayward (1992) surveyed physicians at a university teaching hospital to determine which factors affect drug choice for medications with similar side-effect profiles and efficacies. While 49% of physicians rated cost to the patient as extremely or very important in selecting a particular agent in general, the number decreased to 24–31% when physicians were asked to identify which factors influenced recommendations within a particular therapeutic class.

The authors proceeded to test the physicians' knowledge of drug prices for their first and second drug choices (Safavi & Hayward, 1992). The median physician estimate was outside the range of actual prices at local pharmacies for four of the five chemical entities listed by the authors. For these four agents, only 16–38% of physician estimates were within $10 of the actual cost of a month's supply. This finding complements previous research on physicians' knowledge of prices, which has demonstrated that physicians seldom have a precise idea of the prices of products they prescribe (Lowry, Lowry, & Warner, 1972).

While physicians do not seem to be sensitive to actual drug prices, one study examined whether they responded to perceived drug prices (Ryan, Yule, Bond, & Taylor, 1996). A group of general practitioners in Scotland were asked to provide estimates of the prices of drugs they commonly prescribed. The authors then tracked the actual prescribing behavior of these physicians and estimated the elasticity of demand to the estimated prices of the selected drugs and their substitutes. While the price estimates were poor (between 10–62% of the guesses were within 25% of the actual drug price), they found a significant negative own-price elasticity and a positive estimated price elasticity of competing products, consistent with economic theory. No other variables in the model, such as physician gender, age, or practice characteristics had significant predictive ability.

While physicians generally estimate prescription drug prices inaccurately, their prescribing behavior seems to be malleable to increased information (see, for example, Carter, Butler, Rogers, & Holloway, 1993). Soumerai, McLaughlin, and Avorn (1989) reviewed the experimental literature on interventions that affect prescribing behavior and found that informational effects can have significant effects on prescribing behavior, but much remains to be learned about the efficiency and effectiveness of efforts to improve prescribing behavior.

ADHERENCE

Due to the historical separation between the physician as the prescription writer and the pharmacist as the seller of the final product, the patient has been given a second chance, in a sense, to disagree with the recommended treatment of the medical provider and may choose not to fill the prescription or not to comply with the recommended dose if the prescription is filled. Non-adherence to medications with an established evidence base may indicate that patient preferences are not always in line with physician preferences. Non-adherence also may impose significant *externalities* on others, including family members, communities, employers, and insurers.

Non-adherence is a common occurrence and has received considerable attention in the literature. A portion of non-adherence may be attributed to the failure of the medical establishment to communicate the directions and expectation about symptom reduction and side-effects to their patients (Wilson et al., 2007). While this explanation may be valid, other evidence has shown that adherence may be strongly related to the drug product prescribed. Patients may discontinue therapy because of adverse reactions from specific drug products or simply because they begin to see results and no longer feel a need to continue drug therapy. Regardless of the cause of non-adherence, physicians seem largely unaware of their patients' medication usage patterns (Mushlin & Appel, 1977; Wilson et al., 2007).

While adherence studies generally focus on the patient's deviation from the recommended regime, an often neglected component of non-adherence is the failure to initially fill drug prescriptions, precluding any possibility of consumption-related adherence. It has been estimated that between 9–30% of prescriptions go unfilled (Bazargan et al., 1993; Henry, 1993; Lash & Harding, 1995; Shulman, 1991). The percentage of persons who fill a prescription but do not take the medication (13%) has been estimated to be approximately equivalent to the percent of people who never fill a written prescription (14%) (Lash & Harding, 1995). Factors related to this type of non-adherence are hypothesized as largely economic, as purchases of prescription medication often involve high out-of-pocket payments and time costs. These costs can be especially acute in low-income populations. Few studies have investigated the extent and correlates of this type of non-adherence, largely due to the lack of data which permit this type of analysis.

Non-adherence with psychotropic medication regimes may be a larger problem than in other drug classes. Non-adherence with antidepressant medications has been estimated to be as high as 30% (Henry, 1993) and differences have been observed within this class of medications (Sclar et al., 1994; Wilde & Whittington, 1995). Almost three-fourths of participants in CATIE discontinued their study-assigned antipsychotic medication (Lieberman et al., 2005). Non-adherence, and its causes and consequences, remains an important line of inquiry for pharmacoeconomic research.

Production Issues

Since the price of psychotropic medications influences the level of use, the presence of lower cost generic versions of psychotropic medications should influence the level of use. The two newer classes of psychotropics, SSRIs and second generation antipsychotics, first received approval in the late 1980s and generic alternatives in both classes are now on the market. Intense price competition from generic medications will mean lower prices to health plans and other price sensitive components of the market (Frank & Salkever, 1997), possibly opening the way to greater rates of psychotropic medication use and adherence.

Another production issue important in psychotropic markets is incentives for innovation. While lower drug prices are desirable for current and potential users, higher prices and profits encourage research and development, which leads to more products and choices in the future. Policy proposals that reduce prices may have long-run implications for pharmaceutical innovation (Frank et al., 2005).

Implications for Mental Health

There are a number of challenges that will be analyzed and debated in the pharmacoeconomics arena. The implementation and payment mechanisms in Medicare Part D, the largest public insurance expansion in recent history, is one of the most urgent of these issues. Many facets of the current design of Part D are under debate, including the suggested use of current medications to select among dozens of private plan options, each with their own formulary design and costs to subscribers (Domino, Stearns, Norton, & Yeh, 2008), and whether negotiation of discounts by the federal government with drug manufacturers should be allowed (Frank & Newhouse, 2008). Other components of Medicare Part D that have received attention in pharmacoeconomic analyses are whether the large number of choices of Part D plans is beneficial or merely confusing to subscribers, the use of HMO-like Medicare Advantage plans as a means of receiving prescription drug coverage, and the impact of Medicare Part D on patterns of care for those dually enrolled in the Medicaid program who previously received prescription drug coverage from potentially more generous Medicaid plans.

Another area of pharmacoeconomic inquiry relates to the spillover effects that psychotropic medications have on other sectors, such as employment, education, and criminal justice. These issues may be more acute with regard to treatments for mental health than in other disease areas due to the substantial effect that mental illness has on these areas. Researchers are only beginning to quantify the implications that variations in the use of medications have on these other human resource sectors, and much remains to be learned. Understanding these spillover effects, or externalities, of psychotropic medication use has implications for budgeting because in many cases, changes in the budget for psychotropic medications in one sector can have implications for future expenditures in other areas.

Finally, the much anticipated area of personalized medicines may be especially beneficial for psychotropic medication users, since as noted above, responses to psychotropic medication are highly individualized and very difficult to predict. The ability to know ahead of time who would respond to which medications may result in greater response to medication and greater adherence, but brings with it substantial costs. Armed with training in economics and the perspective of public health, the field is well posed to contribute to the debates surrounding these challenges.

References

Banthin, J. S., & Miller, G. E. (2006). Trends in perscription drug expenditures by Medicaid enrollees. *Medical Care, 44*(5), 127–135.

Baye, M. R., Maness, R., & Wiggins, S. N. (1997). Demand systems and the true subindex of the cost of living for pharmaceuticals. *Applied Economics, 29*(9), 1179–1190.

Bazargan, M., Barbre, A. R., & Hamm, V. (1993). Failure to have prescriptions filled among black elderly. *Journal of Aging and Health, 5*(2), 264–282.

Bloom, B. S., & Jacobs, J. (1985). Cost effects of restricting cost-effective therapy. *Medical Care, 23*(7), 872–880.

Briesacher, B., Limcangco, M., Simoni-Wastila, L., Doshi, J., Levens, S., Shea, D., et al. (2005). The quality of antipsychotic drug prescribing in nursing homes. *Archives of Internal Medicine, 165*(11), 1280–1285.

Carter, B. L., Butler, C. D., Rogers, J. C., & Holloway, R. L. (1993). Evaluation of physician decision making with the use of prior probabilities and a decision-analysis model. *Archives of Family Medicine, 2*(5), 529.

Coffey, R. M., Mark, T., Kind, E., Harwood, H., McKusick, D., Genuardi, J., et al. (2000). *National Estimates of Expenditures for Mental Health and Substance Abuse Treatment, 1997*. Rockville, MD: Center for Substance Abuse Treatment and Center for Mental Health Services.

Congressional Budget Office. (1998). *How Increased Competition from Generic Drugs Has Affected Prices and Returns in Pharmaceutical Industry*. Washington, DC: Author.

Domino, M. E. (2008). *A Flexible Functional Form for Diffusion Research: Applications to the Diffusion of Psychotropic Medications*. Unpublished manuscript, University of North Carolina, Chapel Hill.

Domino, M. E., & Salkever, D. S. (2003). Price elasticity and pharmaceutical selection: The influence of managed care. *Health Economics, 12*(7), 565–586.

Domino, M. E., Stearns, S. C., Norton, E. C., & Yeh, W. S. (2008). Why using current medications to select a Medicare Part D plan may lead to higher out-of-pocket payments. *Medical Care Research and Review, 65*(1), 114–126.

Domino, M. E., & Swartz, M. S. (2008). Who are the new users of antipsychotic medications? *Psychiatric Services, 59*(5), 507–514.

Duggan, M. G. (2005). Do new prescription drugs pay for themselves? The case of second-generation antipsychotics. *Journal of Health Economics 24*(1), 1–31.

Farley, J. F., Cline, R. R., Schommer, J. C., Hadsall, R. S., & Nyman, J. A. (2008). Retrospective assessment of Medicaid step-therapy prior authorization policy for atypical antipsychotic medications. *Clinical Therapeutics, 30*(8), 1524–1539.

Frank, R. G., Conti, R. M., & Goldman, H. H. (2005). Mental health policy and psychotropic drugs. *Milbank Quarterly, 83*(2), 271–298.

Frank, R. G., & Newhouse, J. P. (2008). Should drug prices be negotiated under Part D of Medicare? And if so, how? *Health Affairs, 27*(1), 33–43.

Frank, R. G., & Salkever, D. S. (1997). Generic entry and the pricing of pharmaceuticals. *Journal of Economics & Management Strategy, 6*(1), 75–90.

Frank, R. G., & Zeckhauser, R. J. (2007). Custom-made versus ready-to-wear treatments: Behavioral propensities in physicians' choices. *Journal of Health Economics, 26*(6), 1101–1127.

Gold, M., Siegel, J. E., Russell, L. B., & Weinstein, M. C. (1996). *Cost-effectiveness in Health and Medicine*. New York: Oxford University Press.

Goldman, D. P., Joyce, G. F., Escarce, J. J., Pace, J. E., Solomon, M. D., Laouri, M., et al. (2004). Pharmacy benefits and the use of drugs by the chronically ill. *Journal of the American Medical Association, 291*, (19), 2344–2350.

Goldman, D. P., Joyce, G. F., & Zheng, Y. (2007). Prescription drug cost sharing: Associations with medication and medical utilization and spending and health. *Journal of the American Medical Association, 298*(1), 61.

Hartung, D. M., Carlson, M. J., Kraemer, D. F., Haxby, D. G., Ketchum, K. L., & Greenlick, M. R. (2008). Impact of a Medicaid copayment policy on prescription drug and health services utilization in a fee-for-service Medicaid population. *Medical Care, 46*(6), 565–572.

Henry, J. A. (1993). Debits and credits in the management of depression. *British Journal of Psychiatry, 20*(Suppl.), 33–39.

Huskamp, H. A. (2003). Managing psychotropic drug costs: Will formularies work? *Health Affairs, 22*(5), 84–96.

Huskamp, H. A. (2006). Prices, profits, and innovation: Examining criticisms of new psychotropic drugs' value. *Health Affairs, 25*(3), 635–646.

Huskamp, H. A., Deverka, P. A., Epstein, A. M., Epstein, R. S., McGuigan, K. A., & Frank, R. G. (2003). The effect of incentive-based formularies on prescription-drug utilization and spending. *New England Journal of Medicine, 349*(23), 2224–2232.

Jones, P. B., Barnes, T. R. E., Davies, L., Dunn, G., Lloyd, H., Hayhurst, K. P., et al. (2006). Randomized controlled trial of the effect on quality of life of second- vs first-generation antipsychotic drugs in schizophrenia: Cost utility of the latest antipsychotic drugs in schizophrenia study (CUtLASS 1). *Archives of General Psychiatry, 63*(10), 1079–1087.

Kessler, R. C., Demler, O., Frank, R. G., Olfson, M., Pincus, H. A., Walters, E. E., et al. (2005). Prevalence and treatment of mental disorders, 1990 to 2003. *New England Journal of Medicine, 352*(24), 2515–2523.

Landsman, P. B., Yu, W., Liu, X., Teutsch, S. M., & Berger, M. L. (2005). Impact of 3-tier pharmacy benefit design and increased consumer cost-sharing on drug utilization. *American Journal of Managed Care, 11*(10), 621–628.

Lash, S., & Harding, J. (1995). Abandoned prescriptions: A quantitative assessment of their cause. *Journal of Managed Care Pharmacy, 1*(3), 193–199.

Lieberman, J. A., Stroup, T. S., McEvoy, J. P., Swartz, M. S., Rosenheck, R. A., Perkins, D. O., et al. (2005). Effectiveness of antipsychotic drugs in patients with chronic schizophrenia. *New England Journal of Medicine, 353*(12), 1209–1223.

Ling, D. C., Berndt, E. R., & Frank, R. G. (2008). Economic incentives and contracts: The use of psychotropic medications. *Contemporary Economic Policy, 26*(1), 49–72.

Lowry, D. R., Lowry, L., & Warner, R. S. (1972). A survey of physicians' awareness of drug costs. *Journal of Medical Education, 47*, 349–351.

Mark, T. L., Coffey, R. M., Vandivort-Warren, R., Harwood, H. J., King, E. C., & Team, a. t. M. S. E. (2005). U.S. spending for mental health and substance abuse treatment, 1991–2001. *Health Affairs, 24*(Suppl. 1), W5.133–142.

Mark, T. L., Levit, K. R., Buck, J. A., Coffey, R. M., & Vandivort-Warren, R. (2007). Mental health treatment expenditure trends, 1986–2003. *Psychiatric Services, 58*(8), 1041–1048.

Medical Expenditure Panel Survey: Prescribed Drug Estimates; 2008. Available online at http://www.meps.ahrq.gov/mepsweb/data_stats/summ_tables/hc/drugs/2005/hctcest_totexp2005.shtml. Accessed July 8, 2009.

Motheral, B. R., & Henderson, R. (1999–00). The effect of a closed formulary on prescription drug use and costs. *Inquiry, 36*(4), 481–491.

Mushlin, A. I., & Appel, F. A. (1977). Diagnosing potential noncompliance: Physicians' ability in a behavioral dimension of medical care. *Archives of Internal Medicine, 137*, 318–321.

Novartis. *Pharmacy Benefit Report: Trends & Forecasts, 1998 Edition.* (1998). East Hanover, NJ: Author.

Paulose-Ram, R., Safran, M. A., Jonas, B. S., Gu, Q., & Orwig, D. (2007). Trends in psychotropic medication use among U.S. adults. *Pharmacoepidemiology and Drug Safety, 16*(5), 560–570.

Radley, D. C., Finkelstein, S. N., & Stafford, R. S. (2006). Off-label prescribing among office-based physicians. *Archives of Internal Medicine, 166*(9), 1021–1026.

Reekie, W. D. (1978). Price and quality competition in the United States drug industry. *Journal of Industrial Economics, 26*(3), 223–237.

Rosenheck, R. A., Leslie, D. L., Sindelar, J., Miller, E. A., Lin, H., Stroup, T. S., et al. (2006). Cost-effectiveness of second-generation antipsychotics and perphenazine in a randomized trial of treatment for chronic schizophrenia. *American Journal of Psychiatry, 163*(12), 2080–2089.

Ryan, M., Yule, B., Bond, C., & Taylor, R. J. (1996). Do physicians' perceptions of drug costs influence their prescribing? *Pharmacoeconomics, 9*(4), 321–331.

Safavi, K. T., & Hayward, R. A. (1992). Choosing between apples and apples: Physicians' choices of prescription drugs that have similar side effects and efficacies. *Journal of General Internal Medicine, 7*, 32–37.

Scherer, F. M. (2000). The pharmaceutical industry. In A. J. Culyer & J. P. Newhouse (Eds.), *Handbook of Health Economics* (vol. 1B, pp. 1298–1336). Amsterdam: Elsevier.

Sclar, D. A., Robison, L. M., Skaer, T. L., Legg, R. F., Nemec, N. L., Galin, R. S., et al. (1994). Antidepressant pharmacotherapy: Economic outcomes in a health maintenance organization. *Clinical therapeutics, 16*(4), 715–730.

Semla, T. P., Palla, K., Poddig, B., & Brauner, D. J. (1994). Effect of the Omnibus Reconciliation Act of 1987 on antipsychotic prescribing in nursing home residents. *Journal of the American Geriatric Society, 42*, 648–652.

Shah, N. R., Hirsch, A. G., Zacker, C., Taylor, S., Wood, G. C., & Steward, W. F. (2009). Factors associated with first-fill adherence rates for diabetic medications: A cohort study. *Journal of General Internal Medicine, 24*(2), 233–237.

Shulman, N. B. (1991). Economic issues relating to access to medications. *Cardiovascular Clinics, 21*, 75–82.

Sommers, J. P. (2008). Prescription drug expenditures in the 10 largest states for persons under age 65, 2005. *Medical Expenditure Panel Survey STATISTICAL BRIEF.* Available online at http://meps.ahrq.gov/mepsweb/data_files/publications/st196/stat196.pdf. Accessed July 10, 2009.

Soumerai, S. B. (2004). Benefits and risks of increasing restrictions on access to costly drugs in Medicaid. *Health Affairs, 23*(1), 135–146.

Soumerai, S. B., McLaughlin, T. J., & Avorn, J. (1989). Improving prescribing in primary care: A critical analysis of the experimental literature. *Milbank Quarterly, 67*(2), 268–317.

Soumerai, S. B., McLaughlin, T. J., Ross-Degnan, D., Casteris, C. S., & Bollini, P. (1994). Effects of limiting Medicaid drug-reimbursement benefits on the use of psychotropic agents and acute mental health services by patients with schizophrenia. *New England Journal of Medicine, 331*(10), 650.

Soumerai, S. B., Zhang, F., Ross-Degnan, D., Ball, D. E., LeCates, R. F., Law, M. R., et al. (2008). Use of atypical antipsychotic drugs for schizophrenia in Maine Medicaid following a policy change. *Health Affairs, 27*(3), 185–195.

Stern, S. (1995, November). *Product Demand in Pharmaceutical Markets.* Presented at the Department of Economics, University of Illinois Urbana-Champaign.

U.S. Public Health Service. *Mental Health: A Report of the Surgeon General.* (1999). Rockville, MD: U.S. Department of Health and Human Services, Substance Abuse and Mental Health Services Administration, Center for Mental Health Services, National Institutes of Health, National Institute of Mental Health.

Wang, P. S., Schneeweiss, S., Avorn, J., Fischer, M. A., Mogun, H., Solomon, D. H., et al. (2005). Risk of death in elderly users of conventional vs. atypical antipsychotic medications. *New England Journal of Medicine, 353*(22), 2335.

Wilde, M. I., & Whittington, R. (1995). Paroxetine: A pharmacoeconomic evaluation of its use in depression. *Pharmacoeconomics, 8*(1), 62–81.

Wilson, I. B., Schoen, C., Neuman, P., Strollo, M. K., Rogers, W. H., Hong Chang, H., et al. (2007). Physician–patient communication about prescription medication nonadherence: A 50-state study of America's seniors. *Journal of General Internal Medicine, 22*(1), 6–12.

Zeber, J. E., Grazier, K. L., Valenstein, M., Blow, F. C., & Lantz, P. M. (2007). Effect of a medication copayment increase in veterans with schizophrenia. *American Journal of Managed Care*, *13*(6, Pt. 2), 335–346.

Zuvekas, S. (2005). Prescription drugs and the changing patterns of treatment for mental disorders, 1996–2001. *Health Affairs*, *24*(1), 195–205.

Chapter 22

THE COMPLEXITY OF MENTAL HEALTH SERVICES RESEARCH DATA

Ardis Hanson, MLS; and Bruce Lubotsky Levin, DrPH, MPH

Introduction

Mental health services research is a multidisciplinary area of study that evolved during the 1980s. Those who participate in mental health services research examine the organization, financing, and delivery of mental health services and its implications for cost, quality, access, and outcomes (Scallet & Robinson, 1993). While the broad field of mental health services research has continued to rapidly evolve over the past 30 years through research, services, and training, there has been an accompanying exponential growth in the amount and type of data as well as research generated from numerous public and private sources.

This chapter will examine the complexity of data that are being generated by a multitude of individuals and organizations within the various areas of mental health and substance abuse services research. It will also examine the role of technology in the complexity of services research and in accessing research databases. In addition, this chapter will identify some of the major databases in mental health services research and illustrate the complexity of collecting, organizing, and accessing information from a vast array of data collection sources.

The Role of Technology

The complexity of services, research data, and research sources in mental health delivery systems has contributed to the development of mental health informatics. This section will explore the enormity of mental health delivery systems in the United States, its stakeholders, and the many technologies required to manage information within these systems.

The de facto mental health system (Regier et al., 1993) in America is character-ized as having distinct sectors, organizational settings, financing streams, and differ-ences in the type and duration of care. It is comprised of public sector services, private sector services, and increasingly hybridized services crossing over both pub-lic and private sectors. The existing delivery systems provide acute and long-term care in homes, communities, and institutional settings. In addition, these systems provide services across the specialty mental health sector, the general primary care sector, the voluntary care sector, and various other sectors including the military, the Veterans Administration (VA), long-term care facilities, and in jails and prisons.

Furthermore, there are multiple stakeholders involved in these systems, from providers to clients. There are numerous federal and state agencies, professional licensing and accreditation organizations, managed care provider organizations, advocacy and regulatory agencies, and health care policymaking entities involved with impacting policy and services delivery. Stakeholders also include service users of all ages, their families, and their caregivers (including family members, advo-cates, guardians *ad litem*, and ombudsmen). Providers include clinicians such as psychologists, psychiatrists, psychiatric nurses, and primary care providers, phar-macists, supportive services personnel, the clergy, vocational and rehabilitation staff, administrative and clerical staff, among many others in the prevention, inter-vention, and treatment of individuals with mental disorders. The number and variety of interested stakeholders, in turn, contribute to the complexity of collect-ing, maintaining, and accessing data in mental health and substance abuse service delivery systems.

Collecting data and using technology to develop information systems in mental health service systems are not new initiatives. Rosen and Weil (1997) described the use of electronic office management and psychological assessment software in clinical practice. Sujansky (1998) wrote of the need for decision-support tools embedded in the electronic health record to make it more than just a paper analog. Sujansky (1998) also viewed bibliographic retrieval systems, such as PubMed, as facilitating clinical decision-making. Today, informatics hardware and software handles in-house administrative tasks, such as billing and scheduling, as well as many functions within the managed care environment, such as certifica-tions, authorizations, treatment plans, medication evaluation forms, treatment summary forms, and outcome assessments. However, a closer inspection of the technologies used in mental health should include "soft" technology strategies, such as evidence-based practice.

Some of the mental health services quality problems are attributed to the long-standing delays in the application of services research to clinical practice, which often takes between 15 to 20 years for actual implementation (President's New Freedom Commission, 2003). Further, the rapid change in behavioral health technology over the past decade has brought even more volatility to research and practice settings. For example, not only are "soft" behavioral health service tech-nologies particularly vulnerable to problems of fidelity in implementation (Aarons, 2005), there also are significant challenges to implementing and sustaining compre-hensive mental health service programs at consumer, provider, program adminis-trator, and developer levels (Gotham, 2004; Chambers, Ringeisen, & Hickman, 2005; Gold, Glynn, & Mueser, 2006). These challenges include transportability issues surrounding innovations (such as treatment effectiveness and treatment context), standardization of terminology to reduce ambiguity, and building an improved health information and practice infrastructure. Thus, today's multiple systems for the delivery of mental health and substance abuse services represent an increasingly diversified, interrelated, and complex information framework where data are collected, information is synthesized, and treatment, law, and policy decisions are made based upon the available data.

Federal, State, and Academic Data

Lumpkin (2003) suggested that the terms *data, information,* and *knowledge* have been misused in the information sciences and public health fields. While *data* are measurements of personal characteristics that are the primary focus of an information system, *information* is data placed within a specific context after analysis. Lumpkin (2003) concludes that "knowledge . . . is the application of information by the use of [specific] rules" (p. 18).

Data are gathered in many formats. They can be textual, visual, spatial, and numeric as well as primary or secondary data. Federal agencies collect data in numeric form. Through analysis, numeric data become statistical data. Applied researchers use statistical data to write papers that describe, evaluate, or substantiate programs, interventions, and outcomes. Directory information is also data, namely, who treats what and where. Spatial data, used in epidemiologic research as well as in community assessments, provide data to researchers to analyze the best site to place a new treatment center. Hence, it is important to remember that, when looking at data in mental health services research, data come in a variety of forms.

Through evolving methods of data collection and data analysis, health information systems have gradually emerged in the fields of public health and mental health. For example, the emergence of vital statistics in the early twentieth century included the establishment of birth and death records in the United States. The collection of vital statistics at the local and state levels of government, together with a clearer understanding of the impact of immunization, sanitation, and nutrition upon the health of individuals and communities, led to significant progress in the control of infectious diseases in the United States.

According to O'Carroll (2002), *The Future of Public Health* (Institute of Medicine, 1988) reframed public health practice into three core functions: 1) the identification or assessment of public health problems; 2) policy development through a realization of the necessary effort and resources to address problems; and 3) assurance that the needed services will be provided. The essential component in each of the three public health core functions is the availability and quality of information, since the objective of using information systems is to improve the quality of health and mental health programs and services. There is a significant need to develop high quality data standards that provide the basis for uniform, comparable, and good quality data for mental health services. However, given the amount and types of data collected by a variety of public and private health and mental health organizations, data are collected and utilized for very different purposes. Thus, information systems remain disparate in their structure and function.

Federal Data

Currently, there are numerous agencies, regulatory bodies, legislative initiatives, and surveillance programs all collecting health and mental health data at the federal level. For example, the Department of Health and Human Services (DHHS) contains 13 organizational units. Each of these units may address some aspect of mental health and substance abuse. These components include 1) the Office of the Secretary; 2) the Administration for Children and Families; 3) the Administration on Aging; 4) the Agency for Healthcare Research and Quality; 5) the Agency for Toxic Substances and Disease; 6) the Centers for Disease Control and Prevention (CDC); 7) the Centers for Medicare and Medicaid Services; 8) the Food and Drug Administration; 9) the Health Resources and Services Administration; 10) the Indian Health Service; 11) the National Institutes of Health (NIH); 12) the Office of Inspector General; and 13) the Substance Abuse and Mental Health Services Administration (SAMHSA). There are also 16 oversight offices in addition to the 13 administrative components. Each agency or office may have any number of interrelated initiatives with other agencies and offices within DHHS as well as initiatives and partnerships with agencies outside of DHHS. For example, within the NIH, there are 27 institutes and centers, including the National Institute of Mental Health (NIMH) as well as 12 oversight offices and divisions. Within SAMHSA, there are three centers: 1) Mental Health Services; 2) Substance Abuse Prevention; and 3) Substance Abuse Treatment. The amount of information each agency and office collects, synthesizes, and disseminates can be overwhelming and somewhat duplicative, as well as targeted to different audiences for different purposes.

As an example, within SAMHSA, the Center for Mental Health Services (CMHS) provides the biennial publication, *Mental Health United States*, the Mental Health Statistics Improvement Program, and numerous mental health technical report series, statistics, directories, and publications. CMHS also has oversight over the National Mental Health Information Center (NMHIC). The NMHIC is now part of the SAMHSA Health Information Network (SHIN), along with the National Clearinghouse for Alcohol and Drug Information (NCADI). The NCADI provides access to a number of databases, including the Substance Abuse and Mental Health Data Archive, the National Survey on Drug Use and Health, the Drug Abuse Warning Network, the National Treatment Improvement Evaluation Study, the Treatment Episode Data Set, the Uniform Facility Data Set, and the Services Research Outcome Study. It also provides access to the Substance Abuse Treatment Facility Locator, the Alcohol and Alcohol Problems Science Database (ETOH), and the Substance Abuse Information Database (SAID). It also links to another DHHS agency, namely, the National Library of Medicine's bibliographic database, PubMed, which links to PubMed Central, a repository of free online research articles in refereed press.

There are other resources in SAMHSA that are not linked to SHIN, including the National Registry of Evidence-Based Programs and Practices, an online registry of independently reviewed mental health and substance abuse interventions that have been deemed evidence-based practice. However, it is important to note that not all national data on mental health and substance abuse are directly linked to SAMHSA or the National Institute on Alcohol Abuse and Alcoholism. For example, the National Center for Health Statistics, which is another primary agency for data on health and mental health, is located within the CDC. Further, if the focus shifted to substance abuse and mental health issues in criminal justice, one would need to examine data within the White House Office of National Drug Control Policy, which maintains the Federal Drug Data Sources datasets on drug abuse, consequences of drug abuse, treatment of individuals who abuse substances, the source and volume of illegal drugs, enforcement, and drug offenders. The Bureau of Justice Statistics within the U.S. Department of Justice maintains data related to mental health, drug abuse, and crime. This is a very simple example of the interrelatedness and extent of federal data housed in numerous federal agencies within and outside of DHHS.

State Data

This same complexity of collecting data also exists at the state level. For example, states collect mental health and substance abuse data in a variety of categories. These categories include the estimated number of adults with serious mental disorders, the estimated number of children and adolescents with serious emotional disturbance, sources of funding for treatment of individuals with mental and substance use disorders, state per capita expenditures, and the number of publicly funded state and county inpatient beds. States compile and report to various federal agencies, including the Center for Mental Health Services. In addition, states provide data to other national associations, workgroups, task forces, and compliance agencies, including the National Association of State Mental Health Program Directors and the National Conference of State Legislatures.

However, states have developed highly decentralized information management, infrastructure, technology, and operations to meet the needs of state agencies independent of one another. Many of these systems lack interoperability and transferability of information across disparate platforms and are comprised of new as well as legacy systems requiring complex conversion activities for data exchange. At a minimum, health and mental health state data are comprised of agency, regulatory, administrative, oversight, and financial datasets required by each state, reported to federal agencies as required for Medicaid, Medicare, and other public entitlement programs.

Academic Data

Academic data have their own level of complexity. First, much of the academic research borrows primary data from federal and state sources, gathers its own data, and merges the groups of data together, thereby creating proprietary datasets. Academics publish analyses in academic journals, which may or may not be openly accessible. Projects funded through NIH contracts and grants eventually are published in PubMed Central. However, many health services research projects end up as gray, or fugitive, literature through conference presentations. PowerPoints are often posted on the internet or in annual grant reports, which are not widely disseminated.

Caveats of Mental Health Services Research Data

It is important to keep in mind three types of data: 1) primary data; 2) secondary data; and 3) tertiary data. Primary data are original data (e.g., numeric, spatial, or interview data). Secondary data are analyses run on primary data (e.g., tables, charts, spreadsheets, or coded data). Tertiary data are the reports that take numbers or geography and place them within a specific context within mental health services research. However, mental health services research is complex. Often a research project or research data may address only a very specific portion of a larger issue. There are bits and pieces of data from multiple carriers/vendors across different time frames and in different formats. Further, there are numerous disciplines that work within mental health services research.

For example, data are collected for a variety of federal data-sets and organized into very different information formats (e.g., numeric, spatial, and textual) and contexts (e.g., clinical, statistical, and services delivery). The data are collected based upon specific objectives established for data collection and are based upon the specific plans for the utilization of that data-set. Thus, while there are a significant variety of data-sets in mental health and substance abuse at the federal level, they do not always exist in formats immediately usable for all individuals accessing these databases.

The problems with publicly accessible datasets and predefined tables include the following: 1) the granularity of data one may be seeking is not available through these resources; 2) the combination of variables one is seeking may not be available; and 3) the age of the data may make them unusable in their current context. These three problems plague many of the publicly available federal and state data sources as well as the academic data sources, such as the Interuniversity Consortium for Political and Social Research, which provides access to its collection of downloadable data to other researchers and academicians.

In addition to research dissemination through publications and outreach, the numeric data in federal datasets may be actual datasets or predefined tables of variables. Data also may be repurposed from primary data into secondary data analyses or tertiary data sources, such as reports and white papers. Information on how data are collected or characteristics of state mental health agency data systems for federal systems should always be reviewed to ensure the relevance and accuracy of the data to researchers and practitioners. Reports, such as *Characteristics of State Mental Health Agency Data Systems* (Lutterman, Phelan, Berhane, Shaw, & Rana, 2008), provide information on what researchers and practitioners may or may not find in agency data systems.

Federal and state governments are moving to digital-only data and documents available on the Internet. Public domain data and public sector data are not interchangeable (Abresch, Hanson, & Reehling, 2008). Public domain is a legal status, that is, items in the public domain are copyright-free. Public domain material may be modified, giving the person who did the modification both intellectual property rights and copyrights for the *modification*, not the *original* product. Public sector data, however, are data produced by a public sector body. These data may either be in the public domain or be protected data. Governmental and institutional policies determine access, which potentially vary. Since constitutional, federal, or state law may govern access to public sector information, changes in access to government information, particularly after passage of the Homeland Security Act, potentially affect content and access (Abresch et al., 2008).

There are licensing and distribution issues associated with the use of primary and secondary data-sets, such as data size, format complexity, and potential use restrictions. These restrictions may be due to copyright, access, or license agreements created by either public or private data producers. There are also intellectual property rights, liability issues, distribution methods, and data management practices to address in the acquisition, use, repurposing, and publishing of data and its results. Cho (2005) describes legal risks related to numeric and spatial data and analysis tools, including models, methodologies, and services, based upon the data and tools. Defective data used in decision making may have consequences at a planning or population-based level of policy or practice. Since mental health services research often uses personal data obtained with informed consent, there may be restrictions and authorizations required for its use, with de-identified data used in the final product.

Accessing Mental Health Data

Health services research aims to be inclusive of all relevant information, both in terms of a grounded appreciation of the positive and negative benefits of a specific therapeutic intervention and a statement of the implications for the service. The need for reliable data on clinical- and cost-effectiveness and a range of other contextual information requires practitioners and academics to accommodate "research" as part of everyday practice.

The Research Process

In today's information intensive environments, the research process is often defined in seven steps. The first step is to define and conceptualize the research question. This is critical in determining the languages of the disciplines where the answers may be found. The next step is browsing, where the user examines the literature. Decision making then occurs. The user selects and deselects articles based upon keywords in titles, abstracts, and subject headings, or by recognition of the author(s) names. After selection, retrieval of relevant materials occurs. Items may or may not be immediately available, creating a lag in the next steps of the research process. Once the items are retrieved, distillation occurs. A more thorough examination of the literature ensues as the user reads and digests articles, again selecting and deselecting materials based upon additional and more stringent decision points. The next step, synthesis, helps to identify common themes as well as gaps in information crucial to building a case. Here the process starts again, to frame how the missing information may be described or named and where it may be found. Finally, after the gaps are identified, a research product is accomplished, for example, in the form of a journal article, research report, book, or book chapter.

Hence, a complex process occurs every time a researcher or practitioner formulates a new research question against a backdrop of complex systems of resources that may (or may not) contain the data necessary to answer that specific research question. As practitioners, academicians, or graduate students, the need for data and information that allows us to engage in translational research means that one will be moving across disciplinary silos, across agency boundaries, and through organizational territories. To do so, one must keep aware of current and emergent research in fields that draw from multiple disciplines, such as mental health services research. In an academic setting, one is urged to use proprietary databases, such as PsycInfo, Medline, and the Social Science and Science Citation Indexes. Too often, databases and resources created by federal and state agencies are ignored by research and teaching faculty. However, outside of an academic environment, these resources become nearly impossible to access for practitioners who do not have access to the proprietary, academic databases. From a community mental health perspective, one might examine a few selected open access databases considered pertinent to the study of mental health services research.

Selected Databases Outside of SAMHSA

The National Library of Medicine within NIH provides access to numerous resources on health and mental health services research, including PubMed, Health Services Research Projects in Progress (HSRProj), Health Services and Sciences Research Resources (HSRR), and PubMed Central. PubMed, also known as the academic database Medline, has more than 19 million citations from the fields of medicine, nursing, public health, and the preclinical sciences, indexed by the Medical Subject Headings (MeSH). PubMed Central is a digital archive supported by NIH of biomedical and life science journal literature. Since 2008, all articles published with support by NIH must be archived in PubMed Central for open and free access.

The Healthcare Cost and Utilization Project (HCUP), sponsored by AHRQ, is a national information resource of patient-level health care databases. Created from state agencies, hospital associations, private data organizations, and the federal government, HCUP also provides access to tools and software for decision-making, a searchable publications database of the published literature (not full-text), as well as numerous reports targeted to specific populations, disorders, and methods. HCUP provides data on incidents involving persons with mental illnesses who were hospitalized in non-psychiatric settings or examined in emergency rooms.

From an epidemiologic perspective, sources such as the *Mortality and Morbidity Weekly Report* (*MMWR*) and the Web-Based Injury Statistics Query and Reporting System (WISQARS™) provide more current statistics and offer customized injury-related mortality data and nonfatal injury data, respectively. The *MMWR's* five series, *Weekly Report, Recommendations and Reports, Surveillance Summaries, Supplements,* and *Notifiable Diseases,* contain state and territorial health department data as well as reports on infectious and chronic diseases, environmental hazards, disasters, occupational diseases and injuries, and intentional and unintentional injuries. The *MMWR Recommendations and Reports* addresses policy statements on prevention and treatment. *Surveillance Summaries* provides detailed interpretation of surveillance trends and patterns. *Supplements* provide overviews of special topics, such as the importance of behavioral and social sciences in public health. *Notifiable Diseases* is an annual report, providing information on numbers of persons affected by specific diseases, such as HIV/AIDS.

WISQARS™ (Web-based Injury Statistics Query and Reporting System) is an interactive database system that provides customized reports of injury-related (morbidity and mortality) data. In addition to injury reports and leading causes of death reports on WISQARS™, Years of Potential Life Lost and the National Violent Death Reporting System provide information on suicide, self-injurious behaviors, and homicide.

Prevalence data play a major role in policy and funding decisions. The Behavioral Risk Factor Surveillance System (BFRSS) has been tracking health conditions and risk behaviors since 1984, such as binge drinking and overall alcohol consumption. The CDC also adds specific modules attuned to gathering relevant information on specific outbreaks, such as the H1N1 flu outbreak. All of the surveys are available, including optional modules for each state. Within the BRFSS, there are additional tools to run logistic and regression analyses. Users are also able to generate maps of metropolitan and micropolitan statistical areas for analysis or to inform policy decisions.

Another survey of interest is the National Health Interview Survey (NHIS), which provides early release data on serious psychological distress. Since 1998, the Healthy People program has used NHIS data to track progress toward the 71 objectives and 111 measures of Healthy People 2010. One example is objective 06-08, Disability and secondary conditions, which tracks employment parity for persons with disabilities. In concert with the NHIS data, there is the State and Local Area Integrated Telephone Survey, which supplements current national data collection strategies by providing in-depth state and local area data. In 2007, SLAITS performed the Survey of Adult Transition and Health (SATH) as children aged out of the children's mental health system and into the adult mental health system. Survey instruments and datasets are available on the site.

Evidence-based practice and clinical guidelines are essential in practice and in research. SAMHSA's National Registry of Evidence-Based Programs and Practices (NREPP) is a searchable database of interventions for the prevention and treatment of mental and substance use disorders. Although it is relatively small (approximately 150 measures), NREPP accepts submissions for review.

AHRQ's National Guideline Clearinghouse has merged with the National Quality Measures Clearinghouse to tie evidence-based clinical practice guidelines and related documents with associated measures for diseases and mental disorders. For example, there are 183 measures in the Behavioral Disciplines and Activities class. By selecting specific measures, users can generate a comparison table of chosen measures.

Another source is the Child and Adolescent Mental Health Survey Measures Catalog of the NCHS. This catalog provides an overview of the measures of child and adolescent mental health and mental health service use in the NCHS data systems. In addition to disorders, one may also search for service use or needs. In a quick search of unmet needs for mental health care, three measure summaries appeared in a comparison chart: 1) the National Survey of Children with Special Health Care Needs; 2) the National Survey of Early Childhood Health; and 3) the National Survey of Children's Health. A survey description was also available as well as a link to survey questionnaires, data files, documentation, and other information. Many of the survey measures are available online with a public release data file.

Systematic reviews are essential guides to evidence-based practice. A systematic review (SR) is a more rigorous literature review since it tries to reduce bias by identifying, appraising, selecting, and synthesizing *all* quality research evidence relevant for that question. Each SR follows a peer-reviewed protocol based upon the Cochrane Collaboration protocol for systematic reviews. For a review of clinical studies, the rigor of a systematic review addresses method of analysis and reasons for excluding or including studies.

There are two locations for open access to systematic reviews: 1) the Cochrane Collaboration; and 2) PubMed. The Cochrane Collaboration provides free access to the abstracts of its reviews. Abstracts have both the clinical review and a plain language review. Access information to the full text is provided. Unlike the Cochrane Collaboration, PubMed's *Systematic Reviews* is full text. Within PubMed is its own Systematic Reviews search option. This search option allows users to find a variety of resources, including systematic reviews, meta-analyses, and clinical trials reviews. Evidence-based practice, consensus development conferences, and guidelines are also available. The Systematic Reviews option is in the advanced search feature under the selection Subsets. One example retrieved using the Systematic Reviews option was "Improving the Quality of Mental Health Care," which describes the work of 100 experts from 46 countries in an analysis of international best practices in mental health.

For those individuals who are interested in a more global approach to mental health services research, the World Health Organization has two foci: 1) mental disorders; and 2) mental health. Mental disorders focuses on assessment and diagnosis, treatment, and disorder management. Mental health addresses activities directly or indirectly related to mental well-being as defined by the WHO, such as promotion, prevention, services delivery, and rehabilitation. The WHO's Communicable Disease Global Atlas will provide a single point-of-access for data, reports, and documents on the major diseases of poverty. Its Global Information System on Alcohol and Health provides global epidemiologic surveillance of alcohol use, alcohol-related problems, and alcohol policies. The WHO Statistical Information System provides national statistics on 70-plus core indicators on mortality, morbidity, risk factors, service coverage, and health systems. It also provides the Global Burden of Disease analysis as well as the National Burden of Disease toolkit that estimates mortality and burden of disease for WHO Member States. Health metrics and service availability mapping tools are available from the WHO site as well. Two important classification schemas available from the WHO for health services research include 1) the International Classification of Diseases; and 2) the International Classification of Functioning, Disability, and Health.

Implications for Mental Health

In this chapter, the authors have illustrated the complexity of information in mental health and substance abuse practice and research. There are multiple players, for example, agencies, and departments at federal, national, regional, state, and local levels, who collect data and create information designed to answer specific questions or fulfill reporting requirements. These numerous data and information systems have created an increasingly intricate and often arcane system of health information. As these discrete information systems become part of the emerging health information infrastructure, they are both helped and hampered by the growing and insistent demand for technology to solve the problems of access and barriers. Technology expectations are changing consumer preferences and disrupting traditional health communication methods, particularly as health services research and practice continue to move toward global concerns.

Federal standards, initiatives, and architecture try to make sense of these concerns and issues. The Federal Health Architecture and the Office of the National Coordinator for Health Information Technology are critical to the development and implementation of the Nationwide Health Information Network (NHIN) infrastructure as outlined in the American Recovery and Reinvestment Act. Its focus is to ensure that federal agencies can seamlessly exchange health data between and among themselves; with state, local, and tribal governments; and with private sector health care organizations. To do so, infrastructure efforts address standards harmonization; certification; nationwide network, privacy, and security issues; and health IT adoption.

However, national data on mental health and substance abuse services are incomplete at best. In addition to the suggestions offered in Chapter 16 in this volume, a single data resource shared by numerous federal and state agencies of high-quality data on diagnosis, health risk behaviors, comorbidity, health services use, quality of care, specific care received, medications, after care, and supportive services would simplify findings. This would also utilize current, accurate, and specific mental health services research data. Data on specialty care and primary care organizations, staffing patterns, referral patterns, evaluation, and outcomes would support ongoing research on the interrelationship of services delivery, services structure, and services utilization. Such data would augment the field's understanding of emergent organizational structures and systems of care.

Therefore, the authors suggest that it is time for a national health services research infrastructure that integrates the gargantuan amount of information collected and disseminated by federal agencies, state agencies, and academics to be available for practice and research.

References

Aarons, G. A. (2005). Measuring provider attitudes toward evidence-based practice: Consideration of organizational context and individual differences. *Child and Adolescent Psychiatric Clinics of North America, 14*(2), 255–271.

Abresch, J., Hanson, A., & Reehling, P. (2008). Collection management issues with geospatial information. In J. Abresch, A. Hanson, S. J. Heron, & P. Reehling, *Integrating Geographic Information Systems into Library Services* (pp. 202–238). Hershey, PA: Information Science Publishing.

Chambers, D. A., Ringeisen, H., & Hickman, E. H. (2005). Federal, state, and foundation initiatives around evidence-based practices for child and adolescent mental health. *Child and Adolescent Psychiatric Clinics of North America, 14*, 307–327.

Cho, G. (2005). *Geographic Information Science: Mastering the Legal Issues*. Hoboken, NJ: John Wiley & Sons.

Gold, P. B., Glynn, S. M., & Mueser, K. T. (2006). Challenges to implementing and sustaining comprehensive mental health service programs. *Evaluation & the Health Professions*, 29(2), 195–218.

Gotham, H. J. (2004). Diffusion of mental health and substance abuse treatments: Development, dissemination, and implementation. *Clinical Psychology: Science and Practice*, 11(2), 161–176.

Institute of Medicine. (1988). *The Future of Public Health*. Washington, DC: National Academy Press.

Lumpkin, J. R. (2003). History and significance of information systems and public health. In P. W. O'Carroll, W. A. Yasnoff, M. E. Ward, L. H. Ripp, & E. L. Martin (Eds.), *Public Health Informatics and Information Systems* (pp. 16–38). New York: Springer.

Lutterman, T., Phelan, B., Berhane, A., Shaw, R., & Rana, V. (2008). *Characteristics of State Mental Health Agency Data Systems*. DHHS Pub. No. (SMA) 08-4361. Rockville, MD: Center for Mental Health Services, Substance Abuse and Mental Health Services Administration.

O'Carroll, P. W. (2002). Introduction to public health informatics. In P. W. O'Carroll, W. A. Yasnoff, M. E. Ward, L. H. Ripp, & E. L. Martin (Eds.), *Public Health Informatics and Information Systems* (pp. 3–15). New York: Springer.

President's New Freedom Commission. (2003). *Achieving the Promise: Transforming Mental Health Care in America; Final Report*. DHHS Pub. No. SMA 03-3832. Rockville, MD: Author.

Regier, D. A., Narrow, W. E., Rae, D. S., Manderscheid, R. W., Locke, B. Z., & Goodwin, F. K. (1993). The de facto US mental and addictive disorders service system: Epidemiologic catchment area prospective 1-year prevalence rates of disorders and services. *Archives of General Psychiatry*, 50(2), 85–94.

Rosen, L. D., & Weil, M. M. (1997). *The Mental Health Technology Bible*. New York: John Wiley & Sons.

Scallet, L. J., & Robinson, G. K. (1993). Opportunities in mental health services research. *Health Affairs*, 12(3), 240–250.

Sujansky, W. V. (1998). The benefits and challenges of an electronic medical record: Much more than a "word-processed" patient chart. *Western Journal of Medicine*, 169(3), 176–183.

Chapter 23

EVALUATING MENTAL HEALTH SYSTEMS AND SYSTEMS CHANGE

H. Stephen Leff, PhD; and Crystal R. Blyler, PhD

Introduction

From a public health perspective, achieving positive mental health outcomes requires continuously evaluating and improving mental health systems so that effective services can be implemented and sustained and ineffective ones avoided or discarded. In this process, formative evaluations of systems are important for clarifying means and ends and for tracking implementation, while summative evaluations are critical to discovering attributes of systems that contribute to desired outcomes. There are many excellent sources detailing the principles that should be considered in evaluating individual mental health services and programs. These principles, with some tailoring, can be applied to evaluating mental health systems. This chapter does not attempt to recapitulate what is better addressed in these sources. It does address the tailoring. Readers are encouraged to consult the sources cited for detailed discussions of the principles.

What Is a Mental Health System?

Mental health systems are composed of individuals with mental health problems; relatives and friends of these individuals; organizations and providers delivering mental health and related services to solve or ameliorate the problems; the services themselves; policymakers and administrators who plan, regulate, manage, and evaluate these components; and payers who in various ways finance the services. Systems broadly conceived can be dauntingly complex, as illustrated by Figure 23.1 (taken from O'Leary & Meyers, 2008).

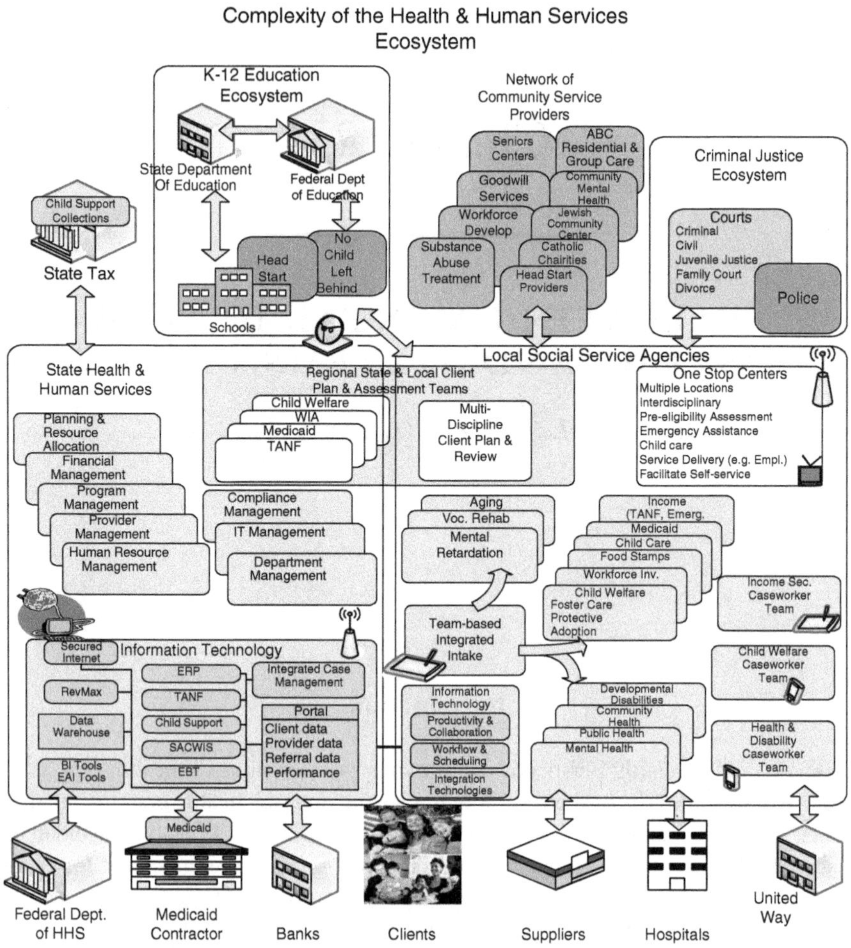

Figure 23.1 Complexity of Mental Health and Related Systems. (Reprinted with permission of O'Leary and Meyers [2008].)

Evaluating Mental Health Systems

Evaluations of mental health systems can describe existing systems to explicate system functioning or discover areas for system improvement. Evaluations of this type are not the focus of this chapter. Instead, this chapter focuses on mental health system evaluations to compare the impacts of different types of systems on outcomes or evaluate the effects on outcomes of systems change interventions designed to improve systems. In these cases, the scientific requirements for evaluating the impacts of mental health systems on outcomes are similar to, but not identical to, those for evaluating individual services or practices.

Consumer-Driven Evaluation

The New Freedom Commission on Mental Health (2003) stated emphatically that "Consumers of mental health services must stand at the center of the system of care. Consumers' needs must drive the care and services that are provided" (New Freedom Commission on Mental Health [NFCMH], 2003, p. 27). The Commission envisioned a transformed mental health system in which "consumers . . . actively participate in designing and developing the systems of care in which they are involved" (NFCMH, 2003, p. 8). This vision explicitly included the involvement of consumers and families in evaluation, as the Commission stated that "Local, State, and Federal authorities must encourage consumers and families to participate in planning and evaluating treatment and support services" (NFCMH, 2003, p. 37). Before embarking on designing any mental health system evaluation, therefore, evaluators should recruit and hire mental health service users to serve as partners in all phases of designing and conducting the evaluation, as well as analyzing, interpreting, and presenting the evaluation results.

Del Vecchio and Blyler (2009) provided detailed examples of how priorities for study, outcomes of interest, and evaluation methodology are substantially altered when consumers are involved in designing and directing research efforts. As recognized by the New Freedom Commission on Mental Health (2003),

> In the past decade, mental health consumers have become involved in planning and evaluating the quality of mental health care and in conducting sophisticated research to affect system reform. Consumers have created and operated satisfaction assessment teams, used concept-mapping technologies, and carried out research on self-help, recovery, and empowerment. (p. 37)

Wallcraft, Schrank, and Amering's *Handbook of Service User Involvement in Mental Health Research* (2009) provides ample guidance on the value to be gained by including consumers in leadership roles from the inception of mental health systems evaluations.

Theory-Driven Evaluation

Evaluations, generally, and mental health services evaluations specifically, are thought to provide higher quality information if they are "driven" by a priori theory (Chen & Rossi, 1983). Such evaluations avoid capitalizing on chance and test constellations of hypotheses that allow for interpreting patterns of results or pattern matching for construct validity (Trochim, 1985). Below, the authors present a theory of mental health systems to guide mental health systems evaluations. This theory is intended to specify the elements that must be detailed to evaluate the impacts of systems on outcomes (Hargreaves, 1986).

A logic model for the proposed mental health systems theory is presented in Figure 23.2. Logic models help to clarify theories by graphically depicting them

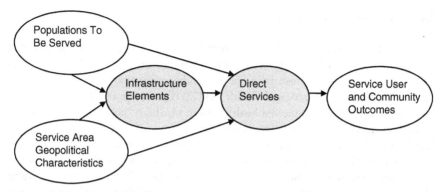

Figure 23.2 Mental Health Systems Theory Logic Model: Mental Health System Elements Shown in Gray.

and are recommended for both services and systems evaluations (Hernandez, 2000; Millar, Simeone, & Carnevale, 2001).

As the logic model in Figure 23.2 shows, the authors' theory considers mental health systems to consist of infrastructure elements and direct services (Dennis, Steadman, & Cocozza, 2000; Donabedian, 1988). Effective services solve or ameliorate mental health problems. Infrastructure elements influence whether the services available in a community are responsive to service user preferences;[1] accessible; high in quality; coordinated; delivered in a cost-efficient manner; and ultimately affordable and sustainable.[2] This view of systems is similar to Donabedian's (1988), which posits that health system quality is a function of structure, process, and outcomes (Isett et al., 2007; Lambert & McGuire, 1990; Magnabosco Bower, 2001; Magnabosco, 2006). Evaluations qualify as systems evaluations if they analyze the roles of both infrastructure elements and direct services in affecting service recipient and community outcomes.

In addition, as this logic model shows, the authors hypothesize that direct service delivery is influenced by infrastructure elements. System evaluations should analyze not only the impacts of infrastructure elements and direct services on outcomes, but also the impacts of infrastructure elements on direct service delivery.

Finally, the logic model in Figure 23.2 also shows that the authors hypothesize that infrastructure elements and direct services are influenced by characteristics of

---

[1] Service users are also referred to as consumers, patients, and service recipients. The authors will use the term *service users* in the interest of clarity, recognizing that many persons who have used mental health services prefer to be called consumers. The authors will not use the terms *patients* or *service recipients* because of the connotations of passivity consumers and advocates do not find acceptable (Campbell-Orde et al., 2005).

[2] Research suggests that services can achieve positive outcomes, at least in limited sites for limited periods of time, even in the context of systems that are not effective. However, studies of mental health systems discussed in this chapter (e.g., Bickman et al., 1995; Goldman et al., 2002) suggest that the reverse is not true: systems with characteristics thought to be effective may not be associated with positive outcomes when the systems provide ineffective services.

populations to be served and service area geopolitical characteristics (Rosenheck et al., 2001). By geopolitical factors the authors mean geographic, political, socio-economic, and cultural aspects of system environments. Evaluations should consider population and service area characteristics in explaining why systems perform as they do and control for these characteristics when comparing systems. Below, the authors describe in detail the elements of this theory in the order in which they are presented in the logic model.

Populations to Be Served

In the logic model, populations to be served are those individuals who public policies or contractual arrangements require mental health systems to serve. Systems evaluations should measure salient baseline characteristics of persons that influence their service needs and their outcomes. These characteristics should include clinical and socio-demographic variables as well as measures of global functioning and baseline recovery status (see discussion of recovery and resiliency below). Clinical variables should include measures such as diagnoses and symptom status. Socio-demographic variables should include measures related to the constituencies and policies mental health systems should address such as age, gender, race, ethnicity, and indicators of socioeconomic status.

Geopolitical Characteristics

Depending upon geopolitical context, the same types of mental health systems may perform differently, or different types of systems may perform similarly (Isett et al., 2007; Lambert & McGuire, 1990; Magnabosco Bower, 2001; Magnabosco, 2006; Raghavan, Bright, & Shadoin, 2008; Rosenheck et al., 2001). In evaluating different types of mental health systems, geopolitical characteristics, therefore, should be considered in explaining system performance, and in system comparisons they should be controlled.

Geopolitical characteristics include characteristics such as continuity of personnel in key political positions; trends in state fiscal conditions; type(s) of environment served (e.g., urban, suburban, rural, frontier); baseline commitment to mental health and human services (e.g., budgeted amounts); performance characteristics of relevant governmental units (state, county, local); political stability; and dominant political orientation.

Infrastructure Elements

Infrastructure elements of mental health systems, as referred to in the logic model, include governmental and non-governmental structures and processes that support or influence the nature of direct service delivery. Provider organizations, governmental funding agencies, and regulatory agencies are a few of the types of bodies that establish or constitute aspects of the infrastructure (Raghavan et al., 2008).

Although recent evaluations have found that infrastructure measures by themselves are not strong predictors of outcomes, evaluators continue to believe that combined with direct service variables, they do impact outcomes and are important to study (Isett et al., 2007; Lambert & McGuire, 1990; Meyer & Massagli, 2001; Sinaiko & McGuire, 2006).

More specific infrastructure elements and illustrative studies or useful discussions of these elements are listed below:

- Value orientations as expressed in plans, policies, and similar materials (Isett et al., 2007; Lambert & McGuire, 1990; Sinaiko & McGuire, 2006);
- Amounts and types of resources available (Bruns, Suter, & Leverentz-Brady, 2006; Frank & Glied, 2006);
- Organizational structures and levels (Bickman, Lambert, Andrade, & Penaloza, 2000; Isett et al., 2008; Magnabosco, 2006);
- Governance structures that determine communication, participation, and decision-making among stakeholders and between organizational levels (Frank & Glied, 2006; Hargreaves, 1992);
- Technologies for system administration including information technology and project management tools (Lagoe & Westert, 2006);
- Quality assurance mechanisms including ones for regulating, monitoring, and evaluating services and assuring the training of providers either directly through offering training or indirectly through licensing and certification (Hermann, 2005; Hermann, Leff, & Lagodmos, 2002; Meyer & Massagli, 2001; Stetler et al., 2006);
- Inter-organizational arrangements (Morrissey et al., 2002; Rosenheck et al., 1998; Rosenheck et al., 2001); and
- Leadership qualities (Corrigan, Lickey, Campion, & Rashid, 2000; Hargreaves, 1998; Isett et al., 2008).

The authors postulate that systems can be categorized or profiled in terms of their direct service delivery characteristics and these infrastructure elements. Evaluations should compare the effectiveness of systems that differ in or change direct service delivery and/or infrastructure elements, in order to produce evidence about effective system models and improvements. Eventually this evidence should be used to produce fidelity measures for assessing the extent to which systems have effective infrastructure elements and services.

Direct Services

By direct services in the logic model, the authors refer to interventions of any type delivered to individuals. Services may be delivered once or over time as a process of care. Persons with severe mental illness typically use service packages consisting of multiple services delivered over time. Hence, systems evaluations should investigate the effects of service packages delivered over time. These evaluations should investigate the effects of types and amounts of services used and the manner in which services are delivered (Hermann et al., 2002). The manner of service delivery refers to the attitudes and expectations caregivers communicate to service users (Donabedian, 1988; Leff, Mulkern, Lieberman, & Raab, 1994). The consumer movement in mental health has advocated assessing the recovery orientation of services as a process measure. Recovery is discussed further below. In addition to examining the effects of direct services on individuals, mental health systems evaluations should investigate the effects of infrastructure elements on types and amounts of services utilized, service quality, service coordination, and service cost-efficiency (Leff et al., 1994; Lehman, 1995; Rosenblatt & Woodbridge, 2003).

Service User and Community Outcomes

Direct services delivered to individuals, as indicated in the logic model, can address specific consumer outcomes, such as symptom remission or employment. Community oriented interventions also can target specific community outcomes, such as reduction in stigma (Raghavan et al., 2008). In these cases, outcome measures targeting these practice-specific outcomes should be used in evaluations as primary impact measures, although these evaluations also can address and use measures of more multifaceted outcomes, such as global level of functioning, quality of life, and recovery (discussed below). If collected routinely on populations, practice-specific outcome measures also can be used in systems evaluations. The Substance Abuse and Mental Health Services Administration's (SAMHSA) National Outcome Measures (Center for Mental Health Services [CMHS], 2007) are examples of outcome measures that can be used for both practice-specific and system level evaluations.

In addition, however, multifaceted or global outcome measures are particularly appropriate as primary impact measures for evaluations of systems that incorporate a variety of services addressing diverse outcomes (Bruns, Burchard, Froelich, Yoe, & Tighe, 1998; Hargreaves, 1986; Leff, Lieberman, Mulkern, & Raab, 1996; Moos, Nichol, & Moos, 2002). Such evaluations, for example, may measure outcomes such as global level of functioning or quality of life (Lehman, 1995).

Currently, users of mental health services have stressed the importance of evaluating mental health systems in terms of "recovery" outcomes. Recovery outcomes are complex outcomes reflecting the hope and meaning consumers find in their lives (Campbell-Orde, Chamberlin, Carpenter, & Leff, 2005; CMHS, 2005). Now that numerous instruments developed for measuring these outcomes are available (Campbell-Orde et al., 2005), recovery outcomes should be included in mental health systems evaluations (see Chapter 20 in this volume for additional information on the recovery movement).

When appropriate, mental health system evaluators should also use outcome measures collected periodically on populations by survey efforts that are not focused specifically on persons with mental illness. Examples of such measures are the Centers for Disease Control's Behavioral Risk Factors Surveillance Survey (Centers for Disease Control and Prevention [CDC], 2004), the National Comorbidity Survey (Kessler & Merikangas, 2004), and SAMHSA's National Survey on Drug Use and Health (Jordan, Karg, Batts, Epstein, & Wiesen, 2008; Substance Abuse and Mental Health Services Administration [SAMHSA], 2007). These measures are particularly useful because they provide both population and time series data.

In the future, the Internet almost certainly will be an important vehicle for what the authors have termed "direct to stakeholder" systems evaluation (Best & Krueger, 2002; Bethell, Fiorillo, Lansky, Hendryx, & Knickman, 2004; Bowling et al., 2006; Braithwaite, Emery, De Lusignan, & Sutton, 2003; Couper, 2000, 2007; Duffy, Terhanian, Bremer, & Smith, 2005; Duncan, White, & Nicholson, 2003). Web-based evaluations can reach large populations without burdening providers and risking provider bias in the selection of respondents (Bethell et al., 2004). In addition, research suggests that even hard-to-reach populations can be contacted using such methods (Duncan et al., 2003). Although methodological issues related to the generalizability of samples and validity of data remain to be resolved, methodologists are developing approaches to these problems (Couper, 2007). These include recruiting respondent panels comprised of members with desired characteristics and selecting respondents from non-probability samples based upon sociodemographic characteristics that mirror desired populations.

As examples of the use of the Web to obtain consumer and family perspectives, the National Alliance on Mental Illness conducted a Web-based survey, seeking input on experiences with state mental health systems. "Using a 'snowball sample,' in which mental health system users participated and were then asked to forward the survey to other eligible people, more than 13,000 responses were received in about two months from across the country" (Aron et al., 2009). As an example of another evaluation Web application, the cross-site evaluation for the Mental Health Transformation State Incentive Grant Program has provided a publicly accessible Web site (Transformation Tracker Explorer) featuring a searchable database of grant supported state transformation activities that visitors to the Web site can comment on and rate in terms of transformative potential (http://mhtsigdata.samhsa.gov).

Efficacy versus Effectiveness

Studies that evaluate single mental health services and practices under laboratory-like conditions and control all independent variables except for the ones under study are referred to as efficacy studies. Studies that measure mental health interventions as they are implemented in actual clinical situations are referred to as effectiveness studies. The difficulties inherent in implementing entire mental health systems solely for evaluation purposes and the desire to develop effectiveness interventions for real world application mean that most evaluations of mental health systems will be effectiveness studies of actual mental health systems operating under real world conditions. The scientific methods used in these effectiveness studies should address the same causal issues faced by efficacy studies of individual services or practices, modified for real world constraints (Campbell, 1969; Roy-Byrne et al., 2003; Wells, 1999a, 1999b). These are discussed below.

Evaluation Designs

For classic descriptions of evaluation designs and the threats to causal inference they address, readers are referred to Campbell (1969) and Shadish, Cook, and

Campbell (2002). Below, the authors discuss the application of these analyses to mental health systems evaluations in particular.

As noted above, some mental health systems evaluations will be descriptive ones, conducted to explicate the functioning of a single mental health system or to discover areas for system improvement. For evaluations of this type, case study designs are useful. Yin, Bickman, and Rog (1998) and Sechrest, Stewart, Stickle, and Sidani (1996) are good sources of guidance on how to conduct case studies. However, case studies are not the strongest designs for comparing the effectiveness of different types of systems or assessing the effectiveness of interventions for improving systems (Campbell, Stanley, & Gage, 1963; Shadish et al., 2002), which is the authors' focus. Consequently, the authors will not discuss case study methods further, although the authors do discuss the collection and use of qualitative data to complement quantitative methods.

Campbell (1969) suggests three evaluation designs that are particularly suited for mental health systems evaluations: 1) randomized control group experimental designs; 2) time series designs; and 3) control series designs.

Randomized control group experimental designs require random assignment of persons to different conditions. Some geographic areas may be served by several health and/or mental health systems (e.g., public and private systems) or sub-systems of larger systems (e.g. different community mental health centers). In such areas, random assignment of persons in need to different types of systems or to systems receiving vs. not receiving systems improvement interventions is the preferred evaluation design. When a specific systems improvement intervention is being tested, random assignment of comparable systems to receive or not receive the intervention is also a strong design for evaluating the intervention (Wells, 1999a).

However, in many geographic areas, there is only one mental health system that individuals desire to evaluate, comparison systems must be found outside the service area, and random assignment of individuals to conditions is impossible. Under these conditions, time series or controlled series designs should be used. Time series data examine system variables over time and provide more observations for comparison. If a system improvement intervention is being implemented, trends before and after the intervention can be compared. Comparing trends provides a much stronger basis for inferring a causal relationship between the intervention and outcomes than differences between single observations before and after a change (Campbell, 1969).

A control series design compares time series data for different groups. Such designs combine the strengths of time series designs and non-equivalent control group designs (Campbell, 1969). Non-equivalent control group designs compare groups (or systems) that are matched or statistically control for group differences (Shadish et al., 2002). Control series designs are the strongest design for most mental health systems evaluations and should be employed whenever possible. Delaney, Seidman, and Willis (1978) provide an example of such a design. They compared trends in quarterly admissions to state hospitals in two subzones in Illinois, one of which implemented a crisis intervention program and one of which did not. Trends were compared for two years before and two years after the program was implemented, using cross-sectional, rather than longitudinal, data; either type of data can be used in control series designs.

Implementation and Fidelity Measurement

The evaluation of individual mental health services has taught the authors that one cannot be certain that service interventions will be implemented as planned and that it is necessary to measure the fidelity of intervention implementation to explain evaluation results. If service interventions are not implemented with fidelity to plans or models, expected outcomes will not occur or will be less positive than expected (Bond, Evans, Salyers, Williams, & Kim, 2000). This is equally true for mental health systems evaluations. Both comparative and system improvement mental health systems evaluations should measure the implementation of infrastructure elements and services so that degree of implementation and fidelity to plans and models can be taken into account in interpreting evaluation results. Bond, Evans, Salyers, Williams, and Kim (2000) provide guidance for developing fidelity measures.

Unlike single services and practices, systems cannot easily be construed as occurring at a point in time. Mental health systems are complex, involving multiple infrastructure and service elements. Even when evaluations focus on just one system characteristic, e.g., integration of two or more types of services or two or more agency efforts, the characteristic is usually comprised of multiple activities. These different activities tend to occur over time so that systems act in different dimensions and incrementally, sometimes over multiple years. One implication of this is that it is useful to categorize systems in terms of stage of implementation. Magnabosco (2006), for example, categorized state level service implementation activities as pre-implementation, initial implementation, and sustainability planning.

Given this, analyses of systems interventions should track implementation trends in different dimensions of activity over time and address the question of when a system intervention is sufficiently implemented to reach a "tipping point" and impact process and consumer outcomes. Tipping points are accretions of smaller changes that result in qualitative or more dramatic changes in entities (Gladwell, 2002). Since the field does not have a substantial body of research on how to predict systems change tipping points, in most cases this should involve observing empirical correlations between trends in types and amounts of activity completion with outcome trends, assuming different lag times between implementation and outcomes (Miles & Huberman, 1994).

Another approach that should be explored is comparing pre-implementation outcomes with outcomes after implementation has stabilized for a specified period of time. In those cases in which sufficient theory and evidence exist to identify tipping points a priori, this should be done.

Qualitative Data Collection

As indicated by the preceding discussion of implementation and fidelity, systems evaluations have described and should describe the various infrastructural and service aspects of systems in detail (Isett et al., 2007; Magnabosco, 2006). There are already instruments that describe and/or rate desired aspects of systems. In 2005, Rivard reviewed seven such measures. Typically, methods for characterizing systems and measuring the implementation of system changes require content analyses of information in policies, plans, reports, brochures, and Web sites; open-ended interviews conducted in-person during site visits or by telephone; and mailed surveys (Isett et al., 2008; Magnabosco Bower, 2001; Randolph et al., 2002). In her study of state level data from the U.S. Evidence-Based Practices Project, for example, Magnabosco (2006) analyzed data from site visit key informant interview notes for individual and group interviews; site visit debriefing meeting notes; and background information collected from documents and Web sites describing state organizations, services, emerging policy issues, consumers served, fiscal resources, consumer issues, information management systems, and the research and evaluation conducted. Two methods frequently used in the analysis of qualitative data are grounded theory (Yin et al., 1998) and concept mapping (Jackson & Trochim, 2002) (although concept mapping, as developed by Trochim, involves quantitative methods). Both methods are useful for translating qualitative data into concepts and variables (Jackson & Trochim, 2002).

Best practices for analyzing qualitative data require that these data be analyzed in a transparent, systematic, and reliable manner (Miles & Huberman, 1994; Sechrest, Stewart et al., 1996). More specifically, it calls for coding data to capture important themes and related variables; demonstrating that coded data meet criteria for reliability; and sorting data by theme, source, organizational level, and other variables. Data sorted in these ways can be used to investigate trends in themes by data source and other variables taken singly and in combination (Isett et al., 2007; Magnabosco, 2006). This is made easier by the development of specialized software for analyzing qualitative data (Lewins & Silver, 2007). Qualitative measures developed with attention to these methodological issues should be combined with quantitative data on service use and service user outcomes to provide explanatory detail and case illustrations for system evaluations. Blasinsky et al. (1998) and Pope, Mays, and Popay (2007) provide guidance for integrating qualitative and quantitative data in project level databases.

System Scale and Complexity and Follow-Up Time Periods

Mental health evaluations of single services and practices can focus on the effectiveness of services in specific locations provided to a limited number of service users after relatively short periods of time. In contrast, evaluations of mental health systems must investigate the effects of systems on multiple services delivered to large numbers of service users in service areas that can be as large as one or several counties or states.

Typical follow-up periods for evaluations of mental health services range between six months and one year with two-year follow-ups considered lengthy. The logic of studying systems suggests that data from more sources over longer periods of time should be collected. This can capture different perspectives, put random fluctuations in context, and, particularly in the case of evaluations of system improvement interventions, give full implementation an opportunity to occur and the impacts of system changes time to emerge.

On the basis of the foregoing, it has been argued that systems improvement evaluations should investigate outcomes for more than the standard two years or less that is typical in studies of individual services and treatments (Behar, 1997). The authors are unaware of a review or synthesis of studies showing typical times for finding such changes. However, several studies of systems' outcomes have focused on 3–5 year outcomes (Bickman et al., 2000; Drake et al., 2006).

If the mental health systems involved in comparative studies are stable, one can assume that characteristics that differentiate the systems are fully distributed throughout the systems and have had time to cause system-wide impacts on process and consumer outcome variables. For this reason, comparative evaluations of stable systems may be cross-sectional in nature or involve shorter follow-up periods than those for system change or improvement evaluations.

Mental health systems change or improvement evaluations need to be carefully timed to focus on where and when outcomes are likely to occur within study time frames. Evaluations with longer time horizons can test for system-wide changes. Studies with shorter time frames, however, may have to focus on specific areas of systems that are likely to change sooner than others; we have labeled such evaluations "proof of concept" studies.

MEASURING OUTCOMES

As noted above, individual mental health services characteristically address a small number of specific outcomes referred to as primary outcomes. Choosing a measure for these outcomes involves finding measures of desired constructs with acceptable psychometric properties. Mental health systems consist of multiple mental health and related services implemented in multiple sites and addressing a variety of outcomes. For this reason, mental health systems evaluations should include multiple individual measures addressing different outcomes; multifaceted measures that include multiple subscales for a variety of outcomes (e.g., quality of life instruments); or global measures that combine multiple dimensions of functioning (e.g., global measures of functioning, measures of recovery) (Drake et al., 2006; Leff et al., 1996). These measures should also have acceptable psychometric properties. If multiple measures are used, statistical analyses should correct for alpha inflation.

COMPARISON SYSTEMS FOR DEMONSTRATING EFFECTIVENESS

When they are initially evaluated, mental health services and practices ideally are studied by comparing them to no service or placebos. Placebos are manipulations designed to provide the impression of a service, but not a full complement of active ingredients (Strayhorn, 1987). This is done under the principle that since services consume resources and might be harmful in some ways, it is important to show that they are "better than nothing" and not "the lesser of two evils" (i.e., doing the least damage compared to no service). Once some service has been established as more effective than no service or placebo, other service options can ethically be compared to that service.

Although it can be argued that some amount of system is present whenever a mental health service is delivered since there is at a minimum a service recipient and a provider, one can conceptualize some amounts of system as so minimal as to be like placebo manipulations. Therefore, more robust mental health systems should be compared with minimal or placebo-like systems in a manner that is similar to how individual services and practices are initially evaluated. As with service and practice evaluations, once some system configuration has been established as more effective than a minimal one, other system options ethically should be compared to it since it has been shown to be "better than nothing" and not "the lesser of two evils."

If mental health systems evaluations focus on differences in or changes to particular infrastructure elements or services, comparison systems should be selected that are similar in other infrastructure elements and services. In addition, recall that the systems theory hypothesizes that mental health systems are influenced by geopolitical factors and populations to be served. These hypotheses are supported by empirical research (Hermann, Rollins, & Chan, 2007; Lambert & McGuire, 1990; Magnabosco Bower, 2001; Rosenheck et al., 2001). Given this, evaluations that compare mental health systems should either select systems that are comparable with respect to populations to be served and salient geopolitical characteristics other than those being investigated or statistically control for differences in these factors.

COST-EFFECTIVENESS AND COST-EFFICIENCY

Like services evaluations, systems evaluations should address not only effectiveness, but also cost-effectiveness and cost-efficiency. Cost-effectiveness refers to the relationship between costs and outcomes and is measured in cost per unit of outcome. Cost-efficiency refers to the relationship between cost-effectiveness for an intervention being evaluated and some standard, usually either a comparison intervention as discussed above, or a value constructed in some fashion for an ideal or particularly efficient intervention (Hargreaves, 1998; Leff et al., 2005; Thomas, 2006).

System evaluations of cost-effectiveness and cost-efficiency differ from those for services in having to consider a wider range of costs and outcomes than service evaluations. Typically, evaluations of individual service and practice cost-effectiveness and cost-efficiency focus on the costs and outcomes associated with giving a particular group of persons a fairly narrow range of specified services. System evaluations should investigate population impacts and system-wide impacts on service costs and quality (Hargreaves, 1998; Sinaiko & McGuire, 2006). For example, cost-effectiveness or cost-efficiency evaluations of the service assertive community treatment (ACT) might focus on the impacts of ACT on the outcomes of ACT service users and on the use and cost of a variety of other mental health services provided to these service users, perhaps even extending to one or a few other services, such as criminal justice system services, provided to ACT service users.

A systems evaluation, in contrast, should focus on the impacts that providing ACT to a subset of service users has on all persons with serious mental illness served by the system and the impacts not just on mental health services provided to the larger population, but on a wide variety of services provided to people served by the system, such as physical health services, criminal justice services, welfare services, and so on (Sinaiko & McGuire, 2006). There are no rules for precisely which services should be included in a systems evaluation; it is true that some mental health service evaluations investigate the impacts of changes in mental health services on non-mental health services (Weisbrod, Test, & Stein, 1980). Nevertheless, mental health systems evaluations should always cast a wide net, whereas individual service and practice evaluations need not and typically do not.

FORMATIVE AND SUMMATIVE EVALUATION

Mental health services and systems evaluations can be summative and formative. Summative evaluations focus on outcomes and are usually produced after an intervention is considered "implemented," at least according to study plans. In addition to outcomes, formative evaluations typically investigate the extent to which interventions are implemented and report findings intended to be helpful in strengthening interventions at designated points during the course of evaluations (Stetler et al., 2006).

Formative mental health systems evaluations should report on infrastructural processes, not just services and they should investigate whether non-mental health services and organizations are performing as planned. Relatedly, formative feedback should be provided not just to mental health system administrators and staff, but also to representatives from non-mental health services and agencies.

ACCOUNTABILITY/QUALITY AND EFFECTIVENESS EVALUATIONS

Evaluations of both mental health services and systems can be accountability and quality oriented. Accountability and quality evaluations focus on whether interventions are implemented according to plans, rules, regulations, or guidelines. Ideally, the plans, rules, regulations, or guidelines are ones proven to promote effectiveness. However, the evidence base for these requirements, particularly in the case of mental health systems, can be limited to expert judgment or the opinions of administrators or public officials. For this reason, mental health systems accountability and quality evaluations should be effectiveness as well as accountability and quality focused, adhering to as many of the requirements for effectiveness studies as possible.

METHODS OF ANALYSIS

Since mental health system outcomes will occur in multiple services and sites it will be necessary to summarize outcomes across services and settings. This task may be made more complex if different services and settings use different outcome measures. One way of dealing with this is to convert outcomes to effect size measures (Leff et al., 2005). Another way is to conduct calibration studies that estimate the relationships among measures so that outcomes on different measures can be adjusted to be comparable (Sechrest, McKnight, & McKnight, 1996). Mental health systems evaluations should be multi-level and measure trends. Since systems should be studied over time, some independent variables and co-variates may be time varying.

Considering this, three statistical approaches should be considered for mental health systems evaluations: 1) hierarchical linear modeling (Bryk & Raudenbush, 1992); 2) random regression (Gibbons et al., 1993); and 3) multiple random effects analyses that analyze data by level of analysis and time period and then synthesize it to test higher order effects (DerSimonian & Laird, 1986). The basic rationales for these approaches are presented in Gibbons et al. (1993).

Implications for Mental Health

This analysis of the requirements for mental health systems evaluations indicates that it is possible to modify existing guidance for evaluating individual services and practices to meet the unique demands of evaluating mental health systems. Hopefully, evaluations of this type eventually will provide the evidentiary base for identifying "evidence-based" mental health system features and system interventions that are particularly effective in causing recovery oriented changes in services and in service user and community outcomes.

Future Challenges

System level evaluations are demanding in terms of expertise and resources. Evaluations of system interventions are more demanding than ones that simply compare existing systems since resources are required for the system interventions as well as the evaluations.

Future progress in system level evaluation will require continued support for such evaluations and system change efforts. In addition, systems level evaluations will require that federal and state governments continue to support the collection of statewide data on services and service user and community outcomes, expanding these efforts to include explicitly recovery oriented information. It is difficult to imagine how the required studies can be conducted without federal and state support. While foundations might support some system evaluations, it is unlikely that their support alone will be sufficient to identify evidence-based mental health system features and interventions.

One area in particular that needs to be developed is system-wide measurement of recovery and/or resilience in individuals and recovery and/or resilience orientation in services. Science is a cumulative activity. Comparing and synthesizing the results of different evaluations are facilitated when the same outcome measures are used or when the interrelationships between measures are known. The field does not as yet have instruments that have been accepted by evaluators and other stakeholders as "gold standard" measures of recovery and resilience. While candidate instruments exist (Campbell-Orde et al., 2005), research is needed to further investigate the psychometric properties and the interrelationships of these measures.

The National Consensus Statement on Mental Health Recovery, produced by the SAMHSA Center for Mental Health Services (2005, and available at http://mental health.samhsa.gov/publications/allpubs/sma05-4129/), can serve as one standard against which measures of recovery can be validated for use in evaluating systems across the United States. However, it should be noted that definitions of recovery and resilience may differ for different groups of service users.

Another challenge is ensuring that the results of system evaluations are optimally used. There have been a number of informative evaluations of mental health systems arrangements and changes addressing topics such as community support systems (Grusky & Tierney, 1989), systems integration (Randolph et al., 2002; Wolff, 2002), managed care (Hargreaves, 1992; Leff et al., 2005), and major systems improvements (Bickman et al., 1995). Among the most noteworthy are the Fort Bragg (Bickman et al., 2000) and ACCESS (Goldman et al., 2002) studies. Nevertheless, reviews of system change efforts suggest that each new cycle fails to fully exploit evaluation information from previous cycles, ignoring lessons learned (Dennis et al., 2000; Goldman & Morrissey, 1985).

The reasons why prior systems evaluations have not been optimally exploited are not fully known. One reason may be that many policymakers and administrators are not aware of the results of past systems evaluations. There has not been a movement to disseminate the evidence on effective system elements or improvements equal to the one for evidence-based practices. An additional reason may be that systems and system improvements are intended to impact goals such as equity and efficiency rather than effectiveness, making effectiveness evaluations less salient to policymakers and administrators (Rosenblatt & Woodbridge, 2003). A different reason may be that stakeholders are reluctant to give up energizing concepts, even after evaluations have failed to support them (Festinger, Riecken, & Schachter, 1964). Another may be that policymakers and administrators do not want to dampen the momentum for change (and the new resources this brings) with discomfiting facts about the cost and limitations of system improvements (Campbell, 1969). Yet another reason may be that policymakers and administrators may feel that they have abilities or access to technologies that will enable them to succeed where others have failed.

Mental health systems change often occurs in the context of optimism about new treatments and practices (Goldman & Morrissey, 1985). While in some cases this may be warranted, cognitive psychology and behavioral economics have identified a predictable "planning fallacy": a "systematic tendency towards unrealistic optimism" (Thaler & Sunstein, 2008).

Additional research is needed on 1) the reasons why systems evaluations may not be optimally used in planning systems improvements and reforms, and 2) methods for increasing the use of evaluations in program planning (see for example, Hermann, 2005; Nadler, 1977; Trochim, Cabrera, Milstein, Gallagher, & Leischow, 2006). In addition, federal, state, and sub-state programs designed to improve systems should reflect evaluation findings and require that proposals, to be funded: 1) show an awareness of previous system evaluations; 2) include evaluation components that follow accepted methods; and 3) promise to increase our understanding of system features and enhancements that advance direct services and consumer and community outcomes.

References

Aron, L., Honberg, R., Duckworth, K., Kimball, A., Edgar, E., Carolla, B., et al. (2009). *Grading the States 2009: Report on America's Health Care System for Adults with Serious Mental Illness.* Arlington, VA: National Alliance on Mental Illness.

Behar, L. B. (1997). Fort Bragg evaluation: A snapshot in time. *American Psychologist, 52*(5), 557–559.

Best, S. J., & Krueger, B. (2002). New approaches to assessing opinion: The prospects for electronic mail surveys. *International Journal of Public Opinion Research, 14*(1), 73–92.

Bethell, C., Fiorillo, J., Lansky, D., Hendryx, M., & Knickman, J. (2004, January 20). Online consumer surveys as a methodology for assessing the quality of the United States Health care system. *Journal of Medical Internet Research, 6*(1), e2.

Bickman, L., Guthrie, P. R., Foster, E. M., Lambert, E. W., Summerfelt, W. T., Breda, C. S., et al. (1995). *Evaluating Managed Mental Health Services: The Fort Bragg Experiment.* New York: Plenum.

Bickman, L., Lambert, E. W., Andrade, A. R., & Penaloza, R. V. (2000). The Fort Bragg continuum of care for children and adolescents: Mental health outcomes over 5 years. *Journal of Consulting and Clinical Psychology, 68*(4), 710–716.

Blasinsky, M., Cohen, B., Goldman, H., Hambrecht, K., Johnsen, M., Landow, W., et al. (1998). *Integrating Process and Outcome Evaluation.* Cambridge, MA: The Evaluation Center@HSRI.

Bond, G. R., Evans, L., Salyers, M. P., Williams, J., & Kim, H. W. (2000). Measurement of fidelity in psychiatric rehabilitation. *Mental Health Services Research, 2*(2), 75–87.

Bowling, J. M., Rimer, B. K., Lyons, E. J., Golin, C. E., Frydman, G., & Ribisl, K. M. (2006). Methodologic challenges of e-health research. *Evaluation and Program Planning, 29*(4), 390–396.

Braithwaite, D., Emery, J., De Lusignan, S., & Sutton, S. (2003). Using the Internet to conduct surveys of health professionals: A valid alternative? *Family Practice, 20*(5), 545–551.

Bruns, E. J., Burchard, J. D., Froelich, P., Yoe, J. T., & Tighe, T. (1998). Tracking behavioral progress within a children's mental health system: The Vermont Community Adjustment Tracking System. *Journal of Emotional and Behavioral Disorders, 6*(1), 19–32.

Bruns, E. J., Suter, J. C., & Leverentz-Brady, K. M. (2006). Relations between program and system variables and fidelity to the wraparound process for children and families. *Psychiatric Services, 57*(11), 1586–1593.

Bryk, A. S., & Raudenbush, S. W. (1992). *Hierarchical Linear Models: Applications and Data Analysis Methods.* Thousand Oaks, CA: Sage.

Campbell, D. T. (1969). Reforms as experiments. *American Psychologist, 24*(4), 409–429.

Campbell, D. T., Stanley, J. C., & Gage, N. L. (1963). *Experimental and Quasi-Experimental Designs for Research.* Boston: Houghton Mifflin.

Campbell-Orde, T., Chamberlin, J., Carpenter, J., & Leff, H. S. (2005). *Measuring the Promise: A Compendium of Recovery Measures* (vol. 2). Cambridge, MA: Evaluation Center@HSRI.

Center for Mental Health Services. (2005). *National Consensus Statement on Mental Health Recovery* [Brochure]. Publication No. SMA05-4129. Rockville, MD: Substance Abuse and Mental Health Services Administration, U.S. Department of Health & Human Services.

Center for Mental Health Services. (2007). *CMHS NOMs: Adult Consumer Outcome Measures for Discretionary Service Programs.* OMB No. 0930-0285. Rockville, MD: Substance Abuse and Mental Health Services Administration.

Centers for Disease Control and Prevention. (2004). *Behavioral Risk Factor Surveillance System: Frequently Asked Questions* [Online]. Available online at http://www.cdc.gov/brfss/faqs.htm. Accessed August 24, 2009.

Chen, H.-T., & Rossi, P. H. (1983). Evaluating with sense: The theory-driven approach. *Evaluation Review, 7*(3), 283–302.

Corrigan, P. W., Lickey, S. E., Campion, J., & Rashid, F. (2000). Mental health team leadership and consumers satisfaction and quality of life. *Psychiatric Services, 51*(6), 781–785.

Couper, M. P. (2000). Web surveys: A review of issues and approaches. *Public Opinion Quarterly, 64*(4), 464–494.

Couper, M. P. (2007). Issues of representation in eHealth research (with a focus on Web surveys). *American Journal of Preventive Medicine, 32*(5), S83–S89.

Delaney, J. A., Seidman, E., & Willis, G. (1978). Crisis intervention and the prevention of institutionalization: An interrupted time series analysis. *American Journal of Community Psychology, 6*(1), 33–45.

del Vecchio, P., & Blyler, C. R. (2009). Topics: Identifying critical outcomes and setting priorities for mental health services research. In J. Wallcraft, B. Schrank, & M. Amering (Eds.), *Handbook of Service User Involvement in Mental Health Research* (ch. 8, pp. 99–112). Hoboken, NJ: Wiley.

Dennis, D. L., Steadman, H. J., & Cocozza, J. J. (2000). The impact of federal systems integration initiatives on services for mentally ill homeless persons. *Mental Health Services Research, 2*(3), 165–174.

DerSimonian, R., & Laird, N. (1986). Meta-analysis in clinical trials. *Controlled Clinical Trials, 7*(3), 177–188.

Donabedian, A. (1988). The quality of care. How can it be assessed? *Journal of the American Medical Association, 260*(12), 1743–1748.

Drake, R. E., McHugo, G. J., Xie, H., Fox, M., Packard, J., & Helmstetter, B. (2006). Ten-year recovery outcomes for clients with co-occurring schizophrenia and substance use disorders. *Schizophrenia Bulletin, 32*(3), 464–473.

Duffy, B., Terhanian, G., Bremer, J., & Smith, K. (2005). Comparing data from online and face-to-face surveys. *International Journal of Market Research, 47*(6), 615–639.

Duncan, D. F., White, J. B., & Nicholson, T. (2003). Using internet-based surveys to reach hidden populations: Case of nonabusive illicit drug users. *American Journal of Health Behavior, 27*(3), 208–218.

Festinger, L., Riecken, H. W., & Schachter, S. (1964). *When Prophecy Fails: A Social and Psychological Study of a Modern Group That Predicted the Destruction of the World.* Oxford, UK: Harper Torchbooks.

Frank, R. G., & Glied, S. (2006). *Better But Not Well: Mental Health Policy in the United States Since 1950.* Baltimore: Johns Hopkins University Press.

Gibbons, R. D., Hedeker, D. R., Elkin, I., Waternaux, C., Kraemer, H. C., Greenhouse, J. B., et al. (1993). Some conceptual and statistical issues in analysis of longitudinal psychiatric data: Application to the NIMH Treatment of Depression Collaborative Research Program dataset. *Archives of General Psychiatry, 50*(9), 739–750.

Gladwell, M. (2002). *Tipping Point: How Little Things Can Make a Big Difference.* Boston: Back Bay Books.

Goldman, H. H., & Morrissey, J. P. (1985). The alchemy of mental health policy: Homelessness and the fourth cycle of reform. *American Journal of Public Health, 75*(7), 727–731.

Goldman, H. H., Morrissey, J. P., Rosenheck, R. A., Cocozza, J., Blasinsky, M., & Randolph, F. (2002). Lessons from the evaluation of the ACCESS program: Access to community care and effective services. *Psychiatric Services, 53*(8), 967–969.

Grusky, O., & Tierney, K. (1989). Evaluating the effectiveness of countywide mental health care systems. *Community Mental Health Journal, 25*(1), 3–20.

Hargreaves, S. (1998). Role of commissioners in promoting clinical effectiveness in everyday psychiatric practice. *Psychiatric Bulletin, 22*(6), 368–369.

Hargreaves, W. A. (1986). Theory of psychiatric treatment systems: An approach. *Archives of General Psychiatry, 43*(7), 701–705.

Hargreaves, W. A. (1992). A capitation model for providing mental health services in California. *Hospital & Community Psychiatry, 43*(3), 275–279.

Hermann, R. C. (2005). *Improving Mental Healthcare: A Guide to Measurement-Based Quality Improvement*. Washington, DC: American Psychiatric Publishing.

Hermann, R. C., Leff, H. S., & Lagodmos, G. (2002). *Selecting Process Measures for Quality Improvement in Mental Healthcare*. Cambridge, MA: Evaluation Center@HSRI.

Hermann, R. C., Rollins, C. K., & Chan, J. A. (2007). Risk-adjusting outcomes of mental health and substance-related care: A review of the literature. *Harvard Review of Psychiatry, 15*(2), 52–69.

Hernandez, M. (2000). Using logic models and program theory to build outcome accountability. *Education & Treatment of Children, 23*(1), 24–40.

Isett, K. R., Burnam, M. A.,Coleman-Beattie, B., Hyde, P. S., Morrissey,J. P.,Magnabosco,J., et al. (2007). The state policy context of implementation issues for evidence-based practices in mental health. *Psychiatric Services, 58*(7), 914–921.

Isett, K. R., Burnam, M. A., Coleman-Beattie, B., Hyde, P. S., Morrissey, J. P., Magnabosco, J. L., et al. (2008). The role of state mental health authorities in managing change for the implementation of evidence-based practices. *Community Mental Health Journal, 44*(3), 195–211.

Jackson, K. M., & Trochim, W. M. K. (2002). Concept mapping as an alternative approach for the analysis of open-ended survey responses. *Organizational Research Methods, 5*(4), 307–336.

Jordan, B. K., Karg, R. S., Batts, K. R., Epstein, J. F., & Wiesen, C. (2008). A clinical validation of the National Survey on Drug Use and Health Assessment of Substance Use Disorders. *Addictive Behaviors, 33*(6), 782–798.

Kessler, R. C., & Merikangas, K. R. (2004). National Comorbidity Survey Replication (NCS-R): Background and aims. *International Journal of Methods and Psychiatric Research, 13*(2), 60–68.

Lagoe, R. J., & Westert, G. P. (2006). Community wide electronic distribution of summary health care utilization data. *BMC Medical Informatics and Decision Making, 6*, 17.

Lambert, D. A., & McGuire, T. G. (1990). Political and economic determinants of insurance regulation in mental health. *Journal of Health Politics, Policy, and Law, 15*(1), 169–189.

Leff, H. S., Lieberman, M., Mulkern, V., & Raab, B. (1996). Outcome trends for severely mentally ill persons in capitated and case managed mental health programs. *Administration and Policy in Mental Health, 24*(1), 3–11.

Leff, H. S., Mulkern, V., Lieberman, M., & Raab, B. (1994). The effects of capitation on service access, adequacy, and appropriateness. *Administration and Policy in Mental Health, 21*(3), 141–160.

Leff, H. S., Wieman, D. A., McFarland, B. H., Morrissey, J. P., Rothbard, A., Shern, D. L., et al. (2005). Assessment of Medicaid managed behavioral health care for persons with serious mental illness. *Psychiatric Services, 56*(10), 1245–1253.

Lehman, A. (1995). *Toolkit on Evaluating Quality of Life for Persons with Severe Mental Illness*. Cambridge, MA: Evaluation Center@HSRI.

Lewins, A., & Silver, C. (2007). *Using Software in Qualitative Research: A Step-by-Step Guide*. Los Angeles and London: SAGE.

Magnabosco, J. L. (2006). Innovations in mental health services implementation: A report on state-level data from the U.S. Evidence-Based Practices Project. *Implementation Science, 1*, 13.

Magnabosco Bower, J. L. (2001). An evaluation of state public mental health system performance for adult persons with serious mental illness: Effects of state political culture and state mental health planning and implementation characteristics on state public mental health system comprehensiveness. *Dissertation Abstracts International: Section B, The Sciences and Engineering, 62-02,* 0775.

Meyer, G. S., & Massagli, M. P. (2001). The forgotten component of the quality triad: Can we still learn something from "structure"? *Joint Commission Journal of Quality Improvement, 27*(9), 484–493.

Miles, M. B., & Huberman, A. M. (1994). *Qualitative Data Analysis: An Expanded Sourcebook* (2nd ed.). Thousand Oaks, CA: Sage.

Millar, A., Simeone, R. S., & Carnevale, J. T. (2001). Logic models: A systems tool for performance management. *Evaluation and Program Planning*, 24(1), 73–81.

Moos, R. H., Nichol, A. C., & Moos, B. S. (2002). Global assessment of functioning ratings and the allocation and outcomes of mental health services. *Psychiatric Services*, 53(6), 730–737.

Morrissey J. P., Calloway, M. O., Thakur, N., Cocozza, J., Steadman, H. J., Dennis, D., et al. (2002, August). Integration of service systems for homeless persons with serious mental illness through the ACCESS program: Access to Community Care and Effective Services and Supports. *Psychiatric Services*, 53(8), 949–957.

Nadler, D. (1977). *Feedback and Organization Development: Using Databased Methods*. Reading, MA: Addison-Wesley.

New Freedom Commission on Mental Health. (2003). *Achieving the Promise: Transforming Mental Health Care in America; Final Report*. DHHS Pub. No. SMA-03-3832. Rockville, MD: Substance Abuse and Mental Health Services Administration.

O'Leary, W. D., & Meyers, D. (2008, June). U.S. Public Sector Connected Health and Human Services (white paper). Microsoft Corporation. [Accessed online at http://www.microsoft.com/industry/government/health/hhs.aspx on March 9, 2010.]

Pope, C., Mays, N., & Popay, J. (2007). *Synthesizing Qualitative and Quantitative Health Evidence: A Guide to Methods*. New York: McGraw-Hill.

Raghavan, R., Bright, C. L., & Shadoin, A.L. (2008). Toward a policy ecology of implementation of evidence-based practices in public mental health settings. *Implementation Science*, 3, 26.

Randolph, F., Blasinsky, M., Morrissey, J. P., Rosenheck, R. A., Cocozza, J., & Goldman, H. H. (2002). Overview of the ACCESS Program: Access to community care and effective services and supports. *Psychiatric Services*, 53(8), 945–948.

Rivard, J. C. (2005). *Measures of Organizational Readiness*. Alexandria, VA: National Association of State Mental Health Program Directors Research Institute.

Rosenblatt, A., & Woodbridge, M. W. (2003). Deconstructing research on systems of care for youth with EBD: Frameworks for policy research. *Journal of Emotional and Behavioral Disorders*, 11(1), 25–35.

Rosenheck, R., Morrissey, J., Lam, J., Calloway, M., Johnsen, M., Goldman, H., et al. (1998, November). Service system integration, access to services, and housing outcomes in a program for homeless persons with severe mental illness. *American Journal of Public Health*, 88(11), 1610–1615.

Rosenheck, R., Morrissey, J., Lam, J., Calloway, M., Stolar, M., Johnsen, M., et al. (2001, August). Service delivery and community: Social capital, service systems integration, and outcomes among homeless persons with severe mental illness. *Health Services Research*, 36(4), 691–710.

Roy-Byrne, P. P., Sherbourne, C. D., Craske, M. G., Stein, M. B., Katon, W., Sullivan, G., et al. (2003). Moving treatment research from clinical trials to the real world. *Psychiatric Services*, 54(3), 327–332.

Sechrest, L., McKnight, P., & McKnight, K. (1996). Calibration of measures for psychotherapy outcome studies. *American Psychologist*, 51(10), 1065–1071.

Sechrest, L., Stewart, M., Stickle, T. R., & Sidani, S. (1996). *Toolkit for Effective and Persuasive Case Studies*. Cambridge, MA: Evaluation Center@HSRI.

Shadish, W. R., Cook, T. D., & Campbell, D. T. (2002). *Experimental and Quasi-Experimental Designs for Generalized Causal Inference*. Boston, MA: Houghton Mifflin.

Sinaiko, A. D., & McGuire, T. G. (2006). Patient inducement, provider priorities, and resource allocation in public mental health systems. *Journal of Health Politics, Policy and Law*, 31(6), 1075–1106.

Stetler, C. B., Legro, M. W., Wallace, C. M., Bowman, C., Guihan, M., Hagedorn, H., et al. (2006, February). The role of formative evaluation in implementation research and the QUERI experience. *Journal of General Internal Medicine*, 21(S2), S1–S8.

Strayhorn, J. M., Jr. (1987). Control groups for psychosocial intervention outcome studies. *American Journal of Psychiatry, 144*(3), 275–282.

Substance Abuse and Mental Health Services Administration. (2007). *2008 National Survey on Drug Use and Health*. Contract No. 283-2004-00022, Project No. 9009. Rockville, MD: Author.

Thaler, R. H., & Sunstein, C. R. (2008). *Nudge: Improving Decisions about Health, Wealth, and Happiness*. New Haven, CT: Yale University Press.

Thomas, J. W. (2006). *Hospital Cost Effiency Measurement: Methodological Approaches*. Prepared for the Hospital Value Initiative sponsored by the California Public Employees' Retirement System and the Pacific Business Group on Health.

Trochim, W. M. (1985). Pattern matching, validity, and conceptualization in program evaluation. *Evaluation Review, 9*(5), 575–604.

Trochim, W. M., Cabrera, D. A., Milstein, B., Gallagher, R. S., & Leischow, S. J. (2006). Practical challenges of systems thinking and modeling in public health. *American Journal of Public Health, 96*(3), 538–546.

Wallcraft, J., Schrank, B., & Amering, M. (Eds.) (2009). *Handbook of Service User Involvement in Mental Health Research*. Hoboken, NJ: Wiley.

Weisbrod, B. A., Test, M. A., & Stein, L. I. (1980, April). Alternative to mental hospital treatment: II, Economic benefit-cost analysis. *Archives of General Psychiatry, 37*(4), 400–405.

Wells, K. B. (1999a). Design of partners in care: Evaluating the cost-effectiveness of improving care for depression in primary care. *Social Psychiatry and Psychiatric Epidemiology, 34*(1), 20–29.

Wells, K. B. (1999b). Treatment research at the crossroads: The scientific interface of clinical trials and effectiveness research. *American Journal of Psychiatry, 156*(1), 5–10.

Wolff, N. (2002). (New) public management of mentally disordered offenders: Part II, A vision with promise. *International Journal of Law and Psychiatry, 25*(5), 427–444.

Yin, R. K., Bickman, L., & Rog, D. J. (1998). The abridged version of case study research: Design and method. In L. Bickman (Ed.), *Handbook of Applied Social Research Methods* (pp. 229–259). Thousand Oaks, CA: Sage.

INDEX

Page numbers followed by "f" indicate figures, those followed by "t" indicate tables.